Defy Your Doctor and Be Healed

A book by Sarah C. Corriher and C. Thomas Corriher

Health Wyze Media

ISBN-13: 978-0615238340

Revision 24

The information provided herein is intended to be a truthful, corrective alternative to the advice provided by the medical industry and most media sources. It is intended to diagnose, treat, cure, and prevent disease. It is intended to save you.

Copyright Notice

Table of Contents

Preface

"And they said, 'Is not this Joseph's son?' And [Christ] *said unto them, 'Ye will surely say unto me this proverb, Physician, heal thyself. Whatsoever we have heard done in Capernaum, do also here in thy country. Verily I say unto you, no prophet is accepted in his own country'."*

-- The Gospel of Luke, 4:22-4:24 (King James Bible)

Most people cannot be healed. They walk about wounded because the health topics of today are as polarized as any system of political parties. As researchers of both alternative and orthodox medicine, we quickly learned that there are no neutral parties, and fewer who are innocent. We shall nevertheless continue onward, because we have nothing to lose.

Our being extraordinarily honest in the completion of this work shall not lose us any friends, because all of our peers have abandoned us. They consider us to be the bad guys of alternative medicine, because we dare to question the unquestionable, which is blasphemy. However, religion and science need not be enemies, and whenever one dogma is threatened by the other, then lies can be found in at least one of them. Real science is not afraid of investigation, and all medicine should be made to withstand scientific scrutiny. Very little medicine, either alternative or mainstream, can withstand being thoughtfully scrutinized. Most of the progress that the public believes has been made was built upon a foundation of lies, and an elaborate system has been constructed to distract us away from this core truth.

Our health research began with a humble blog in 2006, followed by a print magazine in 2008. Nobody had done anything like it before. Nobody had the guts, and we soon learned why. With *Naturally Good Magazine,* we had plenty of supportive peers. We spiritedly wanted to fight against the gross malpractices of a medical establishment that kills more Americans every year than any war in its history, and that is only counting the *properly prescribed* medications. Due to our old fashioned, investigative approach to exposing industry corruption, the magazine survived for less than six months. Our retailer unexpectedly began destroying our magazines, and told us that they could no longer communicate with us. We shall never know all the details; but judging from the terror in the woman's voice, we suspect that someone at corporate got a threatening telephone call from someone. We lost the first of many friends whom we would come to lose in the coming years. We knew that our magazine could not last, but we had assumed that we would get at least two years. Even we were surprised by the swiftness of the reaction.

Any sincere examination of the corrupt state of health affairs should rightfully begin with a painfully honest assessment of our own community. If we cannot be honest about ourselves, then we shall never effect positive changes in others. Alternative medicine is almost entirely made of fair-weather friends. The lofty ethics, ideals, and science dissipate the moment that they are critically analyzed. This overwhelming desire to have always been *right* supersedes seeking real truth or helping others. This common behavior shows that much of alternative medicine is likewise built upon lies. Cultish ideology is a destructive one, which has diseased our society to a level that exceeds comprehension. We have witnessed alternative practitioners telling the most grotesque of lies to prevent patients from visiting a standard doctor, just as we have been informed of regular doctors who tried to medically kill their non-compliant patients, just to disprove an alternative therapy. Make no mistake: these behaviors are quite normal, so the hero worship that is felt by most patients is assuredly not deserved. Evil hides wherever we least expect to find it.

The story of Suzanne Somers is an example of the politics and dishonesty on all sides. The famous actress supposedly cured her cancer using alternative medicine. Since then, she has written numerous books about dieting, and one in particular about curing cancer. Her high-profile success story was so threatening to the lucrative cancer industry that the American Cancer Society began issuing desperate press responses that told the public not to believe Somers. During this period of institutional panic, they carelessly released some statistics that they normally hide from the public.

> *"We're finding that about 25 to 30 percent of some cancers stop growing at some point, that can make some treatments look good that aren't doing anything. Until doctors figure out how to identify which patients have cancers that won't progress, the only option is to treat everyone."*

> -- Dr. Otis Brawley, the American Cancer Society's Chief Medical Officer

They were hoping that we would not notice that a 25% survival is *significantly better* than the success rates of standard therapies (4% for long-term survival). It means that cancer victims who do absolutely nothing have a 6.25 times better chance of living a longer and better life than those who get orthodox therapies. Avoiding standard medicine improves a cancer patient's chances by 625%, as shown by the industry's own statistics. Only the most dangerous and reckless of alternative treatments could compete with such failure.

On the other hand, the promotion of Suzanne Somers in the alternative community paints an unflattering picture of it too. Somers was not really saved with alternative medicine, and she is unqualified to write about medicine of any kind. These are the facts about Suzanne Somers' therapy:

- Somers took radiation, and had surgery to remove a cancerous tumor.
- Then she "medicated" with poisonous mistletoe extract, instead of chemotherapy. The cancer had already been removed. Mistletoe is not an accepted alternative medicine.
- She now uses "bio-identical hormones", which are synthetic hormones that are offered by the pharmaceutical industry.
- She rails behind stem cell therapy as a way to grow back limbs "in the near future", and fix damage resulting from surgery.
- She promotes Dr. Stanilaw Burzynski, a doctor whose cancer therapy is injecting patients with extracts of human urine.

The *Science* of Modern Medicine

Understanding the science of modern orthodox medicine requires a study in the psychology of mass manipulation, because there is very little science involved. Take for instance that hundreds of people have been imprisoned for shaken baby syndrome (i.e. child abuse), due to the way that many infant brain injuries allegedly indicate that they had been shaken violently. Absent from the news reports and the medical reports is that the type of brain swelling seen mimics the brain swelling that is caused by vaccines. In almost every case, the deaths happened soon after vaccinations.

We have been researching long enough to know what has really been happening, but it will be forever impossible to prove. No researcher will ever commit the professional suicide of raising this hypothesis. We know how politically incorrect it would be, and so do they. Vaccines must not be questioned. They are beyond reproach. If a courageous researcher were willing to partake in such self-destruction, it would alas be an endeavor in futility, and this is not just because he would be institutionally ignored. It would also be futile because controlled testing of vaccines is unthinkable. Valid scientific study would require the presence of a test group and a placebo group, in order to isolate the results from the test against the results of the placebo (control) group. Any researcher who conducted a valid vaccine study would have to publicly admit that he had murdered children for the sake of science, because the control group would have to be allowed to die.

Test subjects are not willing to be infected with polio for the sake of learning if the vaccination will stop it, so the polio vaccine was never actually tested for effectiveness. However, the polio vaccine was cunningly released at the time of the epidemic's natural die-off, in order to ensure that the public saw a connection between the vaccine's release and the end of the epidemic. It is the same pattern for the release dates of all the major vaccines. As soon as the infection rate dramatically plummets, then "Eureka!". They suddenly have the vaccine ready for release.

The public, and quite a few doctors, were distracted away from the fact that silver medications were a safe treatment, which effectively killed polio quickly, as well as virtually every other virus known. Prior to the entire smoke-and-mirrors routine, silver medicines were recognized for doing what the establishment now claims is impossible. Had silver medicine not been stripped from the market, the polio epidemic never would have occurred. Today's huge vaccine and antibiotics markets would never have come into being. Silver had to go. Just to stack the dishonest vaccine marketing even more, the F.D.A. and the American Medical Association began promoting tonsillectomies for all children at the same time, while knowing that the tonsils are the only organ in the human body that produces polio antibodies.

The vaccine proponents have said that due to physical and ethical restraints, they must use alternative scientific criteria to evaluate vaccines. What this shows is that they cannot follow their own rules and still get the results that they want, so they change the rules. If they must redefine how appraisals of tests are determined, then it is not science anymore. It is instead politics, and it is ultimately a very murderous form. In all of history, there has never been an independent, peer reviewed, double-blind study of any vaccine. There is not a shred of

4

evidence proving that vaccines do more good than harm, or even that they do any good at all.

Every vaccine was released to the public at a time when its target disease was already in its natural dying-off phase -- making it impossible to learn anything from the statistics. The vaccines were conveniently put into usage just after the epidemics had begun their natural dying-off process that all epidemics undergo. The inevitable dying-off process is why the epidemic of the Black Plague and thousands of other biological terrors no longer exist, and it has historically happened without the assistance of vaccines. The end of modern epidemics that were supposedly defeated by vaccines had successes that were mirrored in countries which did not use any vaccines, and which usually had faster rates of die-off. These statistics are institutionally ignored for the sake of vaccine political correctness in the Western world.

The lack of science is everywhere. For instance, the allopathic establishment cannot, and does not, test cancer medications in double-blind studies. Doing so would mean refusing to give treatments to dying patients (while lying to them about it), and then experimenting on another group with only an experimental treatment. Only the drug manufacturers test the drugs for safety and effectiveness, but they never really do. Valid scientific research (as accepted everywhere else) would require tests that ultimately get subjects killed in a much more direct manner than the industry is accustomed to. The manslaughters would be much more obvious, and much more prosecutable.

The corruption and brokenness of the medical system is not just relegated to cancers and vaccines. It is in every area of medicine. Let us consider a medical example that is easy to visualize. We have all seen defibrillators in action, whether in-person or in our entertainment. We have been led to believe that if doctors electrocute someone's heart enough, then they can raise the patient from the dead like Frankenstein's monster. Few people have paused to consider the ridiculousness of it all.

Now let us consider the science of defibrillators. How did they test those? Where did they find test subjects for electrocution testing? Did they inform test subjects that they would receive an electrocuting pulse of up to 2,000 volts (same amount used by electric chairs) through their hearts for the sake of science? More importantly: where exactly are the statistics proving that these electrocutions save more people than they kill? How would one prove it, other than bringing people back from the dead and then attempting other methods? Of course, they have us believing that they do bring people back from the dead, just like Dr. Frankenstein. Whether a given patient survives this insanity or not, the doctors are always thanked for having the heroism to electrocute their already dying patients. The proponents of defibrillators boast of a 40% survival rate, but what exactly is this compared to? How do they establish a baseline for comparison, unless they admit to having ignored a certain group of dead patients who got no treatments at all? What about the 60% of patients who die while being electrocuted? Is a 60% failure rate really a measurement of success? How do we establish what percentage of that 60% were killed by the electrocutions? Is there any real evidence whatsoever that they are not killing more people than they are saving? Defibrillators are just one of hundreds of examples that we could have used, but the overall point is that the so-called "science" of allopathic medicine is virtually non-existent. It is largely a business of showmanship.

Medical History and the Present

"None are more hopelessly enslaved than those who falsely believe they are free."

-- Johann Wolfgang von Goethe

The popular system of medicine now practiced by doctors world-wide was funded and engineered by the Rockefeller Foundation in the early twentieth century. The foundation continues to maintain very close ties to the F.D.A. and the American Medical Association. Truly conventional therapies were scrapped about a century ago, and replaced with experimental petrochemicals. The medical schools were persuaded to adopt the new pharmaceuticals as a stipulation for obtaining the Rockefeller grants, and surgery was also promoted for the next generation of medicine. These were set to become the two pillars of medicine. Entire libraries of truly conventional medicine were discarded. The first allopathic surgeons were literally butchers, who had been hired from meat plants.

The Rockefeller family had monopolized the entire petrochemical industry at that time, which was positioned to become the only source of medicine in the future. Such has come to pass. The man behind it all, John D. Rockefeller, was unwilling to use the new medicines on himself. He instead used traditional treatments throughout his life: the same ones now known as "alternative" medicine. As a result, his own family was spared the blights that decimated the rest of the population, such as polio and tuberculosis.

It was the Rockefeller Institute that first identified the polio virus. According to records from Rockefeller University, the organization began work on making polio more contagious in the 1940's; not long before the polio epidemic struck. We have no way of knowing if it was unleashed to bolster its new industries of vaccinations and antibiotics, or if this bio-weapon was released by mistake. We do know that the medical industry immediately began taking steps to perpetuate polio, using the following two methods: 1) removing the tonsils of all children, which happens to be the only organ in the human body that produces polio antibodies, and 2) by having the F.D.A. suppress the use of silver medicine, which was the only known medicine that effectively kills polio.

American readers will be especially stunned to learn that the Food and Drug Administration does not work for the American people, or even the U.S. Government. The overwhelming majority of its income is actually derived from *private* regulatory fees and from medical device approvals. In fact, the organization's total income from public money (taxation) is a measly 3%. Its pharmaceutical partners provide 97% of F.D.A. funding. The same shenanigans exist behind the scenes in countries with socialized medical systems, whereby money buys the medical policies. Pharmaceutical companies in the U.S. offer cooperative and high-ranking F.D.A. employees lavish job positions, where a surprising percentage of former F.D.A. administrators can be found. These rewards are a standard industry practice. The biggest perk of being an F.D.A. employee is entry into the next job, where the pay will be obscene; assuming that all the *right* regulatory decisions were made.

"The FDA protects the big drug companies, and is subsequently rewarded, and using the government's police powers, they attack those who threaten the big drug companies. The thing that bugs me is that the people think the FDA is protecting them. It isn't. What the FDA is doing, and what the public thinks it is doing are as different as night and day."

-- Dr. Herbert Ley, former Commissioner of the F.D.A.

Consider all of the research foundations that are searching for disease cures, and all of the various fundraisers that have been implemented to feed the disease industry. Whether it be "pink ribbon" campaigns or walking for cancer cures, we see it everywhere with well-meaning people who are trying to help. Our research has taught us about the futility of it all. The reason why no cures are being found, or ever will be, is because research foundations and other medical industry players are not allowed to find cures. At least in the United States, all therapies require approval from the government (F.D.A.) for doctors to avoid lawsuits, arrest, loss of licensure and imprisonment. In the past century, no cure for any disease has ever been approved. All of those research foundations are researching cures that will never be legal for anyone to practice. Cures have already been found for the diseases that plague us, many times over.

Since the F.D.A. has never approved any cure for any disease, it is illegal for a doctor in the United States to cure any disease. To even suggest vitamin B-17 therapy for cancer, a doctor is required to submit a written confession to the F.D.A. for disciplinary action against him; as if he had committed a crime for using a cheaper, dramatically more effective, and considerably safer therapy. It is how the system works, by design. The pattern is the same for every disease condition. The word "cure" has been removed from the medical vernacular, for every condition is "treated" perpetually. Instead of your healer, your doctor is your dealer.

The approved treatments are designed to *worsen* the underlying conditions, while temporarily suppressing the most unpleasant symptoms through immunosuppression. Over time, the real underlying health issues snowball as a result, and that is the business plan. Standard procedures are literally processes of slow poisoning to ensure that patients never heal; in much the same way that unlicensed drug dealers foster addictions. To demonstrate the appropriateness of this comparison, every addictive street drug was once classified as a "safe and effective" pharmaceutical, and prescribed by doctors. For example, Heroin from Bayer Pharmaceuticals was the industry's best seller of all time. Patients were dishonestly told that Heroin would cure their addictions to other "medicines", such as morphine, which too had been prescribed. Many pharmacies in the United States still keep cocaine in stock. The "street drugs" only became dangerous after the patents on them expired, when the pharmaceutical industry could no longer monopolize profits from them. This is why governments will never be allowed to stop the drug war, because the drugs represent unpatentable market competition. It is the real reason why cannabis (marijuana) is so "dangerous"; for it may well be the most useful plant in the world, and thereby the most dangerous financially. It too was prescribed.

Examples of Standard Care

- Cholesterol drugs that supposedly prevent heart disease actually cause heart disease after long-term use, and they likewise cause fatal heart attacks in people with no history of heart problems. This can be verified in the drug information. They call these "side effects". Cholesterol-lowering drugs are used most often with the middle-aged and the elderly, but a lack of cholesterol in these older populations is the leading cause of death from complications, such as internal bleeding, and ruptured heart vessels. Kidney failure and liver failure are other well-known fatal side effects.

- The use of standard heart medications combined with doctor recommendations to avoid beneficial saturated fats is the reason why heart disease is the medical industry's biggest failure, and the biggest killer for over six decades.

- The new generation of synthetic insulins cause pre-diabetics to become full-blown diabetics. These chemical insulins destroy the pancreas over time to ensure perpetual dependence upon the drugs, so that curing becomes impossible. The F.D.A. banned all-natural insulin products, which neither worsened diabetes nor caused addiction problems. It did it the same year that Eli Lilly patented its chemical version, and now it allows only Eli Lilly to exclusively produce it -- providing Eli Lilly with a monopoly on diabetes treatments. Since then, Eli Lilly has become a revolving door allowing F.D.A. employees to find new jobs at salaries many times higher.

- Standard cancer treatments are therapies that are known to spread and feed cancers (radiation, chemotherapy, surgery). The results are so bad that the long-term cure rate is a depressing 4%, which is actually lower than the percentage of survivors amongst people who got no treatments at all. The cancer chapter explains how the statistics are manipulated to keep the lucrative cancer industry propped-up, despite its actual results. Alarming percentages of oncologists (cancer doctors) have admitted that they would never give their own medicine to themselves or to their own families. The cancer business is so lucrative that it alone is the 5th leading cause of bankruptcy in the United States. Medicine overall ranks as number one for bankrupting Americans.

The examples in the above list represent the best of the best of modern experimental medicine, for these categories are the most funded by research, and they are the most profitable areas of medicine.

The Food and Drug Administration

The F.D.A. began life in 1906 as the Division of Chemistry, and it was later renamed to the Bureau of Chemistry, long before changing its name to the Food and Drug Administration. Its name was changed to conceal its pro-chemical industry mission. Its true purpose is to provide legal immunity for companies that put chemicals into foods, and those who manufacture pharmaceuticals; by means of its chemical substance "approvals". Approvals are designed to leave citizens without legal recourse against the chemical industry. Safety is not the purpose behind the approval process. The agency's true job was, and still is, to officially sanction products from the chemical industry, and to thereby legally shield the industry from *us* by pre-emptively declaring what is "safe". Little has changed since its early days when it was called the Bureau of Chemistry. No jury in the land will vote any F.D.A. approved drug as malpractice, and that is the point of it all. An F.D.A. approval literally translates into a license to kill.

> *"I never have and never will approve a new drug to an individual, but only to a large pharmaceutical company with unlimited finances."*

> -- Dr. Richard J. Crout, Director of the F.D.A.'s
> Bureau of Drugs (Spotlight Magazine, Jan. 1982)

The F.D.A. *privately* gathers data to share with its chemical industry partners, helping them to mitigate liability. These records are kept confidential in direct violation of U.S. law, sometimes followed by claims that it must respect the effected corporation's proprietary secrets. There is no such requirement, and the law specifically forbids them from censoring governmental documents. This industry assistance often occurs with food contamination cases and especially with drug problems. Poisoning problems are treated as public relations issues.

Deadly pharmaceutical products are usually removed from the market *voluntarily* by the manufacturers, without so much as a slap from the F.D.A. The organization seems to only ban competing natural supplements in the majority of cases whenever it actually takes action, and these are normally *mandatory* recalls.

Meanwhile, the organization suppresses natural medicines that their industry cannot legally control and monopolize with patents. Natural substances can never be patented. This is why every natural and non-toxic therapy is automatically called "quackery" by the F.D.A., its chemical industry, and the medical establishment. Only unnatural (e.g. non-organic and toxic) chemicals can be patented, and thereby, all non-toxic medicines are a threat to the *business* of medicine.

The F.D.A. tried to block sales of unprocessed red yeast rice and its supplemental extracts, because they compete with patented cholesterol drugs, which are actually based upon a compound from the same rice. This food has been consumed for thousands of years. The rice was conveniently reclassified as a "drug", so that the F.D.A. could impose arbitrary bans by fiat. It has become a common trick ever since the U.S. Congress forbade the F.D.A. from regulating supplements; in lieu of its abusive history. Nowadays, any supplement that they target for having competed with their lucrative industry is simply reclassified as a "drug" to bypass the congressional rules. The F.D.A. claimed to be suddenly concerned about the safety and effectiveness of eating rice, but it was not worried about the equivalent pharmaceuticals, which cause liver failure (death). It is a familiar story. When a group of cherry farmers made it public knowledge that concentrated cherry supplements were proven, by multiple independent tests, to be far better than the most expensive arthritis medications -- the agency swiftly responded by literally threatening to shutdown the entire cherry industry of the United States, if it were necessary to stop the reporting of those scientific findings. It warned that it was willing to reclassify cherries as unapproved drugs, if necessary. American doctors are not allowed to tell their arthritis patients that a $10 bottle of cherry extract from a health food store would be safer and more effective than the $3,000 per month regimen of standard pharmaceuticals. Cherry therapy would not contribute to liver dysfunction, like arthritis drugs do, to eventually make the condition worse.

Pathological Medicine

When doctors went on strike in Israel in 1983, and again in 2000, the mortality rate fell by approximately 50%. In 1976, the number of deaths fell by 18% in Los Angeles when doctors went on strike for merely a month. This pattern has been mirrored in the 5 other major doctor strikes around the world.

This book will be paradigm shifting for most people. Simple facts that should have always been self-evident will finally become evident. One of the first of these is that the human body is never dysfunctional unless it is made to be broken. The human body is perhaps the greatest marvel in all the universe. It was designed to repair itself; not to naturally succumb to random diseases. When the body is broken, it is broken by abuse and neglect. It does not fail unless our actions or inaction have directly caused the failure. States of being at dis-*ease* are when the harmonious balance of millions of simultaneous reactions, which work together like a symphony, are disrupted. To truly accept this paradigm means accepting personal responsibility for whatever state you are in. All diseases, and all bad medicine, stem from a population that is unwilling to take personal responsibility, and its cowardly inability to take ownership of what was always theirs for the taking. Both the patients and the doctors have taken the politically correct logic of blameless diseases to such an extreme that they are routinely blaming the innocent DNA for diseases that are now labeled as "genetic disorders", as if the problem was God all along. Our crimes against him and our very bodies were never his fault. We did it willingly, and with a smile on our faces, all the way to the morgue. Our bodies and our lives are gifts that we so callously squander, and then we are arrogant enough to conclude that it was God's fault for having shoddy engineering. The engineering is sound, for disease is not actually the normal state of the human body. We destroy our bodies with our abominable food products, the vaccines, our terrible lifestyles, and then whenever the inevitable diseases finally appear, we have the doctors poison us. Our grandchildren will someday look back at the insanity and wonder how we could be so unable to reason. They will see us as we view the cavemen, and we shall deserve the scorn and mocking. They will wonder in amazement at how our society could believe that diseases are caused by drug deficiencies, and that undetectable chemical imbalances somehow require that we routinely harm ourselves through chemical warfare.

Our modern medicine is better suited for a study in pathological psychology than either medicine or science. Remember that one indication of insanity is doing the same thing repeatedly and expecting differing results. We are reminded of the millions of people who have allowed themselves to get burned by cancer-causing radiation to supposedly stop cancer, or take pancreas-destroying synthetic insulins to supposedly stop diabetes, or those who have taken heart-destroying and liver-destroying anti-cholesterol medications to supposedly stop the inflammation that causes heart disease. It is like setting one's car on fire to ensure that it never wrecks.

Our faithful forefathers lived much happier and healthier lives, and they would have had double our life expectancy if they had our hygiene, our food production capabilities, and our heating systems. We would not last a week if we had to trade places with them. Have we really gained a better living through chemistry? Do people still live naturally and die peacefully, or do we live diseased and silence a dying person's agonizing screams with even more drugs, as they waste away in a hospice? This is not hypothetical. This is normal, and yet we manage to congratulate ourselves for our ingenuity.

The word pharmaceutical is derived from the ancient Greek word "pharmakeia". It meant sorcery. A person only needs to comparatively study the history of alchemy (ancient chemistry) with the occult practices of sorcery to discover that they intersect at many points, and that we have been cunningly deceived into accepting what was always unacceptable. People have replaced their faith in God's natural medicines with a faith in new-age sorcery that has been euphemistically renamed to chemistry. The consequences upon health (emotionally, physically, and spiritually) have always been the same. Future generations will recognize that our faith in such failed methodologies created a second dark age of death on par with the original Dark Age. We are as blind to the severity of our plight as the sufferers of the original Dark Age were.

The science of medicine is discussed frequently throughout this book, with a great emphasis upon the perverted science that is used to justify poisoning patients endlessly. However, it is not really science that matters most to people. Faith matters more, because people make their important, life-changing decisions based upon their faith; irregardless of what science proves. That faith is most often as misguided as it is betrayed. People are poisoned and butchered by their doctors, of whom they unquestioningly believe are basing decisions upon the soundest of scientific principles, without any indecent agendas. This misplaced faith is why medical treatments are the biggest killer in the U.S., as shown by the industry's *own* mortality statistics.

You may find this book to be your greatest hope someday, if you first make the appropriate leap of faith that is required to unlock its potential. If you do, then this book will help you to unlock the incredible power of God's medicine. The answers are in plain view, and they always have been. We can save you from the lies, but only you can save you from yourself. If you take that important step, then please read this book in its entirety, for a *little bit* of knowledge can be a dangerous thing. Drink deep or taste not.

Depression

A Sick Industry

Writing for the B.B.C., Dr. Joanna Moncrieff explained that anti-depressants do not cure depression or make people happy. They merely numb people into drug-induced emotional comas, until the emotions are repressed to the point of forcefully reappearing: often explosively. She noted that the chemical imbalance hypothesis has never been proven, and moreover; it's wrong.

> *"Psychoactive drugs make people feel different; they put people into an altered mental and physical state. They affect everyone, regardless of whether they have a mental disorder or not... If we gave people a clearer picture, drug treatment might not always be so appealing. If you told people that we have no idea what is going on in their brain, but that they could take a drug that would make them feel different and might help to suppress their thoughts and feelings, then many people might choose to avoid taking drugs if they could."*

-- Dr. Joanna Moncrieff

Antidepressant Drug Effects and Depression Severity was a 30-year research study utilizing the results of 6 clinical studies. It was published in the Journal of the American Medical Association (J.A.M.A.) in 2009, revealing that S.S.R.I. (selective serotonin reuptake inhibitor) anti-depressants, in the overwhelming majority of cases, are no more effective than placebos. Their admission is ironic, because the same medical establishment routinely ridicules alternative methods as not having been proven effective in official studies.

The general public believes that pharmaceuticals are judged on a risk versus benefit basis. The pharmaceutical marketers and their regulatory partners in government have sworn that this is really the case for the drug approval process. So when the risks of suicide ideation and psychosis are introduced by pharmaceuticals, then it seems unthinkable to the uninitiated that these same medications would not at least provide a benefit above that of a placebo. Anti-depressant medications for the depressed are like medicating diabetics with sugar pills, for the aftermath is blamed on the original organic condition. As a consequence, depressions tend to get worse with long-term medication, business gets more profitable, and survivors are unable to prove a connection.

S.S.R.I. pharmaceuticals have been the most commonly used drugs in the United States for decades, yet there is still little evidence demonstrating their efficacy. There is, however, overwhelming evidence of their horrific side effects, including suicide ideation, anxiety, and homicidal impulses. Anti-depressant drugs *cause* suicidal tendencies, in addition to a litany of physical effects. This entire class of drugs is required to come with a special Black Box notice about the high risk of suicide when taking them. The fact that anti-depressant using patients are killing themselves in significantly higher numbers than unmedicated patients clarifies the effectiveness of these drugs.

The F.D.A.'s Black Box Warning

Suicidality in Children and Adolescents

Antidepressants increase the risk of suicidal thinking and behavior (suicidality) in children and adolescents with major depressive disorder (MDD) and other psychiatric disorders. Anyone considering the use of [Drug Name] or any other antidepressant in a child or adolescent must balance this risk with the clinical need. Patients who are started on therapy should be observed closely for clinical worsening, suicidality, or unusual changes in behavior. Families and caregivers should be advised of the need for close observation and communication with the prescriber. [Drug Name] is not approved for use in pediatric patients except for patients with [Any approved pediatric claims here]. (See Warnings and Precautions: Pediatric Use)

Pooled analyses of short-term (4 to 16 weeks) placebo-controlled trials of nine antidepressant drugs (SSRIs and others) in children and adolescents with MDD, obsessive compulsive disorder (OCD), or other psychiatric disorders (a total of 24 trials involving over 4,400 patients) have revealed a greater risk of adverse events representing suicidal thinking or behavior (suicidality) during the first few months of treatment in those receiving antidepressants. The average risk of such events on drug was 4%, twice the placebo risk of 2%. No suicides occurred in these trials.

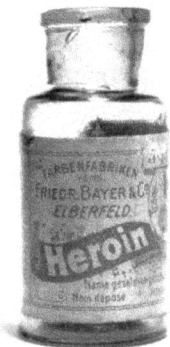

These drugs also cause severe addictions, which the pharmaceutical industry flippantly calls "discontinuation syndrome" to carefully avoid using the words addiction and withdrawal. These word games are both for marketing and legal liability reasons. By labeling the anti-depressant addictions as a disease possessed by the victims, it is another way for the chemical industry to pass the blame onto its victims, in much the same vein as 'bad' genes are now being blamed for the results of pharmaceutical toxicity and artificial foods. These mitigation strategies are beloved by lawyers world-wide. Discontinuation syndrome is their code phrase used throughout medical literature, which is used to hide the fact that these drugs cause terrible withdrawal symptoms. The withdrawal symptoms are frequently worse than those from illegal narcotics. It is important to note that all addictive illegal drugs were originally created by the pharmaceutical industry and sold as safe medications. Take for instance that Bayer's wonder drug for treating drug addictions in yesteryear was Heroin (diacetylmorphine). Heroin is still reverently remembered as the pharmaceutical industry's best seller of all time.

S.S.R.I. drugs have only been shown to be partially effective in those with major depressive disorders. Those who go to a psychiatrist seeking a happy pill due to an episode of mild to moderate depression will not get any appreciable relief. Such patients represent the overwhelming majority of cases for which these drugs are prescribed. For major depressions, psychiatrists mix and match dangerous cocktails of psychogenic drugs like a game of Russian roulette, even though the drugs are not supposed to be mixed. No testing is ever done on drugs combined with other drugs. In fact, such tests are automatically disqualified as invalid by the industry and regulators.

The First Anti-depressant

Modern psychiatry has endeavored to hide the fact that cocaine was its first anti-depressant. It began in 1884, when Doctor Sigmund Freud published a series of papers praising cocaine for its use as a treatment for depression, alcoholism, and addictions. The psychiatric community has gone far to suppress the fact that cocaine and opium derivatives (like Bayer's Heroin) were its first medications, so history has been rewritten to state that Thorazine was the first pharmaceutical anti-depressant. This revised version of history claims that such drugging did not begin until the 1950's. The revisionists likewise neglect to mention that Thorazine's use greatly diminished soon after it caused America's first school massacre (Texas State University), in much the same way that Luvox sales took a dive after being linked to the Columbine massacre.

The real history is quite incriminating, regarding the psychiatric industry's wanton recklessness, its willful tendency to foster drug addictions, its general lack of ethics, and its institutionalized use of torture methods (electro-shock) -- even on toddlers. Psychiatry has never been the squeaky-clean and science-based industry that it portrays itself as being. Its journals never mention the connections between it and school shootings, or how patient records always 'disappear' after the incidents.

Cocaine cannot be patented by drug companies because it is a naturally-occurring substance. This is the main reason why cocaine was made illegal. Dozens of other naturally-occurring medicinal plants (so-called "drugs") were likewise banned for the same anti-competitive reason. Being natural, the coca (cocaine) plant was a threat to the business of the petrochemical industry, for it allowed people to freely treat themselves without paying industry royalties.

Cocaine is so safe in its natural form that coca was once the most notable ingredient inside the original Coca-Cola formula. It is where the drink's name came from. The company still uses coca leaves, which supposedly have their narcotic component neutralized. Their P.R. people claim that coca is kept in the formula for its flavor, but it is really there to stop competition; for who else is allowed to import cocaine into the United States? Now you know the true meaning of the slogan, "Have a coke and a smile". To grasp the magnitude of the governmental corruption and the overall dishonesty of the drug war, be advised that the Illinois-based Stepan Company imports truck-loads of "non-narcotic" coca into the United States every year for the Coca-Cola corporation, while this is flatly ignored by law enforcement and the U.S. media.

As is the case for all other pharmaceutically-extracted, mind-altering compounds, the variety of cocaine that is synthesized by the chemical industry has been concentrated and designed for maximum addictive properties. Natural cocaine, as used by indigenous peoples, has never been addictive. The same thing happened in the case of Heroin. Heroin is a chemically modified variant of opium. Bayer marketed Heroin as the cure for morphine addictions to make sure that patients never really escaped, and morphine had been previously marketed as the cure for the significantly less addictive, and all natural, opium. Heroin was Bayer's biggest profit-maker of all time. L.S.D. was also a standard medication of psychiatry, for which the embarrassing history has also been carefully obscured. In every case, each subsequent medication was proclaimed to be safer, less addictive, and more effective than what came before, and the public always believed it.

Akathisia

"Every child in America entering school at the age of five is insane because he comes to school with certain allegiances to our Founding Fathers, toward our elected officials, toward his parents, toward a belief in a supernatural being, and toward the sovereignty of this nation as a separate entity. It's up to you as teachers to make all these sick children well -- by creating the international child of the future."

-- Dr. Chester M. Pierce, Psychiatrist

The large media houses, working in tandem with their biggest advertisers, have concealed the fact that the entire class of S.S.R.I. anti-depressant drugs cause a dangerous condition that is known as akathisia. Because of the mainstream media's ties with the pharmaceutical industry, most people have never learned of this neurologically degenerative, drug-induced, psycho-pathological and physical disease. In the official pharmaceutical literature of today, akathisia is most often referenced as an "emotional blunting", and what this means in plain language, minus the mitigating marketing, is that the victim of this condition experiences a suppression of *all* emotions; subsequently causing something of a zombie state. The significance of this is that a person's conscience, and his ability to recognize consequences are derived from his ability to empathize with the needs of others, and to experience fear. A patient, or anyone else for that matter, becomes a dangerous person whenever the emotions behind his conscience are chemically neutralized for the sake of suppressing inconvenient emotions. Altering people's mental state to eliminate emotions produces drug-induced sociopaths. Our conscience is, after all, an emotional reaction. The ability to empathize with the suffering of others requires emotions. Mercy itself requires them. Akathisia is the connection between psychiatric drugs, sociopathology and psychopathology.

For a small percentage of the population, akathisia produces a dreamy state, or more aptly, it's a nightmare state whilst being partially awake. In these special cases, it becomes a type of psychiatric drug-induced sleep walking, whereby the victim unconsciously acts in a sociopathic or a psychopathic manner. Friends and family may suddenly become monsters who should be exterminated. For these tragic cases, akathisia is like being possessed by a demon, except that the patient is actually possessed by a chemical. Akathisia is known to occur with every S.S.R.I. anti-depressant, and certain other psychiatric medications; particularly the anti-psychotics.

The irony of anti-depressants causing suicides, and anti-psychotics causing psychosis is hard to miss. The F.D.A. still refuses to label any drugs with a homicidality risk, although it was eventually willing to issue a Black Box suicidality warning for all S.S.R.I. anti-depressants; but this was only after immense public pressure from people who had lost loved ones.

The whole charade is easier to understand and accept once one learns that the F.D.A. actually works for the drug companies, because its drug approval process is where the organization gets most of its funding. The F.D.A.'s average profits for a single drug approval is $800,000,000.00. The agency gets a measly 3% of its income from taxes. The total yearly income that it *privately receives* for medical and drug approvals is $109,800,000,000.00. That's a hundred and nine billion dollars.

Since the 1950's, the definition of akathisia has been changing in an Orwellian sense, so that in the modern medical literature, it has either been redefined to mean only the so-called "emotional blunting" that was mentioned earlier, or only a type of motor dysfunction, which manifests itself like Parkinson's disease. In the latter cases, the drug-induced nerve damage causes bizarre and socially-awkward twitching that remains for an average of two years after the drug is discontinued, but it is permanent for a small percentage of patients.

A joint study by the North Wales Department of Psychological Medicine and United Kingdom Cochrane Centre, in 2006, attempted to correct this deceptive redefinition by citing the original and true description of akathisia from the 1950's. The study's authors noted that, in actuality, akathisia is much more than what is currently being reported throughout modern drug literature.

> *"The first few doses frequently made them anxious and apprehensive. They reported increased feelings of strangeness, verbalized by statements such as, 'I don't feel myself' or 'I'm afraid of some of the unusual impulses I have'."*

The researchers were professionally courageous enough to reestablish the link between akathisia, suicides, general violence, and homicides. Their study also demonstrated the close connection of akathisia to somnambulism, which is otherwise known as sleep walking.

Every school massacre in the United States can be traced back to psychiatric drugs; and in the overwhelming majority of cases, the drugs were anti-depressants, anti-psychotics, or cocktails combining them. The combinations were never tested together, and none of these drugs were ever approved for pediatric use. The media does not report this, and there has been no disciplinary action against any doctor or any pharmaceutical company that had a connection to a school massacre. In almost every relevant instance, the psychiatric records *disappeared* when requested by independent media sources or attorneys, including the Virginia Tech massacre. One of the doctors involved in the first U.S. school massacre, at Texas State University, came forward to admit the massacre's connection to Dexedrine. Nothing like that has ever been allowed to happen since. Now the pharmaceutical companies pay lawyers millions of dollars to halt drug intoxication defenses and to keep these cases hushed from the public. The pharmaceutical companies have been known to send their own legal teams to local courts to ensure that the drugs are never put on trial. More about this will be detailed later.

The Texas State University Massacre

The first school massacre in the United States happened on August 1st, 1966, at the University of Texas, in the city of Austin. The killer was Charles Whitman, a former U.S. Marine sniper and Eagle Scout. To get an ideal location to randomly sniper his victims, he climbed to the top of the school's clock tower. From there he rained bullets on pedestrians. He had already murdered his mother the night before. Prior to the 2007 massacre at Virginia Polytechnic Institute, the University of Texas at Austin massacre by Whitman was the worst school shooting in American history, in both deaths and injuries.

Charles Whitman had seen multiple psychiatrists at the university, and he was given prescriptions for both Valium and Dexedrine by university doctors to cope with his violent impulses. Dexedrine was used as an anti-depressant in the late 1960's, and it is known for causing akathisia. It is a condition which increases the risk of violent behaviors; whereas unmedicated depressives tend to be significantly less violent than average.

After Whitman's shooting rampage, the University of Texas was repeatedly petitioned to make its medical records for Whitman public. The university's administrators refused with claims that the release of Whitman's records would be an ethics violation of confidentiality; regardless of the fact that the patient was certifiably dead. In other words, after the university's psychiatrists had prescribed a violent patient a psychosis-inducing drug, they did not wish to be held accountable for this negligence, the patient's death, or the deaths of his sixteen victims.

The university had suddenly become more concerned about ethics than experimenting on people. In the university's defense, it was later discovered that Whitman had a brain tumor, which may have influenced his actions somewhat. Although no brain tumor has ever been attributed to any massacre, before or since Whitman's rampage.

The large media houses cooperated in the cover-up, by merely reporting Whitman's psychiatric visits, in order to convince the public that it was his organic mental problems that were to blame; instead of the censored psychiatric treatments. This is a journalistic pattern that has been repeated thousands of times in reports of violent crimes. Such omissions by our media corporations support their biggest sponsors, and are terribly convenient in promoting an agenda of disarming the American public.

Charles Whitman wrote a farewell note just before his shooting rampage, wherein he spelled-out his growing psychiatric problems. We shall never know with certainty if it was the brain tumor, or the Dexedrine which played the greatest role in getting so many people killed; but it was almost certainly a combination of the two.

One university doctor, Dr. Heatly, was honorable enough to come forward with his records on Whitman, despite the university's threatening posture. Dr. Heatly observed that Whitman became hostile with a minimum of provocation, had violent impulses, and that he had made vivid references to "thinking about going up on the [clock] tower with a deer rifle and start shooting people". The university psychiatrists had literally been given a face-to-face verbal warning by Whitman after their drugging campaign began.

After killing his mother the night before, Whitman sat down to write his farewell letter. He calmly explained that he had been a victim of irrational and unusual impulses that were hard to resist. He wrote of his plan to kill his wife as painlessly as possible, so that she would not suffer with grief after his death, and he noted his constant aggressive impulses. His lack of understanding of his own thoughts, rapid changes in mood, impulsivity, and vivid thoughts of violent acts were all characteristic of psychiatric drug intoxication; but in all likelihood, the doctors increased his dosage in response to his bad reaction, which is a standard procedure in psychiatry.

The Columbine High School Massacre

The most infamous of all school shootings was the one that happened at Columbine High School, in 1999. Columbine is a word that still sends chills through the spines of most Americans. After the massacre, the media thoroughly distracted and misdirected the public away from the pharmaceutical connections. People who remember the years following the massacre at Columbine High School will remember the blame being shifted onto school administrators, gun ownership, rock music, and even video games. Michael Moore wanted his slice of the propaganda action, and used his documentary, *Bowling for Columbine* to present the real problems as: Americans having too many freedoms, capitalism is bad, and that we need to be disarmed by a socialistic police state.

In all the news reports and documentaries immediately after the massacre were glaring omissions. Investigating the massacre is now fraught with challenges, and technically, such investigative journalism in the Columbine case is potentially illegal. This is due to the fact that U.S. District Judge, Lewis T. Babcock, ordered that records relating to Columbine litigation attempts be sealed for no less than 20 years. In all of our research, we had never before seen a court seal all of the records for anything, nor censor records for 20 years after a case's closure. Such an order is virtually unheard of, and very legally questionable. Most amazing is that the records were sealed for a dismissed case that never saw a jury. Thus, there were no actual proceedings to be disclosed; just shrouded evidence that would never be allowed in any trial or news report. Columbine victims will not be given access to the evidence until after the statute of limitations runs out. The pharmaceutical defendants could not have asked for better legal immunity. By fiat, and the stroke of a pen, Judge Lewis T. Babcock made it a violation of a federal court order to hold the drug companies responsible for what happened at Columbine.

We know from our Littleton sources that both Eric Harris and Dylan Klebold were using high, ever-changing doses of powerful anti-depressant medications, until the time of the massacre. We also know from the autopsy report of Eric Harris, who led the massacre, that he was still taking Luvox at the time of his death. Solvay Pharmaceuticals, the maker of Luvox, temporarily pulled Luvox off the market just two months after the massacre. The company claimed that it needed to revise its manufacturing process at that time.

The most damning element of the Columbine tragedy is perhaps the fact that the local government had been *forcefully* medicating Eric Harris, as part of a court-ordered anger management regimen. Therefore, there is a strong likelihood that Judge Babcock was protecting his judicial friends with his 20-year gag order on Columbine-related evidence.

At the core of the Columbine school massacre were apparently two teenage psychopaths, who suddenly began shooting down their peers, and even their personal friends, without any fear, and whilst laughing about it. Even the most hardened criminals would have had trouble being so fearless and carefree as the world around them crumbled. Whatever possessed those two boys was a bit more powerful than a video game.

Despite what most of us have been led to believe, Eric and Dylan were very typical teenage boys. Neither of them were mentally ill, and neither of them was ever in serious legal trouble. In fact, both of them were former scouts, and Eric in particular, was just short of his Eagle Scout rank. Both of them were intellectually gifted and fluent in multiple foreign languages. They were not the abnormal and hopeless wash-outs that the media presented them as. It is a myth that has been perpetuated for the sake of easing our fears, and subduing all honest investigations as to why the massacre really happened. It is most convenient for everyone involved that we merely believe that the boys were monsters by some genetic fluke. Of course, there is also video games, rock music, and teenage angst to shift the blame onto, but none of these things have ever caused sudden homicidal psychoses. However, such tendencies are actually known side-effects of the new generation of psychiatric pharmaceuticals. Yet the media companies avoid this connection, for the benefit of an industry that pays it more in advertising than all other industries combined.

It is rather common for teenage boys to fantasize about warfare, including playing war games or having secret plans of armed assault upon known targets. Boys will be boys. It is fairly common for boys to dream about blowing-up their own high-schools, and this writer is no exception to that. We know that the boys participated in mock war games for months, and possibly years before the real attack took place. It is unlikely that they ever seriously intended to conduct a real military-style attack during any of that time. Unfortunately, due to the emotional blunting (akathisia) effect of the drugs, the lines between dreams, fantasies, and reality blurred on April 20th, 1999. It happened on Hitler's birthday. In better times, losing one's emotional touch with reality was considered a terrible thing, yet this is exactly the intended design of modern psychiatric drugs; because reality is, after all, sometimes depressing.

The media industry reported, at best, fluff concerning the boys' mental state, and the topic of their psychiatric drugs was categorically censored by news agencies. People who did try to report about the drugs, or who tried to take legal action against the responsible medical parties were dealt with. John DeCamp was one of those people who were dealt with.

The Interview with John DeCamp

The following excerpt is from our upcoming documentary, *Prescription For Manslaughter*. Thomas Corriher interviewed John DeCamp. Mr. DeCamp is a former Senator and a practicing attorney. He is the author of *The Franklin Cover-up*. DeCamp was clearly afraid to answer certain questions during the interview, which speaks volumes about the power of the drug companies in suppressing the disclosure of facts about their products, and their culpability in violent acts. Unfortunately, DeCamp's nervous tone of voice cannot be replicated in print.

DeCamp represented families who had been brutalized by the Columbine High School massacre, in their thwarted attempt to sue Solvay Pharmaceuticals. The case was blocked by a federal court before it ever reached a jury. The records for the case were then sealed by Judge Lewis T. Babcock for twenty years. No media network covered this judicial cover-up, or the case itself. The mainstream media flatly ignored everything that was really happening in Littleton, the fact that the victimized families had identified the pharmaceuticals as the cause of the rampage, and that the families were actively attempting a lawsuit. The media instead reported that nobody had any clue about the cause of the massacre, and that the blame probably laid with violent video games or rock music. The same pattern has happened with every school massacre.

John DeCamp: I have been involved in a number of super high-profile cases since first edition of *Franklin Cover-up* came out, but perhaps the most frightening to me has been the Columbine case, where I represented various victims of the massacre and/or their families. I believe as a result of those cases, I am the only lawyer to have taken the depositions of the Harris boy's mother and father, and I am one of the only victims' lawyers to have seen certain Columbine materials and tapes. I have reached certain conclusions on Columbine which I feel obligated to put into print here in hopes it will some day make a difference. More court action has been done to keep everything secret and destroy the depositions than anything I have seen in my forty years of court activity. So, for my own personal and legal safety and protection, let me say simply that everything, absolutely everything, I say here is simply "my opinion and belief", and not done to violate any court orders or sealed records, but say these opinions and beliefs, I must. Number 1: I believe the first crime committed at Columbine was the slaughter of the children, Harris and Klebold's classmates, by Harris and Klebold. Number 2: Just as surely I do believe the second crime of Columbine has been the continuing and strong suppression of the information and evidence by the legal system which keeps parents and the public from really ever knowing the truth, or at least having a real opportunity to make judgments as to what the truth is, by having available all the information from which to make judgments. Number 3: I believe as sure as I believe anything on this Earth, the claim I made in a lawsuit in federal court, in which I alleged on behalf of the Columbine children, that the Harris boys actions, including particularly and especially his final act of suicide were caused or influenced to occur by the anti-depressant drugs he was taking. Number 4: Remarkably enough, within a year or so after I dropped out of the lawsuit, and the lawsuit was dismissed by the federal judge, it became public information and knowledge that certain of these anti-depressants do in fact cause suicidal behavior, particularly in children and teenagers, and now this fact must be put on the drugs when they are sold or prescribed to children. But of course, when I had this lawsuit going, none of this information was public knowledge, but it was all denied by the drug company, and one of these days, soon, when I get a legal comfort level to do so without getting punished by the legal system, I intend to blow it out all straight on the real Columbine truth. In the case, of.. what's his name? Harris, or Klebold, whichever... Anyway, I happen to have... I've got to be careful what I say. Remember all the depositions I took, plus all kinds of stuff is sealed, never to be accessed. You are aware of that, right?

Thomas Corriher: Erm, I have heard that.

John DeCamp: The judge ordered that, and I condemn that, but anyway.

Thomas Corriher: What was his...

John DeCamp: You'll discover if you had access to that, for example, you would discover that, it had gotten to the situation where he didn't have to go even though (pause) officially these drugs were given to him via a doctor, certified to give drugs, a nurse, and er... anyway... it was very open access and he was doing very excessive amounts and had weird conduct and behavior going on, but that's clearly documented in those... (pause)

Thomas Corriher: Sometimes, these psychotic reactions only happen after the drug is discontinued, like immediately afterwards. They go through a...

John DeCamp: That's also involved in the information in those.

Thomas Corriher: Can you tell us, what was the actual court order? I mean, I'm not a lawyer, and I'm not that familiar with how these things work, but can you tell us, what did the judge actually say? I mean, about being quiet.

John DeCamp: Said they're sealed, and I'm not supposed to talk about them. They actually sent some friggin' team of whatever here to supposedly go through my records and make sure I turned over everything I was supposed to. I think I might have mentioned that somewhere in my book. You said I mentioned it in that statement...

Thomas Corriher: Yeah, but by maintaining those confidential records, like you're supposed to as a representing attorney, you're not committing any crime whatsoever. What gives them the authority to come and snatch your records? To me, that doesn't sound legal.

John DeCamp: Good question. I don't know.

Thomas Corriher: To me, that sounds like a direct violation of the Bill of Rights, to just come -- snatch what they want.

John DeCamp: Under the legal system, judges can... anyway, do about what they want and get away with it.

Thomas Corriher: Whether it's legal or not, technically, right?

John DeCamp: Pretty much. You must know that.

Thomas Corriher: This isn't normal behavior, is it? I mean like, for instance, I'm sure courts ask attorneys to turn over stuff to the court all the time, but they don't show up with hired guns usually to do it, do they?

Decamp laughs nervously

Thomas Corriher: I mean, you know, it's...

John DeCamp: I guess you better speak to lawyers other than me. I don't know what all they do, because I was kind of shocked and didn't think they'd do this.

Thomas Corriher: Yeah, I mean, didn't they show up with the Federal Marshals?

John DeCamp: I have... I can't remember right now.

Thomas Corriher: Okay. I'm sorry.

John DeCamp: And that's 500 miles away, they came to show up. Here! Nebraska! My office!

Thomas Corriher: Whichever agency, they were definitely law enforcement personnel who showed up?

John DeCamp: I probably have some records or something on it.

Thomas Corriher: Okay.

The Depression Business and F.D.A. Science

There has never been a recorded case of any drug ever successfully curing depression. Every study that shows better results with pharmaceuticals than traditional psychological methods was sponsored by the maker of the drug. However, there are numerous documented cases whereby the depressive disorders were worsened in the long term by the drugs, and this is why psychiatrists are now desperately prescribing cocktails of various anti-depressants in a shotgun approach to medicating. The drugs are never approved for such mixed use, or tested for interaction dangers.

According to the May 2004 issue of the British Medical Journal, and a twin article in the New York Times, Allen Jones had been appointed to be a lead criminal corruption investigator for the Pennsylvania Office of the Inspector General, in July of 2002, after it uncovered evidence of payments into an off-the-books account. This mystery account was earmarked for "educational grants". It was funded, in large part, by Pfizer and Janssen Pharmaceuticals. Withdrawals from the account went specifically into the private bank accounts of drug regulatory agents, who were officially developing governmental guidelines recommending experimental, on-patent drugs over older, cheaper drugs that had better safety records.

On April 28th of 2004, Allen Jones was escorted out of his workplace immediately after state officials accused him of leaking information to news agencies. In his subsequent lawsuit against the Pennsylvania State Government, Jones reported that he had been harassed by his superiors and Pennsylvania governmental institutions, in order to suppress his constitutional rights of free speech and freedom of the press. He also stated that the campaign of aggression against him was intended to, "cover-up, discourage, and limit any investigations or oversight into the corrupt practices of large drug companies and corrupt public officials who have acted with them". We attempted to make contact with Allen Jones, but he has apparently found refuge in a log cabin that he built, and he has (perhaps wisely) made reaching him a challenge.

One method used by the establishment to manipulate drug studies is the handling of patients who die during drug trials. Test subjects who die are flatly ignored, as if they had never existed. This standard policy is justified by claims that the dead individuals did not complete the studies. Having dead test subjects might *bias* the safety conclusions of the study, after all. There are also in-place official policies at the pharmaceutical companies, which disallow suicidal patients in any of their anti-depressant studies. In practice, this ban translates into encompassing all depressed patients, since depressed patients always test to have stronger suicidal tendencies than the general population. So, in the vast majority of cases, official anti-depressant drug trials are never actually conducted on depressed subjects. It ensures that all subjects will not be suffering from depression at the end of the trial, because none of the subjects had actually experienced depression in the first place. Moreover, all drug studies are privately performed by the same pharmaceutical companies that are seeking approval, so the private research scientists have compelling reasons to get only the 'right' results. That is, if they hope to keep their prestigious careers. Doctoring the results in these ways are the standard procedure of the pharmaceutical industry, and it is officially F.D.A. approved. They call it "science".

Anti-depressants, and particularly S.S.R.I.'s, have been the subject of a large number of court cases, due to the drugs having caused patients to act irrationally, impulsively, and as if they had no conscience. Emotional blunting, in other words. Patients are never warned of these issues. Lawsuits have provoked certain drug companies to publish so-called "Defense Manuals" that are covertly provided to prosecuting attorneys. These manuals provide attack strategies for the prosecutors in cases involving psychiatric drug intoxication. They have been designed to ensure that the drugs are never put on trial, even when their relationship to the crimes has been established.

A Zoloft-specific defense manual was unintentionally made public, due to its use in the Chris Pittman trial. It was obtained and publicized by Court TV. The Zoloft Defense Manual dishonestly claims that Zoloft reduces violent behaviors, and that nobody has ever been given a reduced sentence due to Zoloft intoxication. This is despite precedent-setting cases to the contrary, which is something that the pharmaceutical legal departments know. Pfizer's defense manual states that previous trials concerning S.S.R.I.s, such as Prozac, are irrelevant; ignoring the similarities of these cases. These defense manuals are intended to manipulate agents of the courts, in order to shift blame from the pharmaceuticals onto the unwitting victims of the intoxications. The manuals are very appealing to prosecutors who wish to appear tough on crime.

Something is inherently immoral, and likely illegal, if it involves secret evidence meant to satisfy corporate agendas at the expense of due process. Our inquiries have shown that, in most cases, prosecutors cooperate with the drug companies to the point of illegally concealing these manuals, in direct defiance of lawful discovery procedure requirements.

The fears plaguing most of the expert witnesses make defending oneself in such cases nearly impossible. The expert witnesses know that their testimony could suggest that they have drugged patients into criminal activities too. Such an admission would be a terrible career move, in the very least. Thus, the experts are ironically the least credible witnesses in these cases, due to their need for self-preservation. It is similar to the way in which Mafia organizations stop members from witnessing. If everyone is made to have a skeleton in the closet, then nobody is going to speak publicly about the crimes.

S.S.R.I. Drugs Are Not Selective

"We can choose to use our growing knowledge to enslave people in ways never dreamed of before, depersonalizing them, controlling them by means so carefully selected that they will perhaps never be aware of their loss of personhood."

-- Carl R. Rodgers, former President of
the American Psychological Association

Contrary to what the public has been led to believe, the prevailing theories concerning serotonin and serotonin-effecting drugs did not originate from either doctors or scientists. They began life as intensive pharmaceutical marketing programs, which promoted fabricated scientific facts so successfully that they became facts in the minds of doctors, regulators and the general public. Understanding modern serotonin science requires a psychological study of mass manipulation.

Serotonin is a hormone that effects emotions, appetite, digestion, and the central nervous system. It was first noted for its effects on the cardiovascular system, particularly relating to constriction of the blood vessels. In more recent times, it is most often referenced as a neurotransmitter; meaning that it aids in the transmission of electrical signals inside the brain. Eighty percent of serotonin is used by the gastrointestinal system and only 10% of serotonin is used by the brain.

Due to the fact that serotonin is primarily used (80%) for the absorption of nutrients in the gastrointestinal tract, it is likely that serotonin's primary function inside the brain is likewise to keep brain matter nourished. This rather obvious conclusion points to the too-often-ignored evidence that depression is usually linked to malnutrition, nutrition loss through pharmaceutical drug use, or other sources of toxicity, such as heavy metals. Psychological depression is often the result of a physical metabolic depression that is caused by starvation hormones that are triggered by the aforementioned factors.

The presiding dogma of depression is that serotonin should be freely floating throughout the brain, particularly around the neurons. With depressed people, serotonin is allegedly assimilated too quickly by the neurons. It is said that this somehow neutralizes the serotonin, and this phenomena is labeled "re-uptake". When serotonin is absorbed too quickly, it simply vanishes and depression ensues -- goes the hypothesis. These drugs attempt to slow the absorption of serotonin, thus allowing it to remain stagnant inside the brain, mysteriously keeping people happy by not being actually used.

We can test for serotonin levels in the blood, but never in the brain of a living person, where the results would be meaningful. There are no methods of testing for the re-uptake of any neurotransmitter, or even if re-uptake actually happens as presented. The entire science is literally founded on a marketing fairy tale. Modern psychiatry dishonestly purports that the chemical imbalance hypothesis is hard core science, but it has never been proven in any study, ever. In fact, most of the independent depression studies that are available actually *disprove* the hypothesis of serotonin imbalance.

If low serotonin caused depression, then depression could be induced on any person by reducing his serotonin. This has been tested, and depression could not be reliably produced. Some studies have proven that depressed people already have higher serotonin levels, while others show that serotonin levels may actually be different in different areas of the brain. In truth, the methods of testing serotonin change from one study to another, because there is no accurate way to measure chemical concentrations in a living person's brain. Using current technology, accurate and meaningful testing would require surgery that would be fatal to the test subject.

Attempts have been made to study the serotonin levels in the blood of already depressed people and compare the results with those from healthy people. There has been absolutely no relationship found between depression and serotonin in the blood. There are approximately the same number of studies demonstrating high serotonin levels in depressed people as there are demonstrating low serotonin levels.

There is a reason why psychiatrists do not perform lab tests prior to diagnoses, or even prior to prescribing powerful drugs that are supposed to fix chemical imbalances. There are no tests for chemical imbalances of the brain. We do not even know what a healthy chemical balance would be, if we discovered it.

If the problem was simply that a neurotransmitter is needed to fix depression, then depression could be alleviated in less than 24 hours after taking a drug that increases it. Yet, S.S.R.I.'s take 5-6 weeks before they have any effect upon even the most severe depressions. Their horrible side-effects can occur within days, or even hours.

In studies that compared either nutritional therapies or exercise against drug therapies, the drug therapies were always the least effective. Furthermore, placebos are generally as effective as anti-depressants for the overwhelming majority of patients. Independent (non-industry) studies show that placebos are more effective, and they are absent of the dangerous drug complications.

The acronym S.S.R.I. is an abbreviation for "selective serotonin re-uptake inhibitor". Even the name for this category of drugs is, in itself, fraudulent. There is nothing selective about which serotonin in the body is effected, and most of the body's serotonin is not inside the brain. Most of a body's serotonin is used by the gastrointestinal tract, which means that the main effect of these drugs is causing nutritional imbalances. The drugs attack the body uniformly (opposite of selective), and their common ingredient, fluoride, suppresses systems throughout a body without regard to serotonin levels. There is no physical evidence that re-uptake in the brain is effected by these drugs, or proof that re-uptake even happens.

The Real Anti-Depressant Side Effects

"The machinery looks good, the technology seems nice, the stainless steel is shiny, everything smells like isopropyl alcohol; I mean they are the greatest salesmen in the world. We're going to go look back at this century and we're going to laugh eventually, but we'll cry first. This is one of the most barbaric periods. It's going to be called the Dark Ages of Medicine."

-- Dr. Richard Shulze, N.D., M.H.

Anti-depressant drugs carry massive risks, not only to the brain, but also to the heart, kidneys, liver, and central nervous system. Scientific research that is independent of the pharmaceutical industry has repeatedly shown that S.S.R.I. drugs can cause severe kidney and liver damage. These drugs also have the potential to cause cardiac arrest and a Parkinson's-like syndrome. Doctors are not required to advise patients of these risks, and they rarely do.

Serotonin works in conjunction with insulin to regulate the blood sugar, so an increase of serotonin in the blood causes the blood sugar to drop. Due to this, people taking S.S.R.I. drugs often get extreme cravings for sugars and carbohydrates. This perpetuates a cycle whereby people turn to junk food to satisfy these cravings, so the more direct weight gain that is caused by anti-depressant usage is compounded by the new bad diet. This is why these drugs cause a 2-to-3 times increase in a person's risk of developing diabetes.

The effects of S.S.R.I. drugs upon blood sugar can make stopping serotonin-altering drugs nearly impossible. Quitting the drug means that the regulator of the blood sugar is eliminated, yet the cravings continue, due to blood sugar instability, habit, and addiction. Thus, the addictions to S.S.R.I. anti-depressants are quite similar to alcoholism. We do not fully understand how these relationships work, but the bigger problem is that *nobody understands*.

Some people are more likely to experience side effects because they lack the liver enzyme: CYP2D6. This enzyme is necessary for the proper elimination of S.S.R.I.'s from the body. Without it, this class of drugs accumulate, in ever-increasing amounts, inside the body of a patient. A simple test for the enzyme can detect whether a person is deficient, to determine if there is a significantly increased risk of a bad reaction; but the test is never done prior to prescribing the drugs. One in every ten people lack this liver enzyme; meaning that every S.S.R.I. drugged individual has about a 10% chance of an accidental drug overdose that could eventually lead to organ failure or psychotic episodes. It is not unusual after S.S.R.I. murders for defendants to be found to have 10-to-20 times the dosage that they were prescribed in their systems.

Depression is exaggerated by nutritional deficiencies, which in turn means that depression can be exaggerated by these nutrient-robbing drugs. Serotonin plays a role in the absorption and assimilation of basic nutrients, and through alterations of the blood sugar, serotonin can alter food cravings. Thus, these drugs are dangerous because they inevitably lead to a state of malnutrition, which is often compounded with severe weight gain. This is one reason why a huge percentage of patients become more suicidal after being medicated, due to the subsequent explosion of weight gain.

Elevated levels of serotonin in the body leads to the poor absorption of zinc, a mineral that is crucial for proper immune system function, along with maintaining skin, hair, and nail health. S.S.R.I. drugs also reduce the usable calcium in the body to thereby make magnesium unusable; since magnesium and calcium are interdependent. Magnesium is believed to play a vital role in the release and re-uptake of serotonin, so the relationship between S.S.R.I.'s and fluctuations in magnesium have been documented by the psychiatric community. People with low magnesium levels are at an increased risk of heart attacks, strokes, seizures, personality changes, anxiety, hyperactivity and agitation. It has been shown that depressed people are already low in magnesium, and depression can sometimes be alleviated through magnesium supplementation alone. S.S.R.I.'s can also cause brittle bone disease by inhibiting the usability of calcium in the body. This has led to increases in broken or fractured bones in the elderly; whom S.S.R.I. drugs are frequently prescribed to, inside of nursing home settings.

According to the Boston Globe, Paxil gives women a 7 times (700%) increase in the risk of breast cancer. In the United States, 1 in 8 women will get diagnosed with breast cancer at some point. Therefore, a woman who uses Paxil for long enough is virtually guaranteed to get breast cancer. According to our statistical calculations, a woman has approximately an 87% chance of getting breast cancer if she uses Paxil for a decade.

> *"The FDA encourages studies in pediatric patients. Clinical trials involving children and orphans are therefore legal and not unusual."*

> -- GlaxoSmithKline, message to DemocracyNow

On April 4th 2011, David W. Freeman of C.B.S. News reported that anti-depressant drugs cause human arteries to dramatically thicken over time, irreversibly increasing the likelihood of heart attacks and strokes. Normal hardening of the arteries is slowly reversible with lifestyle changes, but anti-depressant induced arterial damage is permanent.

> *'"There is a clear association between increased intima-media thickness and taking an antidepressant, and this trend is even stronger when we look at people who are on these medications and are more depressed.', lead investigator Dr. Amit Shah, a cardiology fellow at Emory University in Atlanta."*

> -- C.B.S. News

S.S.R.I. drugs damage the liver, sometimes inducing a condition that mimics hepatitis C. The fact that the main ingredient of these drugs is fluoride also means that they dramatically increase the likelihood of thyroid disorders, particularly hypothyroidism, and these drugs weaken the bones throughout the body. Hypothyroidism can cause permanent hormonal imbalances that lead to countless other diseases, or new psychological disturbances.

Serotonin syndrome (also called serotonergic syndrome) is a life-threatening condition that occurs when serotonin levels in the body rise too high. This condition can only be induced by S.S.R.I. drug usage. It often occurs when people are prescribed multiple S.S.R.I. drugs, as is common in children. The symptoms of serotonergic syndrome include: restlessness, diarrhea, rapid heart beat, hallucinations, increased body temperature, loss of coordination, nausea, overactive reflexes, rapid changes in blood pressure, and vomiting. The agonizing muscle spasms can cause complete muscle breakdown throughout the body, and the waste products then cycle through the body to toxify the kidneys. The strain can cause kidney failure. Serotonin syndrome is rarely cited among the long list of side-effects that are listed with anti-depressant drugs. This well-documented and potentially deadly condition is not known of by most doctors, and the F.D.A. has been working to ensure that doctors remain ignorant of it. In fact, the F.D.A. routinely deletes documentation on this topic, despite attempts by its parent organization, the National Institutes of Health, to publish it.

S.S.R.I. anti-depressant drugs are known to alter the electro-chemical transmissions within the prefrontal cortex area of the brain. The prefrontal cortex is what was severed or scrambled by the lobotomies of yesteryear. Destroying the prefrontal cortex is what makes people passive and compliant to authorities, so it was once considered the ideal treatment for undesirables in U.S. mental institutions. The practice was eventually stopped because the movie, *One Flew Over the Cuckoo's Nest* had graphically showed the public that the surgeries were inhumane and violated the human rights of the patients. Yet, S.S.R.I. drugs have been studied and found to alter the same area of the brain, essentially doing the same thing with chemistry, minus the ice pick. While surgical lobotomies were abandoned decades ago, they were simply replaced with their chemical counterparts. The chemical versions seem less gruesome and barbaric, but they have the same effect upon the brain, thereby creating *the appearance* of more humane treatment.

The ability of these psychiatric drugs to cause aggression is routinely hidden under other names. For example, the U.S. National Institutes of Health admits that S.S.R.I. drugs can cause "hyperarousal", which is better known as the "fight or flight" response. The N.I.H. documentation recognizes that these drugs can cause people to become violently dangerous, by stimulating archaic instincts. Some side-effect labels are now even including the term, "akathisia". Although the chemical companies involved are towing the party line by maintaining that akathisia is merely a minor motor dysfunction. Wyeth Pharmaceuticals (now a division of Pfizer), the maker of Effexor, was the only company that was willing to list "homicidal ideation" alongside "psychosis" on their drug labeling.

In 1998, Patricia Gerber *et al.* from the University of British Columbia published a research study titled, *Selective Serotonin Reuptake Inhibitor-Induced Movement Disorders*, demonstrating that S.S.R.I. anti-depressants can cause multiple types of motor dysfunction. The most frequent of these syndromes is Parkinsonism. There is debate as to whether it is actually Parkinson's disease or just a syndrome mimicking Parkinson's. The occurrence of the condition is usually treated as being coincidental, as if the drugs had no involvement in the condition's development. Medical professionals have historically overlooked the causal relationship between the drugs and Parkinsonism, either willfully or through ignorance. This often results in increased dosages, or the addition of more medications. In *Prescribed Drugs and Neurological Complications*, the British Medical Journal reported that S.S.R.I. drugs are more likely to cause Parkinson's syndrome than the older class of tricyclic anti-depressants. Ironically, the newer S.S.R.I. drugs are preferred because they have been marketed to be safer than the older anti-depressants.

The older class of tricyclic anti-depressants created effects that were more likely to be personally bothersome for doctors; such as ticks, shakes, and other disturbing neurological symptoms. These effects made psychiatrists very uncomfortable, which led to a dramatic reduction in their use. The newer S.S.R.I. drugs are more likely to trouble the patients, by inducing zombie-like states, or making them feel out of control. They make the patients more compliant and suggestible, which is appealing to the psychiatrists. The most dangerous physical effects of the newer class of drugs are drawn out over an extended period; causing conditions like diabetes and cancer, which are less likely to be disturbing to the prescribing doctor than a convulsing patient, as sometimes happened with the older drugs.

S.S.R.I. anti-depressants are prescribed to some pregnant women to suppress depressions caused by normal hormonal fluctuations that are an expected part of their pregnancies. It took thirteen years of Paxil being on the market before the Food and Drug Administration released a warning about Paxil causing birth defects, in December of 2005. A class action lawsuit against GlaxoSmithKline, the maker of Paxil, resulted in the pharmaceutical company paying $1 billion to settle over 800 cases, which was filed by parents of children with birth defects.

Every S.S.R.I. drug has been linked to a wide range of birth defects, and some of them are deadly. The most common S.S.R.I. birth defects are atrial septal defects and ventral septal defects, both of which are holes in differing areas of the heart. These are most likely to occur whenever the mother is given these drugs during her first trimester of pregnancy. When the drugs are used later in the pregnancy, persistent pulmonary hypertension of the newborn (P.P.H.N.) is common, whereby blood cells do not get adequate oxygen. In July of 2006, the F.D.A. warned that women who use S.S.R.I.'s after their 20th week of pregnancy have a six times greater risk of delivering a child with P.P.H.N. Other known birth defects include club foot, craniosynostosis (a skull defect), and infant omphalocele (abdominal wall defect). Kaiser Permanente published the study, *Antidepressant Use During Pregnancy and Childhood Autism Spectrum Disorders* in November of 2011, showing that anti-depressant drugs taken during pregnancy doubled the risk of autism.

Discontinuation syndrome is a phrase that was coined to describe the withdrawal symptoms which are experienced by people who attempt to quit S.S.R.I. drugs. The World Health Organization reported that the phrase "discontinuation syndrome" was a way to obscure the proper association between addiction and these drugs, in order to cover-up the fact that these drugs are extremely addictive. The psychiatric establishment originally gave it the name "anti-depressant withdrawal", after it was discovered that between 20% and 80% of S.S.R.I. drug patients experience it. The percentage depends on the particular drug used. Recognition of anti-depressant withdrawal became a serious marketing problem in the 1990's, so "withdrawal" was renamed to "discontinuation syndrome" at a symposium in 1996 that was sponsored by Eli Lilly.

The most dangerous periods of S.S.R.I. drug usage are when users are first starting, changing dosage, or quitting. During these periods, people are unusually prone to becoming violent, suicidal, and homicidal, even more so than when they were taking the drugs at a stable dosage. It is when extreme akathisia is most likely to occur. For a large percentage of patients, the torture of so-called "discontinuation syndrome" is more extreme than illegal drug withdrawal, and more dangerous. Discontinuation syndrome is often so severe that people are unable to completely quit the drugs, or they become suicidal because their physical and emotional suffering is so great. Withdrawal symptoms often include electrical brain zaps, sensations of electrocution, hot flashes, random pains throughout the body, food poisoning-like symptoms, extreme fatigue, dizziness, anxiety, irritability, panic attacks, decreased concentration, and insomnia.

Anti-depressants are not just prescribed for depression, but rather for a whole host of chronic diseases, including fibromyalgia, chronic fatigue syndrome and arthritis. These drugs are frequently prescribed for conditions that physicians cannot explain, because the drugs make troublesome patients easier to manage. This happens despite risks that the patients may kill themselves or others, and a small percentage will experience a complete loss of identity requiring institutionalization. This usage is completely off-label and irresponsible; for there is no research showing that these drugs assist in suppressing the symptoms that they are being prescribed for. It is entirely about patient management for the convenience of physicians. The drugs are sometimes euphemistically referred to as "happy pills" when used in this manner, because the agenda is to keep the patient artificially appeased, in spite of the fact that his condition is worsening.

S.S.R.I.'s are prescribed for nicotine addictions too, ironically replacing the addiction to tobacco with a more dangerous one from the pharmaceutical industry. If you must choose one addiction over the other, choose the much safer tobacco addiction.

Military personnel are being used as a testing group for these dangerous drugs. There are several rarely known side-effects of these drugs, which have proven especially beneficial to the military's chain of command. An effect of anti-depressants is that they generally make people more submissive to authority, and this is the primary reason why these drugs are being given to children with attention deficit disorder, for the drugs are not truly being given for the benefit of the kids. The real motivation is that the drugs help authorities maintain better control over the patients, whether those authorities be teachers, parents, care home nurses, or military commanders. Such usage is more about power and control over patients who are in no position to give informed consent. Take for example the drugs' wide use in nursing homes, schools, and in the military, which is significantly greater than for the remaining population. As further demonstration of this unofficial agenda, children in the public school system are given fluoride treatments at school, typically without parental consent or notification, and military bases throughout the United States *mysteriously* have had fluoride in their water at such high levels that soldiers have been warned to stop drinking the tap water. This is not happening by accident, and fluoride is an active ingredient in all S.S.R.I. drugs, due to its pacifying effect.

In the past, the military has done experiments with ecstasy, L.S.D., and anti-psychotics. Using these drugs, the command structure intended to make soldiers into better warriors. Soldiers were to become fearless and aggressive. For this change to take place, the drugs must first numb the conscience. Now, massive numbers of military personnel are taking S.S.R.I. medications, and as a result, military suicides are at record highs.

The Mothers Act

It is hard to forget the past horrors of thalidomide whenever we think of pregnant mothers taking anti-depressants. S.S.R.I. anti-depressants have been tied to birth defects, including club foot, persistent pulmonary hypertension, craniosynostosis (skull deformity), infant omphalocele (abdominal wall defects), and congenital malformations. Despite this, there has been a push to force expectant mothers to be screened for mood disorders, and then to undergo *mandatory* "treatment" for them. Has any pregnant woman in history not had severe mood swings? A bill titled, *The Mothers Act* was introduced twice in the U.S. House of Representatives, but it never made it out of the committee in either case. It would have forced pregnant women to undergo screenings for mood disorders, and then it would have forced them to take prescription anti-depressants when they inevitably tested positive. This bill would enshrine into law the practice of forced drugging of all pregnant women, since pregnancy itself causes hormonal changes that lead to mood irregularities. While the bill has already failed twice, it is likely that another bill will appear in the future with the same demands.

> *"Principles of mental health cannot be successfully furthered in any society unless there is progressive acceptance of the concept of world citizenship* [one world government]. *World citizenship can be widely extended among all peoples through applications of the principles of mental health."*

> -- National Association for Mental Health, 1948

The Fluoride Connection

Notice the "fluo" part in Prozac's chemical name, fluoxetine. It denotes the drug's main active ingredient: fluoride. Fluoride is an active ingredient of all modern S.S.R.I. anti-depressants, and the trend of medicating depressed patients with high doses of fluoride began with Prozac. Fluoride robs people of their will; and therefore, it makes people easier to control for both authorities and psychiatrists. This is why these drugs have become so popular for supposedly treating attention deficit disorder, and the newly popularized, oppositional defiant disorder -- revealing that there is an agenda more related to social control than the legitimate practice of medicine. As one might expect, these drugs have become extremely popular in the military and the prisons.

In the 1930's, Germany's NAZI party envisioned a one world government, dominated and controlled by the NAZI philosophy of pan-Germanism. The German chemists produced an ingenious and far-reaching plan of mass-control that was adopted by the German General Staff. The plan was to control the population of any given area through forced mass-drugging with fluoride, via the drinking water. Through this method, they could pacify the populations of entire regions, reduce populations by water medication that sterilizes women, and so on. In their scheme of mass control and population control, sodium fluoride occupied a prominent place.

The following excerpt was reported by Charles Perkins, in 1954. He was an American chemist, who was rebuilding the German infrastructure.

> "Repeated doses of infinitesimal amounts of fluoride will in time reduce an individual's power to resist domination, by slowly poisoning and narcotizing a certain area of the brain, thus making him submissive to the will of those who wish to govern him. The real reason behind water fluoridation is not to benefit children's teeth. If this were the real reason, there are many ways in which it could be done that are much easier, cheaper, and far more effective. The real purpose behind water fluoridation is to reduce the resistance of the masses to domination and control and loss of liberty. I was told of this entire scheme by a German chemist who was an official of the great IG Farben chemical industries and was also prominent in the NAZI movement at the time. I say this with all the earnestness and sincerity of a scientist who has spent nearly 20 years research into the chemistry, biochemistry, physiology and pathology of fluorine."

Fluoride has been shown to accumulate in the pineal gland. The pineal gland is a pine cone-shaped organ near the center of the brain. It is believed to be responsible for melatonin production, and thus the regulation of the sleep cycle. It is also believed to play a role in seasonal depression, because more melatonin is produced in periods of darkness. Brain serotonin appears to be in the highest concentration inside the pineal gland.

In most medical literature, calcification of the pineal gland is expressed to be a natural phenomenon that increases with age. Calcification is when calcium, fluoride and phosphorus combine; until they merge into a hard, rock-like object that is viewable on brain scans. Despite the medical literature's promotion that this occurs normally with aging, pineal calcification is actually only a problem of Western lifestyles; indicating that it is our chemical exposures and diets that cause brain calcification. In West Africa, for example, a hospital that performed 20,000 skull x-ray examinations over a period of 10 years encountered less than 10 cases (less than 0.05%) of patients having pineal gland calcifications. In contrast, calcified pineal glands are visible in about 50% of Caucasian adult skull radiographs, for people over the age of forty in the United States. The rate for American Negroes is 25%.

Fluoride is known to accumulate in the pineal gland in even greater amounts than it does in bone. It increases the uptake of calcium into the cells, which worsens their calcification (hardening), since calcification is predominantly misused calcium. Modern S.S.R.I. anti-depressant drugs are fluoride-based; so they add to the calcification of the pineal gland. The accumulated fluoride attracts calcium. This ironically will worsen depression permanently, by artificially limiting the body's ability to regulate its sleep cycle, and disrupting the production of hormones.

More Effective and Safer Alternatives

Niacin (vitamin B-3) is typically ignored and marginalized, so multi-vitamins and B-complex supplements usually contain negligible amounts of it. Since 1 in 3 people die from heart disease, and depression effects about one in every ten adults, niacin supplementation should be paramount. Niacin is an essential nutrient that Westerners rarely get enough of through their diets, due to depleted soils and processed foods. It can be found in dairy products, poultry, fish, lean meats, and nuts. It is vital for the digestion of food, as well as nerve health and repair. It maintains healthy skin. A condition known as pellagra typically occurs amongst poor populations who are extremely deficient in niacin. It destroys memory and mental health, in as much as it causes chronic physical diseases. It is characterized by gastrointestinal disturbances, skin eruptions, and mental disorders in the worst cases. A niacin deficiency may also cause diarrhea, dermatitis, dementia, hyper-pigmentation, thickening of the skin, inflammations of the mouth and tongue, digestive disturbances, amnesia, delirium, depression, and with extreme deficiency: death.

Niacin is very helpful for the treatment of depression and anxiety, in part because the body can convert it into L-tryptophan. Pellagra sufferers have historically displayed the symptoms of dementia (which is not to be confused with the modern, redefined version of "dementia", which is Alzheimer's disease). This mental condition most closely resembles what we now diagnose as schizophrenia. Only 500 mg. of niacin has been shown to increase short-term memory by 40%. The effects upon long-term memory maintenance could be even greater.

Just like in the case of scurvy (vitamin C deficiency), death from pellagra is much slower in this modern age, and both deficiencies often manifest themselves in the form of heart disease. Niacin protects the arteries from damage and dramatically reduces cholesterol levels, since cholesterol is produced by the body to patch inflamed arteries. It decreases the risk of heart attacks, since it eliminates the conditions that place undue stress upon the heart and the arteries.

Exercise is always more effective than medication for both curing and treating depression, in every independent study ever made which compared them. Diet and exercise only fail in the pharmaceutical industry studies.

Depression is sometimes caused by candida albicans, a yeast that lives in the intestinal tract. Candida can release bio-toxins into the bloodstream that can effect an individual neurologically. It can also prevent the body from being able to properly absorb crucial nutrients from foods. If nutrients are not properly extracted from foods, then depression can result from malnutrition alone. Processed carbohydrates such as white breads, white rice, and pasta that is not whole wheat feed the candida, so limiting these carbohydrates in the diet could be essential. Anything that has been bleached white or minerally depleted, including white sugar and table salt, should be avoided. Yogurt contains flora, a healthy bacteria that fights candida in the body, so plain (preferably organic) yogurt should be added to the diet. Flavored yogurts contain unhealthy sugars, which will feed the candida, and would thus be counterproductive. Yogurt is often homogenized, so supplement with vitamin C and folate (or the inferior folic acid) to protect against inflammation and arterial damage. Read the section about *Allergies and Candida* in the *Alternative Medicine* chapter for more information.

Serotonin, L-Tryptophan, Fructose, and Lactic Acid

L-tryptophan is an essential amino acid that is found in many foods. It cannot be produced by the body itself, so it must be gained through a healthy diet, or through supplementation. It is the compound inside turkey that causes drowsiness, and turkey is the greatest natural source for it. L-tryptophan was a very common dietary supplement before being blocked for a year by the F.D.A. in 1989. It is used as a natural and holistic treatment for depression, and as a sleep aid.

It is widely believed that the body uses L-tryptophan as a building material to produce serotonin as needed. This is technically not true, as will be explained later. There is greater efficacy from L-tryptophan supplements than pharmaceutical S.S.R.I. anti-depressants, because supplemental L-tryptophan helps a body to naturally regulate its own serotonin effectively, so that there will never be too little or too much. It additionally helps the body to produce lactic acid, which has its own effect upon mood regulation.

As a natural substance, L-tryptophan cannot be patented, which became a big concern for the F.D.A. and its business partner, Eli Lilly (maker of Prozac), during the late 1980's. In the fall of 1989, the F.D.A. banned L-tryptophan sales in the U.S., claiming that it caused a rare and deadly flu-like condition known as eosinophilia-myalgia syndrome. The allegation was dishonest, following the usual pattern regarding herbs and supplements. L-tryptophan is merely a naturally-occurring amino acid (protein compound) that is already found inside of our foods. In other words, all of us would be in serious health trouble if the F.D.A. cronies had been telling the truth. Vegetarians would have been the only survivors of the tryptogeddon.

The illnesses reported by the F.D.A. were actually caused by toxic impurities in a specific L-tryptophan product, which was imported by a Japanese manufacturer. The manufacturer was discovered to have been secretly experimenting with a genetically-engineered bacteria, in an attempt to speed the production process and increase the potency of its tryptophan product. The company's mixing of a genetically-engineered neurotoxin with a neurotransmitter precursor like L-tryptophan resulted in accelerated excitotoxin reactions beyond what is normally biologically possible. It was the process of mixing something similar to aspartame with a bioengineered, bio-toxic, nervous system stimulant together: only worse. The deadly end product of this engineering was never truly L-tryptophan, but the perverse product was nevertheless the ammunition that the F.D.A. had been waiting for. The Japanese company was likely paid to taint its own products by the U.S. biotechnology industry, because the biotechnology industry would win regardless of the product's success or failure. Either they would find a way to patent their unnatural "L-tryptophan" to legally kill the natural competition, or they would justify removing the competing natural tryptophan supplements from the market using the scandal.

Eosinophilia-myalgia syndrome was relabeled to "fibromyalgia", because the alleged cause (L-tryptophan) was removed from the market, and yet it occurred anyway. A completely different disease was quickly created by fiat, which conveniently had exactly the same symptoms. This way, L-tryptophan was still guilty of the completely different and yet completely identical disease. No action was ever taken against the Japanese company which was responsible for the poisoned L-tryptophan products, and its involvement was abruptly hushed. Instead of disciplining the manufacturer, or addressing the issue of contaminated products, the F.D.A. completely banned L-tryptophan as an illegal product on March 22nd, 1990.

Prozac was first officially approved by the F.D.A. in December of 1987, but the big marketing scheme had not yet been employed. Just 4 days after the F.D.A. ban on L-tryptophan, on March 26, 1990, Newsweek magazine featured a cover article praising the new anti-depressant drug Prozac. Its cover paid homage to a floating, gigantic green and white capsule of Prozac, with the bold caption: *"Prozac: A Breakthrough Drug for Depression"*. Eli Lilly marketed Prozac as a new "breakthrough" to differentiate it from the older anti-depressants, which had been taken off the market because they were so dangerous.

This four day coincidence went completely unnoticed by media sources, but it is jarring to anyone with a knowledge of how these two substances are believed to work. L-Tryptophan and Prozac are both believed to work with serotonin, which was a relatively new concept for allopathic medicine at the time. Prozac (fluoxetine) is marketed to "enhance" the serotonin that is already present in the brain through some mystical reaction that can only be defined in grotesquely-long marketing buzz words. It made great fodder for waiting room brochures. Prozac was never fully understood, so everyone was fair game.

In contrast, the all-natural L-tryptophan is very well understood. It is used as a building material by the body to produce either serotonin or lactic acid; both of which play large roles in mood regulation. This allows a body to produce the exact amount of natural serotonin and lactic acid that it needs; so that a body neither has too much, nor too little of either. Tryptophan is the body's safety net for an internal balancing act. It safely works with a body, instead of against it; by giving it a tool that is needed, instead of overloading it.

The drug patent on Prozac expired in 2001, which *coincidentally* is the same year that the F.D.A. ban on L-tryptophan was lifted. The F.D.A. was actually helping Eli Lilly again: this time by eliminating would-be competitors. With L-tryptophan again on the market, it was impossible for smaller competitors to successfully profit with generic Prozac, since they would have to compete with Eli Lilly's products and tryptophan at the same time. The F.D.A. was getting flooded by legal actions regarding Prozac at the time, due to the drug's side effects. Eli Lilly soon after re-branded Prozac as Sarafem for the treatment of pre-menstrual dysphoric disorder, in an attempt to illegally extend the patent through deception. Their patent was invalidated in a lawsuit against a manufacturer of generic Prozac, which judicially laid the patent to rest.

The known effects of serotonin on the brain are mostly conjecture. When a patient tells his doctor that he is depressed, there are no tests of his serotonin levels. No such tests exist. Yet serotonin-altering drugs are prescribed, just as surely as antibiotics would be for the common cold. Doctors and other medical professionals are increasingly coming forward to question whether low serotonin levels really lead to depression.

We have done exhaustive research about the mechanisms of L-tryptophan. Those who are lactose intolerant, experience gastrointestinal problems, or who experience fructose malabsorption are likely to experience depression. This is believed to be because L-tryptophan from food sources is not being properly absorbed by the intestines, leading to reduced L-tryptophan in the blood and brain. Thus, supplementation would seem prudent for treating the symptoms. However, there are loopholes in this logic, because both fructose and lactose are metabolized and absorbed differently.

Exercise results in both reduced depression and an increase of lactic acid in the blood. It is this lactic acid that is believed to be responsible for muscular soreness afterward. Exercise has been proven to be equally effective as a treatment for depression as pharmaceutical anti-depressants. Thus, exercise brings about physical changes that can reduce depression, and we will shortly see the clear link between blood-borne lactic acid and mood elevation going beyond the endorphins. Lactic acid is one of the endorphins.

The reason why people with lactose intolerance and fructose malabsorption experience depression may not be a direct result of L-tryptophan deficiency, but of a plasma lactic acid imbalance. Fructose can be converted into lactic acid, but not in the case of someone who is suffering with fructose malabsorption. Those who are lactose intolerant are unable to create their own lactic acid through the usual route of lactose metabolization. This could be remedied by L-tryptophan intake, since lactic acid is metabolized from L-tryptophan reserves. This tells us that lactic acid may well be the cure for non-psychological depressions, but not when it is ingested in a synthetic form. It must foremost be ingested as L-tryptophan or fructose, and then be converted by the body. Without this conversion process, lactic acid is known to produce side effects, which ironically include depression.

Curing is about restoring balance, and the body can do better regulation than any chemist. With that said, lactic acid has long been demonized; especially by ignorant athletes. Recent studies are showing that such attitudes may be backwards. According to the New York Times, new studies show that lactic acid is the main catalyst for muscle repair and re-growth; not an athletic menace causing unnecessary pain and suffering.

The following table shows some of the organic chemical transformations that take place inside the human body. It shows the importance of lactic acid, and that the body can use L-tryptophan whenever it needs to produce either serotonin or more lactic acid, to get the so-called "chemical imbalance" balanced again.

Serotonin	-->	Lactic Acid
Fructose	-->	Lactic Acid
L-tryptophan	-->	Lactic Acid
L-tryptophan	-->	Serotonin

Of course, we are not going to recommend that people start consuming processed sugars or high fructose corn syrup to eliminate their depressions. To the contrary, the lactic acid that is produced from chemically-extracted fructose seems to be much less effective in helping with depression, and it fosters a huge array of very serious disease states. People should also avoid homogenized milk as a source of lactic acid too, because it too will bring long-term health consequences through inflammation, and these consequences include heart disease. Lactic acid from whole milk is nevertheless something of an anti-depressant and calmative, as is shown in its use with young children. Crying over spilled milk is not just a figure of speech.

We recommend L-tryptophan supplementation for those who are suffering with non-psychological depressions, as a method to naturally increase bio-usable lactic acid, but *not necessarily* serotonin. 5-HTP is based upon L-tryptophan, and has very similar effects, but it is not believed to be as effective. The calmative actions of both lead to a much more restful sleep, which is normally a chronic problem for depressed individuals. L-tryptophan will *only* produce more serotonin if it is needed. Only the right balance of serotonin and naturally-produced lactic acid helps to reduce depression. L-tryptophan allows the body to tip the bio-chemical scales in whichever direction they need to go. It demonstrates the difference between new age medicine and God's medicine.

Additional Depression Fighting Supplements

All of the supplements that we recommend to reduce depression *should* be present in a healthy, balanced diet. However, it is becoming difficult to eat a healthy diet, due to our fertilizer-depleted soils, the biotechnology industry, the chemical industry, the pharmaceutical industry, and the nuclear industry. People with well-balanced diets very rarely become depressed.

- Imbalances of zinc and copper have been tied to depression, and they are interdependent in the body. A deficiency of one can cause an unhealthy excess of the other. They should always be supplemented with together, to allow the body to create an ideal balance. *

- Cashews and walnuts are very helpful in stabilizing the hormones that contribute to depression, and provide the B vitamins that improve moods. Peanuts are not very helpful.

- Magnesium (requires vitamin D and calcium). Supplement in very small doses, because an excess of magnesium can cause other nutritional deficiencies.

- White vein kratom (Maeng Da) can be used as an anti-depressant. It is important to know that white vein kratom has entirely different effects to its close cousins, red vein (Thai) kratom and green vein kratom. White vein kratom is known to enhance a person's mood, while paradoxically being a calming stimulant. Some people find that it also improves their drive and overall desire to accomplish. Reference the *Painkillers* section of the *Alternative Medicine* chapter for detailed information about kratom.

- Salvia Divinorum

- Hormone regulating fruits, such as pears, peaches and apples. These work best in combination, so reference the *Hormone Regulator* recipe in the *Juicing* chapter.

- 5-HTP has been gaining a lot of popularity in recent years for its efficacy in eliminating depression. It has been demonstrated to be effective in multiple studies. Start supplementing with 25 mg., and increase the dosage by 25 mg. every four days if it is not having any effect. Do not exceed 100 mg. If you feel anxious, have trouble sleeping, experience nausea, or have diarrhea, reduce the dosage. A lot of people overdose with 5-HTP and thus experience side effects.

  * Some alternative medicine sites sell copper supplements, but oral supplementation with copper is dangerous. Overdosing with copper is very easy to do when using copper supplements, so it is very likely to happen. It leads to liver and kidney failure. For safety, copper must only be orally supplemented with by way of using a chlorophyll supplement. Overdosing with chlorophyll is virtually impossible, and it has other health benefits. Chlorophyll supplementation is the safe way to get extra copper. Transdermal application of copper is likewise safe: just do not drink any copper solution. Chlorophyll concentrate is preferable to more common diluted chlorophyll

products that require drinking large volumes to get any effect, and they contain impurities.

Zinc supplements can be purchased at health food stores, and should only be taken on a full stomach.

Unlike L-tryptophan, supplementing with melatonin can make depression worse or improve it, depending upon the individual. We thus recommend against supplementing with melatonin. Melatonin is produced from serotonin, so the need for melatonin can be fulfilled with L-tryptophan supplementation.

Despite the knowledge and use of L-tryptophan for decades, official studies are still surprisingly scarce, because no company will spend millions on something that they can never patent -- an ingredient of turkey. Nevertheless, there is compelling evidence that it can safely and effectively reduce depression.

Notes About Eliminating Depression

Whenever treating depression, it is critical to remember that depressions are often appropriate for the circumstances. If depression can be linked to an obvious psychological cause, such as the loss of a loved one, a poor work environment, or a relationship that went terribly wrong; you should consider coping with those psychological issues before seeking biological options. To feel depressed in these cases is entirely normal, and not the result of an imbalance.

Try to do something that makes you happy, and perhaps seek a Jungian Analytical Psychologist; for they are the elites in the psychological community. They deal with the root unconscious causes of psychological problems, and they do not prescribe dangerous drugs. Taking L-tryptophan supplements alongside the psychological analysis is an option for some, especially for those whose depressions are severe. For best results, take tryptophan on an empty stomach, because mixing it with foods decreases its effectiveness.

The Avoidance of Pain

Psychiatry is routinely medicating natural conditions with very unnatural results. Depression questionnaires determine if medicating might be of use, but questions determining if the depressions are psychologically appropriate, such as those caused by grief, are not even asked. The prevailing philosophy is that we can chemically turn-off the problematic emotions and worry later about the consequences; in much the same way that most alcoholics began their drinking to suppress depression. Similar to the way a heart attack releases hormones to make a person depressed and slow his metabolism, and post pregnancy depression does the same to force a new mother to slow down, depression is sometimes the appropriate response to overwhelming emotional pain.

Depression causes people to become self-absorbed, and this creates materialistic tendencies; whereby people learn to seek physical items to compensate for their sense of emotional emptiness. They sometimes temporarily fill the void with drugs or alcohol, or even shoes. This materialism feeds back into the depression; because the constant need for more money fuels anxiety, and it eventually increases a victim's sense of emptiness more.

The old-fashioned approaches of psychotherapy and psychoanalysis are proven cures for psychological depression, but no drug has ever been documented to cure any patient. The point of psychoanalysis is to gain a greater acceptance and understanding of oneself, so the analyzed may better relate to others beyond himself. The end result is a process going from selfishness to selflessness. The secret is: if you want to help yourself to recover from depression, then find somebody else to help. It is the surest way to improve someone's sense of self worth, appreciation, and for him to be loved. This code of loving thy neighbor being the most effective cure demonstrates that the problem is usually a moral and spiritual one, instead of a physical one. It is why the famous psychoanalyst, Dr. Carl G. Jung, referred to depression-related disorders, such as alcoholism, as being the product of "spiritual impoverishment".

Alcoholics Anonymous

Alcoholics Anonymous was founded on the basis that faith, and the sense of wholeness that accompanies it are required for people to overcome their alcoholism. It was influenced in large part by Dr. Carl G. Jung. An alcoholic patient of Dr. Jung's was recorded as "Rowland H". Dr. Jung had attempted to cure Rowland of his alcoholism, but in failing to do so, he told Rowland that the only thing that could salvage cases such as his was a spiritual awakening that led to an emotional rearrangement. Rowland passed this message onto others; eventually reaching Bill Wilson, who would later become the founder of Alcoholics Anonymous. Wilson contacted Dr. Jung to ask about the famous psychiatrist's fateful lecture to Rowland, and he received this personal response from Dr. Jung:

Dear Mr. W.;

Your letter has been very welcome indeed.

I had no news from Rowland H. anymore and often wondered what has been his fate. Our conversation which he has adequately reported to you had an aspect of which he did not know. The reason that I could not tell him everything was that those days I had to be exceedingly careful of what I said. I had found out that I was misunderstood in every possible way. Thus I was very careful when I talked to Rowland H. But what I really thought about was the result of many experiences with men of his kind.

His craving for alcohol was the equivalent, on a low level, of the spiritual thirst of our being for wholeness, expressed in medieval language: the union with God.

How could one formulate such an insight in a language that is not misunderstood in our days?

The only right and legitimate way to such an experience is that it happens to you in reality and it can only happen to you when you walk on a path which leads you to higher understanding. You might be led to that goal by an act of grace or through a personal and honest contact with friends, or through a higher education of the mind beyond the confines of mere rationalism. I see from your letter that Rowland H. has chosen the second way, which was, under the circumstances, obviously the best one.

I am strongly convinced that the evil principle prevailing in this world leads the unrecognized spiritual need into perdition, if it is not counteracted either by real religious insight or by the protective wall of human community. An ordinary man, not protected by an action from above and isolated in society, cannot resist the power of evil, which is called very aptly the Devil. But the use of such words arouses so many mistakes that one can only keep aloof from them as much as possible.

These are the reasons why I could not give a full and sufficient explanation to Rowland H., but I am risking it with you because I conclude from your very decent and honest letter that you have acquired a point of view above the misleading platitudes one usually hears about alcoholism. You see, "alcohol" in Latin is "spiritus" and you use the same word for the highest religious experience as well as for the most depraving poison. The helpful formula therefore is: spiritus contra spiritum.

Thanking you again for your kind letter

I remain Yours sincerely;
C. G. Jung

"As the hart panteth after the water brooks, so panteth my soul after thee, O God." (Psalms 42:1)

Alcoholics Anonymous co-founder Robert Smith ("Dr. Bob"), noted that the basic principles of A.A. came directly from the Bible. He wrote that, in particular, the essential passages he considered essential to successfully turn around a person's life were: The Book of James, Jesus' Sermon on the Mount, and Corinthians 13. The act of reading (and taking to heart) these passages is more powerfully life-changing than any pill, and hundreds of thousands of former alcoholics can attest to it.

A.A. records indicate that in Cleveland, Ohio, there was a 93% success rate for recovery in the early 1940's. The group's mission was to provide people with Christian empowerment, and in so doing, free people from alcoholism. Over time, the mission became more watered down, and discussions about God were eventually considered politically incorrect. Today, "God" has been replaced with "Higher Power" and "religion" has become "spiritual". Modern statistics show that the success rate has plummeted to a depressing 5%. The success rate is almost the opposite of what it formerly was, to the degree that avoiding A.A. has a higher success rate than the new A.A. "spiritual" programs.

> *"Over the years a disturbing change began to take place. As an increasing number of alcoholics joined A.A. chapters, many turned out to be misfits who had rejected Christianity, Judaism or the Kiwanis Club. Dogmatic and opinionated in their non-beliefs, they found in A.A. an instrument for a new kind of bigotry. Their only meaning in life was that they had heroically become 'arrested' alcoholics. Arrogant egoists, they soon dominated many of A.A.'s 10,000 chapters. Weekly meetings, once spontaneous and exciting, became formalized and ritualistic. Anyone who questioned A.A.'s principles or even expressed curiosity was handed the slogan, UTILIZE, DON'T ANALYZE, and told to sit down. The desire to help others degenerated. As one disheartened former A.A. member told me, 'I felt nobody cared what happened to Mary W. I felt they were just interested in another alcoholic who would become another notch in their belts. I felt as if I was being pressed into serving their cause and building up their oligarchy.'"*

> -- Dr. Arthur H. Cain

From the earliest records of human history, people have found bio-chemical aids for coping with extreme stress, depression, and grief. The original anti-depressant was wine. It has only been in our recent history that a new generation of synthetic, chemically-engineered solutions have caused mass-murdering rampages coupled with a high rate of suicides. S.S.R.I. drug-induced massacres and suicides tend to be the most vicious and gruesome of killings, which reveals how extreme the psychoses are for people under the influence of these mind-altering drugs.

S.S.R.I. Victim: Kurt Danysh

"I was on Prozac. It's supposed to calm me down, and like level me out, but since I got on it, when something bothers me, it bothers me to [the] *extreme. I just act differently. I don't have the energy or personality I used to. I spend half the time in a trance. I didn't realize I did it until after it was done, and then I realized it. This might sound weird, but it felt like I was left there holding a gun."*

-- Kurt Danysh, police confession

Kurt Danysh was an outgoing 18-year old boy, whose troubles began when he was prescribed Prozac by a doctor who had performed no testing. The teenager quickly became withdrawn, and his emotional instability tail-spinned, making him reckless and violent. His rapid drug-induced deterioration continued; placing him in a fight with his best friend, and later compelling him to intentionally crash his truck into a stone wall. He then vandalized his own kamikazed-truck with graffiti in a manner that was reminiscent of the Charles Manson cult. This era of Kurt's life ended with him fatally shooting his father, at only 17 days after his first dose of Prozac. There was no motive for the crime, and Kurt had no history of violence.

The Court's Shenanigans

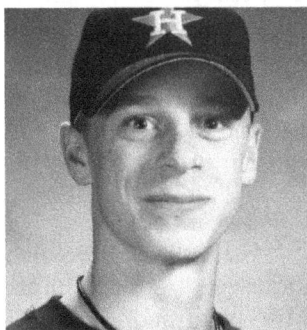

While being incarcerated for eighteen months awaiting a trial that would never come, Kurt refused to plead guilty. He was cruelly taunted by the jail staff with newspaper clippings about him. His attorney, Paul Ackourey, met with Kurt in the county jail, and implored him to plead guilty to third degree murder. The attorney claimed that Kurt's case was hopeless, for there was an apparent lack of evidence linking Prozac to violence. Kurt was refused a trial by jury for eighteen months, where he could have submitted a recount of his experience. The drug had been provided by the sheriff department's doctor, who had met Kurt after a minor offense. It is something that would have looked *really* bad in the press.

On one fateful day, Mr. Ackourey produced graphically disturbing photographs of Kurt's father at the scene of the crime and at autopsy. Kurt was then threatened that if he did not plead guilty, then his family would have to witness the grotesque images at the trial. Mr. Ackourey then left Kurt alone with the disturbing photos. He later returned to find Kurt crying. Kurt finally agreed to plead guilty, and he was immediately driven to the court house to enter a formal guilty plea. After having waited eighteen months, it suddenly took only minutes to get

Kurt into court. That is, once he agreed that there would be no jury, and that the drug that had been provided by the sheriff's department would not be mentioned.

Despite the court having been informed that the state's doctors had been continuing to drug Kurt with two major psychogenic tranquilizers, which are usually reserved for schizophrenic patients, the guilty plea was nevertheless accepted. The court made this decision despite evidence that Prozac had dramatically altered both Kurt's thinking and behavior at the time of his crime, and despite the fact that the state itself was actually giving Kurt even more mind-altering pharmaceuticals at the time of his confession. The Court of Common Pleas, of Susquehanna County, PA., accepted Kurt's "confession" for case number 132-1996 CR. Judge Kenneth Seamans sentenced Kurt to 22.5 to 60 years inside a maximum security prison. Kurt has been incarcerated at SCI Frackville Prison in Frackville, Pennsylvania since 1996.

During his sentencing, Kurt addressed his family:

> *"First and most important, I never meant for this to happen. If I was in control that day, it never would have. I know that doesn't lessen the pain, or the loss, or the anger, but it's the truth. Even though I had no control, I know I did a terrible thing. Words can't begin to describe how I feel. I feel the same hate and anger you do towards myself. The pain I feel will never fade... I am truly sorry for what I have done. I hope my sentence will bring some closure to the family... and to Dad, who I know is watching; I want you to know I always loved you and I never meant to hurt you."*

Kurt later received the expert opinion of Donald H. Marks, M.D., informing him that Prozac can cause violent behavior. Kurt appealed to the court with this newly discovered evidence, including additional complaints about his unlawfully coerced guilty plea, and his being under-represented by an attorney who was unable to uncover the scientific information pertaining to his case. On July 22nd, 2003, the same judge who had originally sentenced Kurt, Judge Kenneth Seamans, denied his appeal and excused this by referring to Kurt's appeal as "untimely". The potential of Kurt having been innocent was irrelevant to the judge, because in his opinion, the evidence was delivered too late. Meanwhile, Kurt waits in prison due to his lack of punctuality.

Eight years into Kurt's conviction, the F.D.A. finally admitted that S.S.R.I. anti-depressants, such as Prozac, cause psychotic suicidal episodes; particularly in adolescents and children. These drugs were never actually approved for pediatric use, and such use is termed as an "off label" use. The F.D.A. now requires that all such (S.S.R.I.) drugs carry a Black Box Warning; citing that they are to be considered dangerous for pediatric patients, due to their unpredictable psychiatric effects. A Black Box warning by the F.D.A. is the last step before an official ban is placed upon a substance, but doctors are actually prescribing S.S.R.I. drugs to young people more often in disregard of the warnings.

Since then, it has been revealed that Eli Lilly & Co. (maker of Prozac) covered up its own data from 1988, which linked Prozac to violence. No disciplinary action was taken against them.

Such cover-ups by the industry are implicitly encouraged by the F.D.A., and it allows companies to conceal negative findings under the guise of "commercial trade secrets". It has obstinately argued that pharmaceutical corporations cannot be compelled to divulge the results of unflattering research, even when the lack of disclosure will result in deaths. Neither will the F.D.A. release its own so-called "proprietary" drug information, and the agency cites that it is compelled to maintain secrecy by law. There is no such law. Pharmaceutical corporations are actually allowed to cherry pick the results that they wish to be made public.

A 1988 document that Eli Lilly held secret for 10 years indicated that 3.7% of Prozac users attempted suicide, which according to C.N.N. is 12 times higher than for other medications. The same document showed that 2.3% of users suffered from psychotic depression, which is double the rate for other anti-depressive drugs. In one paper called, *Activation and Sedation in Fluoxetine Clinical Trials*, the company's researchers reported that Prozac produces nervousness, anxiety, agitation or insomnia in 19% of patients. These research papers were 'misplaced' for approximately ten years, and it appears that Eli Lilly went to great lengths to hide them from the public. They became public only after an anonymous source leaked them to the British Medical Journal, which subsequently published them in December of 2004. Eli Lilly now maintains that they were never missing; and moreover, that they are insignificant. Stamped across each document, is the key phrase, "Fentress Confidential". Fentress is the surname of one of the victims of a Prozac-induced shooting.

Kurt Danysh filed an appeal on October 11th, 2008, citing new DNA evidence that supports the claim that Prozac played a crucial role in his father's death. Genelex Corporation, a laboratory which tests for the liver enzyme CYP2D6, positively identified Kurt as a poor metabolizer of S.S.R.I. medications, such as Prozac. Kurt's inability to properly metabolize such drugs greatly increases his risk of having poor reactions and bizarre side-effects. His liver cannot properly process these drugs, so they accumulate in his body in massive dosages over very short periods of time.

Kurt requested for Judge Kenneth Seamans to be excused from the hearing, due to him having committed glaring errors, and because Judge Seamans has shown an agenda of suppressing the issues surrounding Kurt's drug intoxication. Judge Kenneth Seamans has repeatedly refused to recuse himself from any of the proceedings.

Susquehanna County District Attorney, Jason Legg, filed an opposition to Kurt's right to even have an appeal hearing, because he likewise claimed that Kurt was too "untimely". Mr. Legg alleged that since the DNA test has existed since the year 2000, Kurt should have discovered it earlier (from his prison cell).

For the court of District Attorney Jason Legg, and Judge Kenneth Seamans, destroying someone's life is given less consideration than their more important face-saving measures of political self-service, and protecting their friends in the sheriff's department. As a result, no jury will hear about the Prozac connection to Kurt's crime. It is a repeat of what has happened in thousands of other cases.

"I would estimate that well over half of all defendant's are on some form of medication -- and I have never seen a case where such medication caused a defendant to lack the capacity to enter a guilty plea. There have been occasions when defendant's have appeared in court intoxicated, and, on those occasions, the pleas were rescheduled."

-- Jason Legg, District Attorney
of Susquehanna County, PA

Jason Legg wrote the above statement on his personal blog; regarding the use of involuntary medications being used during confessions. It is concerning that defendants are encouraged to make guilty pleas while being given (forcefully at times) mind-altering drugs. It tends to make getting 'confessions' rather easy. D.A. Jason Legg is not only okay with this, but he openly boasted about it in public, without any sense of shame. Then he noted that if a prisoner *appears* intoxicated, then the confession is rescheduled to a time when it doesn't make the officers of the court look so bad.

The Court Documents

In official documents and letters, the prosecution's own expert stated that Kurt's criminal actions were based on drug-induced insanity, which should have provided Kurt with a concrete defense. The sheriff's department was forcing Kurt to take more of these drugs before and during his confession.

One doctor who evaluated Kurt prior to the confession made the following judgment:

"With regard to his legal dilemmas I find that Kurt Danysh is competent to proceed with his defense. He has killed his father, he has admitted and confessed to the killing of his father. Kurt is severely mentally ill. He has experienced hallucinations, delusions, distortions and illusions. He has been depressed and at least hypomanic. At the time of the crime it is not clear that he was fully conscious of his behavior. There certainly did not appear to be any clear cut motive. Nevertheless he was generally aware of what he was doing... In spite of overwhelming mental illness I do not believe that Kurt Danysh meets the specific criteria for insanity as set forth in M'Naghten. It is clear, however, that his mental illness was the causative factor in the shooting death of his father, and were it not for his mental illness that has chronically impaired his judgment, this crime would not have occurred."

-- Gary M. Glass, M.D.

Hallucinations, delusions, distortions and illusions are classic symptoms of psychiatric drug intoxication. This combination of symptoms only happens through medication or severe head trauma. It never happens organically. Such "impaired judgment" -- not being able to discern right from wrong -- is the very basis of innocence by reason of insanity.

In the reports we received from District Attorney Jason Legg, the doctor questioned whether Kurt was even fully conscious during the murder of his father. He furthermore reported that the crime was completely without malice, without intent, without motive, and without criminal guilt. Nevertheless, Kurt was charged as if he held full responsibility, and he was given the maximum sentence for third degree murder in Pennsylvania.

The Anti-Depressant Legal Defense

The "Paxil Defense" has now been established in court. It has resulted in multiple people being acquitted of criminal charges, or given reduced prison sentences, due to their lack of self-control at the time of their crimes. The "involuntary intoxication" defense has also been used multiple times for other S.S.R.I.'s, such as Wellbutrin and Zoloft.

Herein is an attempt to provide precedent-setting legal information that may help psychiatric drug victims to mount legal defenses. Below is a list of people who were either acquitted, or who received a reduction in sentence, due to the effects of the anti-depressants that they were taking. This list was originally compiled by the S.A.V.E. Project (Stop Anti-depressant Violence from Escalating), but it was not actually placed online.

Cases Resulting In Acquittal

2000: State v. DeAngelo, CR 97 018766S (Milford, CT)

Christopher DeAngelo was acquitted of first-degree robbery, due to anti-depressant (Prozac) intoxication.

COUNSEL: John Williams, Esq. (New Haven, CT)

2000: Louisiana v. Pinckard, No. 2000 CR 286 (35th Judicial District)

Paula Pinckard was found innocent of murdering her 11-year-old daughter by reason of insanity. Her doctors testified that the Prozac she was taking before the shooting caused her behavior, for it acted as a catalyst upon her bipolar condition.

COUNSEL: George L. Higgins (Pineville, LA)

2000: Washington v. Curry, No. 99-1-02073 (Spokane County)

Sharon L. Curry was found not guilty by reason of insanity in the stabbing death of her 8-year-old daughter. The Sanity Commission found that the murder was the result of a drug-induced psychosis, and the court found that the drugs (Paxil and Adderall) were involuntary; since they were prescribed.

COUNSEL: CeCe Glenn (Spokane, WA)

2002: Arizona v. Jodi Lisa Henry, CR 2000-017302 (Maricopa County)

Jodi Lisa Henry was acquitted of trying to murder her two daughters, because she was insane and suffering from delirium, which were caused by her involuntary intoxication from the non-abuse of prescribed drugs (anti-depressants).

COUNSEL: Bernardo M. Garcia (Phoenix, AZ)

2004: California v. Meyers, No. F05187 (Santa Cruz County)

Andrew Meyers was acquitted of attempted murder due to anti-depressant (Zoloft) intoxication.

COUNSEL: Kristen Carter, Public defender (Santa Cruz, CA)

2005: Florida v. Larry J. Smith, No. 2003 CF 016229 NC (Sarasota County)

Larry J. Smith was acquitted of attempted murder by reason of insanity. He was found to have been insane at the time of the crime, because he was involuntarily intoxicated by a prescribed anti-depressant, which caused his violent psychosis.

COUNSEL: Jerry Meisner, Asst. Public Defender (Sarasota, FL)

2006: Washington v. Attwood, No. 05-1-1891-1 (Thurston County)

Eric Attwood, who was charged with attempting to kill his wife, was found legally insane at the time of the offense, because of his psychotic reaction to Wellbutrin.

2008: State v. Witlin, No. CR-07-0159548-T (Stamford, CT)

Eric Witlin was acquitted of attempted murder, assault, burglary, and risk of injury to a child. Two psychiatrists, including one hired by the prosecution, testified that Witlin suffered a psychotic episode, which was brought forth by Prozac and Adderall.

COUNSEL: Wayne R. Keeney (Stamford, CT)

2009: Kansas v. Housworth (Reno County)

Andrew Housworth was acquitted of five counts of battery against correctional officers and two counts of aggravated battery of a corrections officer and a fellow inmate, because Prozac *"caused his aggressive behavior"*.

COUNSEL: Alice Osburn (Hutchinson, KS)

Cases Resulting In Reduced Sentences

2001: South Carolina v. Brooke Jewell, No. 37608 (Charleston County)

Jewell, with no history of violence, committed and pleaded guilty to charges of rape. The judge concluded that Paxil did contribute to the man's crime. Instead of sentencing Jewell to two life sentences, the judge imposed a reduced 21 year sentence.

COUNSEL: Andrew Savage (Charleston, SC)

2001: Regina v. Hawkins, No. [2001] NSWSC 420 (New South Wales, Australia)

David Hawkins strangled to death his wife of nearly 50 years. Hawkins pleaded guilty to manslaughter on grounds of diminished capacity. The judge held that, *"but for the Zoloft which he took... the prisoner would not have committed the crime"*. He imposed a reduced sentence of 3 years.

COUNSEL: Ian Barker (New South Wales, Australia)

2001: Virginia v. John Lowe, No.11-447 & 00-449 (Washington County)

John Lowe shot his estranged wife and a deputy sheriff. A jury sentenced him to 54 years. The judge, relying upon testimony concerning the effects of prescription drugs (Prozac, Remeron, and BuSPAR) upon the defendant's mental condition, reduced the sentence to 19 years.

2002: Washington v. Corey F. Baadsgaard, No. 01-1-00208-5 (Grant County)

16-year-old Corey Baadsgaard took a rifle to his high school and held 23 classmates hostage. Despite being convicted as an adult, of kidnapping and assault, the court found that Effexor and Paxil caused *"prescription drug side effects"* justifying the mitigated sentence of time served (508 days) and 5 years of community custody.

COUNSEL: Tom W. Middleton (Ephreta, WA)

2004: Utah v. Leonard Preston Gall, No. 011919226 (Salt Lake County)

Leonard Gall had just begun taking a cocktail of Paxil and Zyprexa, when he killed his mother with an axe. He was found "Guilty-Mentally Ill" of manslaughter and theft. He received a sentence of 1 to 15 years.

COUNSEL: Stephen R. McCaughey (Salt Lake City, UT)

2006: U.S.A. v. Patrick Henry Stewart, No. 8:06-CR-257-T-30MSS (Florida)

Patrick Stewart was charged and convicted of embezzling $1.8 million. Defense Counsel requested, and was granted a sentence reduction that was based on the "Paxil Defense". Mr. Stewart received a sentence of 12 months of home confinement.

COUNSEL: Kevin Darken; Cohen, Jayson, and Farber (Tampa, FL)

2007: Texas v. Robert Crerar, No. 12521 (Bastrop County)

Robert Crerar, who killed his wife while suffering a violent reaction to Cymbalta, was sentenced to 10 years of probation for his role in the death.

COUNSEL: Art Keinarth and Robert Jenkins (Smithville and Bastrop, TX)

2010: South Carolina v. Christopher Pittman, No. 26339 (Chester County)

12-year-old Christopher Pittman used a shotgun to kill his grandparents. At trial, Pittman attributed his actions to Zoloft, but was found guilty of murder. That conviction was overturned on appeal. As part of a plea deal, Pittman was permitted to plead guilty to the lesser charge of voluntary manslaughter.

2011: Nevada v. Mary Baymiller, No. CR10-0267 (Washoe County)

72-year-old Mary Baymiller stabbed her husband, over 200 times, to death. The court found that Mary's *"conduct was directly and proximately caused by the combination of mood altering medications* [Paxil, Ativan and Ambien] *which she was prescribed"* and imposed a sentence of 5 years of probation.

The Big Psychiatric Picture

The psychiatric industry is perpetuating a fallacy of Eastern religions which corrupted Alcoholics Anonymous. This is namely that rationality combined with a lack of emotions is essential for personal success and growth. It has been modernized in the creed that logic and science shall save us from ourselves, because the underlying belief is that our real illness is our humanity. So at its heart, it is downgrading instead of uplifting. Under the guise of what is widely regarded as "Emotional Intelligence", psychiatry is encouraging people to develop sociopathic traits, to restrain their emotions, and to only exhibit emotions when they are useful for the exploitation of others. It is the warped Machiavellian philosophy of most practicing psychiatrists; most of whom have god complexes, so it is self-evident to them that these socially destructive traits must therefore be good and healthy. After all, their "god" (themselves) feels that this is an appropriate way to "manage" others. No longer is psychotherapy about healing through self-understanding and transferent methodologies that are meant to foster empathy amongst all parties, but it has become the psychology of conditioned responses and domination.

These psychiatric 'principles' were codified in the book *Emotional Intelligence*, by Daniel Coleman, and they were whole-heartedly adopted by the psychiatric community as scientific facts. As a result, new therapies are intended to alter people's personalities, so that patients learn to hide or fake their emotions as deemed appropriate for bending their environments. Emotions become a tool for exploiting others; instead of being bonding factors of personal relatedness and interpersonal warmth. This industry-embraced amorality has been defined as being "adjusted" (healthy) by modern psychiatry, but its replacement of real morality with a self-serving philosophy of deception does not breed functional members for any healthy society. It does the opposite, and the subsequent broken society breeds depression and mental illnesses in a self-perpetuating cycle of evil. These psychiatric policies project a reflection of the psychiatrists' own power drives that are closely linked to their own god complexes. It is always the other people who have "the problem", for not being more like them in controlling others through the careful management of their own emotional responses. Inwardly, they believe that life would be better for the patients if only patients learned to dominate others likewise, and to toy with other people's emotions as necessary for the desired goals. The doctors usually convince themselves that this is the superior method for dealing with life's problems. It *must* be superior, due to the fact that it is used by superior people, such as themselves. With great irony, this degree of narcissism and delusion makes the doctors classic examples of mental illness.

Whenever men have railed for truly uplifting ideals and freedoms throughout history, they have always been wrought with passion. We have no heroes or role models from history who were mediocre or sociopathic. Such people never inspire us, and they are themselves the uninspired. They may successfully manipulate us at times, but this is not the same as leadership, nor does it denote worthy character traits. The health of a society and the health of its individuals suffer equally from enslavement, and manipulative personalities were considered mentally ill in better times. By the old standards, almost every practicing psychiatrist would be considered severely mentally ill and maladjusted. Their reasoning skills are impaired by their illness. For example, their religious adherence to the teachings of emotional intelligence has them confusing "success" with "health", in believing that these are the same; but the two are mutually exclusive whenever a given power structure is itself dysfunctional.

It is emotional bonds that unite us, which are essential for building the free societies that have yielded our inventors, artists and revolutionaries. To care about the freedoms and rights of others requires conscience and passion. Our feelings were never the enemy. Passion is our only hope. The trouble-makers whom psychiatrists seek to drug into compliance are our society's only hope. As society becomes increasingly reason-based at the whims of psychiatry, socialism creeps upon us, as it always has in societies that morally decayed into sociopathology. In the end, the agenda is to destroy our spirit, so that we no longer seek the great ideas, such as our hard-wired programming to seek who is God and peaceably live by his natural laws. These yearnings were the basis of America's founding, and every great nation that has ever appeared on Earth. No decent, moral society has ever thrived being sociopathic, amoral, or while having its spirit destroyed. The countries that have prospered most were those guided by passionate and rebellious trouble-makers. They were blessed because their societies were not crushed by the secular humanistic drive to destroy all that makes humanity great, and they were the great exceptions to history. We should consider what we are sacrificing when we trade away our emotions and individuality, in order to become a compliant workforce; because this is the hallmark of a communistic society. For a century, people world-wide have died trying to escape the slavery that is befalling us, to reach our blessed Western nations. Through the sorcery of modern drugging and the institutional promotion of evil, those blessings are disappearing.

Being a functional, healthy and moral individual frequently means being unsuccessful, due to the efforts of those with lesser degrees of ethics. Nevertheless, greatness is having the character to do what is best for the long-term good, regardless of the consequences; instead of taking the easy path that provides quick satisfaction and less personal risk. According to the philosophy of emotional intelligence, a willingness to embrace necessary failures is not to be honored as a mark of character; but of stupidity. Under this banner, the psychiatric community is not fighting disease, illness or social ills anymore. Their enemy, behind all of their psychological games, is God, our Christian code of morality, and our esteemed Western civilizations. This evil brood has begun its unholy crusade by first targeting our children, our elderly, our military, and we the people are next. There is much more at stake than people realize, as drugging us into compliance becomes even more normal.

Vaccines

Why The Amish Do Not Get Autism

The uninitiated are often confused by the lack of autism in the Amish people. The Amish do not experience autism, or most of the other learning disabilities that plague our technological society. They live in a society that consists of outdated technologies and ideals, at least by contemporary standards. Their diet consists of eating organic, fresh, locally-grown produce, and of course, they do not follow the established vaccination routines. To the dismay of the medical establishment, this has resulted in a healthier people, who are devoid of all of our chronic diseases. Heart disease, cancer, and diabetes are virtually non-existent in Amish villages. Equally non-existent are our modern, chemically-engineered medicines, enhanced (chemically engineered) foods, G.M.O. (genetically engineered) foods, and of course, vaccines. How is it that those who are without the so-called "miracles" of orthodox medicine are healthier? The truth about health, medicine, and how they both relate to the Amish has become an embarrassment to some rather powerful people.

There have been 3 (*yes three*) verified cases of autism in the Amish, and two of those children were vaccinated. No information is available for the third child, who was likely vaccinated himself. The strong correlation between vaccinations and autism is becoming undeniable, unless you work for the medical establishment, the government, or mainstream media.

Proponents of the status quo actually claim that the Amish must have a super gene that makes them immune to autism. They rationalize that autism must be some type of genetic failure, which attacks brains based on religious affiliations. It is truly the best of F.D.A. and A.M.A. science in all its shining glory. Vaccine proponents are willing to espouse any ridiculous explanation, so long as they do not have to accept that their industry is *causing* chronic disease. Due to all their "help", children in the United States have a stunning 2% chance of developing autism, and that percentage is growing rapidly.

Beware When The G' Man Comes Knocking

The Amish are constantly harassed by health officials, who attempt to convince them to vaccinate their children. Whilst most Amish still refuse to vaccinate their children, a small minority are beginning to succumb to the scare tactics. This continues despite the fact that health officials actually have no legal right to visit people's homes and harass them into accepting these poisons. As more of the Amish vaccinate, the autism rates in their community will rise. Fortunately, the majority of the Amish still contend that vaccinations are against God's will, which interestingly enough, does indeed seem to be bringing about many health blessings.

Many of the viruses which children are vaccinated against are no longer circulating. However, fear tactics have led frightened parents to vaccinate their children against these viruses anyway. One of these viruses is polio. The most recent case seen in the Western hemisphere was in Peru, in 1991. The World Health Organization (W.H.O.) declared the Western hemisphere free of Polio in 1994.

On October 14, 2005, the media swung into hysteria after the vaccine-strain of the polio virus was found in the stools of four Amish children. The media declined to mention that it was the chemically-inactivated version, which is only found inside the orally-given vaccine. This means that the source for the 'outbreak' was the vaccine itself. The discovery was sensationally exploited to terrorize parents who had been avoiding vaccines.

Creating the Polio Pandemic

The spread of polio was fueled by the allopathic establishment's across-the-board removal of tonsils, which is the only organ that produces polio antibodies. Around the same time, the newly-created F.D.A. began suppressing the use of silver in medicines, which was the only safe substance that was known to kill viruses (like polio). Finally, "the solution" that industry desired, namely a vaccine, was released at the time when the epidemic was naturally ending, so that the vaccine could be given credit. All of this was orchestrated to manipulate the masses into accepting vaccines, radiation, and chemistry for health.

> *"During the polio epidemics, it was found that people who had their tonsils removed were 3 - 5 times more likely to develop paralysis There were many at that time that suggested that polio was an iatrogenic disease* [caused by the medical establishment]. W*e caused thousands of cases of paralysis. We did not cause the polio, but we converted people who would have recovered from a viral illness into people with a paralytic illness."*

> -- Dr. Mark Donohoe

With vaccinations, we are converting people who might have had natural immune-strengthening infections like the flu, or chickenpox into people who have life-changing disorders like autism. None of the Amish children who had polio in their stools experienced paralysis, or any other horrific symptoms. That fortunate conclusion is likely the result of them lacking the 'miracles' of allopathic medicine.

We must wonder how four Amish children who live in an isolated community managed to become exposed to the unique chemically-inactivated vaccine strain of the polio virus. It is more than likely that such a thing was intentional, especially when the harassment by local health officials is considered. In addition, the vaccine strain that was discovered had not been used for five years, due to the possibility of it causing paralysis. After all, if some Amish children were to get sickened by the polio virus, the Amish may all rush to get their children vaccinated, and the *science* of vaccinations is proven with a wink and a nod.

The manner in which this was reported is very telling. For instance, if the vaccine strain of the polio virus was found in a normal child, would the media have made the story into front page news? Would it even have been reported? The Washington Post explained that both state and federal officials had informed them of the story. Misleading titles such as, "Polio Outbreak Occurs Among Amish Families In Minnesota" were then used to manipulate resistant parents with bioterrorism.

When the Amish are simply left alone, to live free of the chemical toxins that are found in our medicines and foods, they are not plagued with diseases, learning disabilities, or autism. They are categorically more intelligent, with the exception of advanced writing skills, which is explained by the fact that English is not their primary language. Could it be those same Amish "super genes" at work again? Society could learn greatly from their example, if we would only stop poisoning ourselves, and our children on a routine basis.

The Vaccine Information War

Pro-vaccination sources often claim that vaccinations are normal in the Amish community, and so is autism. These are lies. While there may be some small Amish groups which vaccinate, and thus have autism; neither is normal. The United Press, in conjunction with Generation Rescue, published a story about the rates of autism in an Amish community in Pennsylvania.

Reporter Dan Olmsted went searching for the autistic Amish. Statistically, there should have been about 130 Amish with autism in the community he examined. Dan discovered 3 cases. The first was an adopted Chinese girl, who had suffered through all of her vaccinations on the same day. The second developed symptoms within 24 hours after getting vaccinated, and there was no information about the third case. The reporter even spoke with the local allopathic doctor, who the Amish sometimes visit whenever herbs and supplements do not suffice (e.g. broken bones). The doctor admitted that he had never seen autism in the Amish community.

Dr. Max Wiznitzer of University Hospitals in Cleveland is an expert witness for the government, and he fights against families who file for compensation with the National Vaccine Injury Compensation Program. He made a mistake when he admitted that autism rates in the Amish community are somewhere around 1 in 10,000. The rate for the rest of us is currently about 1 in 50, and growing rapidly. The numbers are actually skewed against the Amish, since a tiny portion of their children are secretly being vaccinated now.

Studies which purportedly disprove the link between autism and vaccinations have all been funded by the pharmaceutical industry. No vaccine has ever undergone any independent, controlled, double-blind studies to determine safety and effectiveness. *Seriously.*

Philosophical and religious exemptions are available in almost every U.S. state. The only states that do not allow exemptions are West Virginia and Mississippi. In those two states, children are sometimes home schooled to avoid vaccinations. In the other 48 states, the public schools cannot legally turn people away if they submit exemption forms, so it is crucial that people learn their rights, and use them.

A public education is considered a basic human right in the United States and most of the Western world. Legal threats and court rulings have forced various school systems into funding home schooling with paid tutors or into allowing unvaccinated students admission. The usual excuse that is provided by the school systems for attempting to remove the educational right from unvaccinated children is that such children would somehow endanger the health of vaccinated children. Of course, no evidence is ever cited because there is none. Their hidden admission is that the vaccinated children have weakened immune systems; for there would be no danger to them if the vaccinations provided them with real protection. Why would the vaccinated children be at risk of dangerous diseases? There are already precedent-setting cases that can be used against school boards and their representing attorneys. Most courts would view the ignoring of such precedents as a type of judicial contempt from the opposition, so arm yourself with the knowledge, and let them know that you know. You can beat them, even without an attorney. Hiring an attorney who is beholden to local politics and court protocols may actually hurt your chances of winning.

New and Bizarre Food Allergies

Vaccines are intended to work by forcing a body to overreact to a certain substance, such as a virus. This is accomplished by combining a small amount of the virus with substances that are known to be toxic (adjuvants), thus intentionally increasing the likelihood of a violent immune response. However, instead of merely becoming hyper-reactive to the virus, the body often becomes reactive to other substances in the vaccine. Vaccines are now including peanut oil, latex, soy, eggs, and milk proteins. These are among the most common allergies in modern society, and they are also common ingredients of vaccines. Most of the new and bizarre food allergies are caused by vaccines. People are not just vaccinated against the virus. They are vaccinated against the food ingredients, too. Latex allergies are highest amongst nurses, who are given routine vaccinations which contain latex. More people are being killed every year by these new food allergies than all of the diseases that are being vaccinated against combined. The inclusion of sugars in vaccines, combined with the adjuvant reaction, is almost certainly one of the reasons for the epidemic of type 2 diabetes. The body thereafter falsely associates sugars with an allergen.

Dr. Diane Harper

Dr. Diane Harper was the lead researcher in the development of the human papilloma virus vaccines, Gardasil and Cervarix. She made a surprising announcement at the 4th International Public Conference on Vaccination, which took place in Reston, Virginia on Oct. 2nd through 4th, 2009. Her speech was supposed to promote the Gardasil and Cervarix vaccines, but she instead turned on her corporate bosses in a very public way. When questioned about the presentation, audience members remarked that they came away feeling that the vaccines should not be used.

> *"I came away from the talk with the perception that the risk of adverse side effects is so much greater than the risk of cervical cancer, I couldn't help but question why we need the vaccine at all."*

> -- Joan Robinson

Dr. Harper explained in her presentation that the cervical cancer risk in the U.S. is already extremely low, and that vaccinations are unlikely to have any effect upon the rate of cervical cancer in the United States. In fact, 70% of all HPV infections resolve themselves without treatment within a year, and the number rises to well over 90% in two years. Harper also mentioned the safety angle. All trials of the vaccines were done on children aged 15 and above, despite them currently being marketed for 9-year-olds.

So far, 15,037 girls have reported adverse side effects from Gardasil alone to the Vaccine Adverse Event Reporting System (V.A.E.R.S.) and this number only reflects parents who underwent the hurdles required for reporting adverse reactions. At the time of writing, 44 girls are officially known to have died from these vaccines. The reported side effects include Guillain Barré Syndrome (paralysis lasting for years, or permanently -- sometimes eventually causing suffocation), lupus, seizures, blood clots, and brain inflammation. Parents are usually not made aware of these risks.

> *"About eight in every ten women who have been sexually active will have HPV at some stage of their life. Normally there are no symptoms, and in 98 per cent of cases it clears itself. But in those cases where it doesn't, and isn't treated, it **can** lead to pre-cancerous cells which **may** develop into cervical cancer."*

> -- Dr. Diane Harper

One must understand how the establishment's word games are played to truly understand the meaning of the above quote, and one needs to understand its unique version of "science". When they report that untreated cases *can* lead to something that *may* lead to cervical cancer, it really means that the relationship is merely a hypothetical conjecture. In other words, there is no demonstrated relationship between the condition being vaccinated for and the rare cancers that the vaccine *might* prevent, but it is marketed to do it nonetheless. There is no actual evidence that the vaccine can prevent any cancer.

From the manufacturer's own admission, the vaccine only works on 4 strains out of 40 for a specific venereal disease that dies on its own, so the chance of the vaccine actually saving an individual is about the same as the chance of him being struck by a meteorite. Why do nine-year-old girls need vaccinations for symptom-less venereal diseases that their immune systems kill anyway? Moreover, why are parents not being told that the ingredients in the vaccine are more carcinogenic than the virus that the vaccine is intended to prevent? It harkens back to the 1950's, when doctors were promoting cigarette smoking as a means to obtain better lung health.

Hepatitis B Vaccine

The mandatory hepatitis B vaccine is given to infants at birth for profit alone. It provides no benefit to the infants whom it is administered to. Hepatitis B is as difficult to contract as A.I.D.S. (Acquired Immune Deficiency Syndrome). As with A.I.D.S., the people at risk are drug users and people with multiple sexual partners. It is only transmitted through the following methods:

- Sexual intercourse
- The use of unclean hypodermic needles
- Being born of a mother who is infected

The vaccine is only effective for 7 years, so by the time the child is in a situation in which he could actually be at risk, the vaccine will no longer be effective. With children who have been born of an infected mother, the children already have the disease; and again, the vaccine is of absolutely no use. In order to help these children, completely safe testing could take place before the pregnant mother gives birth. There are options which can be provided to infected mothers in order to stop the transmission of the disease. Instead, the vaccine is given to infants after it is too late to be useful. Finally, it is unlikely that any of the vaccinated children will shoot-up with illegal drugs before their seventh birthday.

Along with being mercury based, the hepatitis B vaccine is said to be one of the primary causes of neurological problems such as A.D.D. and autism, which points toward its degenerative effects upon the brain. The really unlucky children can die as soon as a day after this vaccination. For most children, the risk of a serious vaccine reaction is approximately 100 times greater than the risk of contracting hepatitis B, and the risks are greater for younger children.

The most serious reported adverse effects from the vaccine seem to be restricted to Caucasians. Despite this, the main long-term safety study was conducted with Alaskan natives to avoid statistical and scientific "complications" (e.g. disturbing facts) and other studies typically involved Asians. These sneaky testing policies are representative of pharmaceutical *science*.

In 1996, 54 cases of hepatitis B were reported to the C.D.C. (Centers for Disease Control) in the 0-1 age group. Considering that there were 3.9 million births that year, the likelihood of hepatitis B in that age group was 0.001%. In the Vaccine Adverse Event Reporting System (V.A.E.R.S.) there were 1,080 total reports of adverse reactions from hepatitis B vaccinations in the same year and age group. Forty-seven deaths were officially attributed to the vaccine itself.

For every child with hepatitis B, there were 20 reported to have had severe vaccine complications. Bear in mind that only 10% of the reactions are believed to be reported to V.A.E.R.S., so this means that conventional medicine is harming approximately 200 children for every child it is protecting from hepatitis B. Even more damning is that these numbers assume that the vaccine is always effective, which it is not.

Only 1.3% of those exposed to hepatitis B will develop a serious complication. Coupled with the low risk of hepatitis infection, its small likelihood of causing serious harm, and the well-documented serious dangers of the vaccine: why are we vaccinating all infants for hepatitis B?

The manufacturers of the hepatitis B vaccine are paid over a billion dollars a year for this vaccine. With that money, they sway opinions. A manufacturer of the vaccine was asked at a 1997 Illinois Board of Health hearing to cite evidence that the vaccine is safe for a one-day-old infant. He replied:

"We have none. Our studies were done on 5 and 10-year-olds."

Taste Your Own Medicine

The swine flu hysteria of 2009 compelled the State of New York to enforce mandatory vaccines on all health care workers. The rules mandated both the seasonal flu and H1N1 (swine flu) vaccines. Other states considered following suit, along with select institutions throughout the U.S.

A huge portion of the effected medical personnel spoke out about their opposition to such rules, and many of them threatened to refuse the vaccines; even at the expense of their employment. The Centers for Disease Control surveyed over a thousand health care professionals, finding that most of them did not take the seasonal flu shot. According to the Associated Press:

"The reasons vary from safety concerns to skepticism over vaccine effectiveness."

The Centers for Disease Control found that most doctors considered vaccines to be too unsafe and ineffective for their own use. We can only wonder how many of the health professionals personally avoid the flu shots, in order to protect themselves, and yet hypocritically provide them to others in the name of health. While such legislation is certainly despicable, it is difficult to have much pity for these people who have remained silent, or who have intentionally misinformed the people who placed so much trust into them. How many have lied about vaccine safety and effectiveness to their patients, only to not take the shots themselves or give them to their own families?

Doctors in New York State filed a lawsuit challenging the forced vaccinations. The case was dropped due to a vaccine shortage in New York State, which was very convenient for the pharmaceutical manufacturers, who were trying to avoid the publicity, and having doctors turn against them. Thus, some of the inventory was *misplaced*.

Exemptions for "Mandatory" Vaccines

Although vaccines are frequently said to be "mandatory" in the U.S., almost all of the states have laws offering religious or philosophical exemptions. Parents may wish to consider these as options in order to protect their children. The only states that do not allow such exemptions are West Virginia and Mississippi. The religious exemptions are quite appropriate, because it really is the Christian thing to do. Exempting a child from vaccines is a simple task, and there are a variety of Internet sites that assist parents in crafting exemption forms. Due to the fact that the rules vary for different states, it would not be prudent to include the long list of regulations. In most states, simply creating an official-looking form that contains what follows is enough.

Vaccine/Immunization Exemption Form (example)

We, _____ and _____ the parents/guardians of _____ consider vaccinations (immunizations) to be contrary to our religious and/or philosophical beliefs, and we claim our lawful right as citizens of the State of _____ and county of _____ to exempt _____ from all vaccinations (immunizations) as of this day _____ of the year _____, and henceforth.

Signed: _____ and _____

For maximum impact, cite your state's exemption with its statute number on the form, so they know that you already know your rights, and that you are in a position to ruin their careers if they do not respect your lawful rights; because we have heard some really horrible war stories of school system employees trying dirty tricks. It would be prudent to send copies by registered mail to the school system's headquarters, the school itself, and to the local health department. This way they know you mean serious business, and that you will be in good legal standing to fight.

Dirty Pediatrician Tricks

In 2009, The American Academy of Pediatrics began sending out waiver templates to be given to parents who are resistant to having their children vaccinated. The documents were an attempt to harass and intimidate parents. They were steeped in the language of legal and medical terrorism. One of the documents claimed that children would get cancers without vaccines, despite the nonexistence of cancer vaccines. The forms insinuated that drastically horrible things would happen to children if parents were not compliant, and they included veiled threats that families could be broken-up at some point, due to the parent's alleged medical neglect. Once one of these forms is signed, it provides doctors, lawyers, social services personnel and the courts with what appears to be a written admission that the parents were willfully negligent in the child's care -- admitted child abusers.

Parents may not realize that they were tricked into labeling themselves as unfit parents until the document is used against them in a court of law. If they somehow manage to force you into signing one of these forms, then make certain to note on the document that it was signed under threat and coercion, and write it somewhere near your signature.

The official documents have publicly disappeared from the A.A.P. site after we covered this topic at our site (healthwyze.org), so you may view our archived copy of one of those documents there. At the top of the documents touchingly reads, "Dedicated to the health of all children".

Vaccine Liability

Americans should learn about the U.S. National Vaccine Injury Act before rolling up their children's sleeves.

> *"The NVICA, a 'no-fault' compensation system, was passed in 1986 to shield the pharmaceutical industry from civil litigation due to problems associated with vaccines. Under the law, families of vaccine-injured persons are required to file a petition which may be heard by a Special Master in the vaccine court. Successful claims are paid from a Trust Fund that is managed by the Department of Health and Human Services, with Justice Department attorneys acting as the legal representatives of the Fund. Sadly, it has been reported that less than 25% of those who qualify for a hearing actually receive compensation.*

> *"Processing a claim through the vaccine court can take up to 10 years, and in the end, no blame or culpability is assigned. In the mean time, the heartbreak continues, medical bills pile up and the daily potential for more children to be harmed goes on due to government protection of products that are believed to be the 'sterling backbones' of our country's public health policy.*

> *"Who can parents and vaccine-injured adults hold accountable for injuries caused by vaccines? The system is designed so that no one -- neither a person nor an entity -- can be tagged with accountability: Not the vaccine manufacturer; not the doctor who recommended the vaccines nor the person who administered them; not the Advisory Committee of Immunization Practices members (ACIP) who added the vaccine to the pediatric schedule; not the IOM members (Institute of Medicine) who perpetuate the mantra 'vaccines are safe and effective' and stonewall opportunities for change and improvement. No one is to blame, that is, except the 'defective child' who could not tolerate the immunological onslaught caused by the vaccines."*

-- Dr. Sherri Tenpenny

Accountability in the case of vaccines is legally nullified by the U.S. Government. Any American attempting to litigate against any member of the vaccine industry will have to fight against a team of attorneys from the U.S. Department of Justice, who will endeavor to ensure that the lawsuit fails. American tax dollars are paying them to ensure that justice is not served. The U.S. Department of Justice has officially advertised for these attorney positions on-line. The public posting disappeared immediately after we reported this story, but we had the forethought to keep a copy.

Here are a few excerpts from that D.O.J. job offering page.

> "About the Office: The Civil Division, Torts Branch, is seeking an experienced attorney for a position in the Office of Vaccine Litigation. Trial attorneys in the Vaccine Litigation Group represent the interests of the Secretary of the Department of Health and Human Services in all cases filed in the U.S. Court of Federal Claims under the National Childhood Vaccine Injury Act. The cases involve claims of injury as a result of the receipt of certain vaccines.
>
> "Responsibilities and Opportunity Offered: The position offers a unique experience in public service. The legal and medical issues at stake in each case vary greatly. Attorneys in the section independently manage heavy case loads, and while streamlined procedures are utilized, cases frequently involve complex liability and damages issues. The position involves significant trial practice. Vaccine staff attorneys are obliged to ensure that the Vaccine Trust Fund, from which damage awards are paid, is protected and, where eligibility criteria are met, that fair compensation is distributed to those whom Congress has intended. Attorneys appear frequently before the Office of Special Masters in the U.S. Court of Federal Claims, and also appear before the judges of the Court, as well as in the U.S. Court of Appeals for the Federal Circuit when handling appeals."

The lawyers are salaried up to $133,543 by the Federal Government (using U.S. tax dollars) to make certain that children with disorders, such as autism, never get the assistance that they need, in order to protect the mythology of vaccines. The U.S. Department of Justice described its job of protecting the pharmaceutical industry from child victims as a "public service". Meanwhile, the well-protected pharmaceutical industry is expected to continue making record profits on a yearly basis, and to be the biggest contributor to politicians.

Vaccine Politics

As a reporter for *The Guardian*, Catherine Bennett has been courageously defending society from "vaccine dodgers" and alternative medicine. In the British mainstream media, there has been enormous grandstanding about making the M.M.R. (Measles, Mumps, and Rubella) vaccine mandatory. Vaccinations have never been mandatory in Britain, because the English never believed that forced drugging was moral for a civilized society. This is one of the reasons why water has never been fluoridated in the United Kingdom.

One of our readers sent an article our way, entitled *"It's time we created special schools for MMR dodgers"* by Miss Bennett. That article was an expression of a media agenda to associate those who forgo vaccines with cowards and traitors, instead of the better educated people that they are. Throughout the Guardian's article, insults are piled upon those who have dared to question the wisdom of vaccines, and it was insinuated that society would surely suffer a calamitous failure without more vaccinations.

Bennett's bigoted article provided the revolutionary idea of separating unvaccinated children into quarantine schools for the protection of respectable society. Perhaps society should indeed separate the toxic, dumbed-down, pacified, and obedient families from the unpoisoned, healthy, vibrant, and creative ones; who are better poised to provide society with leadership. Families would be pleased to send their children to these special schools knowing that their children would be surrounded by healthier peers, whose parents were equally well-enough educated to act independently, in the best interest of their families. Such parents would rest easier knowing that the risk of school violence would be extremely low, due to the unlikelihood of any of the children having been given violence-inducing S.S.R.I. anti-depressants, which by the way, have been involved in every school massacre in history. Parents could feel safer sending their kids to school if they were not going to be around kids who emit radiation due to cancer treatments. With this sort of school segregation, we could more easily test which kids score higher in tests, who gets sick the most often, and eventually; which ones are the most successful in the long term. We are able to predict which category of kids would grow up with the best capability to become the leaders of society, and which ones would simply become the drones to be forever condemned to a life of serfdom.

Attempting to provide evidence of the dangers of unvaccinated people, Bennett's article referenced a seventeen-year-old boy who died of measles a year prior. Even with the resources of her major publication at her disposal, she still found only a single death amongst the unvaccinated. She neglected to mention how many more people were killed by lightning or meteors. Of course, she also never mentioned how many *vaccinated* people died of measles that year. Most of the British who catch measles actually get it from the measles vaccination.

The reporter's arguments ignored the fact that the six studies that are routinely cited to promote vaccinations already have well-documented conflicts of interest. All of them were clearly shown to have a high risk of bias by Cochrane's scoring system. Bennett then boldly accused the famous study by Dr. Andrew Wakefield (the first to confirm the M.M.R. vaccine-autism link) of being flawed by a conflict of interest. There are many party-line studies in the U.S.A. and Canada, in which a verifiable collusion with the vaccine manufacturers was ignored, in lieu of assaulting Wakefield's professionalism. The dozens of self-serving studies made by the pharmaceutical industry happened long before the paradigm-shifting study by Wakefield ever made the news. Dr. Wakefield published his findings at great risk to himself and his career.

Below are findings from scientists and researchers concerning the six major pharmaceutically-sponsored pro-vaccine studies:

"The study demonstrates the difficulties of drawing inferences in the absence of a non-exposed population or a clearly defined causal hypothesis." (Taylor 1999)

"The number and possible impact of biases in this study was so high that interpretation of the results is impossible." (Fombonne 2001)

"The Retrospective Person-Time Cohort Study, by Makela, assessed the association between exposure to MMR and encephalitis (EN) aseptic meningitis (AM) and autism (AU) in a cohort of 535,544 Finnish children (95% of the surveillance cohort); the children were aged one to seven years at the time of vaccinations. The authors compared the incidence of disease in the first three months after vaccination with the incidence in the following months and years. They concluded that there was no evidence that vaccines had provided successful inoculation. The study was weakened by the loss of 14% of the original birth cohort, and the effects of the rather long time frame of follow up. What the impact of either of these factors was in terms of confounders is open to debate, however the long follow-up for autism was due to the lack of a properly constructed causal hypothesis..." (Makela 2002)

"The interpretation of the study by Madsen was made difficult by the unequal length of follow-ups for younger cohort members, as well as the use of the date of diagnosis rather than onset of symptoms of autism." (Madsen 2002)

"The conclusion, however, implied bias in the enrollment of cases which may not be representative of the rest of the autistic population of the city of Atlanta, USA where the study was set." (DeStefano 2004)

"In the GPRD-based studies, (Black 2003, Smeeth 2004) the precise nature of controlled unexposed to MMR and their ability to generalize was impossible to determine... The study (Smeeth 2004) appeared carefully conducted and well reported, however, the GPRD-based MMR studies had no unexposed (to MMR)

representative controls. In this study the approximately 4% to 13% seemed to be unexposed controls regarded by the authors as representative. Such a small number may indicate some bias in the selection of controls." (Smeeth 2004)

The drug company that makes the M.M.R. vaccine (Merck) publishes an extensive list of warnings, contraindications, and adverse reactions associated with this triple shot. It may be found in the vaccine package insert that is given to doctors administering M.M.R., and inside the Physician's Desk Reference (PDR)(8,9). However, this information is never given to patients or parents. The original M.M.R. insert is quoted immediately below.

An Excerpt from the Original M.M.R. Drug Insert

The following afflictions affecting nearly every body system -- blood, lymphatic, digestive, cardiovascular, immune, nervous, respiratory, and sensory -- have been reported following receipt of the MMR shot: encephalitis, encephalopathy, neurological disorders, seizure disorders, convulsions, learning disabilities, subacute sclerosing panencephalitis (SSPE) demyelination of the nerve sheaths, Guillain-Barré syndrome (paralysis), muscle incoordination, deafness, panniculitis, vasculitis, optic neuritis (including partial or total blindness) retinitis, otitis media, bronchial spasms, fever, headache, joint pain, arthritis (acute and chronic) transverse myelitis, thrombocytopenia (blood clotting disorders and spontaneous bleeding) anaphylaxis (severe allergic reactions) lymphadenopathy, leukocytosis, pneumonitis, Stevens-Johnson syndrome, erythema multiforme, urticaria, pancreatitis, parotitis, inflammatory bowel disease, Crohn's disease, ulcerative colitis, meningitis, diabetes, **autism**, immune system disorders, and death (Figure 49).(10,11).

The M.M.R. vaccine manufacturer has begun censoring autism from the package insert for its second version of the M.M.R. vaccine ("M.M.R. 2"). Most of the above indications continue to be cited, except for the admission of an autism link, which has been selectively removed. The vaccine manufacturer previously admitted to causing autism, but only in private communications with doctors. Their statements to the public and the media have always been the complete opposite.

Parents in the British medical system are often ignored when they report problems with vaccines, because the doctors act as the gatekeepers. Parents cannot directly report bad reactions to regulators. They must instead go through their doctor, who may refuse, as a matter of protecting himself. Keep in mind that doctors in Britain get monetary bonuses for administering vaccines, which could be considered a conflict of interest.

Examine the following graphs showing the incidence of U.S. disease deaths relative to when the vaccinations for those diseases appeared.

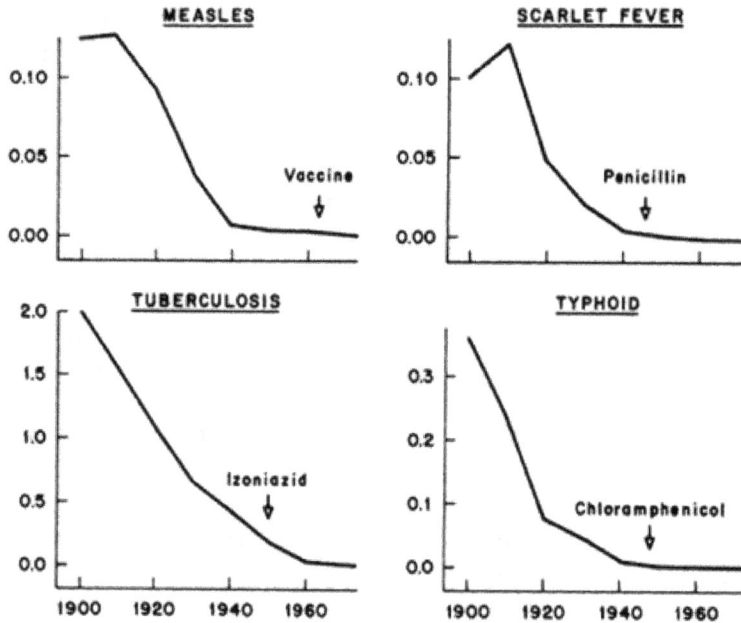

Source: *The Questionable Contribution of Medical Measures to the Decline of Mortality in the United States in the Twentieth Century* by John B. McKinlay and Sonja M. McKinlay, 1977

There is a somewhat inverse relationship in the graphs above. Notice that when the vaccines were implemented that the decreases in disease deaths actually slowed? This means that the vaccinations helped to perpetuate the continuation of the outbreaks.

This will hopefully end some of the delusions that the allopathic establishment has had great scientific breakthroughs which brought about an end to diseases. Measles deaths declined 99.5% before vaccinations, so was it really the vaccine that saved us? Such numbers steer us to ponder if policy makers have been trying to recreate the measles epidemic by injecting the live virus into people at a time when they do not need it. Vaccines should be classified amongst the most toxic and dangerous medicine ever known.

Vaccine Ingredients

There has been much recent concern regarding giving vaccines to children and the related side effects. Particularly concerning is the link between early childhood vaccines and autism. What follows will be a list of known ingredients inside vaccines, and their documented side effects. It will aid you in making informed decisions, which is something that the industry seems to be against. The corporations involved have attempted to suppress this information for decades. Readers are advised that there are additional chemicals and toxins not mentioned, because we had to base this list upon ingredients that are already public knowledge. While the U.S. Food and Drug Administration has made every attempt to suppress the disclosure of vaccine ingredients, much of the information herein was released by the U.S. Centers for Disease Control.

The connection to autism has already been repeatedly established, and there are many other conditions caused by vaccines. Permanent paralysis (Guillain-Barré syndrome) is surprisingly common, for instance. Vaccines are said to prevent certain diseases. However, the chance of catching these diseases is incredibly remote, and the horrid side effects from vaccines are so common that vaccines overall cause much more harm than good. The chance that a particular vaccine will actually offer protection varies between 35% and 90%, and almost all of them lose effectiveness over time. In some cases, vaccines infect patients with the very diseases that they were meant to offer protection from, because they utilize live viral strains.

> *"A single vaccine given to a 6 pound infant is the equivalent of giving a 180 lb. adult 30 vaccines in one day."*

> -- Dr. Boyd Haley

Vaccine Ingredient: Aborted Baby Fetus Tissue and Human Albumin

Did you ever wonder if aborted babies were sold to the pharmaceutical industry? Now you know. From a health perspective, the tissues from another human are foreign tissues, and therefore toxic to the body. One industry-friendly web site matter-of-factly boasted:

> *"The cells reproduce themselves, so there is no need to abort additional fetuses to sustain the culture supply. Viruses are collected from the diploid cell cultures and then processed further to produce the vaccine itself".*

The Liberty Counsel reported:

> *"You may be surprised to learn that some vaccinations are derived from aborted*

fetal tissue. Vaccines for chicken pox, Hepatitis-A, and Rubella were produced solely from aborted fetal tissue".

Vaccine Ingredient: Formaldehyde

This ingredient is used in vaccines as a tissue fixative, and as a preservative. Formaldehyde is oxidized in the human body to become formic acid. Formic acid is the main ingredient of bee and ant venom. Concentrated, it is corrosive and an irritant. While absorbing the oxygen of the body, it may lead to acidosis, nerve, liver and kidney damage. According to the National Research Council, fewer than 20% but perhaps more than 10% of the general population may be susceptible to extreme formaldehyde toxicity, and may violently react to exposure at any level. Formaldehyde is ranked as one of the most hazardous compounds on ecosystems and human health, according to the Environmental Defense Fund. These findings are merely for environmental exposure, and therefore, the dangers are much greater with the formaldehyde included in vaccines, since it is injected directly into the blood. The known effects of environmental formaldehyde exposure are:

- Eye, nasal, throat and pulmonary irritation
- Acute sense of smell due to altered tissue proteins
- Anaemia
- Antibodies formation
- Apathy
- Blindness
- Blood in urine
- Blurred vision
- Body aches
- Bronchial spasms
- Bronchitis
- Burns nasal and throat
- Cardiac impairment
- Palpitations and arrhythmias
- Central nervous system depression
- Changes in higher cognitive functions
- Chemical sensitivity
- Chest pains and tightness
- Chronic vaginitis
- Colds
- Coma
- Conjunctivitis
- Constipation
- Convulsions
- Inability or difficulty swallowing
- Inability to recall words and names
- Inconsistent I.Q. profiles
- Inflammatory diseases of the reproductive organs
- Intestinal pain
- Intrinsic asthma
- Irritability
- Jaundice
- Joint pain
- Aches and swelling
- Kidney pain
- Laryngeal spasm
- Loss of memory
- Loss of sense of smell
- Loss of taste
- Malaise
- Menstrual and testicular pain
- Menstrual irregularities
- Metallic taste
- Muscle spasms and cramps
- Nasal congestions
- Crusting and mucosa inflammation
- Nausea
- Nosebleeds
- Numbness and tingling of the forearms and finger tips

- Corneal erosion
- Cough
- Death
- Destruction of red blood cells
- Depression
- Dermatitis
- Diarrhea
- Difficulty concentrating
- Disorientation
- Dizziness
- Ear aches
- Eczema
- Emotional upsets
- Ethmoid polyps
- Fatigue
- Fecula bleeding
- Foetal asphyxiation
- Flu-like or "common cold" illness
- Frequent urination with pain
- Gastritis
- Astrointestinal inflammation
- Headaches
- Haemolytic anaemia
- Haemolytic haematuria
- Hoarseness
- Hyperactive airway disease
- Hyperactivity
- Hypomenstrual syndrome
- Immune system sensitizer
- Impaired (short) attention span
- Impaired capacity to attain attention
- Pale clammy skin
- Partial laryngeal paralysis
- Pneumonia
- Post nasal drip
- Pulmonary oedema
- Reduced body temperature
- Retarded speech pattern
- Ringing or tingling in the ear
- Schizophrenic-type symptoms
- Sensitivity to sound
- Shock
- Short term memory loss
- Shortness of breath
- Skin lesions
- Sneezing
- Sore throat
- Spacey feeling
- Speaking difficulty
- Sterility
- Swollen glands
- Tearing
- Thirst
- Tracheitis
- Tracheobronchitis
- Vertigo
- Vomiting blood
- Vomiting
- Wheezing

Vaccine Ingredient: Mercury

Mercury compounds are used in vaccines as preservatives. The toxicity of mercury has been repeatedly ignored in the area of vaccines by the medical establishment and oversight agencies. Mercury is the second most poisonous element known to mankind (second only to uranium and its derivatives). Brain neurons rapidly and permanently disintegrate in the presence of mercury within 30 minutes of exposure. Mercury is also known to change a body's chromosomes.

The U.S. Government has known about the potential problems of thimerosal (the mercury-containing preservative) for many years. The World Health Organization expressed concerns about it in 1990.

Mercury is a cumulative poison, which means the body has difficulty removing it, and that levels of it in the body will accumulate significantly over time. Large amounts of mercury can accumulate over a lifetime. During a typical day of routine vaccines, infants sometimes receive the same amount of mercury as the absolute maximum set by the World Health Organization for 3 months of adult exposure.

The following was taken from a website affiliated with the National Institutes of Health:

> *"Symptoms of high exposure to this class of mercury based compounds includes: Aphthous, Stomatitis, Satarrhal gingivitis, nausea, liquid stools, pain, liver disorder, injury to the cardiovascular system and hematopoietic system, deafness and ataxia. Death. Headache, paresthesia of the tongue, lips, fingers and toes, other non-specific dysfunctions, metallic taste, slight gastrointestinal disturbances, excessive flatus and diarrhea may occur. Acute poisoning may cause gastrointestinal irritation and renal failure. Early signs of severe poisoning include fine tremors of extended hands, loss of side vision, slight loss of coordination in the eyes, speech, writing and gait, inability to stand or carry out voluntary movements, occasional muscle atrophy and flexure contractures, generalized myoclonic movements, difficulty understanding ordinary speech, irritability and bad temper progressing to mania, stupor, coma, mental retardation in children, skin irritation, blisters and dermatitis. Other symptoms include chorea, athetosis, tremors, convulsions, pain and numbness in the extremities, nephritis, salivation, loosening of the teeth, blue line on the gums, anxiety, mental depression, insomnia, hallucinations and central nervous system effects. Exposure may also cause irritation of the eyes, mucous membranes and upper respiratory tract."*

Complete intolerance to thimerosal is known to develop from previous vaccines. The vaccines stimulate the immune system and cause a sensitization. The neurologic symptoms caused by mercury compounds have a delayed onset after exposure, so few, if any of these symptoms will be noticed at the time of exposure. The mercury of vaccines causes long-term neurological symptoms like learning disabilities and behavior disorders, which did not exist in previous generations.

Vaccine Ingredient: Antifreeze

Antifreeze (ethylene glycol) is an ingredient of the polio vaccine. It is classified as a "very toxic material". It would take less than a tablespoonful to kill a 20-pound dog with this substance. Pet owners are generally cautious with this dangerous substance, knowing that only a small amount is fatal. For humans, it is directly injected into the blood through vaccinations.

Antifreeze exposure can lead to kidney, liver, blood and central nervous system disorders. It is quite harmful and likely fatal if swallowed. Effects include behavioral disorders, drowsiness, vomiting, diarrhea, visual disturbances, thirst, convulsions, cyanosis, rapid heart rate, depression, cardiopulmonary effects and kidney disorders. It can also lead to liver and blood disorders. It produces reproductive and developmental effects in experimental animals.

Vaccine Ingredient: Aluminum

Aluminum is a carcinogen. It is a cardiovascular (blood) toxicant, neurotoxicant, and respiratory toxicant. It has been implicated as a cause of brain damage, and is a suspected factor in Alzheimer's disease, dementia, convulsions, and comas. It has been placed on at least 2 federal regulatory lists. It is well known in alternative medicine as a toxic and accumulative heavy metal.

Vaccine Ingredient: 2-Phenoxyethanol

This is a carcinogen. It is a developmental and reproductive toxicant. It is also a metabolic poison, which means that it interferes with the metabolism of all cells. This is the primary factor in the formation of cancer cells. It is capable of disabling the immune system's primary response. It also contains phenol (see below).

Vaccine Ingredient: Phenol

This is a carcinogen, and a cardiovascular and blood toxicant. It is also known as carbolic acid. It is a developmental toxin, gastrointestinal toxin, liver toxin, kidney toxin, neurotoxin, respiratory toxin, skin and sense organ toxin. It has been placed on at least 8 federal regulatory watch lists.

Vaccine Ingredient: Methanol

This is a volatile, flammable, poisonous liquid alcohol. It is used as a solvent in industry, and as an antifreeze compound in fuel. In the body it is metabolized into formaldehyde (described earlier). Whilst it can be found naturally in the pectin that is present in some common fruits, the naturally-occurring variant is only in minute quantities, and the organic form is not known to cause any harmful effects.

Vaccine Ingredient: Borax (sodium tetraborate decahydrate)

This was traditionally used as a pesticide. It is suspected to be a cardiovascular or blood toxicant, endocrine toxicant, gastrointestinal toxicant, liver toxicant and neurological toxicant. It was found to cause reproductive damage and reduced fertility in rats. It is already banned in foods in the United States due to its toxicity; but astonishingly, it is still allowed for direct injection into the blood through vaccines. It is toxic to all cells, and it has a slow excretion rate through the kidneys. Kidney retention and toxicity are the greatest. It has a cascading effect after causing kidney impairment, causing liver degeneration, cerebral edema, and gastroenteritis.

Vaccine Ingredient: Glutaraldehyde

Glutaraldehyde is always toxic, causing severe eye, nose, throat and lung irritations, along with headaches, drowsiness, and dizziness. The effects mirror the chemical warfare agent known as nerve gas. It is poisonous if ingested, and it is known to cause birth defects in experimental animals. The effects of direct injection into the blood to bypass the process of digestion are unknown. It is often used to clean medical equipment. In hospital accidents involving environmental exposure, it has been known to cause the following symptoms:

- Throat and lung irritation
- Breathing difficulty
- Nose irritation, sneezing, and wheezing
- Nosebleeds
- Burning eyes and conjunctivitis
- Rash-contact and/or allergic dermatitis
- Discoloring skin (brownish or tan)
- Hives
- Headaches
- Nausea

Vaccine Ingredient: Monosodium Glutamate (MSG)

Monosodium glutamate is a flavor enhancer. In a 1995 report by the Federation of American Societies for Experimental Biology, two groups of people were defined as intolerant of MSG. This includes those who eat large quantities of MSG and those with "poorly controlled asthma". Our research indicates that anyone can suffer after consuming monosodium glutamate; especially if they are deficient in either taurine or magnesium. In the 1995 report, which was contracted by the F.D.A., there was public admission that MSG yields the following symptoms:

- Burning sensation in the back of the neck, forearms and chest
- Numbness in the back of the neck, radiating to the arms and back
- Tingling, warmth, and weakness in the face, temples, upper back, neck and arms
- Facial pressure or tightness
- Chest pain
- Headache
- Nausea
- Rapid heartbeat
- Bronchospasms (difficulty breathing)
- Drowsiness
- Weakness

Note that this is the short list (the one with side effects that the F.D.A. actually admits) and it does not consider the higher toxicity of direct injection into the blood. The long list, which is 15 times longer, includes heart attacks. Injections of glutamate in laboratory animals have resulted in rapid damage to nerve cells in the brain. MSG is in a special class of chemicals called excitotoxins, which are known to directly attack brain cells. In 1978, MSG was banned from baby foods and other baby products that were produced for children who were less than one year of age, because the American Academy of Pediatrics and the National Academy of Sciences expressed concerns. It is now being used in these products again, in addition to being added to childhood vaccines.

Vaccine Ingredients: Sulfate and Phosphate Compounds

These can trigger severe allergies in children, which may last throughout their lives to permanently impair their immune systems.

Vaccine Ingredient: Ammonium Sulfate

This is yet another carcinogen. Ammonium sulfate is prepared by mixing ammonia with sulfuric acid. It is used as a chemical fertilizer for alkaline soils to lower the pH. In the body, it stresses the immune system by causing acidosis. Ammonium sulfate is also a liver toxicant, neurotoxicant, and respiratory toxicant.

Vaccine Ingredient: Gentamicin Sulfate

This is a strong antibiotic that is often used for life-threatening illnesses like pneumonia. The known side effects follow:

- Muscle twitching
- Numbness
- Seizures
- Elevated blood pressure
- Purpura P
- Pseudotumor cerebri
- Photosensitivity when used topically
- Transient irritation
- Vesicular and maculopapular dermatitis
- Stinging
- Bacterial/fungal corneal ulcers.
- Nonspecific conjunctivitis
- Inflammation
- Angioneurotic edema
- Urticaria
- Alopecia
- Burning
- Mydriasis
- Conjunctival paresthesia
- Conjunctival hyperemia
- Conjunctival epithelial defects
- Eyelid itching and swelling
- Itching

Vaccine Ingredient: Neomycin Sulfate

We can only speculate about what damage this causes when injected directly into the blood of infants. It interferes with vitamin B-6 absorption, which is the cause of a rare form of epilepsy, and mental retardation. Adult patients given neomycin as an antibiotic are typically placed under close clinical observation (e.g. hospitalized), so that intensive care intervention is immediately available. Neurotoxicity has been reported, along with nephrotoxicity, and permanent bilateral auditory ototoxicity. Sometimes vestibular toxicity is present in patients with normal renal function when treated with higher or longer doses than recommended.

Vaccine Ingredient: Tri(n)butylphosphate

This is yet another carcinogen. This is a kidney toxicant and a neurotoxicant. It is more hazardous than most chemicals in 2 out of 3 ranking systems. It is on at least 1 federal regulatory list.

Vaccine Ingredient: Polymyxin B

This is another antibiotic. Injection of this is generally avoided by doctors (except in the case of vaccines) due to "severe pain at injection sites, particularly in infants and children".

Known side effects:

- Albuminuria
- Cylindruria
- Azotemia
- Facial flushing
- Dizziness progressing to ataxia
- Drowsiness
- Peripheral paresthesias (circumoral and stocking-glove)
- Apnea
- Signs of meningeal irritation with intrathecal administration

Vaccine Ingredient: Polysorbate 20 / 80 *(Emulsifier)*

This is a known skin and sense organ toxin. It is verified as a cancer agent in animals.

Vaccine Ingredient: Sorbitol *(Sweetener)*

Diabetic retinopathy and neuropathy may be related to excess sorbitol in the cells of the eyes and nerves, leading to blindness. This is another suspected carcinogen. Sorbitol is a gastrointestinal and liver toxicant.

Vaccine Ingredient: Polyribosylribitol

This is an experimental artificial sweetener. The experimentation is ongoing in children, without the knowledge or consent of their parents.

Vaccine Ingredient: Beta-Propiolactone

Documented as a verified carcinogen. It is a gastrointestinal and liver toxicant, respiratory toxicant, skin toxicant, and sense organ toxicant. It is more hazardous than most chemicals earning a 3 out of 3 in ranking systems. It appears on at least 5 federal regulatory lists. It is ranked as one of the most hazardous compounds to humans.

Vaccine Ingredient: Amphotericin B

This can cause irreversible kidney damage, and mild liver failure. It has been known to produce severe histamine (allergic) reactions. There are several reports of anemia and cardiac failure. It is used used to treat fungus infections. Other side effects include blood clots, blood defects, kidney problems, nausea and fever. When used on the skin, allergic reactions can occur.

Vaccine Ingredients: Animal Organ Tissue and Animal Blood

Animal cell lines are used to culture the viruses in vaccines, so animal tissues and impurities are included in the formulation that is injected. Animal tissues are unusable and toxic to the body except for when their protein materials are digested to form amino acids through normal food consumption. There is no digestion process for injections. Injections may also contain many types of animal viruses (see the Animal Viruses section). Animals used include monkey (kidney), cow (heart), calf (serum), chicken (embryo and egg), duck (egg), pig (blood), sheep (blood), dog (kidney), horse (blood), rabbit (brain), and guinea pig.

Vaccine Ingredient: Large Foreign Proteins

In addition to the animal tissue impurities, there are large proteins that are deliberately included, and used for such purposes as adjuvants (substances that aggravate an immune response using their inherent toxicity). Egg albumin and gelatin (or gelatine, obtained from selected pieces of calf and cattle skins, demineralized cattle bones and pork skin) are in several vaccines. Casein (a milk protein) is in the triple antigen (DPT) vaccine. When injected, these normally harmless proteins are toxic to the body. Hence the immune system "response". The immune system is intentionally stressed by this invasion to produce an unnatural sensitization to all of the ingredients. This explains why bizarre allergies such as lactose intolerance, along with egg and nut allergies have suddenly become common in recent history.

Vaccine Ingredient: Latex

Latex is included in the hepatitis B vaccine, which is routinely given to health workers. The high occurrence of latex allergies among nurses is due to their sensitization to latex through the large amount that is injected into them. These vaccines produce a panicked immune response. The nurses will suffer with this allergy permanently. Such allergic reactions can be life-threatening. The hepatitis B vaccine is now routinely given to newborn babies in many countries, including Australia and the United States.

Vaccine Ingredient: Animal Viruses

Some of these can be particularly alien to the human body. The most frequently documented and publicized example is the monkey virus SV40. The virus is harmless in monkeys, but it stimulates rare cancers when injected into humans to produce brain cancer, bone (multiple myeloma), lungs (mesothelioma), and lymphoid tissue (lymphoma). Monkey virus SV40 has only appeared in people born in the last 20 years (The Journal of Infectious Diseases, Sept. 1999), long after the manufacturer claimed to have "cleaned up" the polio vaccines where it was initially found. Such cases include the late Alexander Horwin, whose parents tested negative for SV40. Therefore, recent cases cannot just be blamed on inheritance from parents who received the vaccine. Manufacturers are secretly including the virus again.

Vaccine Ingredient: Human Viruses

The live viruses found in some vaccines are frequently said to be killed, inactivated, or attenuated. This is a myth. The main method used to inactivate viruses is treatment with formaldehyde. Its effectiveness is limited and temporary. Once the brew is injected into the body, the formaldehyde is broken down: potentially releasing the virus in its original state. It is documented in orthodox medical literature that the "crippled" viruses can revert to their former virulence.

The viruses and bacteria included in vaccines are claimed to be in very small volume. However, these quantities are high enough for the diseases to occur in some people. Most of the diseases that people are vaccinated against no longer occur in the Western world, and only ever result from the vaccines. When they do occur, the vaccine-induced cases are always more severe than normal infections of the same pathogens, and these cases are sometimes fatal. Deaths have been reported in the British medical journal, Lancet, from vaccine-induced yellow fever. A susceptible person may succumb to infection when exposed to only a minute dose, especially when it is injected directly into the bloodstream. Conversely, there are other cases in which a healthy person will not succumb, even when exposed to large doses environmentally. It is not the pathogens, but the interaction methods between pathogens and hosts which causes diseases to appear, and ultimately determines their severity.

Most disease symptoms are the visible signs of a body's attempts to defend itself against the infection. With disease injections, many important defenses in the digestion path and mucous membranes are bypassed.

Vaccine Ingredient: Mycoplasma

These are microscopic organisms lacking rigid cell walls and they are considered to be the smallest free-moving organisms. Many are pathogenic, and one species is the cause of mycoplasma pneumonia which interestingly, is noted to occur only "in children and young adults", according to Mosby's Medical Dictionary. This is not simply in vaccines by accident. It is deliberately added as an adjuvant (to increase the immune system's allergic response) to the vaccine.

Vaccine Ingredient: Genetically-Engineered Yeast

This is in the hepatitis B vaccine. Given the controversy over the ingestion of genetically modified foods, how much more dangerous could the direct injection of them be?

Vaccine Ingredient: Foreign DNA

DNA is used from such organisms as animals, viruses, fungi, and bacteria. It has been documented that injecting foreign DNA can cause it, or a portion of it, to be incorporated into the recipient's DNA. The horrendous long-term multi-generational implications defy the imagination.

Final Thoughts

The human body has never experienced such a direct invasion as this before. We hope that you consider this list, and the side effects of vaccines before giving your child vaccinations. We have strong reasons to believe that overall, the risks of horrible and long-term side effects far outweigh the risks of the diseases which vaccines are supposed to prevent.

Human blood is supposed to be, and traditionally was, remarkably sterile. There were few bacteria or organisms present in the bloodstream. With vaccines now being so prevalent, this is no longer the case. Contrary to what we have been told, they weaken the immune system dramatically instead of strengthening it. In the United States, the hepatitis B vaccine is given to a child on the day of his birth, often weakening his immune system for his lifetime. His small body is just becoming accustomed to the germs around him for the first time, and he needs the strong immune system that he was given to remain intact.

Women's Health

The Susan G. Komen Breast Cancer Foundation

It may stun many readers to learn that the Susan G. Komen Breast Cancer Foundation sponsors Planned Parenthood, the "family planning" organization that performs assembly-line abortions. The Komen Foundation is also an organization that conveniently neglects to mention that both abortions and radiation from routine mammograms are methods of inducing breast cancers. The risk of getting breast cancer from either of these activities alone is greater than the risks of smoking and poor diet combined. The Susan G. Komen Breast Cancer Foundation may very well be the greatest cause of breast cancer in the world.

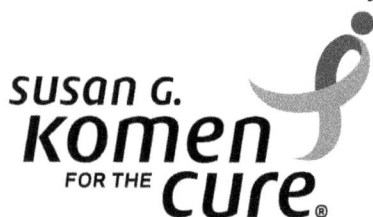

The amount of money that the Susan G. Komen Breast Cancer Foundation has donated to Planned Parenthood is being kept obscured. Life News reported that $730,000 was donated to the abortion organization in 2009 alone, but we are unable to confirm the exact figure. A public relations representative from the Komen Foundation disclosed to The Health Wyze Report that the amount of money annually funneled into Planned Parenthood is "about $700,000", which lends strong credence to the earlier figure. The Komen Foundation boasts that it has "invested almost $2 billion" since its inception in 1982. What the Komen Foundation actually does with that funding is never disclosed. The money is shrouded in secrecy, but it is said to be "energizing science".

> *"Our only goal for our granting process is to support women and families in the fight against breast cancer. Amending our criteria will ensure that politics has no place in our grant process. We will continue to fund existing grants, including those of Planned Parenthood, and preserve their eligibility to apply for future grants, while maintaining the ability of our affiliates to make funding decisions that meet the needs of their communities."*

-- komen.org

The Susan G. Komen Breast Cancer Foundation (alias Susan G. Komen for the Cure) maintains that the money given to Planned Parenthood is specifically earmarked for breast cancer screenings only. They neglect to mention that the money donated for radioactive screenings at Planned Parenthood actually frees Planned Parenthood's funding, so that it can provide more of its *other services*. They carefully omit mentioning the fact that the breast cancer screenings cause breast cancers, due to radiation exposure from the tests. Likewise, the contraceptive pills issued at Planned Parenthood, and the abortions performed -- more than double the cancer risk.

All of these things would be considered horrendous by the pro-life advocates and churches who regularly donate to the Komen Foundation. They are kept ignorant of the special partnership between Komen and Planned Parenthood. Planned Parenthood is scarcely mentioned on the Komen web site. In the event that the partnership is noticed by Christian benefactors, the Komen Foundation has a statement ready from their token Christian, Norman Roberts, who attempts to rationalize funneling donated funds to Planned Parenthood as "moral". The organization considers its fund raising to be moral, despite defrauding its own donors as a routine part of its 'charity' work.

Komen appears to have a policy of partnering with unethical organizations and their pink ribbons never appear on organic foods. They tend to promote only cancer-causing foods and products. The irony of their past support for aluminum-containing (breast cancer causing) deodorants is staggering, and their partnership with KFC was mocked publicly by comedian Stephen Colbert. The organization's partners range from aspartame-laced yogurts to MSG-containing pizzas. Under the banner of saving lives, we find an organization promoting cancer in its every action.

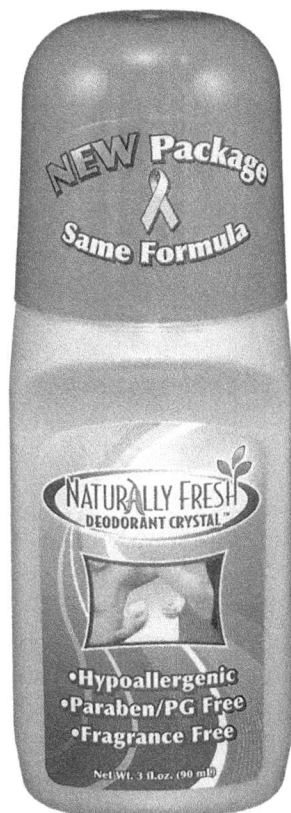

You are likely to find the Naturally Fresh brand of deodorant in Whole Food's Market sporting a Komen pink ribbon emblem. Its ingredient's list includes, "natural mineral salts (potassium alum)". That alum is nothing natural. It is made from aluminum that has been chemically processed. It is an accumulative, carcinogenic, heavy metal compound that is made with aluminum and phosphorus. It was used instead of aluminum chlorohydrate in the product, in order to disguise the fact that the product *still* contains aluminum. Deodorants containing aluminum compounds are one of the leading causes of breast cancer. This is a typical Komen Foundation endorsed product, so buyers should beware of the pink ribbon.

The evidence suggests that the Komen organization has no sincere interest in the cause or cure of cancer. Any success would immediately dry-up its funding, so cures are the last thing that the foundation wants. This is why its members sidestep mentioning any safer or more effective therapies than the status quo. One need not have billions in research funding to discover effective cures or the causes of cancer; for all that is needed is a free card to any public library, or an Internet connection to learn about the 1931 Nobel Prize in medicine discovery of Dr. Otto Warburg. The Komen organization's continued silent complicity with a medical system that easily kills 10 times the number of people who are killed by the cancers themselves is positive proof that maintaining the status quo is their for-profit business model. Meanwhile, as the cancer industry carnage continues, their profits have gone from the millions into the billions, and Komen does not even pay tax.

Where exactly is the two billion dollars of research? After its 31+ years of existence, the organization has yet to show an accomplishment or even a single research paper. On the other hand, it has helped to fund millions of abortions using other people's money without their consent. That could be considered an accomplishment from a certain perspective.

Corporations who market with Komen's pink ribbons do so because they get greater profits due to increased customer sales. It is a con job of legendary proportions that despicably targets the most well intentioned of our society. Awhile, not so much as a finger has been lifted in any honest effort to save any person's life. Readers may wish to begin their own quest to locate any cancer victim who has ever been helped by Komen. The cancer deaths indirectly caused by the products of their corporate partners, and more directly from the Komen-sponsored abortions, are easily into the many millions.

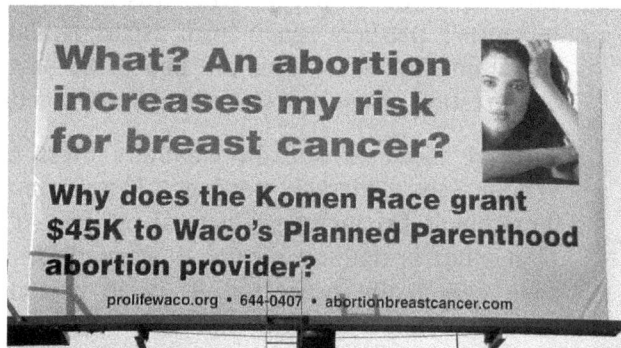

Despite dishonest public comments from Komen's representatives to the contrary, abortion increases the risk of breast cancer. It is not a small increase. For virtually every category of women, in every age group, the chance of getting cancer more than doubles after an abortion. When abortions are combined with birth control pill usage, and radioactive exams (both given by their partner organization) then the long-term prognosis is bleak.

Something never mentioned by Komen or Planned Parenthood is the fact that the surest way to prevent breast cancer is to have a child and then breast feed him. Women become more vulnerable to breast cancer as soon as they become pregnant, showing the unique influence of pregnancy-related hormones, and many researchers believe that a permanent hormonal imbalance is created whenever an abortion interrupts the natural birthing cycle. This explains the correlation between abortion and breast cancers. It is similar to the way in which women with C-sections cannot lose weight afterward, since the natural birthing process was interrupted, which in-turn prevented their hormones from automatically resetting. Following pregnancy, women who breast feed their children are well protected against breast cancer. Cancer resistance is much greater for these woman than for those who did not have children. This is why breast cancer was once referred to as the "Nun's Disease", because only nuns (who were childless) got breast cancer. One might expect these findings to be in Komen's literature, since the organization purports to be so concerned about preventing breast cancers. Instead, the hormone research is a topic that is avoided, but it has been public since the 1970's.

> *"The longer women breast feed the more they are protected against breast cancer."*

-- The Lancet, July 2002

Komen has been under fire from legitimate breast cancer charities, due to its unethical marketing schemes. Particularly highlighted as an example is its partnership with Yoplait, which donated ten cents for each lid that was mailed in by consumers. At the time, postage for this cost 37 cents. Thus, the campaign was largely a farce, but it managed to get people to buy the product at an increased rate, and it required customers to give their address details to Yoplait marketing. This overall pattern of trapping good people through bait-and-switch tactics is seen throughout the huge pink ribbon industry. It is worth mentioning that Yoplait is a yogurt that features high fructose corn syrup, and it also includes the chemically-engineered form of vitamin A to make it 'healthy'.

Komen likes to threaten lawsuits whenever legitimate non-profits use the phrase "for the cure", and it warns companies to never use the color pink in combination with the word "cure". Normally, charities do not legally attack others who have the same altruistic goals, but Komen is not a normal charity; and it is very arguably not even a charity at all. Showing its true character as a business, Komen protects what it perceives to be its trademarks. Jennifer Jenkins, Director of the Center for the Study of the Public Domain at Duke Law School, claims that such threats are typically on "shaky legal ground". Everyday phrases like "for the cure" cannot be trademarked; but so far, no one has challenged this corporate superpower's bogus intellectual property claims of owning everything associated with the color pink and breast cancer.

While they are adamant that they are making a positive difference toward curing breast cancer, most of their public activity involves supporting non-progressive organizations that provide failed, cancer-causing procedures or carcinogenic toxins. There is no mention of the risk of false positives for tests, the dangerous effects of radiation exposure, or the bleak outlook for those who follow the procedures that Komen supports. They especially neglect to mention that avoiding an abortion often saves two lives. There's a killing to be made, after all.

The use of pink in Komen marketing, and the constant female-only imagery shows the unfortunate influence of feminism in our society. For this reason, other news organizations shy away from criticism of Komen, since questioning the organization is an easy way to get labeled as sexist and unsympathetic to cancer victims. Therefore, Komen is relatively immune from criticism and honest coverage about its activities. To most news outlets, this 'charity' is beyond investigation.

Planned Parenthood and the Komen Foundation make surprisingly fitting partners, since they are both militant promoters of a feminist ideology and internally have a death worship culture.

These *ideals* overshadow any amount of compassion for the women who they claim to help. The ultimate product of their agenda is broken families and widespread death. While Planned Parenthood manages to achieve its anti-family and anti-Christian agenda in a direct and obvious manner, the Komen Foundation is more subtle with its own internal strategy groups, such as the *Lesbian, Gay, Bisexual and Transgender National Advisory Council*.

Infertility and Hormones

We have been overwhelmed by requests for help concerning hormonal, fertility, and pregnancy issues. Some of the women have had these sort of problems, despite eating a commendable diet. In this era, chemicals that imbalance the hormones are plentiful, and there is little wonder that both men and women are becoming infertile at higher rates than ever before in history.

The first thing to examine is the water supply. Tap water contains dozens of pharmaceuticals, in addition to the chlorine and fluoride that is ironically added in the name of health. All of these things can imbalance hormones; and fluoride specifically attacks the thyroid, an organ that is responsible for the creation of hormones. Fluoride is likely the biggest reason for the high rates of hypothyroidism throughout America today. Purchasing spring water, or getting a high-quality water filter is essential for avoiding serious disease.

There are plenty of water filters that are found in regular grocery stores, which simply remove the *taste* of chemicals, but not the chemicals themselves. Brita water filters are a good example, and they are actually marketed for removing the chlorine *taste*. Reverse osmosis water filters may or may not remove fluoride; depending entirely upon their engineering. Berkey water filters, with fluoride removal add-ons are the only filters that we trust. A shower filter is important too, because the chemicals and metals from the public water supply absorb through the skin, as well as the lungs by way of the water mist. Gases, such as chlorine, are thoroughly inhaled, which additionally aggravate respiratory conditions such as asthma.

Soy is toxic, and it contains phyto-estrogens that compete with the body's own natural estrogens. In essence, the birth control pill is very similar to soy, because it provides estrogen in order to prevent pregnancy. This is a defense mechanism of the soy plant. In nature, it stops parasitic insects from reproducing. We recommend that all of our readers avoid soy in all forms, and this rule is particularly important for women who are pregnant, or those trying to conceive. For other people, soy's resultant hormonal imbalances will, in the least, make life less pleasant.

The vast majority of cosmetics are toxic, and they are notorious for containing heavy metals, including lead and aluminum. Cosmetics that claim to be natural and organic are usually extremely deceptive. In fact, we have yet to find any off-line source of non-poisonous make-up products. Deodorants and antiperspirants often contain aluminum, which is sometimes hidden under the name "mineral salts" or "alum", even at the health stores in products marketed not to contain aluminum. The chemicals in deodorants and antiperspirants sink through the armpits, accumulating in the breast tissues and lymphatic system, making cancers much more likely. Some of these dishonest products sport the pink ribbon from the Komen Foundation.

Plastics may disrupt the hormones too, especially if they contain bisphenol-A (BPA). People who store their foods, or eat from plastic containers, should ensure that the plastics do not contain BPA. BPA is known for mimicking estrogen in the body (in a similar way to soy) and it thereby causes imbalances of the hormones. Glass and stainless steel containers are ideal whenever possible, but if plastic is necessary, then ensure that the manufacturer does not use BPA. Unless otherwise stated, assume that clear plastics contain BPA, but faded (e.g. milk jug) plastics generally do not.

The majority of retail meats contain hormones, and the meats are furthermore coated with nitrate salts to extend their shelf life. The complete avoidance of meat is neither feasible, nor healthy. Women and children both need plenty of iron, and red meats (beef, venison, etc.) contain nutrients that are not found elsewhere. Instead of avoidance, it is important to purchase grass-fed, hormone-free meat (preferably organic). Hormone-free milk has become fairly easy to find, due to public pressure that has begun to force even the largest retailers to sell pure milk. Non-homogenized milk is preferred, due to the extreme inflammatory damage that is caused by drinking homogenized milk. Our official recommendation is creamline milk, which can be found in most health food stores.

Repairing the Damage

Before trying to have a child, it is important to cleanse the body of toxins. This will make it easier to become pregnant, and more importantly, to have the healthiest possible child. We recommend that all women who are trying to get pregnant first perform a liver and heavy metal cleanse. Do not do any cleanses whilst pregnant, because cleansing will free the heavy metals and toxins from the tissues, which will be absorbed by the growing fetus. Simply supplement with selenium while pregnant to neutralize the toxic effects of most heavy metals.

Pears and peaches have a special ability to regulate the hormones. They are often used in Traditional Chinese Medicine for this purpose. We made a juice that is good tasting and beneficial, which uses both of these fruits. Drink one of these every day, or simply eat the fruits, if you prefer. Reference the *Juicing* chapter for the *Hormone Regulator* drink.

Most Americans are deficient in iodine. It is essential for the thyroid. Never take iodine internally, or supplement with underwater plants for iodine; with the possible exception being red marine algae. Oral supplementation with iodine is dangerous, and most underwater vegetation contains enormous amounts of heavy metals and other environmental toxins. Safe methods of iodine supplementation include eating fresh fish, supplementing with red marine algae, the cautious use of potassium iodide, or applying iodine transdermally, as described in the *Iodine* section of the *Supplements* chapter. Fish should never be fried, and fish should be neither bottom feeders nor shell fish.

Purchase cold-pressed, organic coconut oil. It will stimulate the thyroid, give you energy, provide omega-3, and it will help to balance hormones. It is often recommended by midwives. Consume a teaspoon of it twice a day.

Women with hormonal imbalances should also read the *Hypothyroidism* section of the *Alternative Medicine* chapter to check themselves for the symptoms. If hypothyroidism is confirmed, then treating it should be a priority, using the natural methods cited.

We must reiterate the importance of avoiding fluoride, which includes the use of fluoride toothpastes. The absorbent tissues inside the mouth are one of the fastest pathways into the bloodstream, so every time a person brushes with a fluoride toothpaste, he is essentially drinking fluoride. It is also worth noting that a large percentage of pharmaceuticals contain fluoride too, without having any apparent or disclosed reason for its inclusion. It would be prudent to research any pharmaceuticals that are being used, and this includes fertility treatments. Fluoride has historically been prescribed to patients with hyperthyroidism to cripple the thyroid.

Exercise is important, because it stimulates the body's production of CoQ10, and also because it allows a person to expel toxins through the sweat glands. Exercise is the only way to cleanse the critical lymphatic system (lymph nodes).

Imbalanced hormones may be caused by underlying health issues that took many years to develop. Thus, recovery can be slow. It may require faith and patience.

Consideration should always be given to whether it is the man or the woman in the relationship who is infertile (possibly both). Infertility is now more common in men than in women. The section *Erectile Dysfunction* in the *Alternative Medicine* chapter provides information for men with hormonal issues.

Midwives and Home Birthing

In the early part of the twentieth century, a campaign against midwifery began, which was led by the allopathic establishment. At that time, 95% of deliveries happened in the home with midwives present. The young medical industry was campaigning that midwives were unclean, and that midwives were the last option, reserved for those who could not afford real medicine. The industry jealously spied birthing as a potentially profitable option, so it began a massive marketing blitz. Hospitals were presented as the cleaner and safer option, with supposedly better trained professionals. Every one of these statements was untrue. What made these assertions most disturbing is the fact that doctors in those days received no hands-on training in birthing at all. The attacks against midwives continued for 30 years, despite the statistical proof that midwife-assisted births were categorically safer than those conducted in hospitals. Home birthing is still safer, over a century later.

The slander against midwives was successful. By 1955, only 1% of U.S. births took place in the home. Only 8% of the births in the United States are now attended by midwives, while 70% of the European and Japanese births are attended by midwives. As a result, the United States has the second worst newborn death rate in the developed world. Only Latvia, with six deaths per 1,000 births, has a higher infant mortality rate than the United States. The U.S. also has the highest maternal mortality rates. The safest country to give birth in is Sweden, which has a midwife (or two) at almost every birth, and these same birthing professionals actively involve themselves in prenatal care too. The Swedish do not treat pregnancy as a disease that needs pharmaceuticals, intensive hospital care, and intervention by doctors. Their babies are the better for it.

When preparing for a birth in the United States, doctors present a wide range of choices for the mother, but these options do not materialize on the day of labor. In fact, the great majority of doctors in the United States have never witnessed a completely natural birth. Hospital policies encourage American doctors to always intervene in the birthing process, for the sake of making it as fast and profitable as possible. Thus, American doctors typically seek excuses to intervene, and unnecessary interventions are always dangerous.

During a natural birth, the mother's brain releases a hormone called oxytocin. It is nicknamed "the love hormone", because it fosters a loving emotional bond. It may equally affect the child as much as the soon-to-be mother, but this is impossible to know. This hormone is also believed to induce the contractions that are necessary for vaginal birth.

The chemical marketed as petocin is the drug industry's closest equivalent to oxytocin, but as is usual with synthetic imitations, the body does not react to it in the same way. The pharmaceutical version causes *more* pain, and as is usual for chemical therapies; it comes with an array of side-effects. Petocin is used to induce deliveries prematurely, and such premature births have been made the norm in the United States.

The Hospital Birthing Procedure in the U.S.

1. Petocin is used to induce the delivery prematurely (for doctor's convenience and golf schedule).

2. The petocin causes exaggerated and unnatural pain.

3. An epidural is needed to reduce the agonizing pain caused by the unnecessary pharmaceutical that was previously administered.

4. The epidural then impairs the delivery, so even more petocin is given.

5. The double dose of petocin causes contractions to be much more severe, and last for longer periods of time.

6. This combination begins compromising the oxygen and blood flow to the baby.

7. Women are placed on their backs, in the legs-in-stirrups position, making labor even more difficult for both mothers and babies, but it is more convenient for the doctors.

8. As the baby is increasingly harmed by all of these things, sometimes an emergency C-section becomes necessary.

9. When it is finally over, the doctors then applaud themselves concerning how great their interventions were at saving a child who would have never been in danger in the first place without their 'help'.

At some American hospitals, up to 70% of infants are delivered by way of cesarean section. These unnecessary interventions are the reason why so many American newborns die at birth, or within the first months of life.

> *"The United States has more neonatologists and neonatal intensive care beds per person than Australia, Canada and the United Kingdom, but its newborn [death] rate is higher than any of those countries."*

> -- 2006 State of the World's Mothers Report

C-sections continue to rise in popularity for several reasons. The first reason is that the natural birthing process has been demonized and mocked by the entertainment industry. It has driven terror into expectant mothers. Modern women often expect, and even hope for a C-section well before they enter the delivery room. Whenever a woman demonstrates discomfort with the prospect of having a C-section, or with other interventions, she is told that such interventions are in the best interest of the baby. These are lies in most cases, but doctors know that mothers will always stop questioning once implied threats and guilting about their child's safety are issued.

Statistically, vaginal births are much less dangerous than cesarean sections. C-sections are a major surgery, which often cause infections that do not respond to antibiotics. Despite this, it is the most common surgery performed on women, because it helps doctors to avoid lawsuits. In the event of a lawsuit, the use of a C-section supposedly proves to juries that the doctor "did everything he could" to assist the baby and mother. More often than not, juries believe it.

The cost of giving birth in the United States is at least twice as high as any other country in the world, yet the results are the worst in virtually every category. Here are the current average prices for different births in America:

- C-section: $15,800
- Vaginal delivery: $9,600
- Home birth with a midwife (all expenses): $2,000 - $4,000

After a C-section, women are told that they must continue getting C-sections for every birth thereafter. Thus, each birth doubles the hospital's profit. Each subsequent birth becomes more dangerous for both the mother and child.

Insurance companies often refuse to cover home births, because supporting the alternatives would eventually eliminate our need for health insurance. In other words, the American medical system's prices are kept artificially high, so that customers are forced to buy insurance, which has policies ensuring that medical prices continue being high for the sake of perpetuating its own wealth-generating existence. Insurance companies have an incestuous relationship with the medial establishment, and neither would support anything that might decrease our dependence upon them, or decrease cost. Insurance agents have a tendency to seek only advice from in-system doctors, who predictably claim that home births are dangerous. The statistical evidence overwhelmingly proves the opposite. For example, America has the most births performed in hospitals, but it has the highest infant mortality rate in the industrialized world. Statistics prove that the more medical care a child receives, the more likely he is to die.

Designer Births

"Designer Birth" is a new term that refers to a caesarian-section that is scheduled for a certain day and time, and then a tummy tuck is done immediately afterward. The only part missing is a drive-through. These have become more popular, due to their use by celebrities, such as Victoria Beckham and Britney Spears. Such unnecessary interventions are madness, and they decrease the chance of a healthy mother and child. Regardless, this irresponsible practice is being adopted by a new generation of rich women, who favor glamor over the welfare of their own children.

Allopathic Birthing History In All Its Shining Glory

- In the 1930's, x-rays were used on pregnant women. It was later discovered that these gave the unborn children cancers, so the practice was stopped.

- In the 1940's through the 1960's, morphine and scopolamine were administered successively to induce "twilight sleep". It was believed that this would change the experience of labor forever, by eradicating pain. It merely produced amnesia afterward, so that mothers had no recollection of the traumatic events, and the drug furthermore caused women to lose self-control. Women were routinely placed in straight jackets and strapped down to beds, in order to stop them from hurting themselves. It was common for doctors to leave the new mothers strapped to beds during the drug-induced psychoses, screaming in terror for hours at a time -- sometimes laying in their own feces and urine.

- In the 1960's, the drug thalidomide was given to pregnant women, which resulted in infants who were born without arms and legs, and others with more random deformities. Thus, it too was eventually stopped.

- In the early 1990's, Cytotec (misoprostol) was used to induce labor in women who previously had C-sections. This resulted in thousands of women with ruptured uteruses. This practice was abandoned in 1999, and the drug is now used for abortions.

The track record for Big Medica's interventions with the birthing process is miserable. The doctors still treat pregnancy as a disease, and the unborn children are treated like tumors needing extraction. Perhaps they will eventually stop experimenting on human beings and tampering with God's handiwork. Such a day is unlikely to come until parents start refusing to allow their children to be the test subjects for the industry's current fad, or whatever it finds most profitable.

Cesarean -- "C-Sections"

The Internet is flooded with women who desperately attempt to lose weight following childbirth. The worst cases involve women who experienced cesarean sections. Most women are able to lose the majority of their pregnancy weight, except for the last 20 pounds. However, there are less fortunate women who retain almost all of it, and practically all of these women have had cesarean sections. This is due largely because of the muscles (and sometimes nerves) which were cut during surgery.

The butchery involved can make it impossible for a woman to return to her previous figure. Women who have C-sections never receive warnings about this from their doctors. In fact, these surgeries are usually presented as being safer, and with less complications than vaginal births.

If you can think like typical doctors to understand their special medical jargon, then their statements about C-sections being "safer" make more sense. We'll translate using our medical dictionary.

Safer   *adj., adv.*   **Sāf´ • êr**

1. Having decreased legal liability issues. *(Ex. The jury acquitted the doctor because he had "done everything he could" to ensure 'safety', by employing "surgical intervention" to an "obviously problemed birth".)*

2. More cost effective (more profitable) to the hospital or clinic. *(Ex. The malpractice insurance rates dropped, due to the predictability of the C-section procedures in getting patients discharged fast.)*

3. Conserves time. *(Ex. The doctor was able to attend the golf tournament on time, due to the troublesome mother getting a 30 minute C-section.)*

Now you know. The mother's and child's welfare are lesser issues in deciding the treatments. These are rarely even an afterthought, unless attorneys get involved. If your doctor is an exception, then you are truly blessed to have found him.

Contrasting to a Natural Birth

During a vaginal birth, a set of hormones is released that aids birthing, and these stimulate a nurturing bonding process between the mother and child. Oxytocin, prolactin, the so-called "fight or flight" hormones that are like adrenalin, and beta-endorphin are all produced by the mother. These hormones not only help her throughout the birthing process, but these same hormones later become a signal for her body, indicating that it is safe to return to a state of normalcy (not being pregnant), and to lose weight.

During pregnancy, the frequent hormonal imbalances result in random crying, screaming, or other emotional outbursts in the afflicted lady. To the relief of most new fathers, this drama is usually over following natural labor, but this is not always the case for those who have a cesarean birth. In the latter group, the mothers' bodies are never adequately signaled that their pregnancies are over, and their hormones may remain imbalanced perpetually thereafter. This man-made imbalance sometimes cruelly lasts for the remainder of their lives. Some women in this situation never completely return to normal; living for untold years in states of unrest. It is like taking birth control pills, and some women become completely crazy when their hormones are thusly imbalanced.

Let's not even go into the sheer number of cases of hypothyroidism that these hormonal imbalances cause, or cases of diabetes, heart disease, or adrenal failure. It even effects the cancer risk. It's quite a body count for a 'safe' procedure.

What we find particularly disturbing is that the victimized couples will never know that their marital and parental problems were caused by the surgical intervention in the delivery room. There is absolutely no accountability, even though doctors know from their own medical literature that they are lying about the long-term consequences, and deep-down they must know the true meaning of "safety" and the principle of "first do no harm". There is no way to know how many relationships have ground to a halt because of the effects of cesarean births, and how many lives it has destroyed.

How Birthing Should Be Done

Interventions are necessary in rare and unusual circumstances, but they are exceedingly over-used throughout America. Contrary to America's mythology about how America has "the greatest medical system in the world", Americans actually have the highest maternal mortality rate in the developed world, and the second highest newborn mortality rate. Americans have more C-sections and less midwives than any other country in the world, and the discomforting aftermath is printed in the statistical journals.

The majority of C-sections happen unnecessarily, for the convenience of the doctor. Drugs are given to women during childbirth to speed up the process, and this results in complications like high blood pressure and fetal distress. Thus, an artificial need for a cesarean birth is created by the doctors themselves. C-sections actually provide less complications *for the doctor*, who does not have to wait for the birth, or worry about malpractice lawsuits, since he *obviously* did everything he could. The majority of American doctors have never witnessed a completely natural (drug and surgery-free) birth.

Women who truly embrace natural births sometimes describe the process as one of harmony, when they are in a safe environment to follow their instincts. Instead of laying on a bed with their legs raised, they stand or sit in a position that allows gravity to assist the process, so that they do not have the birthing process hindered by a totally moronic and unnatural position. The standard hospital position is the most convenient *for doctors*, but it is the worst position for both the mother and the child. The standard position specifically hinders the ability of the pelvic ligaments to stretch, as they are supposed to during birth. Those who have natural home births are not only statistically safer, but it is common for them to report a much more fulfilling experience.

Bad Reasons for a C-Section

- "The pelvis isn't big enough". The pelvis stretches throughout pregnancy and during birth, so the only way to really determine if a pelvis is too small is to actually attempt a vaginal birth. There is a large portion of experts who claim that when standing in the upright position, the pelvis is always able to expand as much as needed.

- Being overdue. As long as there are no complications, there is no reason to rush labor. While hospitals like to rush such things, so that they can move on to the next paying customer, heavy birth weights and late arrival times are not legitimate reasons for surgical intervention.

- Taking too long. After the birthing process has started in a hospital, and oxycotin and epidurals have been given, doctors frequently decide that the process is taking too long. For this reason alone, they may engage in surgery.

- Fetal distress. The child is often stressed when the mother is stressed, as a result of the poor environment and the drugs that were administered. Before opting for a C-section, calming the mother, and even getting her to walk a few steps, can dramatically calm a child.

It is important to remember that a C-section is major surgery, and there are massive risks associated with it. It has become so normal in our society, and doctors discuss it with such callousness, that we tend to forget about the implications. The pressure that is placed upon women throughout pregnancy leads many of them to take a path that is not in the best interest of their health or their child's. If doctors have convinced you to take this surgical procedure lightly, then please browse pictures of the actual procedure. It is similar to cutting a woman in half, and it sometimes requires disembowelment.

Endometriosis

Endometriosis is a condition that effects 10 percent of women who are of child-bearing age. It occurs when the tissues that normally grow inside the uterus grow in other locations. It is a notoriously painful condition, which many women have described as being more intense than child birth. Internal scar tissue may eventually develop, which is a known cause of infertility. Medical books provide differing explanations as to why this condition is so incredibly painful, but there are only guesses, and endometriosis is not well understood by the orthodox medical establishment.

Most doctors treat this condition by suppressing its symptoms with painkillers, or by placing women on birth control drugs that cause them to skip their monthly cycle. As a result of such neglect, endometriosis is a leading cause of infertility in the civilized world. The mainstream methods of suppressing endometriosis are usually futile. The only drugs that provide effective relief are extremely addictive, and all surgical attempts are largely failures. The most common long-term treatment is laparoscopic surgery to remove the excess tissues, but the condition has an extremely high recurrence rate despite surgical interventions. Some women get hysterectomies to eliminate endometriosis, but even in these cases, it sometimes returns in different places. Pregnancy is the only thing that reliably cures the condition, and it provides relief even in those rare cases when endometriosis is not completely cured. The condition always stops when menopause begins.

The disease can have a massive impact on the quality of life. Women with endometriosis have an 87% chance of depression, and an 88% chance of having mild to moderate anxiety. Sixty-three percent of endometrial women have severe anxiety problems. Endometriosis sufferers are four times more likely to have allergy problems, and they are also four times more likely to have migraines. Many women with severe endometriosis are forced to go on disability, because their symptoms are so severe. The Internet is riddled with horror stories about those who committed suicide due to their endometriosis pain.

Symptoms of Endometriosis

- Painful Periods
- Painful Intercourse
- Infertility
- Heavy or irregular bleeding
- Painful bowel movements or urination
- Loss of stale menstrual brown blood
- Fatigue
- Depression
- Excessive mood swings
- Lower back pain
- Loss of large menstrual blood clots
- Swollen abdomen

The Causes of Endometriosis

Traditional Chinese Medicine (ancient Chinese medicine) links endometriosis with liver problems. While T.C.M. can seem very confusing upon first glance, we have learned not to underestimate its usefulness. A study titled *Chinese Herbal Medicine For Endometriosis*, at Southampton University revealed that Chinese herbal medicine is more effective for endometriosis relief than mainstream treatments are, with no side effects.

The liver is the primary organ that is responsible for the elimination of toxins. When the liver is unsuccessful at flushing toxins, they sometimes remain in the liver forever. These liver toxins are the most common cause of liver impairment. The liver is responsible for the regulation of the sex hormones, including estrogen, progesterone, and testosterone. Increases in estrogen will make endometriosis more severe, indicating yet another hormonal component of the condition and the condition's relationship to liver health. The fact that this condition is caused by liver dysfunction means that women who opt for mainstream treatments will eventually find themselves in a worse condition after treatments than they were beforehand. This is because all pharmaceuticals stress the liver and increase its toxicity.

The Endometriosis Association has done massive amounts of research on the connection between endometriosis and dioxin exposure. Dioxins are a byproduct of chlorination, which is used to bleach sanitary towels and tampons. The bleaching process is known to release dioxins that remain on consumer products. This exposure, particularly in the case of tampons, could cause endometriosis or worsen it.

It has been shown that alcoholic women (or former alcoholics) are more likely to have endometriosis. Heavy drinking places a massive strain on the liver.

Numerous studies have additionally linked a higher risk of endometriosis with women who have diets which are low in anti-oxidants, or who have above-average "free radicals" (oxidation) in the body. Oxidative damage is indicative of a bad diet overall, lacking in both fruits and vegetables. This can be easily fixed with dietary changes.

The Korean study, *Association of Body Mass Index With Severity of Endometriosis in Korean Women*, has linked endometriosis with small figured women, and the researchers noted that the thinner women are, the more severe the disease. Hormones have a dramatic effect upon a person's weight, and thin women tend to have smaller amounts of the hormone estrogen.

Curing Endometriosis

In the long term, the typical pharmaceutical methods for treating endometriosis will cause the disease to worsen. The prolonged use of either strong painkillers or oral contraceptives is very harmful to the liver.

Areas where endometrial tissue grows in the body become very inflamed, and the long-lasting inflammation prevents the body from properly healing. Therefore, one of the most important things for an endometriosis sufferer to do is reduce the amount of inflammation in the body.

Exercise in the week prior to menstruation can be very beneficial. Sweating is the only way to cleanse the lymph nodes, and endometriosis is a disease that is influenced by toxicity.

Those who are sexually active in healthy relationships are less likely to experience endometriosis attacks, and the attacks are less severe for them. Korean researchers have labeled endometriosis a "working woman's disease" for this reason. This insight has been ignored by the Western press due to political correctness. Intercourse shortly before menstruation will drastically reduce endometrial symptoms. The best effect is achieved when male hormones are directly injected into the patient, but we have opted to not explicitly explain. Becoming pregnant during this time is very unlikely.

Dietary Changes

- Eat organic, grass fed meat. Avoid processed and factory-farmed meats, because they contain growth hormones which will make the problems worse. Iron is essential, so beef must be part of the diet. Iron supplements are less safe and they are poorly absorbed.

- Avoid refined white sugar, white flour, and white rice. The chlorination process used to bleach foods will leave some dioxin residues in the food, because dioxins are always a byproduct of chlorine. The (white) refined variants of these foods are very inflammatory. Read the ingredients and purchase "evaporated cane juice" for sugar. Use only brown rice and whole wheat flour, and do not use any carbohydrates that are not completely homemade.

- Honey is actually an anti-inflammatory sweetener, so it too is recommended. It is the ideal sweetener whenever it is a viable option.

- Do not use homogenized milk. It is one of the most inflammatory food items available. If milk is needed, purchase non-homogenized (creamline) milk from a health food store. In some cases, heavy cream is a perfect substitute for milk, and it is not homogenized.

- Avoid all soy products. Soy contains phytoestrogens, which are compounds that mimic estrogen in the body. They can cause major hormone instability, which will worsen the endometriosis.

- Reduce the intake of processed foods. Virtually all of the chemical additives are inflammatory to the body.

- Dioxins can also be found in municipal drinking water, because it contains chlorine. Women with endometriosis should purchase spring water, or use a Berkey water filter. A shower filter that removes chlorine is prudent, because inhaled chlorine vapors are extremely inflammatory.

Curing endometriosis is a process of providing the body with the nutrients that it needs to heal the liver, while keeping inflammation low, and flushing any toxins out of the body. For information about performing a liver cleanse, see the *Cleansing and Detoxifying* section of the *Wellness* chapter. We furthermore recommend the following supplements for endometriosis sufferers.

Supplement Suggestions

- All of the B vitamins strengthen the liver, and directly assist the body in disposing of excess estrogen.

- Licorice is one of the most commonly used herbs in China, and it is well known for its beneficial effect on the liver.

- Dandelion strengthens the liver and kidneys.

- Milk thistle is renowned for strengthening the liver.

- Selenium has been historically given to cows by farmers to prevent endometriosis. Endometriosis hinders fertility, so farmers work hard to prevent a disease that results in fewer calves. The best single source of selenium is Brazil nuts, followed by tuna, cod, and meats. It can also be purchased in supplement form.

- Vitamin E is known to ensure that animals have healthy uterine linings, and it has been used by farmers since the 1930's. Vitamin E and selenium are believed to work together to prevent damage to cell membranes, and protect against oxidation. Do not take blood thinners like vitamin E during the menstrual period, because they will increase bleeding.

- Due to the link between endometriosis and dioxins, it would be wise to supplement with chlorophyll. Chlorophyll can remove dioxins from the body, and it can be purchased as a liquid concentrate.

- Folate or folic acid. Folate is necessary for the body to make heme (the iron-containing, non-protein part of hemoglobin) for the red blood cells. Too little folate can cause nutritional megoblastic anemia (large red blood cells that cannot transport oxygen well). It is known to help regulate and balance the hormones. Alcohol reduces the absorption of folic acid, and increases the kidney's excretion of it. Folic acid assists in the chelation of lead, and helps the body to properly utilize zinc. There is a strong connection between folate and the liver, because liver disease increases the loss of folate.

- Radishes were used in Traditional Chinese Medicine to cure endometriosis, and to fix liver problems, including jaundice. It would be wise to include them in the diet.

- Alcohol should be avoided, with the exception of an occasional glass of red wine. Greater amounts will weaken an already impaired liver.

- Gelatin is the only common ingredient in endometriosis-related pharmaceuticals. While it is purported to be an "inactive ingredient", many sufferers have noticed that eating foods high in gelatin during menstruation is beneficial. Endometriosis sufferers finally have a bona fide health reason to eat gummy bears.

- Cannabis ("marijuana") is often recommended by doctors in U.S. states that allow medical marijuana use. In addition to helping with the pain, it also seems to reduce the inflammation issues. Some sufferers proclaim that marijuana is more effective in helping with endometriosis than the expensive prescription pain medications. Cannabis does not harm the kidneys, is not addictive, and it helps to suppress the nausea that often accompanies the pain.

Castor Oil Transdermal Packs

At the beginning of menstruation, when the first symptoms of cramping become noticeable, a castor oil transdermal pack can dramatically reduce the severity of symptoms throughout the cycle. This is the basic procedure:

1. A wash cloth should be soaked in pure, cold-pressed castor oil that is obtained from a health food store.

2. The wash cloth should be placed on bare skin on the lower stomach.

3. Put a piece of plastic on top of the cloth, such as a plastic grocery bag.

4. Place a hot water bottle on top of that. The water should be made as hot as possible, so long as the patient can tolerate it.

5. Leave this in place for at least 30 minutes.

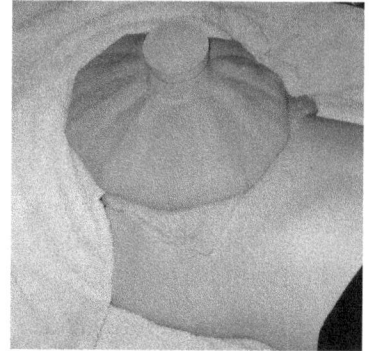

The above procedure can also be done repeatedly during the cycle to provide relief. However, one treatment is usually enough to provide massive relief. Women should use only dioxin-free, unchlorinated feminine products, especially tampons. Consuming Brazil nuts is ideal, because they contain folate, selenium, and magnesium, which have all been shown to reduce menstrual cramps.

Toxic Tampons

Most women with endometriosis will never discover that their problem is greatly aggravated by sanitary napkins and tampons. These products use a semi-synthetic substance called rayon instead of real cotton; in order to achieve maximum absorption. The pads are bleached during the final stage of production. This bleaching process releases dioxins from the rayon as a byproduct. Studies have proven that repeated dioxin exposure leads to reproductive diseases, including endometriosis. Dioxins accumulate in the body's fats over time; and as they gradually build to greater concentrations, so does the list of health conditions that arise as a result.

"In the early 1990's, the Endometriosis Association found that 79% of a group of monkeys developed endometriosis after exposure to dioxin in their food during a research study over ten years earlier. The severity of endometriosis found in the

monkeys was directly related to the amount of T.C.D.D. (2,3,7,8-
tetrachlorodibenzo-p-dioxin -- the most toxic dioxin) to which they had been
exposed. Monkeys that were fed dioxin in amounts as small as five parts per
trillion developed endometriosis. In addition, the dioxin-exposed monkeys showed
immune abnormalities similar to those observed in women with endometriosis."

-- The Endometriosis Association

Dioxins are known for their ability to cause cancer, reproductive harm, hormonal disturbances, and damage to the central nervous system. Endometriosis may just be the latest ailment to add to the long list of health problems that dioxins cause. Thus, it is highly recommended that women seek all-natural, "dioxin-free" options, which are available at health food stores and some grocery stores. If dioxins are not mentioned on the package, then dioxins are present in the product.

These hormone problems are exacerbated by the extreme fluoride exposure that most American women get, combined with iodine deficiencies. Another extremely aggravating factor is the consumption of products containing soybean derivatives and soy cooking oil. The absolute worst soy product is mayonnaise, because it is "cold pasteurized" (saturated with radiation).

Early Puberty

The New York Times reported about a research study that demonstrated puberty is occurring in much younger girls than previous generations. Some girls are growing breasts by the age of 7. This trend has been continuing for a long time, and researchers have been puzzled by it. A 2010 study by the Cincinnati Children's Hospital came close to pinning down the cause.

"It's certainly throwing up a warning flag... I think we need to think about the stuff
we're exposing our bodies to and the bodies of our kids. This is a wake-up call,
and I think we need to pay attention to it."

-- Dr. Frank Biro, Cincinnati Children's Hospital

Chemicals which alter hormones are everywhere. They are in our foods, and the toys that our children play with. Bisphenol-A (BPA) has become very controversial in recent years, because it is known to disrupt the hormones, thus leading to earlier puberty onset, and problematic pregnancies. BPA has also been implicated for causing brain damage, cancer, diabetes, and heart problems. This chemical has been found in the urine of 90% of Americans. It is in drinking bottles, clear plastic containers, aluminum cans and aluminum drinking bottles (they have a clear BPA inner lining). BPA is an ingredient that is never labeled.

Milk that contains growth hormones can also effect development. Avoiding growth hormones can be difficult, and it is not as easy as simply buying milk that is free of rBGH. After all, milk is present in butter, cheese, sour cream, yogurt, ice cream, and more. Most of these products are not easily available with "rBGH free" labeling, which is currently the only way for shoppers to be certain of its absence. It is likewise important for people to buy organic meats, to avoid hormones. Organic meats taste better, are less fatty, and are far more nutritious. It is worth noting that rBGH has been banned throughout the majority of Europe, Australia, New Zealand, Canada, and Japan. Here in America, Monsanto owns the regulators, and it literally has its own attorney on the Supreme Court, Clarence Thomas.

Air fresheners and other fragrances have also been shown to cause hormone disruption, particularly when they contain phthalates. Phthalates are hormone disruptors that are known to cause birth defects, infertility, and reduced sperm production. They are sometimes even found in air fresheners that are labeled, "All Natural" and "Unscented". It is best to avoid perfumes and air fresheners completely, particularly if you have children. In addition, we recommend purchasing laundry detergents which are specifically labeled "Phthalate-free".

Like BPA, pesticides have long been implicated as endocrine disruptors, which means that they destructively mimic human hormones. DDT was first shown to have this effect, but with each subsequent study, modern pesticides are revealing the same traits. This could be due to the fact that a lot of pesticides currently used are derived from DDT. Therefore, buying organic is vitally important, in order to protect your family. Pesticide residues are on conventionally grown produce, and inside it too; due to a new generation of pesticides that are designed to be absorbed into the plants.

Soy is present in almost all processed foods, despite its dangers. It contains estrogen-like compounds which compete with the body's own hormones, causing problems with reproduction and growth. All soy is toxic in its natural state. It is genetically modified and industrially processed into being less-toxic, but the health effects are still unconscionable. It stimulates cancers, as well as hormonal disorders like endometriosis.

Until labeling becomes mandatory for all of these chemicals, children will continue to be exposed to them, without the consent of their parents. It is no mystery why puberty is happening earlier, infertility is common, and breast cancer is on the rise. Worse is the fact that a lack of labeling on products containing these chemicals even make studying their effects difficult.

Low Platelet Counts, Thrombocytopenia, and Pregnancy

Platelets are responsible for blood clotting, and normal levels range between 150,000 and 400,000, but a drop is common during pregnancy. The drop is generally ignored unless it goes below 116,000. Poor testing procedures, in which there is too long of a delay between when blood is drawn and when the testing actually occurs, is a known problem that produces entirely bogus test results. It is common. Thus, it is wise to take at least two tests before making any radical medical decisions concerning the results.

An extremely low platelet count is called thrombocytopenia. It can be caused by a variety of things including A.I.D.S., pharmaceuticals, sepsis, leukemia, and lupus. However, the establishment claims that gestational thrombocytopenia (during pregnancy) has no known cause, and it does not usually result in complications. The standard treatments vary depending upon the perceived severity of the condition. Extreme cases can mean that bleeding will not stop, so there is a threshold at which it may actually become a real problem. Hospitals will usually refuse to provide epidurals if the platelet count is below 100,000.

Pregnancy-related thrombocytopenia is usually caused by malnutrition, and the following recommendations should work to remedy it. This successful nutritional therapy is institutionally ignored, because it lends credence to competing alternative medicine.

Natural Methods to Raise Platelet Counts

- **Astragalus** is a very common remedy for this condition. It has been shown in studies to reduce the platelet damage of chemotherapy, so it has a powerful protective effect. This herb also increases the amount of platelets in the blood. Astragalus can be purchased in supplement form at health food stores or online. It should not be confused with the vegetable asparagus.

- **Vitamin C** has been shown to cause massive increases in platelet counts, and it is likewise beneficial for those with ITP (one of the causes of thrombocytopenia). All pregnant women should supplement with vitamin C to decrease the risk of S.I.D.S., and thrombocytopenia increases their need for it. Vitamin C explains why citrus fruits generate a rise in platelets. A pregnant woman should get, at bare minimum, double the U.S.D.A.'s recommended daily allowance of vitamin C in supplements, in addition to getting it in the diet too.

- **Zinc** is a mineral that all pregnant women should supplement with. Zinc deficiencies have been linked to fetal abnormalities and birth deformities. Zinc deficiencies have also been linked with low platelet counts, and zinc supplementation causes a dramatic rise in platelet aggregation. Reference the *Supplements* chapter for information about the quality considerations of different zinc supplements.

- **Beetroots** (Beets) are frequently recommended by midwives as a dietary method of increasing the platelet count.

- **Meat and Fish** have been shown to increase platelet counts. It is especially important to avoid growth hormones during pregnancy, and to avoid all bottom-feeding fish, due to their heavy metal contamination (think kosher). Also beware of farm-raised fish, which do not have the health benefits that are present in those that are wild caught, and especially beware of fish from China.

- **Vitamin B-12** is essential for the proper production of platelets, along with red and white blood cells. Thrombocytopenia can be caused by this deficiency alone; and therefore, thrombocytopenia is something that is much more likely to occur in vegetarians. B-12 is naturally present in meats, and it can be obtained in dietary supplements. B-12 supplementation should always be purchased in the form of methylcobalamin. Note that B-12 supplements should be crushed and held in the mouth for a minute (or two) before swallowing, so that much of the B-12 will directly absorb into the blood. This is because vitamin B-12 from supplements is almost entirely destroyed by digestion.

- **Chlorophyll** increases the oxygenation of cells, making it easier for the body to function properly. Chlorophyll is strongly recommended.

- **Vitamin K** is essential for proper blood clotting, and thus it is important. Vitamin K is best obtained from green, leafy vegetables. Our Green Drink recipe in the *Nutrition* chapter would be ideal, and supplements are also available at health food stores.

- Avoid alcohol and refined sugars, because these have been shown to reduce the platelet count.

A Poisoned World

Deodorants and Antiperspirants

There are plenty of fraudulent products that are marketed as "natural", which actually poison people chemically or otherwise. We find these cases particularly disturbing because they attempt to target the very people who are trying to be healthy. Among the best examples of this can be found in the industry of natural antiperspirants and deodorants. The leading brands, Crystal and Naturally Fresh both make fraudulent claims at the expense of their customers' health. These products contain a toxic heavy metal, and are dishonestly labeled. A typical example is the boast "No Aluminum Chlorohydrate", with the insinuation that aluminum chlorohydrate is the only source of aluminum for these products. To the contrary, "potassium alum" hides it in plain view in the ingredients list.

Potassium alum is otherwise known as "potassium aluminum sulfate" on honest labeling that is not hiding the presence of aluminum. This alum *can* occur in nature (which is how they manage to claim that it is "all natural"), but that does not make the alum any safer for the human body than any other form of aluminum. Mercury is likewise naturally occurring; as hemlock, strychnine, lead, and cyanide are. All of these ingredients are likewise quite dangerous to human health; especially with long-term exposure. Toxic heavy metals are still toxic heavy metals, regardless of whether they are discovered on the tops of mountains or in the depths of the oceans. Some companies claim that their alum is extracted from volcanic ash, and this makes it both natural and safe. The manufacturing process involves heating alunite rock to over 1,400° Fahrenheit, and then dousing it with sulfuric acid to finalize breaking down its molecular structure. They refer to the resulting chemically-engineered substance as both "all natural" and "unprocessed" alum.

Aluminum has been repeatedly indicated as a cause of breast cancer, Alzheimer's disease, brittle bones, autism, infertility, and generalized permanent damage to the central nervous system. Furthermore, aluminum mimics estrogen to imbalance the hormones; indirectly leading to hypothyroidism, endometriosis, decreased fertility, and virtually every ailment that targets women. Underarm products are one of the greatest causes of breast cancer, since aluminum is absorbed almost directly into the lymph nodes from the armpits. Potassium aluminum sulfate makes up a massive 25% of some antiperspirants, and it cannot be excreted from the body without the intervention of alternative medicine. It accumulates within the body in ever

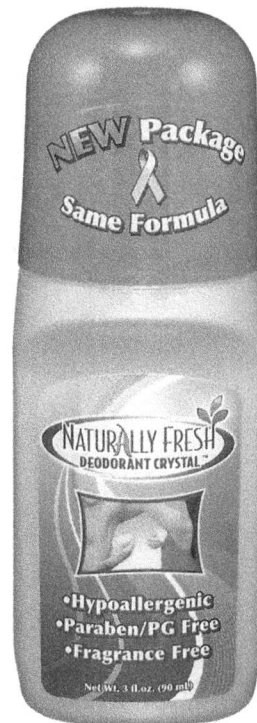

growing amounts throughout a person's life, so that the aluminum becomes more destructive with increased age.

Some of the more principled deodorant companies have begun removing aluminum from their products, while the less scrupulous companies are simply hiding it with dishonest labeling. Ironically, the same companies producing aluminum-based antiperspirants frequently boast about their "breast cancer awareness" by placing pink ribbons on their products. Of course, these products help to make many new customers for the breast cancer industry, so these business partnerships are somewhat understandable, albeit reprehensible.

Why Use Aluminum?

Many reasonable people may wonder why aluminum would ever be added to underarm products. There are two main reasons. The first reason is that aluminum kills bacteria that is responsible for foul odors. It is used specifically because of its toxicity, instead of in spite of it. Although, it has never been necessary. A non-toxic (to humans) option could easily be used in place of aluminum, such as silver or copper. Not only are these known to kill virtually all bacteria, viruses, and fungi, but these alternatives are actually known to provide benefits to health. Thus, safe alternatives have always existed for manufacturers.

The second reason for using aluminum is because its molecules sink into the skin to create such toxicity that the sweat glands can no longer function well. It is unknown exactly how this happens, and perhaps that outlines the problem even further. Various hypotheses exist to explain aluminum's ability to stop sweat production, and many of them are ridiculous. The prevailing hypothesis is cited below, and it clearly lends credence to the assertion that aluminum is pulled into the body as a bio-toxin.

> "The aluminum ions are taken into the cells that line the eccrine-gland ducts at the opening of the epidermis, the top layer of the skin, says dermatologist Dr. Eric Hanson of the University of North Carolina's Department of Dermatology. When the aluminum ions are drawn into the cells, water passes in with them. As more water flows in, the cells begin to swell, squeezing the ducts closed so that sweat can't get out."

-- The Discovery Channel's, *How Stuff Works*

The makers of these products attempted to justify their behavior publicly by claiming that the particles of aluminum in their potassium alum are so large that they cannot be absorbed into the body. The particles of aluminum in potassium alum are typically so microscopic that they produce a completely transparent solution when mixed into clear fluids. The particles are so small that they cannot even produce a color change with all but the most complete saturation. The science shows that aluminum *only* works to stop perspiration if it sinks deep into the cells. It means that those "natural" antiperspirants could do nothing if they did not contain truly toxic aluminum that is absorbed by the body.

Are these companies lying when they claim that the particles are so **large** that they cannot react with the body, or are they lying when they state the particles are so **small** that they sink deep to provide effective "protection"? Is either side of their mouths telling the truth?

Brands that are actually aluminum-free usually contain other questionable ingredients, such as propylene glycol, a petroleum derivative. This is the primary ingredient in brands such as Tom's of Maine and Desert Essence. Finding a safe, all-natural antiperspirant from an honest company has become a herculean task. Remember to read the ingredients when shopping for "all-natural" deodorants, and be wary of "alum".

Chewing Gum

People do not typically ingest gum, so they pay very little attention to its ingredients. The assumption is that if the gum is not swallowed, then the ingredients should not be a concern. However, the ingredients in gum travel into the bloodstream faster and in higher concentrations than food ingredients, because they absorb directly through the walls of the mouth, and these ingredients do not undergo the normal filtration process of digestion.

Gum is typically the most toxic product in supermarkets that is intended for internal use, and it is likely to kill any pet that eats it. Commercial gum products contain roughly the same list of toxic ingredients, with differing labeling, which is virtually always designed to mislead.

Common Ingredients of Gum

After looking at several different brands of chewing gum, we found that these were the most common ingredients:

- Sorbitol
- Gum base
- Maltitol
- Mannitol
- Xylitol
- Artificial and natural flavors
- Acacia
- Acesulfame potassium
- Aspartame
- BHT
- Calcium casein peptone-calcium phosphate
- Candelilla wax
- Sodium stearate
- Titanium dioxide

Titanium dioxide is so cancerous that external skin contact is enough to cause cancer. Be reminded that all of these ingredients absorb directly into the bloodstream through the walls of the mouth. Some of these ingredients are explained in-depth, because it is prudent to correct the myth that chewing gum is harmless and even good for you (e.g. "it strengthens the teeth").

The "Sugar-Free" Sugar Alcohols

Sorbitol, maltitol, and mannitol are sugar alcohols. These are usually made from sugar, and they frequently increase the blood sugar just as much as eating sugar. However, manufacturers make deceptive "sugar-free" claims about sugar alcohols, since these ingredients are not *pure* sugar anymore. While such sugar derivatives are *technically* "sugar free" when the manipulative word games are employed, they nonetheless remain dangerous for diabetics, who are the very audience that these gums are marketed to. Let us not forget that the sugar alcohol containing gums are also marketed to improve our dental health. The sugar alcohols are even more chemically processed than white sugar is; and thus much more foreign to the body by virtue of its artificial nature, so we have reason to believe that these forms of chemical-industry sugars will stimulate *even more* weight gain and inflammation than regular sugar. All of the evidence points in this direction. These chemically-extracted sugar alcohols are documented to cause abdominal pains and diarrhea, whilst aggravating various health conditions, such as irritable bowel syndrome. Therefore, the immune system takes a huge hit from exposure to them. This immune suppression will in turn cause greater yeast development in the body, which will lead to cavities and allergies.

Gum Base

Instead of telling customers what they are really chewing, the phrase "gum base" is used to generalize a list of ingredients that is never actually published. As the name implies, it is the foundation agent of chewing gum. We have tried exhaustively to find exactly what modern "gum base" is made from. We found the following babble repeatedly regurgitated by all of the major gum companies. It was obviously meant to derail serious research:

> *"Gum base is produced through a blend of raw materials which can be categorized in five classes:*
>
> 1. *Elastomers, act as the key ingredient and provide elasticy*
> 2. *Resins act as binders and softeners*
> 3. *Plasticizers render the elastomer soft to ensure thorough blending of the gum base*
> 4. *Fillers contribute to the overall texture*
> 5. *Anti-oxidants prevent oxidation of the gum base and flavors during shelf life"*

Since this was repeated identically at all websites that we looked at, we can only assume that all of these companies are actually owned by the same people, or at least they are working together as a cartel to cover-up an honest disclosure of what is in gum. We eventually confirmed that the ingredients of gum base are commercial trade secrets. None of the websites told us the full ingredients. For instance, exactly what plasticizer is used? Are people chewing on super-toxic PVC? The plasticizing agents could contain dioxins, and quite frankly, they probably do.

After much more research, we found one Chinese company who told us about their ingredients. Wuxi Yueda Gum Base Manufacture Co., Ltd. said:

> *"It is made of several food grade raw materials, which are rubber (food grade), glycerol ester of rosin, paraffin waxes, polyvinyl acetates, talc powder and calcium carbonate."*

Glycerol ester of rosin is often made from the stumps of pine trees. It is used industrially to create fast-drying varnishes. The Internet is riddled with stories of people who had severe allergic reactions to it, usually causing a swollen throat that led to difficulty breathing. Glycerol ester of rosin is now being added to soft drinks, though federal limits ensure that its quantity remains under 100 P.P.M. This safety limitation does not apply to chewing gum.

Talc has been linked to lung cancer, ovarian cancer, and fibrotic pneumoconiosis with just transdermal exposure. It is very rarely put into products that are to be consumed. The only other consumable products that we have seen containing talc are diet aids (most are extremely toxic). Talcum powder was once used on small children, but it has now been replaced with cornstarch, due to safety concerns. It is too dangerous to touch the skin, but absorbing it straight into the bloodstream is apparently acceptable.

Polyvinyl acetate is not quite PVC. It is PVA. PVA is frequently referred to as "carpenter's glue" or simply "white glue". Remember that this is not being used as an industrial product, but as something that children are frequently given to chew upon (gum base is in bubble gum too). This ingredient compliments the paraffin wax, which is derived from refined petroleum.

Aspartame is one of the most controversial additives of all time, and it sits alongside MSG and saccharin in terms of both consumer distrust and poor safety. Its presence in foods has nothing to do with safety, but everything to do with politics and money. Aspartame has been linked to just about every health condition known, from seizures to brain tumors. Some epileptic patients have recovered from their condition simply by eliminating this toxin from their diets. It is found in diet foods, diet drinks, and sugar-free products as an alternative to sugar. Aspartame is a solution that remains worse than the problem. Aspartame is an excitotoxin, which means that it over-excites the neurons in the brain, until they burn out, causing lowered intelligence and a host of neurological problems. Aspartame causes diabetes, fibromyalgia, lowered I.Q., obesity, multiple sclerosis, asthma, insomnia, muscle spasms, and a total of 92 known symptoms.

Acesulfame potassium (acesulfame K) has similar properties to aspartame, and it is believed to be a carcinogen. The Center for Science in the Public Interest petitioned the F.D.A. for a stay of approval, due to the lack of testing done on this substance. Studies on animals have shown a correlation between acesulfame potassium and various tumors.

While we would love to be able to provide information about calcium casein peptone (calcium phosphate), we cannot. We simply do not know. Its only appearance is in Trident gum (the worst brand), and we were unable to find studies or any other information about it. It might be a whitening agent. It is important to note that casein is a milk extract that was linked to the Chinese baby formula poisonings. Trust this ingredient at your own risk, but we would never encourage the use of something that has its research censored from the public. That tends to be a bad sign.

BHT (butylated hydroxytoluene) is a preservative that has been linked to cancer. It was banned in the United Kingdom and Japan. It is unbelievably sold as a "dietary supplement", and some people believe that it has anti-viral effects. So do gasoline and rat poison. We do not recommend it, because of the safety implications. It causes kidney and liver damage. Benjamin Feingold (creator of the Feingold Diet) linked it to hyperactivity in children in the 1970's, as a large component of A.D.H.D.

For the sake of brevity, we shall discontinue examining the ingredients in chewing gum. Chewing gum is easily one of the most toxic products available, and it is difficult to ever know exactly what it contains, due to vague terms such as "gum base" and "artificial flavors". These reflect trade secrets, and the ingredients probably are made of hundreds of other ingredients that they are unwilling to disclose. Manufacturers maintain that customers have no right to know.

Natural gum is available, which is made from chicle, a tree that is native to Central America. There was a time when all chewing gum was made from it, but using it incurs more manufacturing expense. Natural gum can be purchased online or from health food stores.

Non-Stick Cookware

People have a tendency to forget security and safety issues whenever a new technology provides a great convenience. This is especially true regarding health and diet products. There are consequences to that carelessness, and people tend to forget about potential consequences until the consequences actually manifest themselves. A good example of this phenomena is the broad acceptance of non-stick cookware. It is quite convenient, but it is far from safe.

If a bird inhales the toxic PFOA fumes that are produced by heated non-stick pans, its lungs will ulcerate and it will suffocate in its own body fluids. This is due to it having inhaled either polytetrafluoroethylene (PTFE) or perfluorooctanoic acid (PFOA). Birds were used for centuries as an early warning system in mines, because they rapidly die whenever they are exposed to even small amounts of poison gas. Polytetrafluoroethylene (PTFE) and perfluorooctanoic acid (PFOA) are both fluoride compounds. Fluoride is a poison that depresses the thyroid, which can cause hypothyroidism, particularly with repeated exposure. It accumulates in the bones, teeth, and the pineal gland. It has been linked to brittle bone disease and cognitive problems. Fluoride is the main ingredient in some rat poisons.

We discovered studies that vastly contradict the marketing of the companies who sell non-stick pans. The E.P.A. reported that PFOA accumulates inside humans for years, and it has been verified to produce cancers in laboratory tests. It noted that the chemical particularly damaged the livers of rats, and it furthermore had a tendency to raise the triglyceride levels in humans. PFOA has been registered with the E.P.A. as a potential human carcinogen.

Dupont, the inventor of Teflon, was sued for withholding safety information about the use of perfluorooctanoic acid (PFOA) in non-stick cookware. The Environmental Protection Agency filed the suit, claiming that "DuPont concealed its own 1981 research". Dupont records demonstrated that traces of this chemical were detected in a pregnant employee's unborn child, which proved that the company knew of the danger, since it had been pre-emptively testing for it in its own employees before anybody supposedly knew of the danger. In 1991, the company likewise omitted reporting its evidence that PFOA had contaminated the water supply of around 12,000 people. It was again sued by eight of the effected families. One of the plaintiffs was a DuPont factory worker, who bore a son with only one nostril and other facial defects. His son has since had about 30 surgeries. He and his spouse have opted not to have further children, lest they risk passing on the condition.

It is impossible to determine exactly what the fumes of the non-stick pans are doing to our bodies, because the research is so sparse. Although, Gary Craig ran into some obvious problems with the pans.

> "About three or four years ago, I began having to urinate too often, including getting up five or six times at night. Gradually it got worse until it reached a peak a few months ago when I was urinating two or three times an hour all day long... [kidney failure] I noticed, however, that the problem went away when I left home to go on a trip. Within 24 to 48 hours of walking out my front door, my system returned to normal... Although I never used high heat (nothing above medium heat) I recalled that three or four years ago (about the time all this started) my mother gave me a Teflon frying pan... which I began using regularly. I stopped using the Teflon frying pan and BINGO! About 24 to 48 hours later the problem vanished."

This is far from the "flu-like symptoms" that many of the producing companies admit will occur when the pans are "overheated". They have defined "overheated" as reaching 500 degrees Fahrenheit (200 degrees Celsius). It is important to remember that 500 degrees Fahrenheit can be reached with merely the medium temperature setting on some stoves, and some pans will emit the poison gases at much lower temperatures than is admitted by the manufacturers.

What Does PFOA Do to the Body?

Perhaps the hushed studies that have been done by DuPont since the 1950's will provide some enlightenment. Studies which used animals as test subjects revealed that non-stick cookware produces health issues in the following categories:

- Children's health and development
- Risks of liver, pancreatic, testicular, and mammary gland tumors
- Altered thyroid hormone regulation
- Generalized damage to the immune system
- Reproductive problems and birth defects

We additionally recommend that people avoid aluminum cookware. Aluminum is a soft metal that will flake toxic metallic particles into foods being cooked with it; especially if metal utensils are being used. Stainless steel is always a better option; both for its low reactivity (low toxicity), and because this hardened steel will practically never output particles into food. Aluminum is an accumulative heavy metal that is known to lead to many degenerative diseases.

Old-fashioned cast iron pans are an even better alternative, and cast iron is naturally non-stick. Its inherent non-stick property means that cast iron is often easier to cook with than stainless steel, and it has the best heat distribution. Men who regularly eat food that is cooked in cast iron cookware should routinely consume something containing resveratrol, such as grape juice or red wine, in order to remove excessive iron from the blood. High quality cookware is essential for cooking healthy food, so special care should be taken when purchasing cookware to ensure that none of it came from China.

Air Fresheners

Unfortunately, the residual chemicals from common cleaning and deodorizing products often result in accidental poisonings to the very people who were supposedly being protected. Some toxic chemicals accumulate in ever-increasing amounts in the human body over a period of years, so the health consequences are rarely attributed to them. Victims sometimes suffer from a strange form of cancer, or they might have some new-age disease like chronic fatigue syndrome; and of course, there is the growing popularity of 'genetic disorders'.

Do you wish to know why your immune system is weak, why you are always fatigued, and why you and your family have all those mystery illnesses and "genetic" disorders? You may find the answers in your cleaning products, medicine cabinet, laundry products, foods, municipal water, in "healthy" products (soy, canola, margarine) and in your air fresheners. There is an endless barrage of unregulated toxic retail products ranging from Clorox wipes to hand sanitizers and air fresheners. The long-term health consequences of these products multiplied together invariably become much worse than any infection or other seemingly isolated ailment.

It is usually assumed that these products must go through rigorous safety testing before placement in retail stores, but this is not true. The cleaning industry is self-regulated, which translates to no regulation. Chemical companies do not need permission from any authoritative body before releasing their latest air fresheners or cleanup wipes. In fact, it took months for the F.D.A. to even warn Clarcon Biological Chemistry Laboratory Inc. that bacteria was living inside its line of supposedly anti-bacterial products. The hand sanitizer was eventually *voluntarily* recalled, but only after the situation became a public relations problem for both organizations. These voluntary recalls are the most common type, and the term "voluntary" indicates that the F.D.A. officially informed the guilty corporation that it would not take any action against them. The phrase "voluntary recall" seriously means this in the food and pharmaceutical industries.

Air fresheners are thought to be even further outside the jurisdiction of regulators than most products. To its credit, the State of California forces labeling of ingredients that are known to cause cancer or reproductive harm, under Proposition 65, but this is the entirety of this industry's regulations. Common chemical products are increasingly shown in studies to cause serious health problems, and it is impossible to test for truly long-term problems.

The Natural Resources Defense Council studied the effects of air fresheners, discovering that they currently undergo no safety testing. The results were disturbing, because they revealed high levels of phthalates, which are known to be especially harmful to children. These chemicals were even present in sprays which were claimed to be "All-Natural" and "unscented". Phthalates were not disclosed in the list of ingredients for any of the products.

> *"Phthalates are hormone-disrupting chemicals that can be particularly dangerous for young children and unborn babies. Exposure to phthalates can affect testosterone levels and lead to reproductive abnormalities, including abnormal genitalia and reduced sperm production. The State of California notes that five types of phthalates -- including one that we found in air freshener products -- are 'known to cause birth defects or reproductive harm.'"*

-- Natural Resources Defense Council

1,4-Dichlorobenzene is a chemical that is found in the blood of 96% of Americans. It has been linked to lung damage, is a known carcinogen, and it is an E.P.A. registered pesticide. Studies found it to increase rates of asthma. It can be found in the majority of air fresheners, toilet deodorizers, and mothballs. It works by attacking the receptors in the nose, and thus eliminating the sense of smell. This is how the new generation of air fresheners actually "freshen". This chemical was introduced into the American market with the Febreze product from Proctor & Gamble. The new generation of air fresheners that were inspired by the success of Febreze are literally using chemical warfare to destroy their customers' sense of smell. That lack of smell is where the illusion of *freshness* comes from. The user only smells these air fresheners for about a minute after they have been sprayed, and then the nose cannot smell most fragrances anymore. This is not a normal adjustment to odors, anymore than a loss of one of the other four senses. The process is the equivalent of using a chemical blinding agent to escape the unpleasantness of a bright light; when that chemical is known to be both poisonous and carcinogenic. By design, the *freshening* chemical causes damage to the mucous membrane, which is claimed to be temporary. However, no long-term studies have ever been done to test the effects of chronic exposure. It is important to remember that anything inhaled is immediately absorbed into the blood through the lungs relatively unchanged.

Dichlorobenzene is, in large part, the reason why so many pet birds die directly after the use of air fresheners. Due to hundreds of reports of bird deaths on the Internet, Procter & Gamble (Febreze manufacturer) funded its *own* internal study into this, and (without surprise) concluded that there are no safety issues whatsoever concerning pet birds or human beings.

Dichlorobenzene is the main ingredient used to manufacture the infamous pesticide DDT, and its cousins, DDE and DDD. Chlorine alone has a tendency to form DDT and DDT-like compounds when it reacts with many other substances. Such chlorine compounds disrupt the endocrine system by destroying hormones throughout a body, in a similar manner to BPA; but in a much more powerful way. Sometimes exposure results in horrific health problems that never completely disappear. It may help readers to put the situation into perspective by being made aware that their use of most air freshener brands is the literal practice of inhaling small amounts of DDT. Inhalation is much more dangerous than oral ingestion of the same amount.

> *"Problems associated with DDT, as well as many chlorinated hydrocarbons, involved their tendency to concentrate in the fat of humans, livestock, aquatic food chains, and wildlife. This latter phenomena, called bioaccumulation, has had, and continues to have, severe adverse effects on many forms of wildlife...*
>
> *"Since implementation of* [the DDT ban]*, residues of the pesticides have significantly decreased in many regions where they were formerly used. However, DDT, DDD and DDE persist in the environment for a very long time. DDT, DDD and DDE residues can still be found in most areas of the United States"...* [80 years later]

-- The U.S. Fish and Wildlife Service

The issues of synthetic fragrances have been around for years, and have led to many companies selling unscented options. Some fragrances cause changes in blood flow, blood pressure, mood, and trigger migraine headaches. A massive 72% of asthmatics cite these fragrances as a trigger in causing asthma attacks, and they have been implicated as a cause for the initial development of asthma. Asthma rates in the United States have doubled since 1980, and the use of air fresheners has doubled since just 2003. Most synthetic fragrances are also known respiratory irritants, which means that they cause inflammation in the lungs, leading to an increased mucous production, and a greater vulnerability to other chemicals, allergens, and infections. Ninety-five percent of synthetic fragrances are derived from petroleum. They include benzene and aldehydes; which are known to cause cancers, reproductive effects, and problems with the central nervous system. These effects on the nervous system result in increased cases of

Alzheimer's disease, multiple sclerosis, Parkinson's disease, and more. A study from 1991 entitled, *Chemical Exposures: Low Levels and High Stakes*, tested the effects of fragrances among test subjects. When asthmatics were exposed to cologne for 10 minutes, their pulmonary function was impaired by 58% from a previous 18% handicap. Of the 60 asthmatics that they surveyed, 57 complained of respiratory symptoms with exposure to common scents.

Phthalates, like those found in air freshener mists, are usually used in the production of PVC plastics. All air fresheners containing phthalates lack any labeling to indicate their presence. Phthalates are also found in air fresheners that are labeled "unscented" and "all natural". With an estimated 75% of consumers using air fresheners in their homes, we strongly recommend improving ventilation systems to dilute these chemicals as much as possible, if they cannot be eliminated altogether. According to the Environmental Working Group, phthalates produce liver cancer, but this link has not been officially acknowledged by regulatory agencies.

The chemicals emitted from air fresheners (and other toxic products) accumulate in the fatty tissues over time, so the danger increases as they build up inside a body. The presence of toxins inside fat can make weight loss difficult. Since the human body uses fat to store certain materials that are too toxic for it to process, breaking down the fat would mean releasing those toxins again, so a body may resist fat loss for self-defense. Thus, fat retention is sometimes the result of an immune system properly responding to a danger.

Sooner or later, society will have to revert to old-fashioned means of cleaning, cooking, and keeping our homes smelling pleasant. That will include the removal of non-stick pans, air fresheners, and hand sanitizers. While they may make certain tasks easier, avoiding them is an essential step to ensure a long, healthy life for your family. Since children are most at risk, we hope that those reading this will dispose of their air fresheners, to minimize the exposure of those who are not able to protect themselves.

MSG and L-Taurine

If monosodium glutamate (MSG) is as safe as its food industry proponents claim, then why do they consistently labor to hide it from us with deceptive labeling?

Many readers will be thrilled to discover that there is an effective, all-natural antidote for MSG poisoning called taurine. It is an amino acid that is naturally produced by the human body. Also known as L-taurine, it is found in proteins, and it is added to many energy drinks, due to its stimulating effect. Taurine supplement capsules can be found in health food stores, and they should be kept ready for MSG or heart emergencies. It effectively neutralizes MSG and it helps to regulate the pulse. The earlier that it is taken during a time of exposure to MSG, the better that it works to neutralize the MSG. If at all possible, it is best to take taurine just before MSG consumption, but please note that we would never recommend the consumption of MSG, even when there is taurine available to neutralize it. Conversely, MSG neutralizes the taurine already present in the body, which is largely its method of causing heart attacks.

Monosodium glutamate is in a special class of chemicals known as excitotoxins. These chemicals cross the blood brain barrier to over stimulate the neurons of the brain. It has the effect of destroying some neurons permanently, causing a variety of mental issues, including a permanent loss of intelligence. MSG poisoning will lower a person's intelligence faster than lead exposure, in addition to causing its better known mental and physical effects. This toxin is especially dangerous when combined with magnesium deficiencies, which are common in the West. MSG and magnesium deficiency is a deadly combination that can lead to sudden heart failure, and this combination is the primary reason why so many high-school athletes in the United States have mysterious heart failures.

MSG is sprayed directly upon crops, because it is a highly-effective insecticide. Nevertheless, the F.D.A. has blessed its usage inside U.S. foods for decades.

> "Cardiovascular signs [of MSG consumption] *include hypotension, shock, and sometimes cardiac arrhythmias, which, if untreated, may precipitate circulatory collapse.*"
>
> -- Handbook of Diseases, 2003

U.S. food regulators and chemical companies are intentionally making it difficult to avoid MSG, by using other names to hide its presence in ingredients lists.

Common Names Used to Hide MSG

- Glutamic acid
- Calcium caseinate
- Hydrolyzed vegetable protein
- Textured Protein
- Monopotassium glutamate
- Hydrolyzed plant protein
- Yeast extract
- Sodium glutamate
- Vegetable protein extract
- Autolyzed plant protein
- Yeast food

- Yeast
- Nutrient
- Gelatin
- Sodium caseinate
- Autolyzed yeast
- Glutamate
- Soy protein
- Hydrolyzed corn gluten
- Natural flavor *
- Artificial flavor
- Spice *

---

* Since the F.D.A. has intentionally left "natural flavor" and "spice" without meaningful definitions, U.S. companies freely use these names to hide ingredients in our foods. This lack of regulation in enforcing honest labeling is by design.

"commercial use is permitted only due to its marketing before the 1958 Food Additive Amendments to the Food, Drug and Cosmetic Act, which in effect grandfathered hundreds of substances which had never been tested for safety, including MSG...

"... Certain neuroscientists have, for years, warned that consumption of neurotoxic amino acids (glutamic acid, aspartic acid, and L-cysteine) place consumers at risk -- with most risk to newborns and young children whose immature blood-brain barriers leave them less well protected than more mature people. There is now additional and growing concern on the part of neuroscientists that the glutamate that we eat may cause or exacerbate neuro-degenerative diseases such as ALS, Parkinson's disease, and Alzheimers disease."

-- Mission Possible Canada

"Industry has begun to proliferate products with the words 'No MSG', 'No Added MSG', or 'No MSG Added' on product labels when the products contain hydrolyzed protein (which invariably contains MSG) -- a practice that is clearly in violation of existing FDA regulations. Hidden MSG is not limited to use in food. MSG sensitive people have reported reactions to soaps, shampoos, hair conditioners, and cosmetics that contain hidden MSG. The most obvious common hiding places are in ingredients called 'hydrolyzed protein' and 'amino acids'. Drinks, candy and chewing gum are also potential sources of hidden MSG... Binders and fillers for medications, nutrients, and supplements, both prescription and non-prescription, including internal feeding materials and some fluids administered intravenously in hospitals, may contain MSG. Reactions to MSG are dose related, i.e., some people react to even very small amounts of MSG while others usually only react to relatively more. MSG-induced reactions may occur immediately after contact or after as much as 48 hours."

-- Aspartame Poisoning Information Canada

The Documented Effects of MSG Consumption

Epilepsy
Vision disturbances
Panic attacks
Heart attacks
Parkinson's disease
Huntington's disease
A.L.S. (Amyotrophic Lateral Sclerosis)
Alzheimer's disease
Brain lesions
Retinal damage
Obesity
Food cravings
Depleted nutrients
Hyperinsulinemia
Stunted growth
Crosses into the fetus
Ocular (eye) destruction
Liver damage
Diabetes
Kidney damage
Vastly increased chance of A.D.D., A.D.H.D.
Asperger's and autism
Severe headaches
Shortness of breath
Chest pains
Asthma
Gastrointestinal disturbances
Poor memory
Swelling
Numbness of hands, feet, or jaw
Chronic bronchitis
Allergy reactions
Irregular heart beat
Unstable blood pressure
Pain in joints or bones
Abrupt mood changes
Tingling in face or chest
Pressure behind eyes
Difficulty swallowing
Anxiety attacks
Explosive rages
Balance problems
Dizziness or seizures
Mini-strokes
Fibromyalgia
Multiple sclerosis
Tenderness in localized areas, neck, back, etc.
Chronic post nasal drip
Sleep disorders
Blurred vision
Chronic fatigue
Extreme thirst or dry mouth
Hypoglycemia
Difficulty concentrating
Slowed speech

Notice the alarming number of diseases caused by, or aggravated by MSG. It is no coincidence that these symptoms match almost exactly those of insecticide ingestion, for MSG is actually used by farmers as an insecticide.

Glutamate occurs naturally in some foods, but the naturally-occurring glutamate does not cause ill-effects. It is believed to always appear in nature with its own antidote(s), for instance, taurine. The kind of MSG added to foods is a type that the F.D.A. allows manufacturers to call a "natural flavor" even though there is nothing natural about it. What follows describes that 'natural' manufacturing process.

"Today, the glutamic acid component of the food additive monosodium glutamate is generally made by bacterial or microbial fermentation wherein bacteria used are often, if not always, genetically engineered. In this method, bacteria are grown aerobically in a liquid nutrient medium. The bacteria have the ability to excrete glutamic acid they synthesize outside of their cell membrane into the liquid nutrient medium in which they are grown. The glutamic acid is then separated from the fermentation broth by filtration, concentration, acidification, and crystallization, and, through the addition of sodium, converted to its monosodium salt."

-- truthinlabeling.org

In other words, the MSG added to our foods is typically produced from the putrid fermenting wastes of genetically-engineered bacteria combined with powerful chemical agents. This whole process is referred to as "natural", at least by the F.D.A.'s unique version of biological science.

We recommend reading, *The Slow Poisoning Of Mankind*, which was an official report submitted to the World Health Organization about MSG.

Bastardized Beef

The many benefits of eating meat are negated when its nutritional value has been corrupted by the chemical industry. Contrary to what is being widely taught, natural beef is not unhealthy, nor is it full of fat. However, when cows are factory-farmed in concrete sheds, in the most repulsive conditions, and they are barely kept alive with pharmaceuticals; then the resultant meat is fatty and unhealthy.

The fat content of beef sold in regular U.S. retailers is 4 to 5 times higher than beef that was sold during the 1950's. It was common for U.S. beef in the 1950's to have as little as 2% fat, but now the fat content is so high in factory-farmed beef that the U.S.D.A. allows ground beef to be up to 30% fat and 15% pink sludge (described later). That means that ground beef in the U.S. is sometimes only 55% real meat.

Factory-farmed beef in the United States is sometimes one-third fat, which is 15 times worse than the historical ratio. Our contemporaries would not have been able to honestly call it meat, because most beef now is a chemically-enhanced fat delivery system. The situation is made worse when the meat is later soaked in toxic solutions, such as nitrate salts, prior to arrival at grocery stores. The purpose of this is to increase shelf life by making the meats so toxic that fungi and bacteria immediately die from contact with it. Thus, the meat is toxic by design.

The Next Generation of Food Preservatives

There is a new generation of chemicals being employed that are intended to deceive us about the quality of meats, instead of merely increasing their shelf life. These new chemicals are engineered to stop meats from changing colors when they rot, so that customers will not know. This disturbing trend has actually become normal with U.S. meat distributors, and all beef sold in regular retailers should be assumed to have these color stabilizing chemicals. An example of these chemicals is propyl gallate, which causes tumors in laboratory test animals. It was never adequately studied before it was embraced by the U.S.D.A., but it is believed to cause liver damage, kidney damage, and be a carcinogen.

Have you ever shopped in the meat section and noticed that the meat had a rainbow appearance when viewed at certain angles to the lights? This is dismissed by most shoppers, but it is a clear sign that the product is chemically coated. Real meat does not produce rainbows. If you look closely at the packaging of meat at regular retailers, you may notice text that reads something like, "Enhanced with up to 8% marinade". It is always printed tiny in the hope that it goes unnoticed. That so-called "marinade" is not usually a marinade at all, because the F.D.A. allows companies to hide ingredients with a label claiming that they are a marinade, including toxic chemicals like propyl gallate. The word game exists to protect the industrial food and chemical industries, who have financial reasons for not disclosing the real ingredients.

Beware of the word "enhanced", and be cautious of the word "enriched". Mentally substitute the phrase "chemically engineered". These words are frequently used to hide things that none of us would willingly consume.

Processed meats are notorious for having sodium nitrate, a known carcinogen. However, most people assume that fresh meats are completely untouched by the chemical industry. Often this is not the case. Most retail meats are gathered from farms that are separated by vast distances, which typically makes the chemical poisoning of meat a business necessity for the largest food corporations.

Our research shows that some manufacturers coat their meats with hydrolyzed gelatin. This is made from de-haired pig skins that were dissolved in industrial acids. As disgusting and unhealthy as this may be, a more troubling fact is that these coatings are sometimes made from an undisclosed group of chemicals. Again, no labeling whatsoever is required, nor is there any public disclosure.

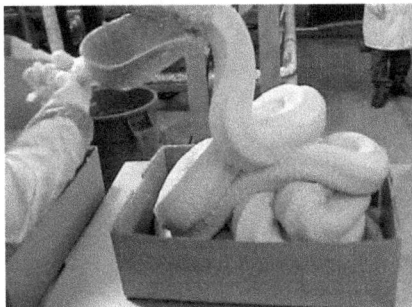

Ammonium hydroxide is being used to sterilize beef that would not normally be considered safe for human contact or consumption. The byproducts of meat processing (waste materials) are put through a high-speed centrifuge, then soaked in an ammonium hydroxide solution, and finally it is ground into a gooey paste. This process produces a pink material that has a slimy texture. The next phase of its processing is mixing it with real ground beef to create the illusion that it is real meat. Following public pressure,

McDonald's restaurants stopped using the disgusting pink slime inside of their burger patties, but the residual ammonia and other incriminating impurities are still being found in retail ground beef. Various groups in the meat industry, including Beef Products Inc., refer to this pink slime by its marketing name, "lean finely textured beef". There is very little real beef in this meat-like product, and independent parties generally consider it to be unfit for human consumption. Neither the F.D.A. nor the U.S.D.A. require any labeling whenever this artificial beef product is sold as real ground beef in U.S. retailers. Approximately, 70% of the ground beef sold in the United States contains this disgusting and substandard beef product, according to an investigation by A.B.C. News.

On February 11th, 2013, Russia banned meat imports from the United States, because so much of the U.S. beef, turkey and pork contain ractopamine. Ractopamine is a dieting chemical that is added to animal feed to make the animals leaner. This chemical can later be detected inside meat products. To place the dangers of this chemical into perspective: the National Institutes of Health warn that after direct human ingestion of ractopamine has occurred, emergency medical personnel should first attempt to control the victim's seizures before implementing life support procedures.

The pervasive use of ractopamine exposes another serious problem in the food chain. Namely, that if factory-farmed animals were given exercise, and if they were not constantly being given toxic foods, synthetic growth hormones, genetically-engineered corn, antibiotics, vaccines and other chemicals that are even worse than ractopamine, then there would not be a fat problem for the ractopamine to eliminate. The policies express the foolishness of using chemicals to compensate for the fact that too many toxic chemicals are already being used. Ractopamine exposure is known to produce cardiovascular abnormalities in humans and hyperactivity. China and the European Union have banned it, due to concerns about its serious health consequences. It is worth a second mention to emphasize that ractopamine is a substance that *even China* banned. As expected, the United Nation's Codex Alimentarius Commission promotes ractopamine, and it gratuitously states that ractopamine has "no impact on human health".

More than ever, we strongly recommend that people only purchase organic meats. Perhaps there will be a time when foods are properly labeled, so that people will be able to make informed choices. Until then, people should only buy range-fed, organic meats. We also recommend that people have their beef well-cooked. The extra cooking will melt away excess fat and it ensures that all parasites are dead. Furthermore, high heat will destroy some chemical impurities too.

Unhealthy Fish

One of our strong suspicions about farmed fish was confirmed by researchers at Wake Forest Baptist University Medical Center. They proved that farm-raised fish are unhealthy, and dangerous with long-term consumption. We have to applaud Wake Forest for this. Through a press release, the university summarized its findings of:

"Farm-raised tilapia, one of the most highly consumed fish in America, has very low levels of beneficial omega-3 fatty acids and, perhaps worse, very high levels of omega-6 fatty acids...

"The researchers say the combination could be a potentially dangerous food source for some patients with heart disease, arthritis, asthma and other allergic and auto-immune diseases that are particularly vulnerable to an 'exaggerated inflammatory response'. Inflammation is known to cause damage to blood vessels, the heart, lung and joint tissues, skin, and the digestive tract.

"They say their research revealed that farm-raised tilapia, as well as farmed catfish, have several fatty acid characteristics that would generally be considered by the scientific community as detrimental. [farm-raised] 'Tilapia has higher levels of potentially detrimental long-chain omega-6 fatty acids than 80-percent-lean hamburger, doughnuts and even pork bacon'... 'For individuals who are eating fish as a method to control inflammatory diseases such as heart disease, it is clear from these numbers that tilapia is not a good choice,'... 'All other nutritional content aside, the inflammatory potential of hamburger and pork bacon is lower than the average serving of farmed tilapia'

"Tilapia is easily farmed using inexpensive [unnatural G.M.O.] corn-based feeds, which contain short chain omega-6s that the fish very efficiently convert to AA [a type of omega-6] and place in their tissues. This ability to feed the fish inexpensive foods, together with their capacity to grow under almost any condition, keeps the market price for the fish so low that it is rapidly becoming a staple in low-income diets."

That last part about the fish's capacity to grow under almost any conditions is telling. What is really being reported is that the fish will survive despite malnutrition, G.M.O. foods, pesticides, chemicals in the water, and being given massive amounts of antibiotics. The use of such pollutants is the cheapest investment for factory farmers. We must ponder what percentage of the fish are themselves genetically engineered.

This is yet another reason why we recommend flax seed oil, instead of fish oil, to supplement omega-3. Fish oils are much more likely to be tainted, toxic, and ineffective. Flax seed oil should always be purchased in capsules that protect it from heat, air, and light. It too can become dangerous if it is not handled properly.

Contrary to what is believed by the researchers at Wake Forest University, our research indicates that the ideal ratio of omega-6 to omega-3 is somewhere between 4:1 and 2:1, with omega-6 being the larger value. This ratio is impossible to obtain through a typical Western diet, which is usually 15:1 in favor of omega-6. It should therefore not be surprising that our Western societies tend to be so sickly.

Precautions Concerning Kelp, Seaweed, and Bladderwrack

Readers should be aware that the kelp, seaweed, and bladderwrack that is sold in supplement form may be from factory farms too. Unless you know the origin of such supplements, it cannot be assumed that these supplements are from the wild, or that they are in their natural form. They too could be contaminated and counter-effective, including man-made contamination from industrialized farms. We advise readers that all such supplements should be considered contaminated. There are shameless companies which promote the consumption of underwater vegetation, and they actually refer to it as "sea vegetables". Beware of these companies and the people behind them.

Even in the best of circumstances, underwater plants are not safe for human consumption, regardless of whether they are in their natural or supplemental form. For more information, reference the *Seaweed, Algae, and Other "Super Foods"* section of the *Frauds* chapter.

Chemical Fertilizers and Modern Produce

For about seventy years, people have been assured that poor quality soil is no longer an issue, so long as they rely on synthetic fertilizer products. Synthetic fertilizers are believed to infuse nutrients into soil, enabling all plants to prosper. However, synthetic fertilizers tend to replenish only nitrogen, potassium, and phosphorus; awhile depleting the other nutrients and minerals that are naturally found in truly fertile soils. Thus, modern farming ironically leads to nutritionally-deficient foods. Most produce is also laced with chemicals; and most troubling, pesticides. Conversely, organically-grown fruits and vegetables have significantly more anti-oxidants, polyphenols, and enzymes. It is not just the soil that is losing out: it is our health.

Omega-3 oils are some of the many nutrients which are rapidly declining in our foods. A lack of omega-3's is known to lead to heart disease, cancers, mental disorders such as attention deficit disorder, and Alzheimer's disease. In earlier times, most of these conditions were rare and merely occurred in society's most elderly.

Another reason behind our nutritional deficiencies is that fruits and vegetables are now being picked prematurely. For instance, non-organic tomatoes are now being made to look red using the chemical ethylene, instead of sunlight.

As far back as 1936, the U.S. Government was already aware that American soils were nutritionally deficient. U.S. Senator Duncan Fletcher, a Democrat from Florida, asked that a document be placed into the Congressional Record during that year. It became *Senate Document No. 264*, which stated:

> *"The alarming fact is that foods -- fruits and vegetables and grains -- now being raised on millions of acres of land that no longer contains enough of certain needed minerals, are starving us -- no matter how much of them we eat!*
>
> *"Laboratory tests prove that the fruits, the vegetables, the grains, the eggs and even the milk and the meats of today are not what they were a few generations ago (which doubtless explains why our forefathers thrived on a selection of foods that would starve us!) No man of today can eat enough fruits and vegetables to supply his system with the mineral salts he requires for perfect health, because his stomach isn't big enough to hold them..."*

The line, "No man of today can eat enough fruits and vegetables to supply his system with the mineral salts he requires for perfect health" is a good explanation for the existence of rampant obesity. Someone who is overweight is never satisfied. His hunger cannot be quenched, because his foods are so lacking in nutrition.

Synthetic fertilizers kill a large percentage of a soil's naturally-occurring microorganisms. These bacteria would normally break down organic matter into plant nutrients, and help convert nitrogen from the air into a plant-usable form. Other useful soil bacteria are "disease organisms" which keep cutworms, chinch bugs, grubs, and other parasites in check. It takes almost six weeks for soil to partially recover biologically from a poisoning by synthetic fertilizer. Considering that many fertilizer producers advise the reapplication of their synthetic fertilizers every three months explains why so many potentially fertile areas of soil are merely wastelands, wherein the essential microorganisms are dead from either fertilizer run-off or direct application. Soil that is deprived of its microorganisms undergoes a rapid decline in soil structure, and it loses its essential ability to retain water, air, and nutrients. Plants grown in such depleted soil are extremely susceptible to damage from diseases, insects, and drought. Healthy soil that is rich in beneficial microorganisms, encourages the natural immune systems of plants, limits the population of plant disease organisms, resists parasitic insects, and creates the ideal conditions for growth.

Organic crops are generally far more flavorful, since they contain many more nutrients. A person's mouth can actually taste the difference between God's goodness and man's sorcery.

For the environmentalists out there, growing organically embraces the ideal that agriculture should meet the needs of the present without harming future generations.

Unfortunately, switching to an organic fertilizer is not a quick fix for soil; especially when the soil has been bombarded with chemicals for years. It can take several years before the soil regains the fertility that it once had, and this may lead some growers into the false belief that organic farming is less productive. Hence, fertilizing with chemicals has become an addiction for farmers.

Organic fertilizer is most often manure from cows, horses, poultry, pigs, and sheep. The problem with manure is that the animals can only make nutrient-rich manure if their food source is also nutrient rich. Because of this, grass-eating animals raised on depleted soil will likewise produce inferior manure. Many organic advocates encourage others to travel to local farms for manure instead of the gardening sections of retailers. This is because the people who sell their products to large stores are likely to be using synthetic products on their fields and crops, because they hope to achieve a quick and easy profit, but their semi-starved animals will only yield depleted manure. Of course, purchasing directly from a farm is not always an option, and taking a risk with commercial manure is far better than using chemicals for the best long-term results and stewardship.

For those who cannot grow their own crops for practical reasons, farmer's markets are usually the next best option. Many of these farmers grow their crops organically, but cannot afford the cost of an official organic certification. Ask to find out.

U.S. Senate Document 264

The document that follows is provided courtesy of Health Wyze Media. It was presented to Congress by U. S. Senator, Mr. Duncan Fletcher on June 1st, 1936. He asked that it be placed into the permanent Congressional Record. The information presented in the following document provides some of the most convincing arguments for nutrition and organic growing ever made. The staff of The Health Wyze Report has taken great pain in obtaining the original document, and recreating it identically. The difficulty was due to the fact that the Internet is riddled with edited copies of this document. It was particularly disturbing that some copies of the document were altered for a political agenda. In particular, we have seen falsified copies of the document, which contained misquotes of all sentences containing the words "men" and "mankind". The history has been reprehensibly *corrected* by militant feminists. We present the document as it really was, for the sake of the value that it provides, and for its historical importance. The different styling, such as the use of italics, were in the original document. All formatting has been preserved to the best of our ability. As with all official U. S. governmental documents, it is not copyrighted, and it cannot be copyrighted. If you use this document or portions of it elsewhere, then we would appreciate being given attribution for our labored contribution to ensuring the survival of this document in its legitimate state. Copies of this document may be found at our website (healthwyze.org) in different formats, for free public dissemination.

MODERN MIRACLE MEN

DR. CHARLES NORTHEN, WHO BUILDS UP HEALTH FROM THE GROUND UP.

This quiet, unballyhooed pioneer and genius in the field of nutrition demonstrates that countless human ills stem from the fact that impoverished soil of America no longer provides plant foods with the mineral elements essential to human nourishment and health!To overcome this alarming condition, he doctors sick soils and, by seeming miracles, raises truly healthy and health-giving fruits and vegetables

(By Rex Beach)

Do you know that most of us today are suffering from certain dangerous diet deficiencies which cannot be remedied until the depleted soils from which our foods come are brought into *proper mineral balance?*

The alarming fact is that foods -- fruits and vegetables and grains -- now being raised on millions of acres of land that no longer contains enough of certain needed minerals, are starving us -- no matter how much of them we eat!

This talk about minerals is novel and quite startling. In fact, a realization of the importance of minerals in food is so new that the textbooks on nutritional dietetics contain very little about it. Nevertheless, it is something that concerns all of us, and the further we delve into it the more startling it becomes.

You'd think, wouldn't you, that a carrot is a carrot -- that one is about as good as another as far as nourishment is concerned? But it isn't; one carrot may look and taste like another and yet be lacking in the particular mineral element which our system requires and which carrots are supposed to contain. Laboratory tests prove that the fruits, the vegetables, the grains, the eggs and even the milk and the meats of today are not what they were a few generations ago (which doubtless explains why our forefathers thrived on a selection of foods that would starve us!)No man of today can eat enough fruits and vegetables to supply his system with the mineral salts he requires for perfect health, because his stomach isn't big enough to hold them! And we are running to big stomachs.

No longer does a balanced and fully nourishing diet consist merely of so many calories or certain vitamins or a fixed proportion of starches, proteins, and carbohydrates. We now know that *it must contain, in addition, something like a score of mineral salts.*

It is bad news to learn from our leading authorities that *99 percent of the American people are deficient in these minerals, and that a marked deficiency in any one of the more important minerals actually results in disease.* Any upset of this balance, any considerable lack of one or another element, however microscopic the body requirement may be, and we sicken, suffer, shorten our lives.

This discovery is one of the latest and most important contributions of science to the problem of human health.

So far as the records go, the first man in this field of research, the first to demonstrate that most human foods of our day are poor in minerals and that their proportions are not balanced, was Dr. Charles Northen, an Alabama physician now living at Orlando, Fla. His discoveries and achievements are of enormous importance to mankind.

Following a wide experience in general practice, Dr. Northen specialized in stomach diseases and nutritional disorders. Later, he moved to New York and made extensive studies along this line, in conjunction with the famous French scientist from the Sorbonne. In the course of that work he convinced himself that there was little authentic, definite information on the chemistry of foods, and that no dependence could be placed on existing data.

He asked himself how foods could be used intelligently in the treatment of disease, when they differed so widely in content. The answer seemed to be that they could not be used intelligently. In establishing the fact that serious deficiencies existed and in searching out the reasons therefor, he made an extensive study of the soil. *It was he who first voiced the surprising assertion that we must make soil building the basis of food building* in order to accomplish human building.

"Bear in mind, " says Dr. Northen, "that minerals are vital to human metabolism and health -- and that no plant or animal can appropriate by itself any mineral which is not present in the soil upon which it feeds.

"When I first made this statement I was ridiculed, for up to that time people had paid little attention to food deficiencies and even less to soil deficiencies. Men eminent in medicine denied there was any such thing as vegetables and fruits that did not contain sufficient minerals for human needs. Eminent agricultural authorities insisted that *all* soil contained all necessary minerals. They reasoned that plants take what they need, and that it is the function of the human body to appropriate what it requires. Failure to do so, they said, was a symptom of disorder.

"Some of our respected authorities even claimed that the so-called secondary minerals played no part whatsoever in human health. It is only recently that such men as Dr. McCollum at John Hopkins, Dr. Mendel of Yale, Dr. Sherman of Columbia, Dr. Lipman at Rutgers, and Drs. H. G. Knight in Oswald Schreiner of the United States Department of Agriculture have agreed that these minerals are essential to plant, animal, and human feeding.

"We know that vitamins are complex chemical substances which are indispensable to nutrition, and that each of them is of importance for the normal function of some special structure in the body. Disorder and disease result from any vitamin deficiency.

"It is not commonly realized, however, that vitamins control the body's appropriation of minerals, and in the absence of minerals they have no function to perform. Lacking vitamins, the system can make some use of minerals, but lacking minerals, vitamins are useless.

"Neither does the layman realize that there may be a pronounced difference in both foods and soils -- to him one vegetable, one glass of milk, or one egg is about the same as another. Dirt is dirt, too, and he assumes that by adding a little fertilizer to it, a satisfactory vegetable or fruit can be grown.

"The truth is that our foods vary enormously in value, and some of them aren't worth eating, as food. For example, vegetation grown in one part of the country may assay 1,100 parts, per billion, of iodine, as against 20 in that grown elsewhere. Processed milk has run anywhere from 362 parts, per million, of iodine and 127 of iron, down to nothing.

"Some of our lands, even in a virgin state, never were well balanced in mineral content, and unhappily for us, we have been systematically robbing the poor soils and the good soils alike of the very substances most necessary to health, growth, long life, and resistance to disease. Up to the time I began experimenting, almost nothing had been done to make good the theft.

"The more I studied nutritional problems and the effects of mineral deficiencies upon disease, the more plainly I saw that here lay the most direct approach to better health, and the more important it became in my mind to find a method of restoring those missing minerals to our foods.

"The subject interested me so profoundly that I retired from active medical practice and for a good many years now I have devoted myself to it. It's a fascinating subject, for it goes to the heart of human betterment."

The results obtained by Dr. Northen are outstanding. By putting back into foods the stuff that foods are made of, he has proved himself to be a real miracle man of medicine, for he has opened up the shortest and most rational route to better health.

He showed first that it should be done, and then that it could be done.

He doubled and redoubled the natural mineral content of fruits and vegetables.

He improved the quality of milk by increasing the iron and the iodine in it.

The caused hens to lay eggs richer in the vital elements.

By scientific soil feeding, he raised better seed potatoes in Maine, better grapes in California, better oranges in Florida and better field crops in other states. (By "better" is meant not only an improvement in food value but also an increase in quality and quantity.)

Before going further into the results he has obtained, let's see just what is involved in this matter of "mineral deficiencies", what it may mean to our health, and how it may affect the growth and development, both mental and physical, of our children.

We know that rats, guinea pigs, and other animals can be fed into a diseased condition and out again *by controlling only the minerals in their food*.

A 10-year test with rats proved that by withholding calcium they can breed down to a third the size of those fed with an adequate amount of that mineral. Their intelligence, too, can be controlled by mineral feeding as readily as can their size, their bony structure, and their general health.

Place a number of these little animals inside a maze after starving some of them in a certain mineral element. The starved ones will be unable to find their way out, whereas the others will have little or no difficulty in getting out. Their dispositions can be altered by mineral feeding. They can be made quarrelsome and belligerent; they can even be turned into cannibals and be made to devour each other.

A cage full of normal rats will live in amity. Restrict their calcium, and they will become irritable and draw apart from one another. Then they will begin to fight. Restore their calcium balance and they will grow more friendly; in time they will begin to sleep in a pile as before.

Many backward children are "stupid" merely because they are deficient in magnesia. We punish them for our failure to feed them properly.

Certainly our physical well-being is more directly dependent upon the minerals we take into our systems than upon calories or vitamins or upon the precise proportions of starch, protein, or carbohydrates we consume.

It is now agreed that at least *16 mineral elements are indispensable for normal nutrition*, and several more are always found in small amounts in the body, although their precise physiological role has not been determined. Of the 11 indispensable salts, calcium, phosphorus, and iron are perhaps the most important.

Calcium is the dominant nerve controller; it powerfully affects the cell formation of all living things and regulates nerve action. It governs contractility of the muscles and the rhythmic beat of the heart. It also coordinates the other mineral elements and corrects disturbances made by them. It works only in sunlight. Vitamin *D* is its buddy.

Dr. Sherman of Columbia asserts that *50 percent* of the American people are starving for calcium. A recent article in the Journal of the American Medical Association stated that out of the 4,000 cases in New York hospital, only 2 were not suffering from a lack of calcium.

What does such a deficiency mean? How would it affect your health or mine? So many morbid conditions and actual diseases may result that it is almost hopeless to catalog them. Included in the list are rickets, bone deformities, bad teeth, nervous disorders, reduced resistance to other diseases, fatigability, and behavior disturbances such as incorrigibility, assaultiveness, non-adaptability.

Here's one specific example: The soil around a certain Midwest city is poor in calcium. Three hundred children of this community were examined and nearly 90 percent had bad teeth, 69 percent showed affections of the nose and throat, swollen glands, enlarged or diseased tonsils. More than one-third had defective vision, round shoulders, bow legs, and anemia.

Calcium and phosphorus appear to pull in double harness. A child requires as much per day as two grown men, but studies indicate a common deficiency of both in our food. Researchers on farm animals point to a deficiency of one or the other as the cause of serious losses to the farmers, and when the soil is poor in phosphorus these animals become bone-chewers. Dr. McCollum says that when there are enough phosphates in the blood there can be no dental decay.

Iron is an essential constituent of the oxygen-carrying pigment of the blood: iron starvation results in anemia, and yet iron cannot be assimilated unless some *copper* is contained in the diet. In Florida many cattle die from an obscure disease called "salt sickness. "It has been found to arise from a lack of iron and copper in the soil and hence in the grass. A man may starve for want of these elements just as a beef "critter" starves.

If *iodine* is not present in our foods the function of the thyroid gland is disturbed and goiter afflicts us. The human body requires only fourteen-thousandths of a milligram daily, yet we have a distinct "goiter belt" in the Great Lakes section, and in parts of the North-west the soil is so poor in iodine that the disease is common.

So it goes, down through the list, each mineral element playing a definite role in nutrition. A characteristic set of symptoms, just as specific as any vitamin-deficiency disease, follows a deficiency in any one of them. It is alarming, therefore, to face the fact that we are starving for these precious, health-giving substances.

Very well, you say, if our foods are poor in the mineral salts they are supposed to contain, why not resort to dosing?

That is precisely what is being done, or being attempted. However, those who should know assert that the human system cannot appropriate those elements to the best advantage in any but the food form. At best, only a part of them in the form of drugs can be utilized by the body,and certain dieticians go so far as to say it is a waste of effort to fool with them. Calcium, for instance, cannot be supplied in any form of medication with lasting effect.

But there is a more potent reason why the curing of diet deficiencies by drugging hasn't worked out so well. Consider those 16 indispensable elements and those others which presumably perform some obscure function as yet undetermined. Aside from calcium and phosphorus, they are needed only in infinitesimal quantities, and the activity of one may be dependent upon the presence of another. To determine the precise requirements of each individual case and to attempt to weigh it out on a druggists scales would appear hopeless.

It is a problem and a serious one. But here is the hopeful side of the picture: *Nature can and will solve it if she is encouraged to do so*. The minerals in fruit and vegetables are colloidal; i. e. , they are in a state of such extremely fine suspension that they can be assimilated by the human system: It is merely a question of giving back to nature the materials with which she works.

We must rebuild our soils: Put back the minerals we have taken out. That sounds difficult but it isn't. Neither is it expensive. Therein lies the shortcut to better health and longer life.

When Dr. Northen first asserted that many foods were lacking in mineral content and that this deficiency was due solely to an absence of those elements in the soil, his findings were challenged and he was called a crank. But differences of opinion in the medical profession are not uncommon -- it was only 60 years ago that the Medical Society of Boston passed a resolution condemning the use of bathtubs -- and he persisted in his assertion that inasmuch as foods did not contain what they were supposed to contain, no physician could with certainty prescribe a diet to overcome physical ills.

He showed that the textbooks are not dependable because many of the analyses in them were made many years ago, perhaps from products raised in virgin soils, whereas our soils have been constantly depleted. Soil analyses, he pointed out, reflect only the content of the samples. One analysis may be entirely different from another made 10 miles away.

"And so what?" came the query.

Dr. Northen undertook to demonstrate that something could be done about it. *By reestablishing a proper soil balance he actually grew crops that contained an ample amount of the desired minerals.*

This was incredible. It was contrary to the books and it upset everything connected with diet practice. The scoffers began to pay attention to him. Recently the Southern Medical Association, realizing the hopelessness of trying to remedy nutritional deficiencies without positive factors to work with, recommended a careful study to determine the real mineral content of food stuffs and the variations due to soil depletion in different localities. These progressive medical men are awake to the importance of prevention.

Dr. Northen went even further and proved that crops grown in a properly mineralized soil were bigger and better; that seeds germinated quicker, grew more rapidly and made larger plants; that trees were healthier and put on more fruit of better quality.

By increasing the mineral content of citrus fruit he likewise improved its texture, its appearance and its flavor.

He experimented with a variety of growing things, and in every case the story was the same. By mineralizing the feed at poultry farms, he got more and better eggs; by balancing pasture soils, he produced richer milk. Persistently he hammered home to farmers, to doctors, and to the general public the thought that life depends upon the minerals.

His work led him into a careful study of the effects of climate, sunlight, ultraviolet and thermal rays upon plant, animal, and human hygiene. In consequence he moved to Florida. People familiar with his work consider him the most valuable man in the State. I met him by reason of the fact that I was harassed by certain soil problems on my Florida farm which had baffled the best chemists and fertilizer experts available.

He is an elderly, retiring man, with a warm smile and engaging personality. He is a trifle shy until he opens up on his pet topic; then his diffidence disappears and he speaks with authority. His mind is a storehouse crammed with precise, scientific data about soil and food chemistry, the complicated life processes of plants, animals, and human beings -- and the effect of malnutrition upon all three. He is perhaps as close to the secret of life as any man anywhere.

"Do you call yourself a soil or a food chemist?" I inquired.

"Neither. I'm an M. D. My work lies in the field of biochemistry and nutrition. I gave up medicine because this is a wider and a more important work. Sick soils mean sick plants, sick animals, and sick people. Physical, mental, and moral fitness depends largely upon an ample supply and a proper proportion of the minerals in our foods. Nerve function, nerve stability, nerve cell building likewise depend thereon. I'm really a doctor of sick soils."

"Do you mean to imply that the vegetables I'm raising on my farm are sick?" I asked.

"Precisely!They're as weak and undernourished as anemic children. They're not much good as food. Look at the pests and the diseases that plague them. Insecticides cost farmers nearly as much as fertilizer these days.

"A healthy plant, however, grown in soil properly balanced, *can and will resist most insect pests*. That very characteristic makes it a better food product. You have tuberculosis and pneumonia germs in your system but you're strong enough to throw them off. Similarly, a really healthy plant will pretty nearly take care of itself in the battle against insects and blights -- and will also give the human system what it requires."

"Good heavens! Do you realize what that means to agriculture?"

"Perfectly. Enormous savings. Better crops. Lowered living costs to the rest of us. But I am not so much interested in agriculture as in health."

"It sounds beautifully theoretical and utterly impractical to me," I told the doctor, whereupon he gave me some of his case records. For instance, in an orange grove infected with scale, when he restored the mineral balance to part of the soil, the trees growing in that part became clean while the rest remain diseased. By the same means he had grown healthy rosebushes between rows that were riddled with insects.

He had grown tomato and cucumber plants, both healthy and diseased, where the vines intertwined. The bugs ate up the diseased and refused to touch the healthy plants!He showed me interesting analyses of citrus fruit, the chemistry and the food value of which accurately reflected the soil treatment the trees had received.

There is no space here to go fully into Dr. Northen's work but it is of such importance as to rank with that of Burbank, the plant wizard, and with that of our famous physiologists and nutritional experts.

"Healthy plants mean healthy people", said he. "We can't raise a strong race on a weak soil. Why don't you try mending the deficiencies on your farm and growing more minerals into your crops?"

I did try and I succeeded. I was planting a large acreage of celery and under Dr. Northen's direction I fed minerals into certain blocks of the land in varying amounts. When the plants from this soil were mature I had them analyzed, along with celery from other parts of the State. It was the most careful and comprehensive study of the kind ever made, and it included over 250 separate chemical determinations. I was amazed to learn that my celery had more than twice the mineral content of the best grown elsewhere. Furthermore, it kept much better, with and without refrigeration, proving that the cell structure was sounder.

In 1927, Mr. W. W. Kincaid, a "gentleman farmer" of Niagara Falls, heard an address by Dr. Northen and was so impressed that he began extensive experiments in the mineral feeding of plants and animals. The results he has accomplished are conspicuous. He set himself the task of increasing the iodine in the milk from his diary herd. He has succeeded in adding both iodine and iron so liberally that one glass of his milk contains all of these minerals that an adult man requires for a day.

Is this significant? Listen to these incredible figures taken from a bulletin of the South Carolina Food Research Commission: "In many sections *3 out of 5 persons* have goiter and a recent estimate states that *30 million people in the United States suffer from it*."

Foods rich in iodine are of the greatest importance to these sufferers.

Mr. Kincaid took a brown Swiss heifer calf which was dropped in the stockyards, and by raising her on a mineralized pasturage and a properly balanced diet made her the third all-time champion of her breed! In one season she gave 21,924 pounds of milk. He raised her butterfat production from 410 pounds in 1 year to 1,037 pounds. Results like these are of incalculable importance.

Others besides Mr. Kincaid are following the trail Dr. Northen blazed. Similar experiments with milk have been made in Illinois and nearly every fertilizer company is beginning to urge use of the rare mineral elements. As an example I quote from statements of a subsidiary of one of the leading copper companies:

> Many States show a marked reduction in the productive capacity of the soil... in
> many districts amounting to a 25 to 50 percent reduction in the last 50 years...
> some areas show a tenfold variation in calcium. Some show a sixtyfold variation in
> phosphorus... authorities... see soil depletion, baron life stock, increased human
> death rate due to heart disease, deformations, arthritis, increased dental caries, all
> due to a lack of elemental minerals in plant foods.

"It is neither a complicated nor an expensive undertaking to restore our soils to balance and thereby work a real miracle in the control of disease," says Dr. Northen. "As a matter of fact, it's a money-making move for the farmer, and any competent soil chemist can tell him how to proceed.

"First determined by analysis the precise chemistry of any given soil, then correct the deficiencies by putting down enough of the missing elements to restore its balance. This same care should be used as in prescribing for a sick patient, for *proportions are of vital importance*.

"In my early experiments I found it extremely difficult to get the variety of minerals needed in the form in which I wanted to use them but advancement in chemistry, and especially our ever-increasing knowledge of colloidal chemistry, has solved that difficulty. It is now possible, by the use of minerals in colloidal form, to prescribe a cheap and effective system of soil correction which meets this vital need and one which fits in admirably with nature's plans.

"Soils seriously deficient in minerals cannot produce plant life competent to maintain our needs, and with the continuous cropping and shipping away of those concentrates, the condition becomes worse.

"A famous nutrition authority recently said, 'One sure way to end the American people's susceptibility to infection is to supply through food a balanced ration of iron, copper, and other minerals. An organism supplied with a diet adequate to, or preferably in excess of, our mineral requirements may so utilize these elements as to produce immunity from infection quite beyond anything we are able to produce artificially by our present method of immunization. You can't make up the deficiency by using patent medicine.'

"He's absolutely right. Prevention of disease is easier, more practical, and more economical than cure, but not until foods are standardized on a basis of what they contain instead of what they look like can the dietician prescribe them with intelligence and with effect.

"There was a time when medical therapy had no standards because the therapeutic elements in drugs had not been definitely determined on a chemical basis. Pharmaceutical houses have changed all that. Food chemistry, on the other hand, has depended almost entirely upon governmental agencies for its research, and in our real knowledge of values we are about where medicine was a century ago.

"Disease preys most surely and most viciously on the undernourished and unfit plants, animals, and human beings alike, and when the importance of these obscured mineral elements is fully realized the chemistry of life will have to be rewritten. No man knows his mental or bodily capacity, how well he can feel or how long he can live, for we are all cripples and weaklings. It is a disgrace to science. Happily, that chemistry is being rewritten and we're on our way to better health by returning to the soil the things we have stolen from it.

"*The public can help; it can hasten the change.* How? By demanding quality in its food. By insisting that our doctors and our health departments establish scientific standards of nutritional value.

"The growers will quickly respond. They can put back those minerals almost overnight, and by doing so they can actually make money through bigger and better crops.

"It is simpler to cure sick soils than sick people -- which shall we choose?"

Sodium Benzoate In Soft Drinks

One of the dirty secrets of the soft drink and processed food industries is sodium benzoate. It is a benzene compound that is produced by mixing benzoic acid with sodium hydroxide. It is a common preservative. It has been associated with a vast array of health problems, including all of our major epidemics. Sodium benzoate is considerably more toxic than either processed sugar or high fructose corn syrup, yet it gets very little media coverage. It is a *bona fide* poison. Outside of our foods, benzene is the main ingredient of Liquid Wrench, various paint stripper products, rubber cements, and spot removers, due it its highly destructive and solvent qualities. It was discontinued in rubber manufacture in the U.S. because it caused a large percentage of the workers to get leukemia.

Countries throughout Europe have been pressuring the food industry to voluntarily remove sodium benzoate from products, before more aggressive action is taken. Several European media outlets have called for an absolute ban on this toxic preservative due to concerns about children's developmental safety. The U.S. Government and media have remained disturbingly silent. As usual, there have been no studies in the U.S. about the chemical's effects upon children, but it is studied elsewhere. The chemical industry in the United States is well protected, and studying sodium benzoate's effects upon children in the United States would be career suicide for any researcher, as has happened with many researchers of fluoride. Meanwhile, thousands of children are dying of leukemia.

Like many other food industry chemicals, it was originally found in an organic form. Trace amounts of the organic form can be found in blueberries, apples, cranberries, plums, and cinnamon. However, sodium benzoate has no known negative effects in its organic form. Only the synthetic version has toxic effects. Perhaps the organic form occurs with its own biological neutralizers, as is frequently the case with organically-occurring food toxins; or the organic form is somehow different from the sodium benzoate that is made in chemical laboratories. The natural version does not have any preservative action, because it has no toxicity. It is only when sodium benzoate is produced inside a chemical laboratory that the result is a cheap, toxic agent that destroys living organisms.

There are many chemical additives that present health hazards, but sodium benzoate is especially dangerous because it is able to destroy parts of the DNA. This means that the sodium benzoate consumed today may still be causing problems in future generations. Sodium benzoate is known to specifically attack the mitochondria of DNA. The mitochondria use oxygen to produce energy. They also control the cell life cycle and cell growth. Whenever there is a change in the DNA or overall genetic structure, the effects on the organism are unpredictably random. Sodium benzoate and DNA damage have already been linked with

Parkinson's disease, liver problems, and these just scratch the surface of the possibilities.

Our confused medical establishment increasingly labels new diseases as spontaneous and genetic in origin, while ignoring that poisons like sodium benzoate are known to cause genetic mutations. The link to genetic mutations explains why benzene is so incredibly carcinogenic, and it likewise explains why radiation is so carcinogenic; for radiation exposure induces the formation of benzene compounds inside proteins.

> *"Once again, the FDA has sided with big food companies and misled consumers about the problem of benzene in beverages, withholding data and issuing public reassurances that are contradicted by their own test results."*
>
> -- Richard Wiles, Environmental Working Group

Whenever sodium benzoate is exposed to vitamin C, it forms pure benzene. It is astounding that our chemical industry found a method through which they could make vitamin C dangerous. Virtually all soft drinks currently have added vitamin C in the form of ascorbic acid, as if that would make the drinks healthy. This leads to the inevitable creation of dangerous benzene. Its inclusion causes a decrease of red blood cells, a severe depression of the immune system to produce generalized allergy symptoms, leukemia, various other blood cancers, and pre-cancerous blood conditions.

The amount of benzene in soft drinks is not even known. Benzene content increases in correlation with shelf-life, heat, and light exposure. A study of diet Orange Crush by Cadbury's in 1990 revealed that benzene levels "off the shelf" were 25 P.P.B. (parts per billion) and it rose to 82 P.P.B. after exposure to heat and light. U.S. federal safety rules limit benzene levels in drinking water to 5 P.P.B.; but regulators made a special exception for soft drinks, which made the manufacturers immune from this safety regulation. Some soft drinks tested to have well over 100 P.P.B. of benzene at the point of purchase -- 20 times greater than the maximum safe level for human consumption. By the safety standards set for drinking water, a six-pack of Mountain Dew could develop 120 times the safe level of benzene. Is that Mountain Dew really worth the risk of having a leg-less grandchild, or one having low intelligence?

The clear connections between benzene formation, sodium benzoate, and vitamin C were discovered in the early 1990's. The findings were ignored in the United States, and debate about them has been avoided by the soft drink industry. Sodium benzoate is one of the most dangerous preservatives available, but it is the cheapest. Coca-Cola confirmed that alternatives exist when they reformulated Diet Coke in the U.K., following public outrage about sodium benzoate. Despite being knowledgeable of the risks involved, public pressure on soft drink manufacturers is not yet great enough for them to reformulate in the United States. Corporations which seek to profit through immoral actions are nothing new, but far more sickening is the way in which the Food and Drug Administration has ignored the dangers of benzene in soft drinks, and it has even worked to hide the studies from the public, according to the Environmental Working Group.

Researchers at Southampton University noted that tests have shown sodium benzoate to lower the I.Q. by up to five points in children. Britain's Food Standards Agency has even warned parents that sodium benzoate is a primary cause of hyperactivity in children, along with artificial colorings.

"Sodium benzoate is the most effective preservative currently authorized."

-- Richard Laming, British Soft Drinks Association

A preservative is a chemical suitable for killing bacteria, fungi, and anything else that could otherwise live inside a product. Preservatives do not keep foods "fresh" as marketers contend. They are instead toxic enough to ensure that nothing in a food item can survive. Therefore, if sodium benzoate is the most effective preservative currently authorized, it must also be the most poisonous one.

There have been truly natural preservatives available for decades, which include grape seed extract, pine bark extract, stevia, colloidal silver, organic nitrates from celery, and raw honey. There are also the older techniques of using vinegar, salt, and smoking; which actually improve flavor. With the possible exception of salt, none of these pose any risk to health, but they are more expensive. The natural alternatives do not sponsor the chemical industry, which funds the U.S. Food and Drug Administration; whose approval is necessary for American food distribution. Thus, companies are strongly encouraged not to use any natural preservatives -- that is, if they wish to stay in business. The situation produces a double whammy for the public, because the petrochemical industry first profits by creating toxic chemicals for foods, and then it profits by selling the drugs to treat the resultant diseases.

Anti-Bacterial Soaps and Hand Sanitizers

The Washington Post reported that the F.D.A. has finally found fault in a chemical. The chemical is found in the urine of more than 75% of Americans, and research has shown for years that it is dangerous. New research has grabbed the attention of the E.P.A., F.D.A. and C.P.S.C. The chemical is so widely used that it falls under the jurisdiction of all three federal agencies.

Triclosan is an anti-bacterial and anti-fungal chemical. Astute readers may already be making the connection that anything which is poisonous to organisms is, well, poisonous. The poison is added to anti-bacterial soaps, pesticides, toothpastes, cleaning agents, shaving creams, and mouthwashes. In recent years, it has been infused into children's toys, bedding, and some clothing. From observing the history of the chemical industry, we are making bets amongst ourselves as to how long it will be before it is a component of vaccines and infant formula.

> *"But the FDA, which oversees its use in personal-care products, medical devices and products that come into contact with food, has been working for 38 years to establish the rules for the use of triclosan but has not completed that task."*

-- Washington Post, April 8th, 2010

For approximately four decades, the Food and Drug Administration has not managed to decide if triclosan is safe. Meanwhile, people are washing their hands and brushing their teeth with this chemical; with direct absorption into the blood through the mouth tissues.

Current research shows that triclosan is damaging to the endocrine system. The endocrine system is made up of glands that are responsible for mood regulation, metabolism, and growth. Therefore, we have quite a disease-inflicting cocktail when this is mixed with fluoride in oral care products. When these crucial glands begin to fail, diseases emanate. Failure of the adrenal glands, for instance, can quickly result in the onset of diabetes or Cushing's syndrome. Failure of the thyroid gland can result in hypothyroidism and diabetes. Meanwhile, the establishment does not seem to know why these are epidemics.

The F.D.A. claims to be re-evaluating triclosan, but they have been willfully blind to all of the dangers for the past four decades. Will they suddenly find them now? The fact that the press has drawn attention to this poison is probably the only reason why the F.D.A. has finally shown the issue lip service. As usual, the involved companies will be paying the F.D.A.'s research costs to ensure that their products are found to be safe.

To exemplify how unsafe and ineffective this chemical is, some leading brands of triclosan-based hand sanitizers were recalled in 2009, after they were found to contain high levels of multiple strains of bacteria. The F.D.A. admitted that some of the bacteria were only found in "particularly unsanitary conditions". It warned that the subsequent skin infections could be so severe as to need surgical attention, and result in permanent damage.

Most commercial toothpastes should already be avoided, because of the fluoride and sodium lauryl sulfate. The use of anti-bacterial soaps are the equivalent of taking an antibiotic several times each day. Chemicals that are placed on the skin will often sink directly through the skin and into the bloodstream. Not only do we generally recommend against antibiotics, but it has also been shown that anti-bacterial soaps are no more effective than regular soaps in killing bacteria. The risk of illness actually increases with their usage, because of how the immune system is weakened by exposure to such toxins.

Skin Health and Lotions

Many people use commercial hand lotions to make their skin softer and moister. This is especially true throughout the winter months, when less moisture is present in the air. Commercial lotions seem to provide some short-term relief for skin dryness, but they actually make the problems worse in the long term. This phenomena is similar to what we have seen with pharmaceuticals and dieting aids, which ultimately exaggerate the root problems.

People rarely use hand lotions in moderation. Lotion becomes an essential accessory, which is applied generously several times daily, for years at a time. This necessity seems to be by design from the industry. The great majority of hand lotions contain chemicals which accumulate in the liver and fatty tissues, causing long-term problems. The chemicals accumulate in ever greater amounts in the body over time in a snowballing reaction. Many of the common chemicals used in hand lotions are known to cause skin dryness and skin irritation with extended use, which coincidentally happens to be great for business. When people start experiencing long-term dryness after using hand lotions, they eventually become dependent on these lotions for their quick-fix. None of this is accidental.

Lotion Ingredients

Common ingredients in commercial hand lotions include parabens (propylparaben, ethylparaben, methylparaben), alcohols, mineral oil, other petroleum products, and aluminum. Most people seem oblivious to the fact that chemicals placed on the skin are frequently absorbed directly into the bloodstream. If this were to become common knowledge, then most of the cosmetic companies would be driven out of business. Cosmetic products are not regulated at all, so formulations are made at the whims of manufacturers.

Parabens bio-accumulate in the liver, breasts, and fatty tissues. They are known for causing skin irritation, dry skin, sensitizing the skin, and they trigger allergic reactions to weaken the immune system. Much controversy has surrounded this set of chemicals in recent years, due to the fact that some studies link their use to breast cancer. A study conducted by St. Joseph's Hospital in September 2008, monitored girls who used cosmetic products containing parabens, and contrasted them with girls who did not. They found higher rates of cancer in the girls who were exposed to parabens. Animal studies show that parabens reduce sperm counts.

Petroleum has been shown in studies to not only cause cancerous tumors, but also to cause long-term dryness of skin. Petroleum-based creams cannot absorb completely, so some remains on the surface of the hands. The hands then appear to improve, because the layer of oil feels like something of a second skin. The overall condition of the skin is actually worse, whenever the petroleum mask is removed. Meanwhile, the skin remains dry and smothered underneath the oily layer. Mineral oil works in the same way, except that more of it sinks into the bloodstream as a whole-body toxicant.

Amazingly, many hand lotions contain alcohols too, which are known to dry the skin by almost everyone. Why then, would they be added into lotions that are marketed for moisturizing?

Aluminum is a bio-accumulative heavy metal, which cannot normally be excreted by a body. It damages the I.Q., contributes to cancer, as well as causing Alzheimer's disease and multiple sclerosis. The list of disease states caused by aluminum is a very long one. A heavy metal cleanse is necessary to remove the build-up of this toxic metal, and selenium should be used as a neutralizing supplement in the meantime. Always be sure to buy aluminum-free baking powder for this reason. Beware that it is in commercial breads and crackers. It is in almost every commercial product that uses leavened bread. It is in the vaccines too.

Most people never even consider reading the ingredients lists on their cosmetic products. Our analysis on leading brands of moisturizers was horrifying. The long list of chemicals that are found inside modern cosmetics seems endless, and it is perfectly legal for companies to avoid listing some ingredients, under the guise of "trade secrets". This is normal, in fact. If you are one of the millions of people who have been scammed by the chemical industry in regard to hand lotions, then we strongly recommend a liver and heavy metal cleanse; and if still needed, a switch to a natural skin lotion.

We (Health Wyze Media) formulated our own hand lotion and now sell it, because the commercial lotions that were available were all completely unacceptable.

Skin Care Recommendations

- People with extreme skin problems should stay away from direct contact with latex. This includes latex in foods (avocado, bananas, chestnuts, kiwi, and perhaps even tomatoes). Many people have latex allergies because of vaccinations. Latex allergies can have terrible effects upon the skin.

- Topical use of colloidal copper. Copper is important for the synthesis of both collagen and elastin. It has also been shown to increase the thickness of the skin. For a safe oral method of supplementing with copper, we suggest chlorophyll. Otherwise, do not ingest copper because it is dangerous unless it is naturally occurring in foods.

- The benefits of coconut oil seem limitless, and it is extremely useful for dry skin. Orally take a teaspoon or so daily. Buy only organic, cold-pressed coconut oil from a health food store. It is not expensive, and it will help.

- Vitamin C increases collagen and elastin. It is commonly used for the treatment of dry skin.

- Since unhealthy fats disrupt collagen production, there is part of the Budwig Protocol which should be helpful. Purchase flax seed oil capsules and mix the extracted oil with goat cheese. Yogurt can be used instead of goat cheese, but it is not as healthy, because it is usually made with homogenized milk. Make sure the flax seed oil is in dark capsules in a dark container. The oil can quickly become dangerously rancid when it is exposed to heat and light. Do not mix with a metal object. Wood is ideal.

- Get liquid iodine and place about a 2 inch (5 cm.) patch on your skin. Let it sink in throughout the day. Your body will absorb only the amount that it needs. Always avoid povidone iodine. Read the *Iodine* section of the *Supplements* chapter for safety information concerning the oral supplementation of iodine.

- You may have pre-diabetes. Check yourself and treat accordingly after reading our *Diabetes* chapter.

- Try supplementing with niacin at a small dosage, but please read the *Niacin* section of the *Supplements* chapter concerning niacin's strange side effects.

- Zinc supplementation is known to help with a variety of skin, hair, and nail problems. A body cannot properly utilize zinc without copper.

- You may have hypothyroidism if you have severe or chronic skin problems.

- Sunbathing is a helpful treatment for many skin diseases, such as athlete's foot fungus, psoriasis, acne, boils, and impetigo. Sunlight converts cholesterol in the skin into vitamin D-2 to help the liver.

Dangerous Copper Peptide Products

The most common copper-based creams that are being sold are the ones containing copper peptides. Copper peptides are synthetic compounds that are alleged to mimic the biological copper compounds that are inside the human body. However, this belief and the overall science of biochemistry are both largely frauds, because science is still unable to precisely reproduce any nutrient that is found in nature. Exemplifying this, synthesized vitamins are never as effective as those found naturally in foods. Chemists had their best success in creating synthetic vitamin C (ascorbic acid), but it performs differently in the human body to the organic vitamin C that can be extracted from foods, such as the original vitamin C supplement which was extracted from paprika. Various chemists have inadvertently admitted this difference by making arrogant proclamations about how synthetic vitamin C has superior absorption over natural vitamin C. Of course, there could be no differing absorption rate if the two substances were actually identical, as they claim. They still cannot reproduce true vitamin C, awhile being unable to detect any differences chemically. It condemns the science as little more than a game of charades. Whenever the chemical industry boasts that it has created an identical copy of a God-given nutrient, then we can safely assume that it has differences, even when those differences cannot be detected in a laboratory.

Copper Peptides Have Long-Term Side Effects

The following side effects of copper peptides demonstrate that they are damaging to the skin and liver.

- Sagging skin

- Sunken eyes

- Green stained skin

- Loss of elasticity in the skin

Some copper product sellers market that their synthetic copper peptides are identical to the natural copper compounds that a human body produces. The evidence of side-effects clearly shows otherwise; but even if it were true, then it would still not necessarily be a good thing. The real benefit of copper may actually be in the biological transformation processes, whereby a body binds copper with other substances. There may be no benefit in the finished copper compounds that they are trying to emulate. These may simply be another bodily waste product, and yet they are using it like a supplement, despite having absolutely no understanding of it. This sort of "science" reflects the typical stupidity and dishonesty that we have seen from the chemical community in its constant attempts to out-engineer God. The long-term consequences of copper peptide use is yet another example of their failure.

The greatest irony of the copper peptide products is that they yield exactly the opposite effect of what a good copper product should achieve. For example, the products are known to temporarily increase the elasticity of the skin, which is initially favorable; but a projected side-effect of copper peptide exposure is an eventual decrease in skin elasticity that tends to be worse than the original problem. Since we know that true nutrients do not harm the human body (or skin) in any way, it is obvious that the ingredients of these products in no way resemble real nutrients, including organic copper compounds.

In a manner that is typical of the chemical and cosmetic industries, the potential risks of copper peptides are being suppressed by the manufacturers. Companies which produce copper peptides are becoming notorious for only permitting glowing commentary about their products on their websites and forums. As a result, those who have had their skin permanently damaged by such products are congregating elsewhere for discussions. The victims of this sham often describe their skin damage as being like that from malpracticed laser surgery.

The primary reason why we use colloidal copper for our lotion product is because there is no safer way to extract copper than through electrolysis. There are plenty of chemical methods for producing copper solutions that are cheaper, but they are unsafe, and they yield harmful chemical impurities. It is incredible that the copper peptide manufacturers are marketing their products on the basis of having impurities, of which they have not studied for adverse effects; so many people are learning the truth the hard way. It is tragic that the majority of people who search for copper-based skin products are tricked into paying the same chemical industry that caused their health problems.

Sunscreen Lies and Cosmetic Trade Secrets

Everything most people think they know about sunscreen and sunshine is wrong, and part of a clever marketing campaign designed to benefit large industry at our expense. These lies may be putting you on a collision course with cancer. These same corporations have been chemically medicating women through cosmetics for years without their knowledge, consent, and with very little governmental oversight.

Transdermal Medication

The use of patches that are placed onto the skin to administer drugs has become increasingly common in modern medicine. It is recognized that many compounds enter into the bloodstream unaltered through this method of medication. Medication by skin absorption bypasses the digestive system; making medications more potent. These patches are often marketed to people who have difficulty taking large or foul-tasting pills.

With transdermal medications, liquids and tiny particle pastes sink through the skin into the blood, giving the digestive system no chance of neutralizing any ingredients. Human skin eventually absorbs all chemical solutions that are rubbed onto it, or lay resting on it. This realization should make us rather uncomfortable, considering all of the chemicals that are placed upon our skin throughout our lifetimes. These compounds include lipsticks, sunscreens, makeup foundations, and various other cosmetic products.

Most women never consider why lipstick must be reapplied every 4 to 6 hours. Some of it is absorbed by the mouth, tongue, and stomach; but most of it is absorbed straight into the blood through the lips. Contrary to popular belief, only a small portion of lipstick is removed by napkins and drinking glasses. Women absorb up to 6 pounds of lipstick in their lifetimes. This is an enormous amount of lipstick, and the studies cannot even guess the total amount of cosmetics absorbed for all products. Especially alarming is the fact that the majority of lipsticks contain lead, a heavy metal neurotoxin. Lipsticks are the most toxic of all cosmetic products. Test studies of popular lipsticks have demonstrated that they produce birth defects, and mental retardation in particular.

Cosmetics get very little governmental oversight. Cosmetic companies are given broad liberties, and for the most part, may make whatever claims about their products that they wish. They may include practically any ingredient in their products. Unless a product already contains an ingredient that has been banned, cosmetic products do not need approval from the F.D.A. before they are sold; nor do they need to complete any safety testing. The testing is performed on us.

The F.D.A. and F.T.C. actually allow cosmetic companies to hide information pertaining to ingredients, under the guise of "trade secrets". Reading the ingredients of your makeup may prove to be horrifying, but the undisclosed ingredients are worse. Companies can write whatever they want for the ingredients lists of cosmetics, because the lists are never verified. An eyeliner company could list the ingredients for apple pie on the label, and no action would be taken. Consider the ingredients lists for cosmetics to be meaningless.

The Top 10 Trade Secrets of Cosmetics

1. Mercury

2. Lead acetate

3. Formaldehyde

4. Toluene

5. Petroleum distillates

6. Ethylacrylate

7. Coal tar

8. Dibutyl phthalate

9. Potassium dichromate

10. 2Bromo2Nitropropane1,3Diol

Sunscreens

The aluminum found in these products stays in a body forever, as an accumulative, heavy metal toxin. A trace amount of it might do little harm, but aluminum forever accumulates in ever-increasing amounts; because the human body is generally incapable of flushing-out toxic metals without intervention. The risks therefore become cascading, since such metals persistently accumulate throughout a lifetime to cause numerous mysterious dysfunctions, diseases, allergies, and an overall impaired immune system. These conditions in turn make it even more difficult for the immune system to properly cope with additional toxic metals.

Sunscreen products often contain zinc oxide and titanium dioxide as the two active ingredients. These are known carcinogens, which will penetrate into a person's bloodstream. In the past couple of years, sunscreen manufacturers have turned to a worse active ingredient: oxybenzone. It is a derivative of benzophenone, which is well known to attack DNA whenever it is exposed to light, which makes it a particularly interesting choice of chemicals to use in sunscreens. It has been shown to penetrate deep into the skin, where it acts as a photosynthesizer. The chemical reaction causes an increased production of free radicals under illumination, which makes it a photocarcinogen; especially for those with less-than-ideal diets. The Department of Chemistry and Bioengineering at the University of California studied this effect and documented it in the report, *Sunscreen Enhancement of UV-Induced Reactive*

Oxygen Species in the Skin, which was published in June of 2006.

A person should not put anything onto his skin that he would not feel safe eating. Absorbing chemicals through the skin can be more dangerous than ingesting them. This is because they are not decomposed by the potent acid (hydrochloric acid) of the stomach before reaching the bloodstream. Stomach acid works to neutralize many chemical toxins, at least partially; and then the remaining toxins are passed through the normal filtration of the digestive system. In comparison, chemicals absorbed through the skin do not get diluted, filtered, or neutralized at all. They directly enter into the bloodstream, and in doing so bypass digestive safeguards.

None of us would ever consider eating sunscreen. Yet we follow the misguided advice of the medical establishment, which purports that many of us will inevitably suffer from skin cancer without it. The truth is that sunscreen ingredients, such as zinc oxide and oxybenzone, directly cause cancer. This is the predominant reason why people with large amounts of sun exposure statistically have higher rates of skin cancer, for it is their elevated use of sunscreens that is causing the cancers -- not the sun. Sunlight provides an individual with a bountiful supply of all-natural Vitamin D, and it is the kind that a body can actually use (D-3). Vitamin D is one of the most effective anti-cancer vitamins, and most cancers occur in people who do not get enough sunlight exposure, or vitamin D. Prior to the invention of sunscreens, skin cancer was virtually unheard of, and people got significantly more sun exposure in those days.

The Lesser of Evils

It is unfortunate that some situations make sunscreens necessary. Sunscreens containing zinc oxide are always safer than their oxybenzone counterparts. The DNA-altering capabilities of oxybenzone mean that it could have irreversible and unpredictable, life-long effects on you and your grandchildren. Thus, whenever a sunscreen is a necessity, then always choose one that contains zinc oxide instead of oxybenzone.

They Poison You and Blame the Sun

The sunscreen industry is reliant upon keeping us ignorant, and afraid of the sun. If the general public ever realized just how much this industry endangered and defrauded them, then the liability for them would be limitless. The aftermath would make the tobacco lawsuits look tiny in comparison. Unfortunately, the business of these corporations is backed by the same medical establishment that once recommended smoking cigarettes for health.

Vitamin D is known as "the sunshine vitamin", and it is medically referred to as cholecalciferol. It is one of the most important vitamins necessary for warding off diseases. The body converts excess cholesterol in the skin to an inactive form of vitamin D (D-2) which is subsequently converted into the active form (D-3) by the liver and kidneys. These bio-chemical reactions remove excess cholesterol, greatly benefit the liver, and give us vitamin D-3. It is challenging to get adequate amounts of vitamin D from diet alone, and some people cannot absorb the synthetic version at all. Sufficient levels of vitamin D are crucial for calcium absorption in the intestines. Without sufficient vitamin D, a body cannot properly utilize calcium; rendering calcium supplements useless. This will cause unusable calcium to accumulate in the body to cause dozens of other health problems such as kidney stones, osteoporosis, arthritis, and excessive arterial plaque. The proper utilization of calcium is also necessary for the proper use of magnesium.

Current research indicates that a vitamin D deficiency plays a role in causing seventeen types of cancer, as well as heart disease, stroke, hypertension, "autoimmune" diseases, diabetes, depression, chronic pain, osteoarthritis, osteoporosis, muscle weakness, muscle wasting, birth defects, and periodontal disease. Sunlight has been shown to increase our sense of well being and to improve sleep. It is the only cure for certain depressive disorders, such as seasonal affective disorder. Natural ultraviolet light coming into our eyes stimulates the pineal gland, which helps to regulate hormone levels. Since vitamin D from sunlight is essential for the proper handling of calcium in the body, it is critical for the prevention of rickets and adult osteomalacia.

The ultraviolet rays of the sun are antiseptic. They are capable of killing bacteria, viruses, fungi, yeasts, molds, and mites. Sunbathing is a useful treatment for many skin diseases, such as diaper rash, athlete's foot fungus, psoriasis, acne, boils, or impetigo. The warming infrared rays of the sun, or heat from various sources, is useful in the treatment of neuralgia, neuritis, arthritis, sinusitis, and research also has indicated that sunlight increases pain tolerance somehow. The sun's infrared rays help to bring healthful, natural body oils to the surface of the skin, keeping the skin beautiful, smooth, and protected.

Remember Common Sense and Moderation

No article about sun exposure would be complete without mentioning the need for using common sense and exposing oneself to sunlight in moderation. As with all other things, sunlight in the extreme can be harmful. We hope to not insult our readers' intelligence with this polite reminder that excessive sun exposure can be detrimental. The benefits of sunlight do not actually require tanning, because the human body will produce ample amounts of vitamin D before it begins the tanning process. In fact, the human body will generate all of the vitamin D that it can handle for a period of days in only 10 minutes of direct sunlight exposure. A little bit of it goes a very long way. Sunburns, of course, should always be avoided.

There are alternatives to the chemical madness, with products using natural ingredients. As an alternative to facials, many people choose to use coconut butter. It is also reported to make a great alternative to shaving cream. Ground oatmeal makes for a superior facial mask, so does bentonite clay. Oatmeal can be made into a fine powder in any blender and then cooked in water to make a paste. Apple cider vinegar is commonly used for the skin, and it is a remarkable conditioner for the hair. Apple cider vinegar helps replenish the natural acidic oils of the face and hair that the body uses as an anti-fungal and antibiotic defense. Many people recommend placing aloe vera juice on top of apple cider vinegar, and leaving it on the face for around twenty minutes, as an all-natural facial. If used in tiny amounts, our own (Health Wyze brand) colloidal copper lotion has been reported to be an exceptional natural facial product and hair conditioner.

As alternative medicine leads the charge, there will be an increasing supply of natural and organic products, some of which are already available, but not in most regular retailers. Our staff recommends carefully reading the ingredients and doing some research, for these products are often not as natural as they pretend to be.

Most cosmetic products (both natural and synthetic) are designed to make the user look more healthy, while ignoring the fact that there really is no substitute for being healthy. With a healthy diet, the skin and eyes become more radiant, the lips become a deeper color, and the person feels energized and happy. Eating a healthy diet and exercising regularly is the true secret of beauty. Of course, a little sunlight helps too.

Laundry Products

Health conscious people have a tendency to overlook the hazards in their cleaning materials, and manufacturers are not required to accurately list the ingredients of such products. Manufacturers simply do not mention ingredients that they think customers would disapprove of. In other cases, they use vague terms like "brightener", instead of listing the standard chemical names.

Laundry detergents usually contain chemicals that are dangerous to the health and irritating to the skin. A residue of these chemicals remains on clothing after it is washed. Clear evidence of this can be found in scented products, because chemical fragrances would be useless if they were simply washed out. Chemical fragrances are especially bad, and are known for aggravating asthma.

Nonylphenol is a byproduct of a chemical that is used in laundry detergents. According to the U.S. Environmental Protection Agency, it has been detected in human breast milk, blood, and urine. It has been shown in animal studies to cause adverse reproductive and developmental effects. It is so prevalent that it is now being detected in municipal water supplies.

Sodium lauryl sulphate is an industrial degreaser that is found in a wide variety of cleaning products. It is even in most toothpastes. It is known for being a skin irritant. When it breaks down, it releases another chemical, 1,4-dioxane. The National Institutes of Health have warned that 1,4-dioxane is "reasonably expected to be a human carcinogen", because it has been repeatedly shown to cause cancers in animal studies. It is also known for causing kidney, liver, and nervous system damage. Preliminary research is showing that it accumulates in the body over time. It likewise accumulates in the environment, in a manner similar to the infamous DDT pesticide.

Laundry manufacturers sometimes add formaldehyde to their formulas. Formaldehyde is carcinogenic, a skin irritant, and a respiratory poison. The massive list of formaldehyde side effects can be found in the *Vaccines* chapter. Formaldehyde was the main ingredient in hair straightening products that prompted O.S.H.A. to issue a hazard alert about the health risks. Some of the products have been reformulated to remove formaldehyde, because the California Attorney General sued the companies responsible.

Most cleaning products contain phthalates, which are chemicals that are normally used to make plastics softer and malleable. They are often present in laundry products as manufacturing byproducts. Phthalates cause massive hormone disruptions, which makes them particularly damaging to women's health. They also cause cancer, birth defects, and fertility problems. Phthalates are still being studied, but the findings are arriving too late. The Centers for Disease Control reported that phthalates can be found in the blood of most Americans, and the greatest quantities are in women. Women have more contact with cleaning products, which is the main reason for their increased exposure. The breadth of the danger is not yet fully understood, but phthalates are being studied by several government agencies, including the F.D.A., the N.I.E.H.S., and the National Toxicology Program's Center for the Evaluation of Risks to Human Reproduction.

Many people who are searching for alternatives will be tempted to use borax as a natural alternative to detergents. However, borax is neither natural nor is it safe. It is a chemical skin irritant, and its residue on clothing is damaging to the skin. Some claim that it is natural because it contains the mineral boron, but it is a completely different substance, and even boron has been shown to present risks. It is acceptable to use borax on occasion to kill fleas, bed bugs, or other insects, and for bleaching; but laundry should be thoroughly rinsed through a second wash to ensure that none remains. This is especially important for those with sensitive or damaged skin.

The Most Common Ingredients in Fabric Softeners

- Benzyl acetate
- Limonene
- Y-methyl ionone
- Linalool
- A-terpineol
- Methylene chloride

In 1991, the U.S. Environmental Protection Agency released a document revealing that potent carcinogens are present in fabric softeners and dryer sheets. Inside these chemical cocktails is benzyl acetate, which has been linked to pancreatic cancer. Limonene, a known lung irritant, was also prominent. Fabric softeners and dryer sheets are specifically designed to impart chemicals onto clothing, instead of being rinsed away. They lubricate clothing to make it seem softer.

The effects of inhaling these chemicals have not been well studied, but there are people who breathe these chemicals for hours every day, when laundering. People living in apartment blocks are especially vulnerable, because exposure can be persistent when other inhabitants wash their clothes on a rotating schedule. In recent years, there have been increases in work-related lawsuits because of forced exposure to perfumes, which are known to yield asthma attacks, and difficulty breathing. The same chemicals in perfume and cologne products are also used in laundry detergents and softeners.

Safe laundry products may be found on the Internet or in health food stores. Natural laundry soaps typically contain soap nut extract or extracts from citrus fruits. Surprisingly, they are usually as effective as the harsh detergent chemicals. Natural soaps can be less effective in areas with "hard" (mineral rich) water. In such cases, the effects of the minerals can be neutralized with the addition of distilled vinegar. A ball of aluminum can remove static from clothing in the dryer.

Metal Drinking Bottles

In a small victory for consumers, BPA-free water bottles have found their way into regular grocery stores. Researchers and the public already know the dangers of BPA, despite the refusal of the F.D.A. to acknowledge them. However, the new water bottles may not be as safe as people assume. While they may not leach the hormone-destroying bisphenol-A (BPA), a strong plastic taste can still be noticed in water stored in the new generation of bottles.

The chemicals that leach out of plastics are always harmful to health. Oftentimes these chemicals go unnoticed because flavored drinks can mask the chemical taste. As a rule of thumb, plastics should be categorically avoided for food and beverage containers. All plastics leach, but they leach different chemicals at varying levels. Therefore, some plastics may be safer than others, but none are completely safe. The plastics used to make milk jugs are fairly safe. Clear plastics, like those used for soft drinks, are the worst.

Those who realize the dangers of plastic bottles will usually use metal containers. Unfortunately, manufacturers are using extremely dirty marketing tactics to continue poisoning us. A major design problem was found with the cheap aluminum containers, and a more insidious remedy was employed. The problem was that common aluminum drinking bottles normally react with acidic drinks (all popular soft drinks), to cause the drinks to become toxic with heavy metal compounds, whilst the containers themselves decay from the acids. Instead of switching to a non-toxic, more resilient metal like stainless steel; the manufacturers secretly began lining aluminum drink cans with clear plastic, like clear coats that are used on automobiles.

Most of the *safe* metal water bottles are essentially plastic bottles in disguise. While no mention of this is found on the labels, manufacturers have an incredible tendency to boast about the plastic linings on their websites:

"A baked on inner-lining which meets F.D.A. requirements, doesn't impart odors or tastes."

"Contains a strong, taste-neutral bpa-free plastic lining."

"This eco-friendly bottle has a special leach-proof lining."

These companies completely disregard that the primary reason for the purchase of metal bottles is because people do not want plastic. Manufacturers are charging consumers four times the amount that they would charge for a plastic bottle of the same size. They trick customers into buying plastic containers, when customers are specifically attempting to avoid them. The scam is perpetrated by simply adding an aluminum outer layer over the plastic interior, which exists for deception only.

Sigg Brand Bottles

Sigg, a brand which is proudly made in Switzerland, is one of the companies that deceives consumers with this method. In fact, Sigg boasts that they use a "proprietary" lining, which means that they go to special efforts to hide which plastics are used. We paid particular attention to this company, because it is the brand sold in Whole Food's Market. It is a store that most people feel is safe for finding non-toxic merchandise, but unfortunately, this seems to be changing fast.

Modified Food Starch

Selecting healthy foods from grocery stores is very difficult in this era, since so many of the products are actually toxic. Reading the ingredients can be scary, and most people do not understand them. This is intentional. There is one ingredient that recurs often: modified food starch. The only thing this label tells with certainty is that the "food starch" is not really food starch anymore. There is no definitive way to know what the derived substance is, but it is unnatural.

It is most often corn starch that has been chemically treated to change it into a thickening agent, emulsifier, or a stabilizer. It can be chemically treated in many ways, and for different reasons. Many of the foods are now being altered by being fermented with genetically-engineered bacteria. Consumers have no way to know. The F.D.A. believes that people have no right to know; as is the case for radioactive foods, genetically-engineered foods, and so on.

An ingredient simply labeled "modified starch" has been treated with an acid in order to lower its viscosity. The chemical industry apparently believes that acid, especially sulfuric acid, is an essential nutrient. Perhaps that is why U.S.P iron supplements are made with it and it is certainly why iron supplements are so dangerous. The long-term health effects of these things are completely unknown. These modified starches are difficult for a body to digest, and of course, there have been no publicly-released studies about the long-term effects of eating these mystery substances. Modified corn starch often contains about 10% maltodextrin, which is a common term used by industry to hide the presence of monosodium glutamate.

A huge portion of modified starches come from China. The lead poisoning of toys and the melamine poisoning of infant formulas should have resulted in huge concerns over Chinese food supplies, but the F.D.A. treated the poisoned babies as just another public relation's problem, and even coached the companies involved about how to best deal with the media backlash. Modified food starch is in the great majority of processed foods, and if they were to become likewise tainted by the Chinese, then millions of American citizens would die before the source was discovered.

Modified food starch seems to be an all-encompassing term which allows food manufacturers free reign over what they do to their products. There are several different base foods that can be used to produce food starch, including corn (usually labeled as "modified corn starch"), potatoes, tapioca, and wheat.

Hidden Dangers of Tap Water

The water supply in most American cities contains chlorine, fluoride, and varying amounts of dissolved minerals including calcium, magnesium, sodium, chlorides, sulfates, and bicarbonates. It is also common to find traces of iron, manganese, copper, aluminum, nitrates, insecticides, and herbicides. Prescription medications have also been found in the tap water of 41,000,000 American homes. According to the Associated Press, there is a vast array of pharmaceuticals including antibiotics, anti-convulsants, mood stabilizers, and sex hormones in the municipal water supplies. The U.S. Government does not require any testing for drugs in the water supplies; nor does it set safety limits for drug contamination. It will be decades before we know the long-term effects of ingesting random cocktails of partially-digested prescription drugs.

Chlorine

Chlorine bleach in the form of chlorine dioxide is added to practically all U.S. public water supplies as a disinfectant. It is not used because it is safe, but because it is cheap. Adding chlorine limits the liability of the governmental agencies which regulate public water. The side-effects of their chlorine disinfection are difficult to trace and occur only after extensive long-term use. For example, it would be easy for citizens to prove that they became ill from drinking non-disinfected water by simply testing the contaminated water for live pathogens, but it is much more difficult to prove that their heart disease or cancer was created by chlorine byproducts after twenty years of consuming them. Chlorine bleach is used to satisfy certain priorities, whereby saving money is a much higher priority than long-term public health.

When usage of chlorine began in the early 1900's, the long-term effects were unknown, but there are no longer any legitimate excuses that could be used to justify forcing the public to drink bleach. It is not uncommon to find the chlorine in tap water at such a high level that it is unsafe for swimming pools. A simple chlorine test kit from a local retailer will typically yield surprising results.

One troubling quality of chlorine is its tendency to neutralize oxygen. Once inside the body, it has an oxygen-depleting effect, and this shifts the body's pH toward becoming acidic. These effects are disruptive to a person's immune system, which opens him up to a whole host of potential infections, and it makes him much more prone to suffering allergy symptoms. Water occurring in nature always contains a small amount of hydrogen peroxide, which in many ways makes natural water the opposite of "treated" water in pH, oxygen levels, and in overall healthiness. The difference between pure water and chemically-altered tap water is literally the difference between natural rain and acid rain.

The most significant risk with chlorine products, such as chlorine dioxide, come not from the chlorine itself, but from its dangerous byproducts that are known as trihalomethanes (THM's). These are produced whenever the chlorine agents contact organic proteins. An example of a THM is chloroform, a proven cancer-causing agent. Animal studies have consistently shown an association between THM's and cancers of the liver and kidneys. Chlorine and THM's are strong contributing factors in creating colon and bladder cancers, as well as diabetes, kidney stones, and heart attacks.

Chlorine has been known for years to both cause and worsen respiratory problems, including asthma and pneumonia. As a halogen which damages enzymes, chlorine weakens the immune system upon ingestion. Chlorine causes magnesium deficiencies, which can cause migraine

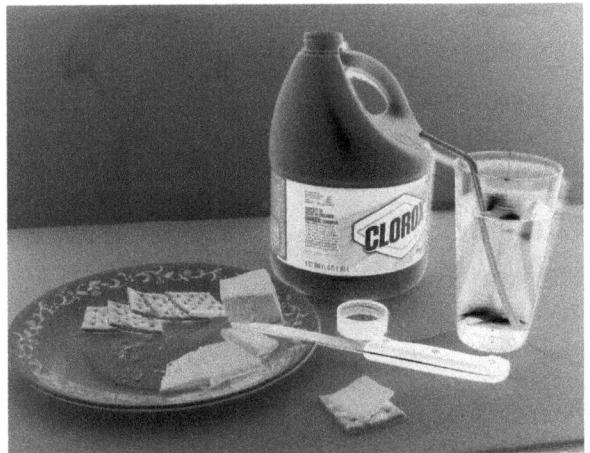

headaches, high blood pressure, chemical sensitivities, and in severe cases, sudden death according to Mark J. Eisenberg, M.D. (especially when it is combined with MSG). Chlorine also decreases the absorption of calcium while increasing its excretion, and the excretion of phosphorus. This increased loss of calcium into the urine can lead to bone-related problems including osteoporosis. Chlorine is known to irritate the skin, the eyes, and the respiratory system.

> *"Chlorine is the greatest crippler and killer of modern times. While it prevented epidemics of one disease, it was creating another. Two decades ago, after the start of chlorinating our drinking water in 1904, the present epidemic of heart trouble, cancer and senility began."*

-- Dr. Joseph M. Price

Dioxins are a byproduct of the chlorination process, and they are known for causing cancers, endometriosis, and neurological damage. Dioxins are present in municipal water as a result of the chlorine dioxide.

Fluoride

The American Dental Association, the F.D.A., and the U.S. Centers for Disease Control all maintain that mercury, a cumulative, toxic heavy metal is perfectly safe to be embedded into our living teeth. Not surprisingly, they also support the fluoridation of public water reservoirs under the guise of improving dental health. The American public has been mass-poisoned with fluoride for more than half a century. It was justified with claims that fluoride produces dental health benefits, even though there has never been evidence that ingestion of it is beneficial. Only topical applications of fluoride have been shown to strengthen teeth. Conversely, there is overwhelming evidence indicating that ingested fluoride is a bio-accumulative poison that attacks the human body systemically, including the teeth. These facts were known long before fluoride was added to tap water.

> *"If this stuff gets out into the air, it's a pollutant; if it gets into the river, it's a pollutant; if it gets into the lake, it's a pollutant; but if it goes right into your drinking water system, it's not a pollutant. That's amazing..."*

-- Dr. J. William Hirzy, E.P.A.

The E.P.A. classifies fluoride as a toxic waste product from aluminum processing, uranium processing, and fertilizer manufacture; but they nonetheless allow it to be added directly into water for human consumption. Instead of the pharmaceutical grade fluoride that is used in toothpastes, it is this left-over industrial waste that is added to water supplies. If a large amount of fluoride is spilled at any location, then it is immediately quarantined as an E.P.A. emergency clean-up site, and all of the clean-up workers are required to wear hazardous materials suits. Nearby communities are evacuated by law enforcement and National Guard units. The risk that they never mention to the public is that if the fluoride truck catches fire, then the fluorine gas released by the heat could kill thousands. The lucky victims would die immediately but the not-so-lucky would die in the following years from horrific bone cancers. Public health authorities could be expected to follow the usual pattern of claiming the subsequent cancers to be mysterious and unexplainable.

Fluorine gas is what eradicated the dinosaurs after a major volcanic eruption filled the Earth's atmosphere with it. However, our regulators are okay with fluoride lacing the public water supplies, and with it being used in infant formulas for babies who are much more susceptible, and who do not even have teeth. Aside from being placed in our toothpaste and various fluoride 'supplements', sodium fluoride is the main ingredient of rat poisons. It is also used in pesticides, insecticides, and fungicides.

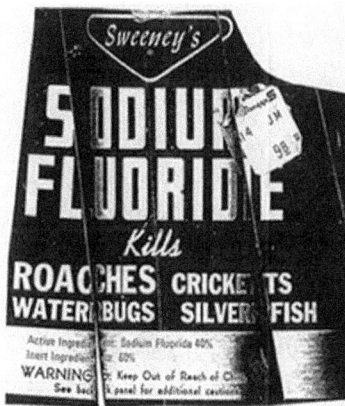

Every form of fluoride has a cumulative effect in the body. Every time a person drinks fluoridated water, eats contaminated produce (produce grown with high-phosphate fertilizers), eats processed foods, or brushes his teeth with fluoridated toothpaste, he is adding to his body's toxic reserves. Even without swallowing any toothpaste, his mouth will absorb up to 1 mg. of fluoride per brushing directly into the bloodstream through skin absorption.

The scientists who originally promoted the use of fluoride are the same infamous ones who promoted adding lead to gasoline, and who performed radiation experiments on unknowing soldiers. They were well endowed by the chemical industry for all of this, and for keeping silent about their most disturbing findings. They were traitors to the practice of medicine, and traitors to their country. These doctors were proud mass murderers, and their experiments are well documented.

Here is some of that history. The top scientist who oversaw the Newburgh Experiment, and the leading voice promoting water fluoridation as safe was Dr. Harold Hodge. Dr. Hodge is still regarded as "the dean" of the science of toxicology in the United States. While selling the use of fluoride for children, he was simultaneously head of the Division of Pharmacology and Toxicology for the Manhattan Project. He was charged with protecting the government from worker and community lawsuits for fluoride exposure, since fluoride was a byproduct of uranium enrichment. Marketing that fluoride was safe in low doses was the Manhattan Project's official policy to reduce the risk of lawsuits against the atomic bomb program. Current fluoride policy is the result of that deceptive marketing. People now believe that it is safe enough to drink.

Since cities purchase fluoride for their water supplies, the fertilizer and nuclear industries have the best corporate welfare programs. Instead of paying billions to neutralize their toxic waste before discarding it, they accept payments for creating the toxic waste at a 20,000% markup. The tax payers are customers of this substance which is poisoning them, whether they like it or not. The industry is really making a killing.

> *"If I were to name one element or chemical compound that would represent the 'Bane of Mans existence on Earth' it would be fluorine or fluoride. Fluorine has caused huge problems for man since the beginning of time due to volcanic events on Earth. Fluorine or Hydrogen Fluoride released from volcanic events or even meteor terminal events is the principle effect for extinction events on this planet... Rising levels of fluoride are directly connected to disruption of enzymes necessary for cell repair (glutathione particularly) and fluoride prevents the removal of toxic metals from the human body. The effect results in the rise of lead, mercury, and other toxic metals in children that impair their I.Q. and long term health. In the elderly, it hastens the onset of gray hair because it is linked to mercury concentrations in the body. It also adds to brittle bone problems, dementia from toxic metals' effects on the brain, and quite literally onset for immune illnesses and death. Fluoride is not a friend to children's teeth, but a deadly cumulative poison where 98 percent of the fluoride ingested goes right to the bone of children to disrupt their health in much the same way that Sr90 from nuclear testing was feared to cause cancer in children. The remaining unabsorbed fluoride attacks the kidneys as they attempt to filter it out of the body, and excrete it through the urinary tract".*

-- Jim Phelps, former Oak Ridge
National Laboratory researcher

A Partial List of the Effects of Fluoride Ingestion

- Brittle bone disease
- Brittle teeth
- Brown, yellow, spotted and discolored teeth
- Cancer
- Heart disease
- Arthritis
- Premature aging

All of these conditions are epidemic in the United States. Fluoride has also been directly linked to osteosarcoma, a rare bone cancer. Fluoride consumption amongst young children results in reduced mental work capacity and a significantly lower I.Q. Fluoridated water effects the hormones in the body, and thus it is a leading cause of the growing infertility rates, and both underweight and premature births. Those who have any doubts about the danger level surrounding fluoride should take another look at their fluoride toothpaste label. The F.D.A. forces toothpaste companies to print the following label on all products that contain fluoride:

> *"If more than used for [normal product use] is accidentally swallowed, get medical help or contact a poison-control center right away."*

Fluoride Was First Utilized by the NAZIs

"In the 1930's, Hitler and the German NAZIs envisioned a world to be dominated and controlled by a NAZI philosophy of pan-Germanism. The German chemists worked out a very ingenious and far-reaching plan of mass-control which was submitted to and adopted by the German General Staff. This plan was to control the population in any given area through mass medication of drinking water supplies. By this method they could control the population in whole areas, reduce population by water medication that would produce sterility in women, and so on. In this scheme of mass-control, sodium fluoride occupied a prominent place.

"Repeated doses of infinitesimal amounts of fluoride will in time reduce an individual's power to resist domination, by slowly poisoning and narcotizing a certain area of the brain, thus making him submissive to the will of those who wish to govern him.

"The real reason behind water fluoridation is not to benefit children's teeth. If this were the real reason there are many ways in which it could be done that are much easier, cheaper, and far more effective. The real purpose behind water fluoridation is to reduce the resistance of the masses to domination and control and loss of liberty. I was told of this entire scheme by a German chemist who was an official of the great I.G. Farben chemical industries and was also prominent in the NAZI movement at the time. I say this with all the earnestness and sincerity of a scientist who has spent nearly 20 years research into the chemistry, biochemistry, physiology and pathology of fluorine."

-- Charles Perkins, Chemist Rebuilding
German Infrastructure, 1954

Reversing the Damage and Neutralizing Fluoride Poisoning

Most Americans experience fluoride poisoning symptoms through various mysterious ailments and aggravated conditions. Iodine and fluoride neutralize one another. Our modern diets are deficient in iodine, which makes the fluoride problem worse. In moderate amounts, iodine will work wonders for most people's immune systems, because most people have under-active thyroids due to the toxicity of their diets, fluoride from pharmaceuticals, and years of miscellaneous fluoride exposure. It is a big part of obesity.

Unfortunately, it is quite difficult to find either iodine or iodide that is safe for human consumption. The largest fraud of alternative medicine is dangerous iodine supplementation, so beware of iodine supplement products. We recommend that readers carefully read the section about *Iodine* in the *Supplements* chapter before attempting any iodine or iodide supplementation. Iodine that is improperly used can quickly destroy the health or kill.

We only provided an analysis of the two main toxins found in U.S. water supplies in this chapter. We neglected the dangers of heavy metals, pesticides, drugs, and various industrial pollutants that are a normal part of municipal water supplies.

The acquisition of a high-end water filter is prudent. For those readers who already filter their water, we regret to inform you that you may not be as safe as you believe. There is only one type of water filter we know of that can remove fluoride, and it cannot be found in retailers. Most water filters are not designed to remove the chemicals that go through them, and instead merely aim to mask the foul taste. Take this as being typical of water filter scams: Brita water filters mask only the chlorine *taste*, but they do not remove the chlorine. The manufacturer would have us believe that drinking chlorine is completely safe -- whose identity is the Clorox Company. We were actually contacted by a company representative, who tried to convince us that chlorine is a health-boosting elixir, after we exposed the Brita filters in one of our audio shows.

Our official recommendations are to either purchase bottled spring water in a safe plastic, drink well water, or purchase a Berkey water filter. Americans should also get the optional fluoride filters. Be forewarned that some spring water is not really spring water. Sometimes, it is tap water that has been filtered through reverse osmosis or other means, then the minerals are added back in (at the chemical factory). Buyer beware, and read the labels carefully.

> *"According to the handbook, 'Clinical Toxicology of Commercial Products',*
> *fluoride is more poisonous than lead, and just slightly less poisonous than arsenic.*
> *It is a cumulative poison that accumulates in bones over the years.*
>
> *"A study by Proctor and Gamble showed that as little as half the amount of*
> *fluoride used to fluoridate public water supplies resulted in a sizable and*
> *significant increase in genetic damage. Epidemiology research in the mid-1970's*
> *by the late Dr. Dean Burk, head of the cytochemistry division of the National*
> *Cancer Institute, indicated that 10,000 or more fluoridation-linked cancer deaths*
> *occur yearly in the United States. In 1989, the ability of fluoride to transform*
> *normal cells into cancer cells was confirmed by Argonne National Laboratories.*
> *Results released in 1989 of studies carried out at the prestigious Batelle Research*
> *Institute showed that fluoride was linked to a rare form of liver cancer in mice,*
> *oral tumors and cancers in rats, and bone cancer in male rats. Since 1991, the*
> *New Jersey Department of Health found that the incidence of osteosarcoma, a type*
> *of bone cancer, was far higher in young men exposed to fluoridated water as*
> *compared to those who were not. In addition to the well documented toxic effects*
> *of fluoride, fluoride even at dosages of 1 part per million, found in artificially*
> *fluoridated water, can inhibit enzyme systems, damage the immune system,*
> *contribute to calcification of soft tissues, worsen arthritis, and of course, cause*
> *dental fluorosis in children. Fluorosis consists of unsightly white, yellow, or brown*
> *spots that are found in teeth exposed to fluoride during childhood. In 1993, the*
> *Subcommittee on Health Effects of Ingested Fluoride of the National Research*

Council admitted that 8% to 51% and sometimes up to 80% of the children living in fluoridated areas have dental fluorosis. Malnourished people, particularly children (who are usually targeted most for fluoridation) are at the greatest risk of experiencing fluoride's harmful effects.

"Surprisingly, the most recent studies do not even show that water fluoridation is effective in reducing tooth decay. In the largest U.S. study of fluoridation and tooth decay, United States Public Health Service dental records of over 39,000 school children, ages 5-17, from 84 areas around the United States showed that the number of decayed, missing, and filled teeth per child was virtually the same in fluoridated and non-fluoridated areas. Dr. John Colquhoun, former Chief Dental Officer of the Department of Health for Auckland, New Zealand, investigated tooth decay statistics from about 60,000 12 to 13 year old children and showed that fluoridation had no significant effect on tooth decay rate. Given all of this scientific information, what is behind this push for universal fluoridation? Prior to 1945, fluoride was properly regarded as an environmental pollutant. It was responsible for many lawsuits against industries, such as the aluminum industry, and the phosphate fertilizer industry, whose waste products contain large quantities of fluoride. This fluoride destroyed crops and animals, leading to the lawsuits. The limited public view was that fluoride was an environmental pollutant that needed to be reduced or eliminated from the environment. As a result of clever public relations campaigns, fluoride was transformed from an environmental pollutant to an essential nutrient necessary for producing healthy teeth. The science was poor, but the P.R. campaign was great. Being against fluoride was like being against motherhood or apple pie. Industries not only made millions from selling this environmental pollutant to water companies and toothpaste companies, but more importantly, it saved billions of dollars that would be required to clean up this environmental pollutant."

-- Michael Schachter, M.D. and Naturopathic Doctor

Fluoride causes irreversible damage to an area of the brain that is known as the pineal gland. This gland is known to release melatonin, and thereby to help regulate the sleep cycle. Over an extended period of time, repeated fluoride exposure causes the pineal gland to calcify and become impaired. Such fluoride-induced damage may result in permanent depression and mood disorder problems. More information about this phenomenon may be found in *The Fluoride Connection* section of the *Depression* chapter.

Most Common U.S. Water Toxins

1) 1,1,1,2-Tetrachloroethane
2) 1,1,2-Trichloroethane
3) 1,1-Dichloroethane
4) 1,1-Dichloropropene
5) 1,2 Dibromo-3-chloropropane (DBCP)
6) 1,2,3-Trichloropropane
7) 1,2,4-Trichlorobenzene
8) 1,2-Dibromoethylene
9) 1,2-Dichloroethane
10) 1,3,5-Trimethylbenzene
11) 1,3-Dichloropropane
12) 1,4-Dioxane
13) 2,2-Dichloropropane
14) 2,4,5-T
15) 2,4,5-TP (Silvex)
16) 2,4-D
17) 2-Hexanone
18) 2-Nitropropane
19) Acetochlor
20) Aldicarb
21) Aldicarb sulfone
22) Aldicarb sulfoxide
23) Alpha-Lindane
24) Aluminum
25) Ammonia
26) Aniline
27) Anthracene
28) Antimony
29) Arsenic
30) Atrazine
31) Barium
32) Benzene
33) Benzo[a]pyrene
34) Beryllium

35) Bromate
36) Bromide
37) Bromobenzene
38) Bromodichloromethane
39) Bromoform
40) Bromomethane
41) Cadmium
42) Carbaryl
43) Carbon tetrachloride
44) Chloroethane
45) Chloroform
46) Chloromethane
47) Chromium
48) cis-1,2-Dichloroethylene
49) Cyanide
50) Dalapon
51) Di(2-Ethylhexyl) adipate
52) Di(2-ethylhexyl) phthalate
53) Dibromochloromethane
54) Dibromomethane
55) Dicamba
56) Dichlorodifluoromethane
57) Methylene chloride
58) Dieldrin
59) Dinoseb
60) Endrin
61) Ethylbenzene
62) Ethylene dibromide (EDB)
63) Heptachlor
64) Heptachlor epoxide
65) Hexachloro-cyclopentadiene
66) Isopropylbenzene
67) Lindane
68) m-Dichlorobenzene

69) Manganese
70) Mercury
71) Metolachlor
72) Monochlorobenzene (Chlorobenzene)
73) n-Butylbenzene
74) n-Propylbenzene
75) Naphthalene
76) Nitrate
77) Nitrates & nitrites
78) o-Chlorotoluene
79) o-Dichlorobenzene
80) Oxamyl (Vydate)
81) p-Chlorotoluene
82) p-Dichlorobenzene
83) p-Isopropyltoluene
84) Pentachlorophenol
85) Picloram
86) Radium-226 & Radium-228
87) sec-Butylbenzene
88) Simazine
89) Styrene
90) Sulfates
91) tert-Butylbenzene
92) Tetrachloroethylene
93) Thallium
94) Toluene
95) Haloacetic acids
96) Trihalomethanes (THMs)
97) Toxaphene
98) Trichloroethylene
99) Trichlorofluoromethane
100) Vinyl chloride

The Smoker Massacre

It is near sacrilege to publish anything that in any way defends smokers. Brace yourself, for you are about to read such a sacrilege. For the sake of political correctness, let us preface by noting that smokers are hellishly evil creatures, for they savagely murder our innocent children with their second-hand death gas. Now we can move on with political correctness satisfied.

As a collective society, we have come to view anything tobacco-related as evil, and its users as needing to be stoned (in the biblical sense). Because of the almost religious anti-tobacco dogma nowadays, what follows might be difficult for some readers to believe.

The first smokers were the American Indians. They also gave us cannabis (marijuana), which was a favorite choice inside peace pipes. For hundreds, if not thousands of years, the American Indians frequently smoked unfiltered and organic tobaccos, for which the smoke was stronger than any cigarette sold now. The Indians did not get lung cancers. They suffered from no major diseases at all. They did not even suffer from allergies, despite living outdoors constantly. It is similar to the situation with the modern-day, unvaccinated Amish. It was not until the English and the Europeans began importing the European diets, long-term food storage, and the overall European lifestyle that serious diseases appeared in Indian tribes. The Old World diseases struck with an ugly vengeance. Entire tribes were wiped-out in days, because the Indians had never needed to develop an immunity against European pathogens.

No Indian was ever killed by tobacco before modern cigarette processing became normal. Our modern killer-tobacco is not the same tobacco that was smoked by our forefathers around camp fires. As an interesting aside, there *still* have been no deaths attributed to marijuana, ever. If marijuana were regulated and 'enhanced' by the same chemical industry partners and governmental regulators that manage our cigarettes, foods, and drugs, then marijuana would become cancerous too. The pharmaceutical industry would not tolerate safe marijuana anymore than it tolerates safe cigarettes. Marijuana is actually a greater threat, because it has potent medicinal qualities, and that is why the public must be made to fear it.

Like our foods and medicines, modern tobacco is 'enhanced' by the chemical industry, and now our foods, medicines, and even tobaccos comprise an unholy trinity of death. In modern cigarette smoke, the chemical compounds outnumber the tobacco compounds over 100-to-1. Every one of these intentionally added chemicals is toxic and most of them are carcinogenic. There is some truth to the belief that most (if not all) tobacco companies are evil, because what they do to their own customers is truly evil. None of it is necessary. We are frankly baffled by the insanity of it all. Cigarettes, like medicines and foods, do not need to be poisoned, but all of them tend to be quite toxic in this era, thanks to adulterations.

Fire Safe Cigarettes

It is getting much worse for smokers in America. Since January of 2010, in 49 out of the 50 states, there has been a legal requirement that a much worse poison be added to all cigarettes. The new state laws require that cigarette manufacturers poison smokers with something worse than we have seen before, like a state-mandated genocide against smokers. Please have the compassion to help us get the message out, even if you personally despise smoking and smokers. It is the right thing to do.

Cigarettes now must contain ethylene/vinyl acetate copolymer, which is literally carpet glue. It is known to cause tumors in mice, but inhalation of its smoke has never been tested on humans. The Material Safety Data Sheet for this substance notes that it produces toxic fumes when exposed to fire. The new "fire safe" cigarettes are made with 3 layers of paper, which requires triple the glue of past cigarettes. They contain what are referred to as "speed bumps" (made from carpet glue) all the way down the shaft. These are designed to reduce oxygen flow, so that the cigarette will quickly extinguish if nobody is inhaling it. This often puts the cigarette out too early, causing the smoker to re-ignite several times throughout a cigarette. It forces smokers to inhale more deeply and more frequently than they otherwise would, whilst they smoke a considerably more toxic cigarette. We call this *deadly by design*.

Activists have been campaigning for decades to get tobacco companies to remove other substances that are toxic when smoked, such as citrates, phosphates and calcium carbonate; which are added to ensure that cigarettes do not self-extinguish. Instead of just removing these burn accelerators, tobacco companies instead added carpet glue. Their logic for appeasing law-makers is hopelessly flawed. Newspaper articles which blame victims for cigarette-induced fires with headlines like "House Burned Down by Reckless Cigarette Use" neglect to mention the fact that cigarettes contain burn accelerators, which should rightly place the blame on the manufacturers. These fire-accelerating chemicals incredibly remain inside the "fire safe cigarettes". It is a similar situation to the one that we have witnessed with the pharmaceutical industry, in which new chemicals are needed to eliminate the side-effects of the chemicals that they provided originally.

The Genocidal Politics of Tobacco

No studies have ever been done on cigarettes containing pure, *organic* tobacco, because such a test might actually prove it to be safe in moderation. Such a finding would not be politically correct science. It would be on-par with questioning Darwinism, and it would destroy careers.

Most anti-tobacco groups are opposed to any sort of harm reduction, such as additive-free or organically-grown tobacco, because they are funded by pharmaceutical and chemical companies. These companies profit from drugs and patches that are alleged to help smokers break their addiction. Those who are unable to quit smoking, or simply do not wish to, are forced to smoke needlessly toxic cigarettes.

Despite all of the campaigns that have been led by politicians who talk about how they are "getting tough" on Big Tobacco, no labeling is yet required for the additives that are in cigarettes. Smokers are unaware that hundreds of chemical compounds are added to most cigarettes. Even fewer have been told that they are legally required to inhale burning carpet glue whenever they smoke.

A study by the Harvard School of Health revealed that tar, carbon monoxide, and naphthalene levels were higher in the new fire safe cigarettes. In fact, according to their study, every chemical, <u>except nicotine</u>, was higher in fire-safe cigarettes. Despite the alarming results, the study's conclusions were actually biased toward promoting fire-safe cigarettes. We can empathize with their good intentions, but this cure is obviously worse than the disease. If the agenda is truly innocent, then why have these 'improved' cigarettes never been reported to the public? Why has there been a media black-out?

Naphthalene is an insecticide and a byproduct of the coal tar industry. It is also a core part of the new "safe cigarettes". Exposure to high amounts of naphthalene can result in irreversible damage to the eyes and liver, according to the E.P.A. It is also a carcinogen, particularly through inhalation exposure. Symptoms of acute exposure include headache, nausea, vomiting, diarrhea, malaise, confusion, anemia, jaundice, convulsions, and coma. It can also cause neurological effects in infants. Thus, it is easy to conclude that normal cigarettes are actually safer than their 'safe' counterparts. These are the effects of just a single chemical. An investigation into the effects of every chemical that is added to modern cigarettes would require a book of its own.

If all of this were not damning enough, these "fire safe cigarettes" are not truly fire safe. In one final move to alleviate themselves from any sort of liability, the cigarette companies admit on their websites that "no cigarette is fire safe". The legislation was supposedly enacted for the purpose of stopping fires, but the very initials that are found on these cigarette packets (FSC) promote a false sense of security that is prone to cause more fires. Even with the misnomer of increased safety, victims may not necessarily be able to sue manufacturers if the cigarettes cause a fire. Even with the existence of their chemical burn accelerators, the corporate lawyers will predictably contend that the addition of carpet glue was a good faith effort to ensure safety, and therefore fires will still be blamed on smokers.

Legislation mandating the sale of only fire-safe cigarettes first went into effect on January 1st, 2010, for certain states. We have heard dozens of reports about the health issues that are being caused by these cigarettes, which seem to mimic the symptoms of naphthalene exposure. All fire safe cigarettes must be labeled on the box. Usually found around the bar code, the letters FSC mean Fire Safety Compliant.

Some smokers choose the American Spirit brand of organic cigarettes, but these are also "fire safe". This company uses organic tobacco, but the glue-coated paper is far from organic. The only way for most American smokers to avoid fire safe cigarettes is for them to roll their own, or to purchase them online from foreign countries. As with all things, organic is of higher quality and safer.

Radioactive Cigarettes

In order to grow what the tobacco industry calls "more flavorful" tobacco, farmers use high-phosphate fertilizers. The phosphate is taken from a rock mineral called apatite, which is ground into a powder and dissolved by sulfuric acid. Hydrogen fluoride is produced as a byproduct of this process, which is then integrated into U.S. drinking water and toothpastes.

Apatite rock contains radium and other radioactive elements, such as lead 210, and polonium 210. Due to these fertilizers, radioactive compounds enter the tobacco through the roots, and from direct contact with the leaves. When a smoker inhales apatite-ridden smoke, radioactive particles enter his lungs, which causes radiation poisoning and lung cancer.

> *"Uranium has a very long half-life and will accumulate in the soil with repeated applications of fertilizer. As a result, modern cigarettes may contain higher levels of Po-210 than those measured 40 years ago."*
>
> -- *The Big Idea: Polonium, Radon and Cigarettes*, The Royal Society of Medicine

The University of Massachusetts wrote to the New England Journal of Medicine in 1982, warning that a person smoking one and a half packs of cigarettes per day would be exposed to a radiation dose in certain areas of the lung at 8,000 mrem per year, which is the equivalent of 300 chest x-rays per year. It has been theorized that the amount of radiation is much greater now than it was when these tests were completed. The only way to avoid this radiation is to use organically grown tobacco. "All natural" and additive-free tobacco may still be radioactive.

Toxic Restaurants

People assume that restaurant plates, utensils, and cups are dried using heat, not chemicals. Few restaurants dry their food utensils after washing them nowadays. They are using so-called "drying agents" on everything except for the tables and chairs, and perhaps we would have cause to shudder if we knew what was being used on them.

Some of the drying agents used are bone phosphate, calcium aluminum silicate, calcium ferrocyanide, calcium silicate, sulfamic acid, calcium stearate, kaolin, magnesium silicate (synthetic), magnesium stearate, potassium ferrocyanide, salts of fatty acids, silicon dioxide, sodium aluminosilicate, sodium ferrocyanide, tricalcium phosphate, and trimagnesium phosphate.

What we found particularly disturbing is that plenty of the major brands refuse to even disclose their ingredients, and jealously guard them as trade secrets. Jet Dry and Cascade, the leading brands of consumer drying agents, claim that their ingredients are proprietary; and therefore, will never be publicly disclosed. Even the Material Safety Data Sheet available from the National Institutes of Health does not list the full ingredients, in order to protect these corporations, in disregard of U.S. law.

Many people, particularly in hard water areas, choose to use rinse or drying agents to avoid blotchy stains on dishes. The fumes are known to cause coughing and dizziness when dishwashers are first opened. People will undoubtedly inhale these chemicals, as well as ingest them from the cookware. As a result of the associated health problems (particularly from inhalation), health-conscious consumers are switching to white vinegar to get the same result. Drying agents are used in the final rinse cycle, so they dry onto the dishes. The residual chemical coating is intentional, as a means to remove water and minerals.

In a restaurant, this applies to every plate, bowl, utensil, glass and even the pans that are used for cooking. The chemicals seem to be far worse in restaurants than those of household drying agents. When eating out, there is no way to avoid consuming the drying agents. While we could find serious negative health implications for virtually every chemical that we discovered in drying agents, we shall focus on a select few for the sake of brevity.

Calcium Aluminum Silicate, Sodium Aluminosilicate, and Kaolin

(Hydrated Aluminum Silicate)

It is amazing that chemists were able to combine three separate sources of aluminum into a single product. Aluminum is a heavy metal toxin that is slightly less toxic than mercury. Like mercury, aluminum in even trace amounts will persistently attack the brain and central nervous system for many years. It is already documented to cause Alzheimer's disease, autism, cancer, lowered fertility, and brittle bones. It particularly reeks havoc in the bodies of older women, since it effects the body like an estrogen substitute. In these women, it causes breast cancer, osteoporosis, and brittle bone disease. Despite being listed in the Hazardous Substances Data Bank as a skin, eye, and lung irritant; sodium aluminosilicate is present in restaurant drying products, and it is placed inside some foods and spices as an anti-caking agent, with the full approval of regulators. Aluminum is particularly bad because it accumulates deep inside the body, causing dozens of disease conditions over time. The body cannot normally eliminate it. Aluminum has become a favorite of the chemical industry, and it has become difficult to avoid. It is in most store-bought breads, some baking powders, pharmaceuticals, vaccines, and even the tap water.

Kaolin causes breathing difficulties, bronchitis, decreased pulmonary (lung) function, cumulative lung damage, and stomach granulama (extreme tissue trauma).

Sodium Ferrocyanide and Potassium Ferrocyanide

The "cyanide" part of these ingredients should be emphasized. Restaurants are actually spraying dishes with cyanide, and allowing it to remain on them. When it contacts an acid, sodium ferrocyanide releases the extremely poisonous hydrogen cyanide gas. This is the infamous zyklon B gas that was reported to have been used by the NAZI's. Sodium ferrocyanide is also used in photography for bleaching and toning. It is highly toxic in the lungs, blood, and the mucous membranes. It is known to cause organ damage with prolonged exposure. It is especially hazardous when ingested. If a truckload of this hazardous material is spilled, clean-up crews are required by regulations to wear full environmental suits with self-contained breathing apparatuses. Nevertheless, it is being sprayed on restaurant plates, glasses, and utensils.

Inhalation of potassium ferrocyanide results in coughing and shortness of breath. Skin contact will cause pain and redness. Any contact should be immediately diluted with large amounts of water. If it is involved in a fire, or if it comes into contact with a strong acid, then it will emit cyanide gas.

Bone Phosphate and Tricalcium Phosphate

Whilst researching these ingredients, we were hoping that "bone" was merely a chemical-industry pseudonym for something that was never alive. Bone phosphate is really made by grinding bones and teeth into a powder. Tricalcium phosphate is a very similar bone-based compound. It is frequently added to spices as an anti-caking agent. If you feel uncomfortable with eating ground up bones, which have been soaked in a hydrochloric acid solution, then we recommend that you avoid bone phosphate, calcium phosphate, and tricalcium phosphate.

Synthetic Magnesium Silicate

The Material Safety Data Sheet for this chemical reads, "Do not swallow". It is a skin, eye, and respiratory irritant. In other words, it should never be in or around foods. Ingesting large amounts can cause convulsions and unconsciousness. Silica dust is a known carcinogen when inhaled.

Sulfamic Acid

Inhalation of sulfamic acid results in laryngitis, coughing, permanent lung damage, bronchitis, and damage to the mucous membranes. As a corrosive agent, ingestion of sulfamic acid burns the mouth, throat, stomach, and can lead to death. There have been no studies on the cumulative effects of ingested sulfamic acid, because it has been assumed that people would not be eating this chemical.

Conclusionary Remarks

It should be evident that restaurant chemical drying agents degrade human health. The use of aluminum in these products is especially disturbing because of its cumulative property. Each exposure increases the aluminum content in a body, thereby increasing the risk of Alzheimer's disease, multiple sclerosis, various cancers, hormonal problems, bone diseases, and it will absolutely reduce a person's I.Q. Save yourself and your family by cooking your own wholesome foods.

High Efficiency Light Bulbs

The new generation of C.F.L. energy efficient light bulbs ("corkscrew bulbs") are so dangerous in so many ways that they had to be designed to satisfy an evil agenda of sickening the population. You will understand that it is no exaggeration by the time you finish this chapter.

According to the U.S. Environmental Protection Agency, the following emergency procedure should be followed in the event of a bulb breakage, due to the poison gas that is released.

The Official E.P.A. Broken Bulb Clean-up Procedure

Before Cleanup

1. Have people and pets leave the room.

2. Air out the room for 5-10 minutes by opening a window or door to the outdoor environment.

3. Shut off the central forced air heating/air-conditioning system, if you have one.

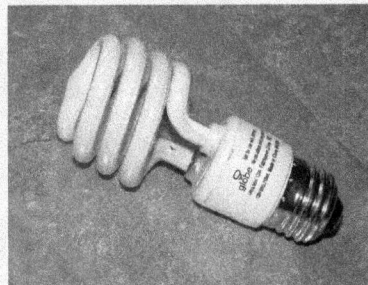

Collect materials needed to clean up broken bulb:

- Stiff paper or cardboard
- Sticky tape
- Damp paper towels or disposable wet wipes (for hard surfaces)
- A glass jar with a metal lid or a sealable plastic bag.

During Cleanup

- DO NOT VACUUM. Vacuuming is not recommended unless broken glass remains after all other cleanup steps have been taken. Vacuuming could spread mercury-containing powder or mercury vapor.

- Be thorough in collecting broken glass and visible powder. Scoop up glass fragments and powder using stiff paper or cardboard. Use sticky tape, such as duct tape, to pick up any remaining small glass fragments and powder. Place the used tape in the glass jar or plastic bag. See the detailed cleanup instructions for more information, and for differences in cleaning up hard surfaces versus carpeting or rugs.

- Place cleanup materials in a sealable container.

After Cleanup

1. Promptly place all bulb debris and cleanup materials, including vacuum cleaner bags, outdoors in a trash container or protected area until materials can be disposed of. Avoid leaving any bulb fragments or cleanup materials indoors.

2. Next, check with your local government about disposal requirements in your area, because some localities require fluorescent bulbs (broken or unbroken) be taken to a local recycling center. If there is no such requirement in your area, you can dispose of the materials with your household trash.

3. If practical, continue to air out the room where the bulb was broken and leave the heating/air conditioning system shut off for several hours.

Radiation from Energy Efficient Bulbs

A new radiation threat is upon us all. In lieu of this, we begin by emphasizing the "radio" and "radiant" links to the word radiation. They ultimately are descriptions of the same phenomena: radiant energy in the form of electromagnetic waves of pulsating energy. So, how does the energy actually radiate itself outward? The truth is, we do not really understand that part. Physicists have pulled their hair out for decades over that question. What we do know is that when things vibrate at a nuclear level or have electrical current changes, then these changes of state -- these frequencies -- cause energy to be radiated outward at the same frequencies. This is how radio transmissions work. Radio transmissions merely mix the audio (voice) signal with a fixed frequency that listening radios are "tuned" to, and viola! Or as my past electronics teachers would have said, in their fancy engineering terms: "It will have imparted intelligence upon the carrier wave". A good analogy of how frequencies operate is remembering the ripples from a time when you dropped a pebble into a small creek or pond. You may recall that the ripples were reflected from the banks at exactly the same rate and distance as the original waves that struck them. The whole point of this is to make clear that the very basis of radiant energy transmissions and all types of radiation on the entire electromagnetic spectrum boil down to one thing: frequencies. Frequencies determine how far the energy travels, how well it penetrates, and how it effects things. The ultra high frequencies of gamma (i.e. nuclear) radiation can quickly destroy a person through burns, cancer, or otherwise; while the low 60 Hz. of standard American power has little effect in typical exposure. Frequency determines if the energy is radio, microwave, infrared light, visible light, x-rays, gamma, or ultraviolet. There is real power in frequencies. As a general rule, the higher the frequency, the more dangerous the energy is. Nuclear radiation is at mindbogglingly high frequencies.

For years, we have heard about how energy-wasting incandescent bulbs are bad for the environment. This made way for a whole new industry of "green" bulbs, marketed to the growing population of people who seek to address environmental concerns. However, these bulbs compromise people's health, and they are ultimately much more harmful to the environment.

Exposure Effects of "Energy Efficient" Light Bulbs

- Dizziness
- Cluster headaches
- Migraines
- Seizures
- Fatigue
- Inability to concentrate
- Anxiety

There are lots of speculations regarding how these bulbs can cause these effects. Very little research has been done. Despite this, European countries are phasing out incandescent bulbs, and forcing the public to switch to the "energy efficient" alternative.

The new light bulbs emit two forms of radiation outside of the light spectrum: ultraviolet and radio frequency. The F.D.A. states that in addition to visible light (UVA), these bulbs also emit UVB, and infrared radiation; but let us not forget the radio transmissions. These bulbs are reported to have a flicker rate of 100-120 cycles per second, which seems low considering the UVB light that these bulbs produce, and of course, radio transmissions. In any case, even a flicker rate as low as 100 hertz is more than enough to trigger severe epileptic seizures. Video games are well known to do the same at a mere 60 Hz. Judging from the multiple bands of radiation released, the flicker rate can be expected to be well beyond 120 hertz (including the light that we cannot actually see), so just start adding zeros to get the point about how likely they are to trigger epileptic seizures. These bulbs have negative effects on people with lupus too, which is something that has baffled everyone so far. They are also known to damage the skin, and thus they must emit high frequency radiation. Watchdog organizations in the U.K. are clamoring about the issues mentioned above, and the fact that these bulbs also aggravate eczema and porphyria.

We have been doing this work long enough to spot the pattern. The radiation from these bulbs directly attacks the immune system, and furthermore damages the skin tissues enough to prevent the proper formation of vitamin D-3. This will cause major cholesterol problems in time, and cripple the liver by preventing it from converting the cholesterol reserves inside the skin tissues (vitamin D-2) into usable vitamin D-3. This has the potential to cause or aggravate, not dozens, but hundreds of disease states. All that they had to do was shift the frequencies of otherwise benign light bulbs, and suddenly we have this mess. It is as if the whole mess with fluorescent light bulbs gave somebody inspiration for how to radiation poison us, while tricking us into begging for it.

The Energy Efficient Scam

One of my first lessons while studying electronics was that energy efficiency is effected more by heat than any other factor. That is why super conductors are always super cooled, and why your oven uses about 60 times more power than your television. Heat equals wasted power. It is written in stone. Amazingly, standard light bulbs manage to be extremely energy efficient, despite the heat that they produce, and despite the fact that their light comes from heated elements. In fact, they manage to waste less than 10% of the power applied. This is because the heat resists the current flow in the wire coil -- to the point of practically cutting off the current. You see, heat also increases resistance. This breaking effect upon a bulb's current gives standard incandescent light bulbs their overall high efficiency.

My first engineering project was testing light bulbs with high-end testing equipment, to study this rare property. I remember our teacher gleefully laughing at us as we sat befuddled by the fact that all of our calculations for voltages and power usage contradicted the measurements. The exercise was meant to be a memorable lesson about how heat may dissipate (or conserve) power in such a way that electrical devices appear to bend the rules of physics. An important lesson was that while theoretically incandescent light bulbs ought to be wasteful of energy, they actually increase their own resistance via heat to the point that very little of their energy is wasted. Take for example how long a standard flashlight will produce bright light with one or two small batteries. On the other hand, just try to power an oven with those same batteries for an exercise in frustration.

It shows the breadth of the deception to note that the new generation of bulbs is supposedly designed to save us from a problem that does not actually exist -- inefficient conventional bulbs. The new bulbs, as you may have already noticed, do not produce any noticeable amount of heat. This is because the light from the new generation of bulbs is produced by injecting pulsating electricity (having a frequency) into a chemical gas to radiate light, as in pure radiation. By the types of radiation that the new bulbs emit, they must operate at frequencies astronomically higher than the 120 hertz that they are said to, so somebody is certainly lying about them. Technically, there is no reason for high frequencies to be used. If a lower frequency produces the needed visible light, then why do these bulbs operate at unnecessary higher frequency bands too? These extra frequencies simply could not have been stepped up and oscillated (frequency generated) higher by accident, regardless of whether the oscillation is chemical or electronic. Doing such a thing can make even an experienced engineer's head spin, due to the overall technical difficulties in frequency tuning; especially on the higher end. Furthermore, are we expected to believe that none of the companies or regulators involved ever bothered to test these new light bulbs with an oscilloscope during the testing? It is absolutely ludicrous to believe that they do not know. Thus, the only explanation is that these bulbs produce harmful radiation by design. They are designed to produce radiation outside of the range of visible light, which is known to be harmful to humans, and it is all justified to solve an environmental problem that does not even exist.

The proof is already before you to observe at your leisure -- how these lights interfere with radios, cordless phones, and R.F. remote controls.

It Gets Even Worse

This may be showing my age to some, but I had never heard of "dirty electricity" when I was in college. For those of you with some electronics training, it is similar to the topic of harmonics, but the rest of you need not worry about this point. Here is the quick and dirty about dirty electricity. The new age bulbs do not just directly radiate radiation from themselves, which alone would be a reason for infamy. Believe it or not, these bulbs actually inject frequencies back into a building's electrical supply lines. Thus, the building's normal electricity (at 60 Hertz) has been made "dirty" (contaminated with other frequencies). This means that every wire in the building is also emitting radiation, like a spider web of antennas.

Dr. Magda Havas, of Trent University, cataloged it with empirical data about the frequency ranges for both the radiation coming from the bulbs, and the dirty electricity radiation that pulses throughout entire buildings. She is credited for creating the following charts.

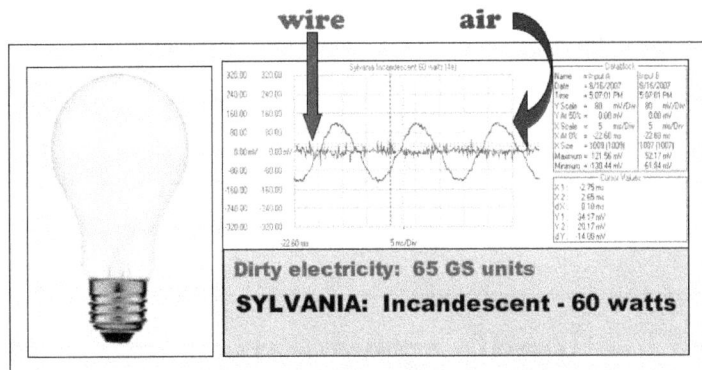

Dirty electricity: 65 GS units
SYLVANIA: Incandescent - 60 watts

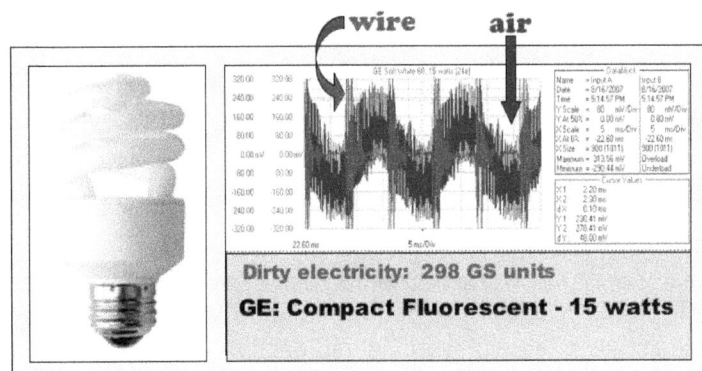

Dirty electricity: 298 GS units
GE: Compact Fluorescent - 15 watts

"The energy efficient compact fluorescent lights that are commercial available generate radio frequency radiation and ultraviolet radiation, they contain mercury - a known neurotoxin, and they are making some people ill. Instead of promoting these light bulbs governments around the world should be insisting that manufactures produces light bulbs that are electromagnetically clean and contain no toxic chemicals. Some of these are already available (CLED) but are too expensive for regular use. With a growing number of people developing electrohypersensitivity we have a serious emerging and newly identified health risk that is likely to get worse until regulations restricting our exposure to electromagnetic pollutants are enforced. Since everyone uses light bulbs and since the incandescent light bulbs are being phased out this is an area that requires immediate attention."

-- Dr. Magda Havas

It is ironic that people buy these bulbs to help the environment, because the bulbs will leak mercury and emit mercury vapors when they break. They are so toxic that we not supposed to put them in the regular garbage. They are literally household hazardous waste. If you break one in a house, you are supposed to open all of your windows and doors, and evacuate the house for at least 15 minutes to minimize your exposure to the poisonous gas.

Our Recommendations

We recommend using either incandescent or L.E.D. bulbs. L.E.D.'s use less power, produce a more natural (and relaxing) light that is less yellow, do not burn out, are not toxic, do not produce harmful radiation, and they operate at a cool temperature so that there is never a fire or burn risk. L.E.D. bulbs are simply a superior technology in every way.

Radioactive Patients

In some countries, cancer patients who are made radioactive are told to avoid contact with children, because radiation exposure is especially bad for children's developing bodies. These ethically-required warnings are never given in the U.S., because radiation is so zealously promoted.

What if our medical people and journalists had the same ethical standards as their peers in other countries? What if they too warned patients to at least stay away from innocent children? The American people would quickly realize that radiation is inherently bad, and that irradiated patients remain radioactive after exposure to radioactive 'medicine'. Think of the financial implications for the U.S. cancer industry, if the same warnings for children were to be given inside the states. The political lie about collateral radiation not effecting close friends and family is a large part of why the United States kills more people with medicine than any other industrialized nation. It is one reason why cancer runs in families now, because the entire family gets irradiated.

The Ugly Truth About Radiation

Radiation is bad -- *really bad*. It attacks the entire body from inside-out, including mutating the DNA, so that birth defects after radiation exposure are not uncommon. It is prudent that a person never try to become pregnant immediately after radiation exposure. Radiation exposure is the surest way to cause cancer, and the cancers from radiation exposure can strike anywhere, and at any random time in the future.

Americans are told that radiation poisoning is advanced medicine, and that being exposed to people who are made radioactive is completely safe. They are sometimes even told that the residual radiation from patients is somehow safer than the radiation from the original source, as if it undergoes a magical transformation inside patients' bodies. They are told that science proves that human-emitted radiation is a 'special' radiation that it is better for them than the ever-dangerous sunlight. The absurdities are akin to childhood fairy tales.

Americans are in their third or fourth generation of being guinea pigs for the nuclear industry, like the army soldiers who were forced to watch A-bomb explosions in the 1950's, which were designed to show how safe and beneficial radiation is. Check the cancer statistics for those men for some enlightenment about their deformed children or their own cancers, if you can stand the heartbreak.

A century of records, dating back to Madam Curie, proves than radiation is never safe. It was radiation that killed her. Radiation is the most toxic thing known, because it will poison without any physical contact.

The sex organs and the thyroid are always the first to be damaged by radiation exposure. Unfortunately, there is little that men can do to protect their sex organs, so the recommendation is to avoid making babies for several weeks after exposure. Women are luckier, because they can use iodine or iodide to protect both their ovaries and their thyroids, somewhat. Men can only protect their thyroids. While symptoms of exposure may vary, an overall feeling of general illness is the most common.

Reference the *Radiation Poisoning* section of the *Quick Tips* chapter for information on natural treatments for radiation poisoning, in the event that you have one of these glowing patients in your family.

A Chinese Christmas

During Christmas time, people tend to be more trusting, and are not as vigilant about protecting their health as they are throughout the year. Yet, there are elevated poisoning risks during Christmas. One of the biggest health threats at Christmas is lead. Lead is present in the cabling of Christmas lights, and in the solder of artificial Christmas trees.

American shoppers may notice this warning on Christmas light packages:

> *"Handling the coated electrical wire on this product exposes you to lead, a chemical known to the State of California to cause birth defects or other reproductive harm. Wash hands after use."*

The lead inside Christmas light insulation is used to stabilize the polyvinyl chloride (PVC plastic) around the wires. Without lead, the PVC would crack and crumble with age. Lead is also a fire retardant for the PVC, because PVC is a fire hazard. Manufacturers employ a flammable plastic with a poisonous metal added to it, in order to reduce its flammability, instead of using a superior material. Slightly less flexible Christmas lights would be a welcome change to lead-free lights, which would also be much less likely to burn down houses at Christmas.

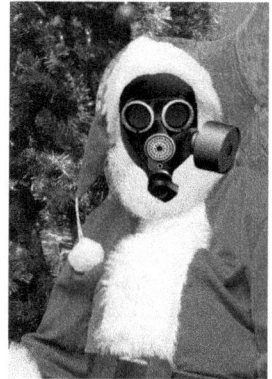

There are safer fire retardants than lead, including calcium and zinc. These are not used because they are more expensive. The claim that these companies are acting on behalf of their customer's well-being is thus patently dishonest. It betrays relentlessly unethical behavior.

When Walmart corporation was questioned in 2007 about their lead-laden lights, Walmart cited the following in its official press release:

> *"It is our understanding that the manufacturers' use of lead in these products is to improve the safety of the lights. We are told that the use of lead is required by Underwriters Laboratory, an organization that certifies the safety of lighting products in the United States. The amount of lead used is a tiny amount and does not exceed any applicable federal guidelines. Our holiday lights meet industry standards and are compliant with state and federal regulations governing their sale."*

We have been assured that only safe levels of lead are present in the cords, but lead is bio-accumulative. It builds up in the liver, and the body cannot normally excrete it. So, there is no safe level, because such a figure would have to be based upon previous exposure. C.N.N. hired Quantex Laboratories in December of 2007 to conduct a study evaluating lead safety. That study proves that even those supposedly safe levels can significantly lower the I.Q. Another study, titled *Low Blood Lead Levels Associated with Clinically Diagnosed Attention-Deficit/Hyperactivity Disorder and Mediated by Weak Cognitive Control* by Michigan State University proved that lead in the blood is a contributing factor to attention deficit disorder.

> *"Even at one microgram/deciliter - the lowest level in a person's blood stream that we can detect - that level has been associated with cognitive impairment in children."*

-- Dr. Leo Trasande, Mt. Sinai School of Medicine

According to the double-standards set by regulators, the "safe level" of lead in Christmas lights is higher than what would be considered safe in children's toys. A study by the independent testing organization, Quantez Laboratories, revealed that surface levels of lead on Christmas lights were far higher than the Consumer Product Safety Commission's recommended limit of 15 micrograms for children. In fact, Walmart brand lights from China were the highest in surface lead. They had levels ranging from 86.6 to 132.7 micrograms.

The Poisonous Chinese Onslaught

Toys that are made in China often contain lead, alongside other poisonous chemicals such as BPA and cadmium. Lead-laced toys are illegal in the United States, but they can be found at almost every U.S. retailer. Lead toys from China suddenly began appearing during the Christmas season of 2007. This sudden inclusion just before Christmas indicates that the poisonings were intentional, so it is recommended that readers choose only toys which have been made elsewhere. This may require extra effort by parents, such as finding gifts online. Lead typically appears in Chinese-made toys at Christmas time, when sales are highest. Lead likewise always appears in Chinese-made lunch boxes at the beginning of every school year. Such coincidences simply do not occur. In more honorable times, this would have been considered an act of war, and the poisoned items would have been immediately removed from retail shelves. Most Americans were either not told about, or were distracted away from the anti-freeze that the Chinese were adding to toothpastes being sold in the United States. The Chinese told U.S. regulators that the anti-freeze was a "sweetener". They were also caught adding the pesticide melamine to 90% of U.S. infant formulas in 2008, which the F.D.A. subsequently helped the food industry cover-up. They claimed that the pesticide was added to artificially increase the protein content of nutritionally-deficient infant formulas.

Cadmium is the newest poisonous material that is appearing in toys from China. Cadmium is being used as a method to continue the poisoning, because of more aggressive lead testing. Cadmium levels are not tested, or even regulated; despite it being more harmful. It is especially difficult to chelate cadmium out of the body. The addition of cadmium establishes that these behaviors are part of an official agenda, because unlike lead with its ability to improve plastics and paints, there is no legitimate reason to include it.

One of the most dangerous attributes of lead is that it absorbs through the skin. Just touching Christmas lights or artificial trees is therefore enough for it to enter into a body. The risk increases for young children who put their hands into their mouths. Those who use lead-laced Christmas lights should wear waterproof gloves when handling the lights, and then discard the gloves. Always keep children away from these lights, and from artificial trees. In light of what has been happening, we have a moral and patriotic duty to not buy from the Chinese, or companies that have betrayed us by relocating operations to China.

Vegetarians Should Consume Hemp Instead of Soy

Vegetarian and vegan diets leave individuals lacking in key nutrients, proteins, fats, and amino acids. Adults have a right to make such decisions for themselves, but parents who keep children on vegetarian diets are guilty of chronic child abuse. Vegetarian diets for children should be illegal, and this is doubly so for vegan diets.

When people choose to be vegetarian or vegan, they generally utilize soy-based products to compensate for their protein deficiency. Soy is horrendous to a body, and it is unfit for human consumption. Infants who are fed soy formulas are far more likely to develop hormonal diseases like endometriosis and thyroid disease later in life. The estrogen-like compounds contained within soy hinder development by mimicking estrogen. They imbalance human hormones; especially in females. The ever-increasing use of soy in today's processed foods is one of the reasons why young girls are starting puberty at younger ages than ever before.

Hemp-based alternatives have become widely available. Hemp does not contain THC, the active narcotic found in its close cousin, cannabis (marijuana). Therefore, hemp products come with no legal liabilities for its possession. It is a miraculous plant that contains similar amounts of protein to soy products, but it comes without any of soy's risks. Shelled hemp seeds are about 31% protein, in comparison to 35% for soybeans. Hemp protein is widely available in higher concentrations. It is produced naturally by simply sieving out the fiber. Hemp contains every important amino acid that science has been able to identify, and high amounts of omega-3, a substance that is lacking in almost every Western diet. Vegetarians should take heed that hemp contains even more omega-3 than walnuts, the most highly acclaimed vegetarian source for it.

Vegetarians frequently have problems with stamina, which has been shown to be massively improved with hemp; especially when combined with iron. Hemp also helps those who are lacking fiber, and those who are embracing gluten-free diets. Readers should be aware that this report does not imply that any vegetarian diet could be considered ideal, but merely that the introduction of hemp as a complete soy replacement would be a very wise health choice. An occasional steak to provide bio-reactive iron that the human body can actually use would be wise too.

Soy Products

The chemical industry perpetually uses devious tactics to con health-seeking people into poisoning themselves. The confusion existing around fats and oils is intentional, and it is designed to prevent us from making healthier choices. The margarine scam of yesteryear presented margarine as a healthier alternative to butter. The medical establishment bought into the lie, and then it advantageously based an entirely new business segment upon eliminating cholesterol. Thus began the lucrative partnership between the food industry and the petrochemical industry, which are conveniently owned by the same people. One group profits from doing the damage, and the other division profits by treating the resultant diseases perpetually.

The epidemic of heart disease began in the mid-twentieth century, after butter and traditional oils were replaced in our diets by the new "healthier" vegetable oils. Leading the health-destroying parade was researcher, Ancel Keys. He is known as the father of the Lipid Hypothesis. Keys cherry-picked statistics to create an international study of heart disease, and presented it to medical publications to prove that natural saturated fats cause heart disease. For Keys' research, the term "international" meant using only the results from the 7 countries which yielded the conclusions that he wanted. He even titled his original paper, "The Seven Countries Study". The data from the other dozen countries was stricken, because the data from everywhere else disproved the Lipid Hypothesis. Most of the data actually showed that there was no relationship between saturated fat and cholesterol, or even cholesterol and heart disease. At the time, many other research scientists were appalled by Keys' shoddy research, but the media and its top clients in the petrochemical industry embraced Keys' findings. Natural fats had to be replaced with chemically-altered fats and highly processed vegetable oils, of which the young biotechnology industry was in the process of perfecting. All of this very conveniently opened the door for industry giants to obtain monopoly patents concerning food preparation. The processes of obtaining naturally-occurring foods, such as butter, cannot be patented.

Keys' scientific swindle was so masterful that the medical establishment is *still* direly warning us about how dangerous butter is. In reality, butter contains a uniquely beneficial spread of nutrients and fats that are critical to heart, brain, dental, bone, and nervous system health. There is little wonder why the Bible foretold that the Christ would be raised on butter and honey, so that he would know the good. Most people now at least know of the dangers of hydrogenated oils, but they are still doctor recommended as the healthy alternative.

Deceptive Marketing about Cooking Oils

Soy oil is still being promoted at some retailers as the healthy choice, despite all of the revelations about it over the past decade. All soy sold is genetically engineered and highly processed. The word "soy" sometimes appears inside the fine print on the back of the so-called *healthy* vegetable oil containers, as if companies are finally beginning to hide it. Even though soy is now known to be an unhealthy oil by most health conscious people, companies are much more willing to alter their marketing than their unethical practices. Some of the oil containers boldly list olive oil in huge text across the front of the bottles; implying that it is the main ingredient, but the labeling often reveals that olive oil is actually the last (least used) ingredient. The real and main ingredients are toxic combinations of highly processed soy and canola oil. A few of the braver companies still emphasize that their product is canola oil, since not everyone knows about canola oil yet. When the dangers of canola become more widely known, we can be certain that it will be the marketing (not the ingredients) that changes. One toxic cooking oil product is even called Omega-3 Oil. This is despite the fact that it is virtually impossible to extract raw omega-3 oil without it immediately breaking down into something completely different, especially whenever heat (from processing) is added. The resultant non-omega compounds are hazardous. The Omega-3 Oil product is actually just canola oil -- which, by the way, loses all of its omega-3 and becomes toxic when heated. Bear in mind that it is an oil intended for cooking.

Pesticides are rarely used on soybean or canola plants, because both plants are so toxic that insects avoid them. Canola oil is officially an E.P.A. registered pesticide, and soy contains compounds that are designed specifically to disrupt hormones.

> *"The amount of phytoestrogens that are in a day's worth of soy infant formula equals 5 birth control pills"*
>
> -- Mike Fitzpatrick, toxicologist

What The Soy Industry Never Told You

There is no such thing as an all-natural soy-based food, because soybeans are toxic in their natural state. Processing is essential for soy foods, because soy is poisonous in its natural organic state (containing natural insecticides), so there are never truly organic soy products for human consumption. When you see a product that is claimed to have "healthy all-natural soy", then make a mental note to never buy anything from that unethical company. It has proven that it will happily hurt you, and lie about it for profit.

Soy must be processed in some manner for it to be safe for human consumption, and even then, it is not truly safe. The fermentation processes historically used by Asian nations are no longer used today, and the overall health of modern-day Asians is rapidly declining. Soy is now made *safe* by chemical engineering in large-scale food processing factories. Putting all of the toxic impurities and alterations from the processing aside, the soy itself retains many of its original poisonous compounds which directly attack the thyroid, such as its hormones that are designed to disrupt fertility. Women are especially prone to experiencing horrific hormonal disorders like endometriosis from soy intake. There is no way to accurately determine how many miscarriages and how many cases of infertility are the direct result of soy consumption.

> "Tofu and other soybean foods contain isoflavones, three-ringed molecules bearing a structural resemblance to mammalian steroidal hormones. White and his fellow researchers speculate that soy's estrogen-like compounds (phytoestrogens) might compete with the bodys natural estrogens for estrogen receptors in brain cells.
>
> "Plants have evolved many different strategies to protect themselves from predators. Some have thorns or spines, while others smell bad, taste bad, or poison animals that eat them. Some plants took a different route, using birth control as a way to counter the critters who were wont to munch.
>
> "'Plants such as soy are making oral contraceptives to defend themselves', says Claude Hughes, Ph.D., a neuroendocrinologist at Cedars-Sinai Medical Center. 'They evolved compounds that mimic natural estrogen. These phytoestrogens can interfere with the mammalian hormones involved in reproduction and growth -- a strategy to reduce the number and size of predators.'"

-- John MacArthur

Soy's Effects on Human Health

- 250% increased risk of developing Alzheimer's disease
- Cognitive impairment
- Brain shrinkage and premature deterioration
- Produces steroidal hormones
- Produces estrogen-like compounds
- Vascular dementia
- Decreases brain calcium-binding proteins
- Early puberty in girls and retarded physical maturation in boys
- Unnatural menstrual patterns in women
- Malnutrition - soybeans have potent enzyme inhibitors
- Reduced protein digestion

- Interference with tyrosine kinase-dependent mechanisms required for optimal hippocampal function, structure and plasticity
- Inhibits tyrosine kinase which impairs memory formation
- Inhibits dopamine
- Movement difficulties characteristic of Parkinson's disease
- Depressed thyroid function
- Infants who receive soy formula are 200% more likely to develop diabetes
- Birth defects
- Due to suppression of the thyroid, fluoride becomes much more toxic
- Inhibits zinc absorption

Mayonnaise and Cold Pasteurization

All commercial mayonnaise is cold pasteurized, because the raw eggs that are necessary for mayonnaise could not be left unrefrigerated for months on store shelves otherwise. Cold pasteurization is the process of saturating a food with radiation to sterilize it. Any "cold pasteurized" food is laced with cancer-inducing radiolytic compounds, in addition to benzene. It is very likely to still be radioactive at the time of sale. Radiolytic compounds and benzene formation are normal, expected occurrences whenever proteins are exposed to high levels of radiation.

In addition to its radioactivity, commercial mayonnaise is made primarily of genetically-engineered soy oil, which is heavily chemically processed. Furthermore, mayonnaise typically contains hydrogenated oils and chemically-engineered additives. Since the toxins in mayonnaise are bound inside various fats, and since the human body protects itself by storing toxins inside fat cells, it is easy to deduce that a body will rapidly convert commercial mayonnaise to body fat.

Canola Oil

Back in the 1960's, the food industry was in search of an oil that could be produced cheaply, but marketed toward health conscious consumers. While olive oil was preferred amongst those who cared about their health, it was never easy or cheap to mass produce. As a result, the food industry began selling rapeseed oil as a supposedly healthy substitute. Serious problems were later discovered with the erucic acid in rapeseed, like the fact that it caused degenerative lesions in the heart muscles. It should not have been surprising to the producers, since rapeseed is so naturally poisonous that insects avoid it. Food companies decided to sell it anyway, even after realizing the serious liability risk.

Starting in 1964, the food industry joined forces with the chemical and nuclear industries to begin work in reducing rapeseed's poisonous erucic acid content, in the hope of producing a less toxic version of rapeseed oil. It had been banned in the U.S. in 1956. It would take the industry over a decade and enormous amounts of genetic engineering to get rapeseed oil back into the U.S. market. The resultant plant from the genetic modifications was originally called L.E.A.R. (low erucic acid rapeseed) and it is sometimes still called that within the food industry. It has been widely renamed to "canola" for marketing reasons, because no company wanted to market a cooking oil that had been officially banned for causing permanent heart damage, and having "rape" in the product name was considered a liability too.

The promoters of canola freely admit that its name was only changed for marketing purposes, which serves only to perpetuate the deception about its true lineage, as if canola were a totally different plant from rapeseed. This Frankenstein plant may be even worse than its parent rapeseed, for canola cooking oil is an E.P.A. registered pesticide. It is far from the natural product of selective breeding that its proponents contend. Canola oil was *invented* in a biotechnology laboratory in 1976, using radiation bombardment techniques to destroy parts of the plant's DNA. This produced the first canola plant that has ever existed in the world.

This comes from the official Canola Council of Canada:

> *"Here are some key facts on growing genetically modified (GM) canola in Canada.*
>
> *"GM or transgenic canola varieties have been modified to be resistant to specific herbicides. They are called herbicide-resistant varieties. The plants are modified, but the oil is not modified. It is identical to canola oil from non-modified or conventional canola.*

"Herbicide-resistant GM canola is grown on about 80% of the acres in western Canada. GM canola was first introduced in 1995."

The figures cited in the previous quotations are dated. About 90% of the canola was genetically engineered to be herbicide resistant at the time this was written. The quotation betrays that canola has been through two separate generations of genetic engineering: first to create the low erucic acid rapeseed that was renamed to canola, and then to further genetically modify it again to make it herbicide resistant. No canola in the United States has any labeling to indicate that it is genetically engineered, or any labeling to indicate that it is a variety of rapeseed.

The following quotes come from the research paper, *Genetic Control of Fatty Acid Biosynthesis in Rapeseed,* which was published in The Journal Of The American Oil Chemists' Society when work on modifying rapeseed began. Here are a couple of snippets from that report, explaining exactly how canola oil (L.E.A.R.) began life:

> *"Self-pollinated seed harvested from each plant was oven-dried, weighed and crushed with a glass rod in a 50-ml Erlenmeyer flask containing 10 ml solution of methanol, acetyl chloride and benzene in the ratio of 20:1:4. The mixture was refluxed under an air condenser for 1 hr to extract and esterify the seed oil. A known wt of internal standard (dibutyl sebacate dissolved in carbon tetrachloride) was added and 0.2-0.4 ~1 of the sample injected into an F and M model 500 gas chromatograph operated at 208c with a helium flow rate of 75 ml / min and using an 8 ft 3/16 in... At the base of each pod, 10 ~1 aqueous solution of radioactive sodium acetate (0.2 ,c methyl labelled) was injected with a Hamilton micro-syringe. A branch from a rapeseed plant bearing 15 pods was excised below the lowest pod, the pods were similarly injected..."*

What was noticeably absent from the procedure was any mention whatsoever of controlled pollination, which the canola marketers have been swearing was at the core of their organic selective breeding process to create all-natural canola. Part of the propaganda used to deceive us about canola oil's safety involves the fact that its manufacturer's laboratory tests have shown it to be a more-or-less healthy cooking oil, until it is actually heated. Then canola undergoes a chemical transformation. Canola is *technically* a healthy cooking oil -- provided that it is never actually cooked. As long as it remains cold and inside its air-tight bottle or test tube -- it tests to be healthy. However, once heated, canola oil produces high levels of 1,3-butadiene, benzene, acrolein, formaldehyde, and other related compounds which become infused into the foods being cooked. All traces of omega-3 are gone.

Canola shares soy's hormone-disrupting tendencies. Canola oil is also noted to produce cancer-causing toxic fumes when heated, and at much lower temperatures than are required to cause equivalent smoking by other cooking oils. Rapeseed and canola oil fumes are the primary reason for the surprisingly high incidence of Asian lung cancers, despite tobacco smoking being a rarity. Canola fumes have been known to kill pet birds, and many readers will remember that canaries were once used in coal mines to detect the presence of poisonous gases.

Dr. Joseph Mercola was the first person who was brave enough to go against the collective grain by attacking the fraudulent canola industry, and he was right to do it. As reported by Dr. Mercola:

> *"Canola oil was developed from the rape seed, a member of the mustard family. Rape seed is unsuited to human consumption because it contains a very-long-chain fatty acid called erucic acid, which under some circumstances is associated with fibrotic heart lesions. It has a high sulfur content and goes rancid easily. Baked goods made with canola oil develop mold very quickly. During the deodorizing process, the omega-3 fatty acids of processed canola oil are transformed into the dangerous trans fatty acids, similar to those in margarine, and possibly more dangerous. A recent study indicates that 'heart healthy' canola oil actually creates a deficiency of vitamin E, a vitamin required for a healthy cardiovascular system. Other studies indicate that even low-erucic-acid canola oil causes heart lesions, particularly when the diet is low in saturated fat."*

Our recommendations include using extra virgin olive oil that is cold pressed for most recipes and using peanut oil for high heat recipes, such as frying. Sunflower oil (not to be confused with safflower) is an acceptable alternative to olive oil. For high-heat cooking and frying, peanut oil is absolutely the safest choice. It is the rapid break down of other oils that make fried foods unhealthy. Butter is good for use with practically every recipe, and natural (preferably organic) butter should be a core component of every diet. Always be watchful of the "smoke point" temperature of an oil, because smoking is an indication of dangerous break-down.

Identifying Poisonous Plastics

This section summarizes the dangers of plastic containers, which we typically assume are safe to eat and drink from. It explains the symbols found on plastic containers, which is useful for identifying the different types of poisons that are leached from them -- from arsenic to petroleum. Plainly labeled on the underside of plastic containers is a number indicating the type of plastic used.

Plastic Identifier: **#1 or PET**

> PET is a plastic that is sometimes distinguished by a #1 stamp. PET is an abbreviation for polyethylene terephthalate. It releases a chemical named antimony trioxide. This chemical toxin has been cited many times as a serious health concern, yet these concerns have been discarded by governments, who have claimed that not enough of this chemical is released to cause problems.

> It is well known that antimony trioxide leaches into drinks that are bottled in PET

plastics, and the longer the shelf life, the more toxic the drinks become. According Canadian studies, typical ground water contains about two parts per trillion of antimony, but freshly bottled water averages 160 P.P.T., rising to 630 P.P.T. within 6 months. Throughout Europe, the average bottled water contains 350 P.P.T. In Germany, PET water that had been bottled for 6 months contained a huge 700 P.P.T. Antimony is very similar to arsenic. In small amounts, antimony poisoning causes headaches, dizziness, and depression. Larger doses produce violent and frequent vomiting, and may lead to death within a few days. Another compound leached by PET plastics is antimony pentafluoride, which reacts with many different compounds. These plastics are produced using hydrogen fluoride and benzene. The chemicals are so toxic during the manufacturing stage that even a small amount in contact with skin can be fatal.

Plastic Identifier: #2 or **HDPE**

HDPE is identified by a #2 stamp. HDPE stands for high density polyethylene, which is a thermoplastic made from petroleum. This is the safest plastic available, because it is very non-reactive.

Plastic Identifier: #3 or **PVC**

This plastic is one of the most hazardous. Poisonous chemicals are released throughout the life cycle of PVC, including mercury, dioxins, and phthalates. When people burn PVC products, they release dioxins producing cancers, respiratory, and reproductive problems. The fumes can cripple the immune system for years. The noticeable smell from a new car or shower curtain is the result of PVC fumes.

In July 2005, the European Parliament banned the use of PVC toys, although they are still legal in America. This material is also used in drinking bottles, and therefore, toxins are inside most bottled drinks. Factory workers who work with this plastic face long-term health risks, including angiosarcoma of the liver, lung cancer, brain cancer, lymphomas, leukemia, and liver cirrhosis. Firefighters also often face similar risks after extinguishing PVC fires, which release hydrogen chloride gas, which forms deadly hydrochloric acid when inhaled.

PVC is not recyclable due to its extremely toxic properties. It is known to leach its poisonous chemicals into drink containers.

Plastic Identifier: #4 or **LDPE**

LDPE is the abbreviation for Low Density Polyethylene. It is virtually identical to HDPE (reference #2 above).

Plastic Identifier: **#5** or **Polystyrene**

> This is one of the *safer* plastics, but safe is a relative term. Since it is manufactured with benzene and petroleum, we recommend avoiding it. Styrene is itself a carcinogen.

Plastic Identifier: **#7** or **Other**

> The "other" literally means unspecified and uncategorized. This plastic could be made from anything, so always avoid these plastics. It is very common for these plastics to contain BPA.

Plastics Containing BPA

Consumer awareness groups have been on the news in recent years decrying the bisphenol-A (BPA) found to be leaching from plastics; especially regarding the plastics used for the drink containers of children and infants. BPA is a chemical which is known to leach out of plastics, disrupting the hormones, as well as causing brain damage, cancer, diabetes and heart problems. The great majority of plastic bottles in use today contain BPA, which some manufacturers claim does not leach into food or drinks. However, the Harvard University study, *Polycarbonate Bottle Use and Urinary Bisphenol A Concentrations* has shown that drinking from BPA-infused bottles increases BPA urine levels by 70%. Imagine the level for an infant who is given formula from one of these containers 6-7 times a day, every day for years, as is normal. This toxin is found in all clear, hard plastic bottles. Cloudy plastics do not contain BPA, such as milk jugs. The F.D.A. has maintained that BPA is safe after having consulted with BPA-industry lobbyists.

We recommend against the use of plastics for the storage of food and drinks. The immune system will otherwise get weakened from coping with added toxicity, in the very least.

Poisoned Food Cans

Those who are knowledgeable about plastic containers and the dozens of toxins that they leach (e.g. antimony and BPA) will often choose canned foods as a healthier alternative. However, aluminum cans, and aluminum water bottles have a secret plastic inner lining. This is because aluminum is known for reacting with either acids or alkalies, and aluminum combines with whatever it reacts to. If no plastic liner were present, people would be getting massive amounts of aluminum in their diets through metal food and drink containers. The plastic liners contain bisphenol-A in practically every case, including the organic options. This is not simply restricted to aluminum drink cans, but it branches out to all aluminum cans, including those that are used to can foods. The baked beans, soups and canned vegetables found at retailers all have it.

Studies testing for the presence of BPA found that it was higher in food containers than soft drink cans. It is presumed that this is because canned foods are processed at much higher temperatures. There is only one brand that is currently claiming to use BPA-free cans, Eden Organic Baked Beans. However, the company still uses BPA for its canned tomato products. Some companies claim that their use of BPA is currently unavoidable for some products. However, there are other options that they could explore, such as glass containers, bees wax coatings, and more resilient metals. Most people would gladly pay a few cents more for alternative containers, if it ensured that their foods and drinks were pure.

The situation is particularly sad, given that people are buying aluminum cans as a safer option to plastic bottles. It is important that health conscious people are made aware of this, so that they may make informed decisions. Due to the great aluminum lie, there are currently very few companies offering BPA-free cans. The food industry is exploiting our ignorance.

Completely avoiding BPA can be difficult, but it can be done. Avoidance is especially important for pregnant women, infants, and young children. Avoiding BPA means avoiding all aluminum cans and hard, clear plastics. When buying plastic containers, use companies which pledge to never use plastics containing BPA, such as Ziplock. Buy foods fresh or frozen, whenever possible, because the foods are usually more nutritious, and the different packaging will eliminate plastic toxins such as BPA.

Infant Formula

Years ago, we went searching for the most unhealthy food item that was available at local grocery stores. To our great shock, infant formula was the worst product. We made the video, *Disturbing Infant Formula Ingredients,* in which we actually repeated the full manufacturing process for an infant formula, with all of the standard ingredients.

Common Infant Formula Ingredients

- Arachidonic acid has been shown to be highly poisonous in animal testing. It is supposed to be omega-6, but this synthetic variant is so toxic that it almost immediately kills lab animals.

- Magnesium chloride is made with ammonia and hydrochloric acid. It is used as a de-icer by state highway departments.

- Potassium hydroxide is used commercially as a cleaner. It may be found in carpet cleaning degreasers, tile cleansers, and even in drain cleaners.

- Cupric sulphate is an algaecide, bactericide, and fungicide. It is used commercially as a herbicide. It is an extremely toxic preservative. Foods that are poisoned with this 'ingredient' should be avoided.

- Carageenan is a seaweed extract that is used as a thickening agent. Consumption of it has been tied with intestinal inflammation and inflammatory bowel disease. It causes gastrointestinal cancers.

- Chrypthecodinium cohnii oil is made from a type of algae. It is typically extracted using the industrial solvent hexane. It is moronically hyped as a health product by some, despite the known heavy metal contamination of algae products, and its industrial solvent byproducts.

- Mono and di-glycerides are chemically-altered fats that are used as emulsifiers. They are hydrogenated, which makes them more damaging. These start the child's life with a significantly greater chance of diseases such as cancer and arterial damage, as well as decreased intelligence by their interference with omega oils.

- Synthetic casein is a carcinogen that has been documented to break down in the stomach to produce the peptide casomorphin. Casomorphin is known to worsen the symptoms of autism and cause difficulty concentrating. It can lead to life-long learning disabilities.

- Soy lecithin is disrupting to the hormones, like all soy products. Hormone disruptors in infant formula can lead to life-long hormonal conditions, such as hypothyroidism and endometriosis.

We knew that we had to spread the word, because people are poisoning their children at an age when children are the most vulnerable. It is everyone's responsibility to protect them. Especially make certain that soy-based formulas (or anything else made with soy) are always avoided, or there will be long-term consequences for the child. Soy is especially destructive to females. Our recommendation is to breast feed. The child will be healthier, and it will prevent the mother from developing breast cancer. Also, avoid all products from China, whether they be foods or toys.

Alternative Medicine

Allergies and Candida

A typical allergy-prone individual has to take a pill every twelve hours endlessly if he trusts orthodox medicine to treat him, and this merely suppresses the symptoms temporarily. What we call "allergies" are actually just symptoms of a body trying to defend itself from perceived threats, so allergies are incurable until the aggravating factors are removed, or the irate immune system is calmed. It is impossible to completely stop the histamine reactions for perceived threats, because these reactions stem from the immune system reacting appropriately. Completely stopping these reactions using standard symptom suppression techniques would mean totally halting the immune system, and it would mean death. It is why most established therapies are ultimately so futile, and why there is no sign of a pharmaceutical cure. Conversely, alternative medicine deals with the root cause of the problems, instead of merely symptom suppression, so there are vastly better options available with holistic methods.

Chronic allergies are caused by the overgrowth of candida albicans. This is a type of yeast that thrives in the gastrointestinal tract whenever the body has an acidic pH. There will always be some of this yeast in every human being, but it is ideally balanced by beneficial bacteria. The beneficial bacteria is commonly referred to as intestinal flora. Intestinal flora helps in the digestion process, and it furthermore aids in removing toxic materials. Conversely, candida is a parasitic yeast, which robs the body of nutrients, and it increases the toxic waste products that a body must eliminate. These two groups of organisms are two warring armies.

With ideal health, the flora bacteria vastly outnumbers and persistently overwhelms the candida yeast; in a similar way to how grass on a healthy lawn will crowd-out weeds. Flora provides immune system support to the dirtiest parts of the human body, where the normal immune system can otherwise become overwhelmed if it is unaided, and it aids in the proper assimilation of nutrients. Our lives depend on those little guys protecting our bodies. If all of the flora dies, then the result is sepsis and death; which has become surprisingly common for patients who get too much medical 'help'. Statistics show this to be an alarming reality.

Whenever an overgrowth of yeast overwhelms the flora, it causes various health issues. Excessive yeast creates a toxic state for the digestive system from its generated waste products, which ultimately trickle into the rest of the body to cause a snowballing effect. Allergies are most often triggered by an immune system that has already been made hyperactive by the rapid growth of the fungal invaders. The results are symptoms of illness. The impaired absorption of nutrients combined with an onslaught of candida waste products (and the related immune responses) begins the vicious cycle of declining health and opportunistic infections. The aftermath can include fatigue, headaches, mood swings, depression, poor memory, lack of concentration, sweet cravings, carbohydrate cravings, and a further weakening of an already compromised immune system as the issues snowball. This sad and sickly state is called "normal" in the Western world.

Candida usually undergoes a massive growth spurt following antibiotic use. This is partly due to antibiotics being more fatal to the good bacteria, which would normally keep candida in check. It has been known for over seventy years that antibiotics are more harmful to the beneficial bacteria than to harmful pathogens, and this rule generally includes even the all-natural antibiotics, such as colloidal silver. Whenever antibiotics are discontinued, the immune system remains weakened for a lengthy period (sometimes years for pharmaceuticals), which places candida in a position of advantage. For someone who has just stopped taking antibiotics, the best thing that he could do for his body is to eat large amounts of plain yogurt (preferably organic) as a natural probiotic. Flavored yogurts contain lots of processed sugars, which will actually feed the yeast, and therefore make the condition worse. Some of the flavored yogurts even contain high fructose corn syrup. Yogurt is usually made with homogenized milk, so also supplement with vitamin C and folate (or the inferior folic acid) to protect against inflammation and arterial damage. Unhomogenized yogurt can often be found at health food stores.

People who eat diets emphasizing carbohydrates tend to experience more allergies and other immune system problems, because processed sugars feed candida. The worst of the sugars are the bleached-white, refined sugars and high fructose corn syrup. The toxicity of these unnatural sugar-like products is enough to massively kill beneficial bacteria, but it feeds pathogenic life forms. These products also aid the fermentation process that keeps yeast thriving. Processed sugar is like fertilizer for the fungal invaders.

The same sugar-loving yeast is the main cause of both dental cavities and bad breath. People who have flora winning the war (who have unimpaired immune systems) rarely get cavities or bad breath. If you ever wondered why bad breath often smells like rotting mushrooms, then you should now understand why. The so-called "breath freshener" products contain ingredients that aggravate the immune system further, which makes the problems worse over an extended period. All of these factors combine in the Western lifestyle to make the common cold so *very* common. For most people, their immune systems are always weakened, aggravated, and overdriven. Unchecked fermentation is how cancer begins in most cases; once all of these factors shift a person's pH too much into the acidic range that cells must themselves begin deriving their energy from a fermentation process too.

Curing Candida

Curing candida through diet is surprisingly easy. It involves the avoidance of foods which are based on yeast and refined (simple) carbohydrates, such as white flour, white rice, processed sugars, white sugar, mushrooms and beer. These foods are never white in nature, and some of them never existed until the 1950's, when the chemical industry decided to *enhance* and *enrich* our foods with chemical processing; including the use of chlorine bleaches that leave behind traces of dioxin compounds. The food remnants of bleaching are incredibly bad for the body, as well as being especially toxic to flora.

For any person wishing to cure his generalized allergies, the reduction of his simple and processed carbohydrates is the first step. The recommended dietary improvements will make a person's life significantly easier, and it will completely eliminate the depressions of some individuals. The elimination of unhealthy carbohydrates is the basis of the very successful Atkin's diet for weight loss, so it will have a double benefit for some. Note that whole wheat foods and brown rice are fine in moderation, because real foods are wholesome until they have been 'enhanced'. However, be aware that commercial whole wheat breads often contain worse chemical additives than white breads.

Eliminate all refined sugars, and replace with fruits whenever cravings for sweets occur. Honey is a great sugar substitute that has compounds to help balance blood sugar levels, and it contains naturally-occurring anti-histamines that are produced by bees to protect themselves from pollen, since they spend most of their lives being covered in it. Local honey is ideal, because the anti-histamines in it are designed to counteract local pollens.

Avoid all soft drinks, and this is the most important of all the suggestions. Soft drinks massively lower a body's pH and thereby its oxygen content. They even release carbon dioxide (from carbonation) into the body, further flushing out the body's critical oxygen. Combining these factors with the artificial sugars and high fructose corn syrup that are found in soft drinks produces an abomination so bad that it would require a separate chapter just to detail. Both the sugars and the carbon dioxide from soft drinks feed the fermentation process that candida uses.

Especially avoid soft drinks with sodium benzoate, because sodium benzoate itself triggers allergies. This substance is in most soft drinks. Tests conducted in 2005, and paid for by a soft drink industry whistle-blower, showed that certain sodas and juices had benzene levels up to ten times higher than the U.S. drinking water limit of five parts per billion. Benzene is classified as a known carcinogen by the U.S. Food and Drug Administration, and it is directly linked to leukemia. Benzene can form in beverages that contain either sodium benzoate or potassium benzoate, when combined with ascorbic acid (erythorbic acid or vitamin C) according to the F.D.A. Heat and light exacerbate the benzene formation in sodas. The benzene limit for drinking water does not apply to soft drinks, which have much less stringent quality standards than municipal water supplies. Sodas with obscenely high benzene content are perfectly legal in the U.S.

Eat plenty of protein, with an emphasis on white meats (preferably free-range and organic), nuts, and beans. As always, include as many vegetables in the diet as possible. They provide core nutrients that are needed by the body in order to fully recover, and vitamins are not a substitute for vegetables. Vitamins can sometimes make things worse, because many of the vitamins are now being extracted using genetically-engineered yeasts, or they contain impurities. These problems are especially likely to occur with vitamins made in China. Most of the vitamins now come from China, and they are deceptively re-branded by domestic companies. Try to obtain vitamins with the fewest non-vitamin ingredients. Most people will need multiple supplements, because finding a trustworthy multivitamin is exceedingly difficult.

For sugar cravings, it is okay to cheat with fruits and *pure* fruit juices without guilt, because the body can handle natural sugars much more efficiently than the engineered sugars. Fruit sugars do not fuel candida growth significantly. Avoid juice cocktails and juices from concentrate because they contain toxic additives, tap water, and sweeteners. One general rule of thumb is that if an ingredient is made in a chemical laboratory, then it is toxic.

The protective and anti-inflammatory properties of omega-3 fatty acids help with allergy problems. We recommend taking flax seed oil supplements daily for allergies, and for overall health. We can find omega-6 throughout Western diets, but there is very little omega-3 in comparison. Much more omega-3 was in our foods before chemical fertilizers depleted the farm lands; and again, it is yet another problem caused by a chemical industry 'solution'. For in-depth information about supplementation with flax oil, see the *Flax Oil* section of the *Supplements* chapter.

> *"Over time, candida grows from a yeast form into a fungal form and starts creating waste products known as mycotoxins. Among the mycotoxins produced is acetaldehyde, a poison that is converted by the liver into alcohol. As alcohol builds up in the system, symptoms associated with alcohol intoxication develop. This is why one of the most common symptoms of candida is brain fog... In its fungal form, candida also grows long roots called rhizoids that puncture the intestinal lining, leading to a condition called leaky gut syndrome. This creates holes in the digestive tract, allowing candida to pass through into the bloodstream."*
>
> -- Brenda Watson, N.D.

Chamomile is an effective natural anti-histamine that can be used alongside these therapies. It can also have a sedative effect. Although this seems to vary greatly between individuals. Do not use chamomile if you have a ragweed allergy. Its anti-histamine properties yield almost instant relief from itchy insect bites, when used transdermally.

A diet with sea salt (not table salt) will help to prevent candida overgrowth. For millenia, diets have been high in mineral-rich salt, and it was glorified for being the life-giving substance that it really is. In modern times, politically correct doctors have labeled salt as a villain, instead of placing the blame on the high-sodium artificial additives that are present in processed foods, which really do cause disease. Table salt roughly has the same toxicity problem that other processed foods do, because all useful minerals are removed. Remember that it is not natural if it is brilliant white. The healthiest sea salts usually have a grayish color, because they are darkened by important trace minerals.

A little coconut oil every day will speed the metabolism, provide an energy boost, be a tonic for the thyroid, and attack yeast in both the mouth (e.g. plaque) and in the gastrointestinal tract (e.g. candida). Everyone should supplement with a small amount of cold-pressed organic coconut oil every day; and of course, it can be added to foods too. Be wary of its inability to withstand high heat; lest it will become rancid and unhealthy.

Most allergy problems can be eliminated with a healthy diet that is low in processed sugars, simple carbohydrates, and chemicals. These therapies, in addition to common sense remedies, such as using high quality air filters, will yield very favorable results in the long term. Allergies are not really normal for the human body, and neither should routine illnesses be. The problems are almost entirely man-made. We have been trained to believe that both are normal, and this has been great for the medical business. The germ theory behind modern medicine has convinced us, and the establishment, that illnesses are more-or-less random events that may strike anyone at anytime, so that the causes of illnesses are either never fully explainable, or as is becoming the belief nowadays, that sickness results from genetic defects. There is a reason for everything that happens, and this rule includes events of the human body. Illness symptoms are a body's way of telling us that someone is doing something terribly wrong; and most often, it is the diet that is the most wrong. Most allergies and illnesses are a result of weakened immune systems, and the problems can usually be corrected without drugs. Following the recommendations cited herein will also help a person to remove toxins, and therefore eliminate other health conditions. The alternative for most people is to continue forever on an expensive treadmill of drugs that suppress the symptoms and the immune system; awhile increasing their overall toxicity, so that disease problems only worsen in time.

The Next Generation Allergies

There is an extraordinary list of new food allergies that have never existed before in history, which are being caused almost exclusively by vaccinations. This ever-growing list of allergens includes peanuts, eggs, milk, latex, and soy. The problem is that these food ingredients are being put into vaccines, and vaccines are specifically designed to trigger a hyperactive immune response. In some cases, the response is life-long. This situation is why health care workers have developed allergies to their latex gloves at an unprecedented level, and why you will not find latex gloves in hospitals anymore. The new generation of potentially fatal food allergies is one of a multitude of reasons why we contend that vaccines do much more harm than good. The only way to eliminate these allergies is a slow process of desensitization, but this process can be dangerous. Readers may attempt to desensitize themselves at their own risk. For those who do, the most important symptoms to be watchful for are respiratory distress and throat swelling. Call for emergency assistance if you experience these symptoms. Such victims may be able to partly subdue their allergic reactions by immediately ingesting activated carbon (activated charcoal) powder. There is information about activated carbon in the *Activated Carbon* section of the *Emergency Medicine* chapter.

Arthritis and Joint Pain

Chronic joint pain is a plague for 47 million Americans, with a large portion of them having become totally dependent upon expensive pain medications. Despite mountains of misinformation, joint pain does not necessarily need to occur with aging, and it can usually be eliminated with much safer alternatives. The human body was designed to heal itself when given the appropriate nutrients.

Arthritis is sometimes caused by a virus. This fact is somewhat ignored in the health industry, because the mainstream establishment is unable to kill the virus with antibiotics. Admitting the impotency of their pharmaceutical arsenal would be admitting failure, so they lie about it. Their lack of success in stopping the arthritis virus is heralded as unquestionable scientific proof that no virus exists. The logic is very circular. The evidence of the medical cover-up begins with the fact that there are some viral conditions which are known to directly cause arthritis, such as hepatitis and Lyme disease. Furthermore, the orthodox explanation of arthritis suggests that it should only occur in regions which have been historically aggravated or injured. If arthritis begins spreading throughout a body like they now admit that it does, then it is obviously not the result of an injury, or of regionalized inflammation. Injuries cannot move about with a will of their own, even if modern medical men claim that they do. Finally, there are alternative therapies that actually kill the (supposedly non-existent) virus, such as colloidal silver; to effect a permanent cure.

Be warned about Internet scoundrels who recommend using toxic borax to kill the virus, because borax is likely to yield long-term organ damage.

Natural Treatment Options

- Glucosamine is a compound that is found naturally in healthy cartilage, but is typically deficient in those with serious joint issues. Glucosamine sulfate has repeatedly been shown to be effective in people suffering from arthritis, particularly of the knees. One study found that the supplementation of glucosamine sulfate resulted in a carry over effect, which means that some of the benefits continued after the supplement was discontinued. We recommend that readers seek vegetarian glucosamine sulfate capsules, else their supplements will be produced from the skeletons of crustaceans.

- Apple cider vinegar is a natural anti-inflammatory agent. Many people have reported remarkable relief, simply through the consumption of 1-2 tablespoons of apple cider vinegar each morning. Unfortunately, no official studies have been done on the effect of apple cider vinegar regarding joint health. However, it is very cheap and worth trying. Never buy vinegar in clear plastic containers, since the vinegar's high acidity will cause the plastic to leach chemicals.

- Curcumin is an extract of turmeric. This supplement is a powerful anti-inflammatory. Do not confuse it with the spice, cumin.

- A 2003 study by The Department of Forensic Medicine in Germany, showed that devil's claw extract was more effective for treating lower back pain than the potent pharmaceutical, Vioxx. Devil's claw is known for its pain relieving and anti-inflammatory properties. It is used by natural medicine practitioners for the treatment of carpal tunnel, as well as arthritis.

- Cherry supplementation significantly decreases arthritis pain. Cherries are natural COX-2 inhibitors, which means that they reduce the enzyme that causes inflammation within a body. Unlike pharmaceutical COX-2 inhibitors, such as Vioxx and Celebrex, cherries do not cause heart attacks, and concentrated cherry supplements tend to be more effective. Concentrated cherry extract pills may be purchased from most health food stores and various online sellers. Eating cherries will be beneficial too, but eating cherries does not provide the same degree of benefit that cherry concentrate does.

- MSM is a sulfur compound that is naturally found in many foods. In dietary supplements, it is sometimes mixed with glucosamine. Studies on the effects of methylsulfonylmethane (MSM) for joint pain, particularly arthritis, repeatedly show massive improvements in pain relief and decreases of inflammation.

- Vitamin C is required for the production of collagen. It is needed to repair and maintain the soft tissues around the joints. Practically everyone is lacking adequate vitamin C, according to the research of the Linus Pauling Institute.

- Muscadine grapes are a natural source of resveratrol. Resveratrol has received a lot of notoriety in recent times for its effect upon joint and heart health. It is present in red wines and dark grape juice. We recommend resveratrol from dietary sources, because only a tiny amount of it is needed for effectiveness, and because resveratrol supplements are shamelessly over-priced. The excessive concentration of resveratrol in supplements also risks chelating too much iron from a body.

- The Budwig Protocol was first used for people with arthritis with great success. The anti-cancer Budwig Protocol is extremely anti-inflammatory, which is likely why it is so effective in treating arthritis, reversing heart disease, and curing cancers. For more information about the Budwig Protocol, reference the *Cancer* chapter.

- Colloidal gold (internally) and colloidal copper (topically) are both helpful. Copper is dangerous for internal supplementation, because only a small amount of copper can cause an overdose that is toxic to the liver. A copper overdose can quickly become a health emergency. Chlorophyll supplementation is the only safe method for oral copper supplementation. Colloidal copper and copper hydroxide may be purchased from disreputable sellers as supplement products, but such products are always dangerous.

- Colloidal silver can cure the condition when it is caused by a virus. The percentage of cases that are caused by viruses is unknown, since the medical establishment refuses to even acknowledge that viruses could be involved. When the condition begins spreading throughout the body, then it is certainly viral. It is rare to find colloidal silver that is acceptably safe and effective, so we encourage readers to reference the *Colloidal Silver* section of the *Alternative Medicine* chapter, in order to make their own. To have it done right, one needs to make it himself.

The supplemental treatments work by correcting deficiencies. People with exceptional diets and lifestyles do not suffer chronic diseases like arthritis. Our soils are now so minerally deficient that even well-balanced diets are not always enough. Always choose organic produce whenever it is available, and read the PLU numbers on produce to avoid genetically-engineered produce. Read the *PLU Numbers* section of the *Biotechnology* chapter for more information about this. Eating wholesome, homemade foods is a primary step in the elimination of health conditions. Society's reliance upon processed foods has left it chronically malnourished and physiologically inflamed.

Pay close attention to the effects of lotions. Most lotions damage the liver to eventually produce cascading health problems. They are one of the many hidden chemical industry gotchas that are found in retailers. For these reasons, we formulated our own copper-based lotion. We could not find anything commercially that we believed was fit for human usage, so we created a copper lotion containing natural ingredients.

When Arthritis is Not Really Arthritis

An entirely different therapy and a parasite cleanse are necessary for an unknown percentage of arthritis cases, because the "arthritis" is sometimes Lyme disease that has been misdiagnosed, or another parasitic condition. Nevertheless, some of the symptom treatments herein may be of use for pain. Reference the *Lyme Disease* section of the *Alternative Medicine* chapter, if you need a detailed Lyme disease treatment protocol.

Asthma

Asthma is a condition that is characterized by shortness of breath, wheezing, chest tightness, pain in the chest, and coughing (especially at night). As with all the other confusing diseases, experimental medicine has recently redefined asthma as a genetic condition. For the uninitiated, the word "genetic" is medical code for "we have no idea" or "we'll blame it on God". Despite medical science's newly discovered genetic cause of asthma, the rates of its occurrence have been increasing disproportionately to population growth each year.

There are many triggers of asthma attacks. Environmental pollution is a major cause for those who live in urban areas. Air fresheners, in particular, have been shown to trigger asthma attacks by dramatically reducing lung capacity. Asthmatics should avoid all scented products, including candles, deodorizers, dryer sheets, scented soaps, and especially all "air fresheners". It is wise for healthy individuals to avoid them too. Allergens stress the body to exaggerate asthma problems, which can provoke terrifying hyper-immune responses. Certain plants may cause these reactions, such as ragweed, along with a new generation of food allergies, which have been artificially created by vaccinations containing food ingredients.

Standard Care

As is the usual pattern, the medical establishment offers no cures, but it offers many options to perpetually treat asthma symptoms at great cost. Doctors have been prescribing steroid-based asthma inhalers for decades. These steroid-based inhalers are intended to prevent future asthma attacks, and this is actually considered preventative medicine. The steroid side effects are dismissed off-hand by doctors, but these frequently include: headaches, joint pain, mental disturbances, nosebleeds, weight gain, frequent infections, growth retardation and adrenal insufficiency. Adrenal insufficiency is the primary catalyst of pre-diabetes, which explains why asthma patients have a high incidence of diabetes. The treatments eventually prove to be highly profitable in the long term from the new diseases that the "preventative medicine" caused.

> *"When steroid drugs are taken by mouth, they substitute for and decrease the body's normal ability to make its own steroids as well as its ability to respond to stress."*

-- Drugs.com

Cortisteroids can accumulate in the body's tissues, resulting in increasing health damage over time. They have been linked to diabetes. In addition to steroid-based inhalers, some asthma sufferers are also prescribed anti-inflammatory pills to reduce asthma attacks. This is particularly sad in the case of children, because the massive amount of pharmaceuticals provided each day, for years at a time, will have long-term health consequences, which will make them forever dependent upon the system. The eventual result is suppressed immune systems that make asthma and a host of other disorders much more likely, and more severe.

One of the latest 'treatments' for asthma is the oral contraceptive pill. The medical establishment never stops creating novel uses for this class of hormone-destroying pharmaceuticals, which are some of the most damaging drugs in existence. The contraceptive pill is one of the reasons for the high rate of thyroid diseases, diabetes, mental illnesses, female hair loss, and strokes. These drugs are especially dangerous because they destroy the natural balance of a body's hormones -- sometimes permanently.

Eliminating Asthma

An extraordinary percentage of asthma sufferers do not seem to know how to breathe well. They have a tendency of breathing through their mouths, instead of their noses. Breathing through the mouth actually causes the constriction of blood vessels, and increases the chances of lung infections, due to the lack of nasal filtering. This constriction can cause the sufferer to require even more oxygen, in a snowballing reaction. The type of breathing exercises that are practiced in Karate are ideal for asthma sufferers to gradually increase their lung capacity. To do this, one must focus on breathing slowly but deeply through the nose only, and out through the mouth slowly. A maximum breath should be taken in during inhalation, and then after a brief pause, some effort should be made to force slightly more air in. This air should be held for about 2 seconds before slowly exhaling as much as possible, and then the process is repeated. This technique of breathing deeper (yet more slowly) should be employed whenever there is physical exertion. Through practice, a person will become trained to breathe more slowly and deeply, and this exercise will actually increase the air capacity of the lungs.

Eating 1-2 tablespoons of honey each day is beneficial, particularly if the honey was produced by local bees. Honey from local bees contains antihistamines that are specific to local plants. It also contains an exceptional set of nutrients, and natural sugars that are not inflammatory.

Vitamin B-12 has been shown to dramatically reduce asthma attacks. The recommended dose is 500 mcg. (micrograms) for children who are younger than twelve, and 1,000-2,000 mcg. for older children and adults. Only use vitamin B-12 in the form of methylcobalamin.

Indian tobacco (lobelia inflata) is known for its therapeutic effects on asthma and other respiratory problems, particularly when it is smoked. Take notice that it is not a true tobacco, despite its name, and it contains no nicotine. Reference the *Indian Tobacco* section of the *Supplements* chapter.

Vitamin B-6 deficiency has been observed in many asthma sufferers, and this is usually caused by the asthma medications, which are known to deplete the body of vitamin B-6. Studies on children with severe asthma showed marked improvement with B-6 supplementation.

Avoid tap water, and start drinking cleaner water instead. Be wary of water filters that are sold at major retail stores, which advertise that they, "remove chlorine taste", and invest in one that actually removes the chlorine.

Acquire a shower filter that eliminates chlorine, because chlorine steam from a hot shower will aggravate the lungs. This may be the most important recommendation. For the same reason, chlorinated water should never be used in vaporizers or humidifiers, because they will output chlorine vapors too. For readers who do not immediately grasp the significance, chlorine gas was a chemical warfare agent that was used during World War I to cause suffocation.

Avoid aspartame, the dangerous artificial sweetener. It is known to stimulate asthma attacks and cause difficulty breathing. It is in chewing gum and diet products.

A high quality air filter that properly eliminates allergens will be very helpful in combating asthma. The E.P.A. reported 10 years ago that indoor air pollutants have a greater impact on health than outdoor pollutants, so it is vital that indoor air be effectively filtered by an anti-allergen air filter, and the filter should be changed monthly (regardless of manufacturer recommendations).

Due to the connection between asthma and allergies, some sufferers may wish to try chamomile. Chamomile is an effective antihistamine that can be purchased in capsule form. It can cause drowsiness, and it is a relative of ragweed. Do not use chamomile if you have a ragweed allergy.

Eliminate all processed foods and simple carbohydrates. Stop eating all of the new "white" foods, including white bread, white flour, white sugar, and white rice. Homemade bread is best, because the whole wheat breads being sold in grocery stores are so perverted that they are worse than the white breads. Start cooking balanced meals, which include some organic proteins, alongside plenty of vegetables and fruits (preferably organic).

Attention Deficit Disorder

There are a lot of people in modern society who have trouble concentrating on seemingly simple tasks. There is an emerging epidemic of people who are having difficulties with organization, memory, and they have a tendency to become easily distracted. In the most problematic cases, it has been blamed on an increased need to multi-task in the workplace or school. However, the workload for most Americans has not actually increased at the same rate as these problems have, and people with low-stress jobs are experiencing these same issues at equally-elevated rates.

A June 2009 C.N.N. article titled, *Why Can't I Concentrate?* blamed A.D.D. as the cause of these problems, pointing to the fact that 5 million female Americans suffer from it, and it is even more common in men. The media ignored the most basic probing questions such as, what is the cause and the cure? Perhaps they were silent on these questions because any mention of curing would have meant that the reporters were risking criminal prosecution for making unapproved medical claims or practicing medicine without a license. Even though they should be immune from such worries as journalists, we can nevertheless imagine the cold chill as they conferenced about this matter with their legal department beforehand.

The truth is that A.D.D. is usually an easily correctable condition, for which there exists no conclusive diagnostic testing. It is simply a diagnosis that is based on a collection of symptoms that naturally occur to lesser degrees within healthy people. The newer and more expensive drugs that are available at the time of diagnosis largely define the overall diagnosis and the treatment strategy. Attention deficit disorder is similar to the case of restless leg syndrome, for which a new disease had to be created (by vote) to sell a pharmaceutical that had no known benefit. They call it "science". The final diagnosis can be A.D.H.D., bipolar disorder, or a whole list of other conditions that are coincidentally appearing at the same rate as the new pharmaceuticals to treat them. The most comical of the new psychiatric disorders is oppositional defiant disorder, whose primary symptom is being a child who dislikes punishment. It is reported to be rampant.

The Causes of Attention Deficit Disorder

A.D.D. may be caused by chemical poisoning combined with malnutrition in childhood. Therefore, A.D.D. is often diagnosed soon after vaccinations (just like autism), because vaccines are known to induce vitamin deficiencies. For more information about this, reference the section about *Sudden Infant Death Syndrome* in the *Wellness* chapter. The condition may also slowly develop for people who have poor diets. A.D.D. *appears* to be a genetic disorder, for poor diet habits and family doctors are cross-generational. While most people do not have A.D.D., they nevertheless experience at least some of its symptoms routinely, due to horrible lifestyles and health.

Children are more likely to get diagnosed, because the foods which are marketed to them are often brightly colored with chemicals, full of artificial flavors, have huge amounts of acids, refined sugars, and artificial sweeteners which greatly exaggerate their symptoms. Artificial colors and several additives have been removed from children's foods in England, due to their well-documented toxicity problems, while in the U.S., the F.D.A. is running interference to keep the chemical companies protected.

Most sources ignore one of the most insidious dangers of poisons. This danger is that they equally attack the brain. Mercury causes autism. Lead causes retardation. MSG lowers the I.Q. and may even cause heart failure. Aspartame causes epilepsy, Parkinson's disease, multiple sclerosis and brain cancer. Most artificial food additives aggravate A.D.D. You will find a plethora of evidence proving these statements if you look to sources outside of the U.S.A. Research is *discouraged* in the Americas, where the chemical industry is well protected.

A prime cause for the initial onset of attention deficit disorders are very severe illnesses that occurred during childhood, such as pneumonias. Life-threatening illnesses at a young age often have a lifetime impact; and such events may hyper-stimulate the immune system, so that it forever overreacts to even the most minor threats. People who are thus afflicted are significantly more vulnerable to chemical toxicity and allergens than average people. In these cases, a patient's cognitive instability stems from his hysterically overdriven immune system, which was trained to react violently to even the most minor of threats. This is exactly what attention deficit disorder is. It is a body that cannot believe it is well.

Curing Attention Deficit Disorder

The cure for this relatively new disorder requires major changes in diet. Sufferers need to reduce (hopefully eliminate) their overall exposure to toxins; like pharmaceuticals, hand sanitizers, corn-fed meat with nitrate salts and synthetic growth hormones, refined sugars, and other bleached white products, artificial colors, artificial flavors, the so-called "natural flavors" that are usually unnatural, artificial fats such as margarine, and even tap water. Getting healthy oils and avoiding damaging fats is particularly important for those with attention deficit disorder symptoms. Soy, canola, and all hydrogenated oils should be avoided. Real butter is a healthy addition to the diet, as is coconut oil and olive oil. Using the Budwig Protocol's mixture of flax seed oil and unhomogenized cheese is likely to have a dramatic effect upon the concentration and it will eliminate some of the allergen sensitivities.

Beware of the new generation of drugs, especially the S.S.R.I. anti-depressants, which typically require that a user slowly be weaned from them. This is extremely revealing about the intentions of the industry, which is legally allowed to create drug addictions at will. The treatment drugs, at best, only suppress some of the A.D.D. symptoms for a short period, before it is time to upgrade to a stronger dose, or to a stronger drug. This is the intent. The effects of the drugs are disastrous; like homicidal violence (discussed in the *Depression* chapter) and the drugs frequently induce fantasies about violent suicides too. Every school massacre in U.S. history had these drugs involved; to put the danger into perspective. The drugs cause the suicide rate to skyrocket from an emotional effect that the pharmaceutical industry callously calls "suicidality".

Some people who exhibit A.D.D. symptoms are introverted, and they actually do better when given more tasks to work with; not because they are diseased, but because they are of a higher intelligence; and therefore, they require more stimulation. The down-side is that they also suffer with increased sensitivity to toxins and unnatural foods. There is a poorly-understood link between attention deficit disorder and high intelligence, so the druggings are actually the pacification of our future leaders.

It really is this simple: detoxify yourself, stop feeding your body poisons, and stop allowing others to poison you. A.D.D. can be transformed into a gift, instead of a disease. There is absolutely nothing wrong with being creative, being a leader, or having individuality. In the not-so-distant past, society rewarded these qualities.

Changing the diet to an all-natural one (preferably organic) will provide enormous assistance for A.D.D. people, without the need for drugs; and it will furthermore greatly help with the patient's overall long-term health.

There are supplements that can help to reduce A.D.D. symptoms. However, these should only be used in combination with the proposed dietary changes. White vein kratom is a supplemental herb that helps with concentration, energy, and motivation. It could be considered a natural version of Ritalin. Kava kava might also be helpful, because it helps to prevent seizures. Note that attention deficit disorder is in part a seizure disorder, but this has been whitewashed by the psychiatric establishment throughout the last decade. To learn more about these herbs, read the *Painkillers* section of this chapter. The following supplements may also prove helpful: gotu kola, ginkgo biloba, guarana, and L-tyrosine (may cause fatigue in some people).

Autism

Autism strikes 2% of all U.S. children, and this rate is rapidly rising. Members of the medical establishment maintain that they cannot ascertain the cure, and claim to not know the cause. The only thing they claim to know with certainty is that vaccinations cannot be the culprit. Vaccines are categorically exempt from all institutional criticisms, and they are paraded as an unquestionable "miracle of modern science". Although the Centers For Disease Control found that approximately half of the physicians refuse to take routine vaccinations themselves, due to safety and efficacy reasons.

Nevertheless, they preach in unison that vaccines are safe for *us* and *our* children. After all, vaccines are said to have ended the polio and smallpox epidemics. *Not exactly*. The vaccines were conveniently put into usage just after the epidemics had begun their natural dying-off process that all epidemics undergo. This dying-off process is why the epidemic of the Black Plague and thousands of other biological terrors no longer exist, and it has historically happened without the assistance of vaccines. The end of modern epidemics that were fought against with vaccines had successes that were mirrored in countries which did not use any vaccines, and they usually had faster rates of die-off. These statistics are institutionally ignored for the sake of vaccine political correctness in the Western world. Not only has medical history been rewritten to categorically favor vaccines, but evidence of their side-effects is routinely suppressed. There is no better example of this than autism.

The Cover-Up

The vaccine industry will make over 34 billion dollars in profits this year, with no foreseeable end in its profit growth. People who have never researched the pharmaceutical industry cannot grasp the corruption of this lucrative industry, its cozy relations with regulatory agents, or its virtual ownership of the media industry. It pays more for media advertising than any other industry; making it the most influential paying client for media organizations; and moreover, the pharmaceutical industry has the biggest political lobby in the United States. In other words, nobody with a voice ever gives the industry, or its practices, serious criticism.

Before grasping the breadth of the industry's influence, one needs to first grasp its history. The international pharmaceutical conglomerates originate from the former petrochemical empire that was once exclusively owned by the Rockefeller family. It was so powerful that the U.S. Government considered it to be a threat to U.S. national security, and thus anti-trust actions were commenced to cripple the empire. However, this dragon was never slain. It is bigger and stronger than ever, to the degree that governments now answer to them, and any reporter who wants to keep his job knows to fear it.

Despite studies showing an unquestionable link between the vaccine ingredient ethyl mercury and autism, the mainstream media favors studies which have shown the opposite. What is interesting is that all of the studies that are used to deny the autism link to mercury poisoning were funded by pharmaceutical companies, doctors who own vaccine patents, or the F.D.A., which gets most of its funding (97%) from the pharmaceutical industry.

The Explosive Growth of Autism

The cure is elusive, we are told, and there is no talk about promising studies concerning treatments for autism. In fact, some claim that autism is an incurable genetic condition. Some scientists have noted that the percentage of autistic children is growing so exponentially fast that autism cannot possibly be explained by genetic causes. Others argue that only the diagnoses of it have increased, whilst the actual percentage of autistic children has not actually changed.

People who work with children have been easily contradicting these gratuitous speculations. Child care workers have made it increasingly clear that autistic children portray some unmistakable symptoms, which have become so common in recent years that the genetics and misdiagnoses arguments explaining its growth are fundamentally flawed. The presiding theories are more a matter of political damage control by the medical establishment than science.

What Parents Need to Know

The truth is that autism can *sometimes* be cured, but only if it is caught in time. There is not enough data to make a statement about what percentage of cases are curable; even for those who begin the treatments early. We know that fast action is prudent, because vaccine-injected mercury does tremendous damage to the brain over time, and to the central nervous system. If the mercury is not removed in a timely manner, then recovery might not be possible. Mercury poisoning for autistic children is a ticking time-bomb, and its eventual payload is permanent brain damage. Young children are the most receptive to a full recovery.

Thousands of families are currently using DMSA, a substance that was F.D.A. approved for the removal of lead. Studies are now beginning to show that it is likewise effective for mercury removal, which explains why this therapy helps autistic children.

Skeptics deny the effectiveness of this protocol, based only on the fact that they religiously believe that no vaccine-autism link could exist. Their bias stems from the fear that successful treatments prove that autism is indeed caused by mercury poisoning, and therefore by modern medicine. Accepting this link would mean committing a career-ending sacrilege for anyone involved with the medical industry. So instead, they ignore data showing the benefits of this therapy, and categorically deride chelation proponents for being "unscientific". We have repeatedly witnessed that the whole vaccine debate is much more about business, power, and politics than science.

When the DMSA cure began becoming popular, James Adams, Ph.D, Professor in the Division of Clinical Sciences at the Southwest Clinic of Natural Medicine, began a study of DMSA, largely because his teenage daughter had autism. N.B.C. News actually covered the story. The conclusion of the study done by Jim Adams was that autism can be reversed safely and effectively in some children. His study was intended to be the starting point for further research, and was conducted on children aged 3 to 8 years. Most people would assume that positive results in one study would lead the way to further investigations by different groups, but this has not been the case. Scientific progress is being thwarted by politics and business agendas at university medical schools. However, at least one other study, published in *Toxicology and Applied Pharmacology* did reveal that not only does the vaccine preservative thimerosal deposit mercury inside the body, but that it is effectively removed with DMSA.

Alternative medicine offers several different forms of chelation (heavy metal removal). These can be used in conjunction with DMSA, and we advise parents to utilize all methods to get the maximum results as fast as possible. The longer the process of removing heavy metal toxins takes, the more brain damage and side effects there will be. Parents of an autistic child should accept that the onset of autistic symptoms indicates a mercury-based time bomb that they are racing against to save their child from a life-long handicap.

Chelation Regimen

- A.L.A. (alpha lipoic acid)
- Cilantro (supplement 100 mg. per 50 lbs. of weight)
- NAC (N-Acetyl-Cysteine)
- Selenium (50 mcg. per 50 lbs.) *
- B complex vitamins
- 5-HTP (Never exceed 100 mg., and do not take alongside anti-depressants.)
- DMSA (3x/day, at 10 mg. per kg. of body weight, taken in pill form. 1 lbs. = 0.45 kg.)
- Garlic
- Regular exercise

  * Excessive supplementation with selenium is dangerous. Children should not supplement with more than 100 mcg.

DMSA can only be found in select herbal stores, and of course, the Internet. We warn readers to not confuse it with DMSO. In the case of autistic children, most parents continue their program for about eight months. While this is an extended period of time, and perhaps longer than necessary; it is nonetheless prudent that the maximum amount of mercury be removed at the earliest time. This may not be a process that can be finished later. Exercise is the only way that the lymph nodes expel toxins, so it is important for best results.

Current research shows that DMSA has difficulty crossing into the brain, so it mostly removes the mercury that is built-up in other tissues. Therefore, for maximum efficacy, alpha lipoic acid (A.L.A.) should also be employed. It is readily available at health food stores. A Hungarian study titled, *Effect of Lipoic Acid on Biliary Excretion of Glutathione and Metals*, showed that A.L.A. supplementation can increase the excretion of mercury by 12 to 37 times. We furthermore know from other studies that A.L.A. crosses the blood-brain barrier. Studies demonstrating its removal of metals from the brain are intentionally sparse, because such politically-incorrect research proves that autism is caused by mercury (and vaccines), and that Alzheimer's disease is caused by aluminum (vaccines too). Researchers, especially those in the U.S., avoid such controversies in lieu of maintaining their research grants and avoiding career suicides with what would be considered institutional blasphemy.

Repairing the Damage

It is wise to stimulate nerve regeneration when treating autism. Vitamin B-12, in the form of methylcobalamin, is known to be helpful for creating and repairing nerves, along with MSM (methylsulfonylmethane). The intake of saturated fats is essential, since nerve repair cannot take place without them. Saturated fats (e.g. dairy products) like real butter are ideal. The patient should supplement daily with omega-3 in the form of flax seed oil; in independent, light-resistant capsules. Never use fish oil or other supplementary sources for the omega-3. Baked fish is the ideal source of omega-3, but it will be impossible to get the needed amount from diet alone. Include a source of dietary sulfur proteins, such as goat cheese or eggs, for best results with omega supplementation. Yogurt can be used too, but it is not as healthy, because it is usually made from homogenized milk. If yogurt is used, then also supplement with folate (or the inferior folic acid) and vitamin C to prevent inflammation and arterial damage.

Mainstream physicians and psychiatrists are likely to tell you that it is impossible to heal nerve damage, especially damage to the brain neurons. Do not assume this to be true, because it is only true for some cases. Young people, in particular, have excellent chances of nervous system regeneration. Just remember that those same *experts* told you that vaccines are harmless, and that there is no cure for autism.

The autism epidemic is sweeping our society, and the medical establishment has remained silent about chelation-based options, which help an unknown percentage of autistic children. It is worth noting that thimerosal is *still* present in some vaccines. It was withdrawn for a brief period, so that manufacturers could claim that it was "removed". Then they put it back into the vaccines and continued making the mercury-free claims based dishonestly upon the fact that it technically *was* removed (at one time). These are the sort of manipulations and word games that one uncovers when studying the pharmaceutical industry.

We strongly recommend that parents consider using a chelation protocol on their autistic children immediately, and avoiding all future vaccines. All states, except for West Virginia and Mississippi have religious or philosophical exemptions to protect those who are in-the-know from "mandatory" vaccinations. Parents from those two states must home school their children in order to avoid vaccinating them, or legally challenge the school systems. If you are beginning to treat your autistic child, then we wish you the best of luck and God-speed. A prayer for help and guidance would probably be the best first step.

The Independent Studies

Here is a sampling of the independent studies that are institutionally ignored. They show an unmistakable correlation between mercury poisoning and autism.

Cell Biology and Toxicology, April 2010: *Induction of metallothionein in mouse cerebellum and cerebrum with low-dose thimerosal injection.*

> "As a result of the present findings, in combination with the brain pathology observed in patients diagnosed with autism, the present study helps to support the possible biological plausibility for how low-dose exposure to mercury from thimerosal-containing vaccines may be associated with autism."

Journal of Toxicology and Environmental Health, 2010: *Hepatitis B Vaccination of Male Neonates and Autism*

> "Findings suggest that U.S. male neonates vaccinated with hepatitis B vaccine had a 3-fold greater risk of ASD; risk was greatest for non-white boys."

Toxicology & Applied Pharmacology, 2006: *Porphyrinuria in childhood autistic disorder: Implications for environmental toxicity*

> "A subgroup with autistic disorder was treated with oral dimercaptosuccinic acid (DMSA) with a view to heavy metal removal. Following DMSA there was a significant ($P = 0.002$) drop in urinary porphyrin excretion. These data implicate environmental toxicity in childhood autistic disorder."

Toxicological & Environmental Chemistry, Volume 91, 2009: *Mitochondrial dysfunction, impaired oxidative-reduction activity, degeneration, and death in human neuronal and fetal cells induced by low-level exposure to thimerosal and other metal compounds.* This study showed the effects of exposure to ethyl mercury on cells, a component that vaccine advocates claim is harmless (unlike methyl mercury which is found in dental fillings, etc).

Journal of American Physicians and Surgeons, Volume 11, 2006: *Early Downward Trends in Neurodevelopmental Disorders Following Removal of Thimerosal-Containing Vaccines*

> "Holmes et al. examined first baby haircuts and determined that autistics had significantly higher body burdens of mercury in comparison to nonautistic matched controls, by demonstrating that the mercury level in hair, and thus the ability to excrete mercury, was inversely proportional to the severity of autism and overall much lower in the autistic group."

Medical Hypotheses, April 2001: *Autism: a novel form of mercury poisoning.*

"A review of medical literature and US government data suggests that: (i) many cases of idiopathic autism are induced by early mercury exposure from thimerosal."

Bell's Palsy

The Politics of *Not* Curing Bell's Palsy

As reported by Gazette.Net:

> *"The 68-year-old Montgomery Village man whose Bells Palsy clinic treated thousands of people over a 20-year period was sentenced to spend the next seven months in county jail after an emotional hearing in Montgomery County [Maryland] Circuit Court last week... Judge Marielsa Bernard sentenced Robert Scott Targan on Nov. 14 to more than 90 years in jail for 24 separate charges, but suspended all but 10 years, then assigned the terms to run concurrently, leaving Targan with a nine-month sentence. Targan received credit for two months he has already spent in jail. Bernard also ordered Targan, who has a host of severe medical ailments, to pay more than $40,000 in restitution and to five years supervised probation."*

Ninety years? What was Dr. Targan's heinous crime? The crime was curing long-term sufferers of Bell's palsy in patients whom other doctors were unable to help. Some desperate doctors were even recommending him to their patients, so that he could do what the American Medical Association had forbidden them from doing.

> *"Eight former patients, including one from South Carolina and one from New Jersey, testified in Targan's support. They said that if not for the treatment they received at the Bells Palsy Research Foundation, their lives would still be in shambles. Brenda Iraola of Laurel broke down into heavy sobs as she recalled her deepening depression as one doctor after another -- 14 in all -- offered little or no help. 'I was literally falling apart in front of these doctors,' she said."*

In the end, the medical establishment and the local prosecutors were so desperate to find any manipulation that would sway a jury that they hounded a former client to accuse him of sexual harassment, and they exaggerated billing mistakes to charge him with crimes such as, "unauthorized use of a credit card", "possession of another's credit card number", among 4 counts of "felony theft", "misdemeanor theft", and "theft scheme". Jurors were distracted away from the fact that all business owners have in their possession the credit card numbers of their customers. The situation with Bell's palsy and this court case demonstrates clearly how competition to the medical establishment is dealt with. Like with many other diseases, Bell's palsy is illegal to cure, because no cures have ever been approved by the Food and Drug Administration. Dr. Targan made the mistake of violating this regulatory law and he was steamrolled for it -- for curing people.

What Is Bell's Palsy?

Bell's palsy is an unexpected temporary paralysis of one side of the face. It can often become so severe that its victims are unable to close one eye, or even smile. There is usually very little warning, and the sudden onset leads some to believe that they have experienced a stroke. Bell's palsy often lasts several months, which can make having a normal life very challenging, and some people never fully recover. It usually begins with a numb sensation and a lack of control of the lips. It then causes an inability to smile properly, the inability to blink with one eye, and eventually the complete paralysis of one side of the face.

Approved Methods and Underground Cures

Conventional medicine uses steroid injections in the face and neck, in a haphazard attempt to help the patient to regain control of his face. This drastic and dangerous treatment is usually ineffective. The following treatment protocol combines our research efforts, and our own experimentation with different treatments. Recovery is often possible within two weeks, using our alternative medicine, whereas recovery normally takes months with standard therapies.

The Health Wyze Protocol

Bell's palsy is related to herpes, a virus which the majority of the population silently hosts without showing any symptoms. It is therefore strongly recommended that the patient's diet be high in L-lysine and low in L-arginine. The herpes virus becomes dormant under high levels of L-lysine, an amino acid that is present in many fruits, vegetables, and proteins. A healthy diet is usually higher in lysine. Use the chart below to ensure that the diet is higher in lysine than arginine. It would be wise to purchase an actual lysine supplement and to take about 1,500 mg. (1.5 grams) of it each day, until the virus becomes dormant.

Foods with Lysine (Encouraged)	Foods with Arginine (Avoid)
All meats	Tomatoes
Fish	Wheat Germ
Yogurt	Brussels sprouts
Cheese	Cashews
Milk	Grapes
Eggs	Pumpkin Seeds
Apples	Pecans
Pears	Blackberries
Apricots	Blueberries
Avocados	Peanuts
Pineapples	Chocolate
Green beans	Sugars
Asparagus	

The B vitamins have repeatedly been shown to help in healing damaged nerves in studies. They are also especially good for brain health, and thereby concentration. Supplementation with the B vitamins is strongly recommended. When buying these supplements, be sure to read the labels. Vitamin B-12 should be in the form of methylcobalamin instead of cyanocobalamin, B-9 should be either folic acid or the superior folate, and also supplement with B-6. These will dramatically speed recovery.

MSM (methylsulfonylmethane) has been shown to assist in the repair of nerve damage. Supplement with 500 mg. of MSM each day.

Alpha lipoic acid is an antioxidant that repairs damaged nerves, even in cases of diabetic neuropathy, which is believed to be impossible by orthodox medicine. Adults should generally take 300 mg. of alpha lipoic acid that is spread throughout each day. Although, more may be needed in some cases. Experimentation may be required to determine the correct amount, but people should never exceed 1.2 grams (1,200 mg.) per day. Take care to not confuse alpha lipoic acid with alpha linolinic acid, which is also abbreviated as A.L.A.

Purchase DMSO (dimethyl sulfoxide) from a health food store and dilute to 60% (40% distilled water). DMSO is known for its miraculous effect on nerves. Make the skin surgically clean, because DMSO has special solvent properties that will drag just about any substance through the skin. Apply it thinly to the injured side of the face with cotton. An itching reaction is normal, but the excess should be removed if it causes burning. Always store in a glass container, to prevent potential chemical reactions with plastics and metals. DMSO can be found at small health food stores, but you will not find it at any major chains. It can also be purchased on the Internet. Caution is recommended, for misuse could result in skin burns, or possible eye injuries in the case of eye contact. Therefore, DMSO may be used AT YOUR OWN RISK. If you use DMSO, remain close to a sink in case an emergency eye wash is required. When used properly, it is very helpful for treating Bell's palsy. You will notice more of a burning sensation in the areas of the damaged nerves, because DMSO is toxic to the invading pathogens and because these areas are already inflamed most.

Massage the paralyzed side of the face regularly, because this will increase the likelihood of regaining complete control of the face after the Bell's palsy.

Niacin will improve circulation in the outer tissues, such as those of the face, to speed recovery. We recommend reading the *Niacin* section of the *Supplements* chapter first, because it can have some frightening effects when it is used improperly.

Some of the luckier people who fall victim to Bell's palsy experience a tremendous improvement from a chiropractic adjustment. For those who it helps, they experience a drastic change and reduction of symptoms within 24 hours. Therefore, it is worthwhile to try, and most chiropractic sessions are cheap. Bell's palsy is aggravated by spinal misalignments, and the virus lives in the spinal column.

Low voltage electro-stimulation on the injured side of the face can result in immediate short-term improvement, and it will hasten the overall recovery time. This is the technique that earned Dr. Robert Scott Targan his 90-year sentence, which testifies to the effectiveness of it. We had success with 12-26 volts D.C. and pulsating D.C. is fine too. It is best to start at 12 volts and increase the voltage gradually, so long as the patient can tolerate it. Some pain will occur, but only when touching the skin at the damaged nerves. It is fascinating how the electrical probes can be used to pinpoint the same problem spots around the paralyzed areas, time and time again; but then change locations as the healing progresses. For the best results, rest the positive probe on the top and center of the head, and then move the negative contact around the paralyzed side of the face. Be cautious with the probes, especially if they are sharp, because the patient may suddenly move by reflex to cause a serious eye injury. Keeping the probes pointing away from the eyes while holding them sideways or diagonally is safest. The improvements brought about by this treatment can be huge, and rapid.

Unusual food cravings often occur, and it is wise to obey them. Craving fats is normal, since fats are required for nerve creation and repair, especially for those inside of the brain. Try to choose the healthiest fats that you can, and supplement with omega-3 in the form of flax seed oil capsules. An ideal dosage of flax seed oil for an average adult is 4 grams (4,000 mg.).

The Solvent Connection

Exposure to solvents can cause Bell's palsy. It may not be possible to remedy the condition if the victim is continually being exposed to them. Chemicals like glues, paints, paint thinners, polyurethane, and lacquer, which emit solvent fumes, should be avoided until the condition subsides. When the paralysis has been relieved, extra measures should be taken to reduce future exposure. We recommend the use of a rebreather mask when working around chemicals, because an effected individual is more vulnerable to chemical toxicity than most people are. The relationship between Bell's palsy and solvent exposure has been ignored by the medical establishment. Allopathic medicine is based upon chemistry, so its experts expend great effort in discounting connections between chemicals and disease states, in order to avoid the otherwise obvious conclusion that most diseases are caused (not cured) by our use of chemistry.

Conclusionary Remarks

This regimen should ensure that recovery is quick, and it is much more successful than the protocol of the orthodox establishment. It is also far cheaper than the usual brutal treatment of 10 steroid injections, which are delivered on multiple return doctor visits to ensure maximum patient bilking. There is no known singular cause for Bell's palsy, but recovery from it can be quick and relatively easy. The sooner that a recovery is made, the more likely that full facial control will be regained, which is why we provided so many options that can be combined to provide fast recovery.

Carpal Tunnel Syndrome

Carpal tunnel syndrome is a condition which occurs with repetitive motions of the wrist, usually arising from excessive computer use. It is caused by pressure on the median nerve, which runs from the forearm into the hand. This nerve controls all sensations on the palm side of the thumb and fingers, along with controlling the movements of them. The carpal tunnel is a passage at the base of the hand, made from bone and ligament, which houses the median nerve and associated tendons. When the tendons become enlarged by inflammation, the tunnel diameter is no longer adequate. This causes the median nerve to become pinched. This results in pain, weakness and numbness in the fingers, wrist, hand, and occasionally the forearm. In particularly bad cases, the sufferer may have trouble making a fist and picking up small objects.

The medical establishment often uses steroids, splints, and even surgery to eliminate the symptoms of carpal tunnel syndrome. However, there are problems with all of these strategies. Steroids cause endless problems, especially when taken perpetually. They cause type 2 diabetes. While a splint is a good solution for a broken bone, using it for muscle and nerve problems results in weakened muscles, which thereby increases the chance of a relapse. Surgery is always a dangerous option, because human error by the surgeon can result in a complete crippling of the hand, which is surprisingly common.

Alternative medicine usually deals with the causes of conditions, but carpal tunnel is a special case. Most people cannot stop the repetitive activities that cause this condition, because these activities are usually a job requirement. However, there are things that make recurrence less likely. If the cause of carpal tunnel is computer-related, using a mouse mat and a keyboard wrist rest can help substantially. These should be used by all regular computer users, because they have been documented to prevent carpal tunnel. Ergonomic vertical mice may also be used to reduce strain on the wrist, because such mice do not require the hand to be tilted in a strenuous manner. Some people experience dramatic improvement from this change alone.

Natural Remedies

- **Cherry Extract**. Cherries are known for their ability to reduce inflammation. Cherry extract is very useful in reducing all carpal tunnel symptoms. We have learned not to underestimate the power of concentrated cherry extract supplements, which can be found at herbal and health food stores.

- **Vitamin B-6** (pyridoxine). Over the past 30 years, there has been a lot of controversy surrounding the use of B-6 for carpal tunnel syndrome. Some studies have shown it to be very effective, whilst others show no difference between it and a placebo. When studies are cast aside, the Internet is full of people who are using vitamin B-6 to effectively treat their carpal tunnel. It is difficult to get enough B-6 through diet, for it is known to dissipate through cooking, it decomposes in long-term storage, and in the case of flour, it is removed by modern milling practices.

- **Devil's Claw**. A 2003 study showed that Devil's Claw extract is more effective for treating lower back pain than pharmaceutical Vioxx. Devil's Claw is known for its pain-relieving properties, and is therefore used for carpal tunnel treatment, as well as arthritis. It is a powerful anti-inflammatory agent.

- **Alpha lipoic acid**. Although it is a relatively new supplement, alpha lipoic acid has already gained a reputation for healing nerve damage. Alpha lipoic acid may be helpful in healing the median nerve in those with carpal tunnel, which would also eliminate the pain. It should not be confused with alpha linolinic acid, an omega-3 fatty acid, which is also commonly abbreviated as A.L.A.

These tips should help you to eliminate the effects of carpal tunnel syndrome, and in some cases; prevent a recurrence. Prevention is always better than cure. We strongly recommend that you try these suggestions before a drastic approach such as steroids or surgery, which could have permanent consequences.

Cluster Headaches

Cluster headaches are otherwise known as suicide headaches, because it is the common fate of many sufferers. These headaches are worse than migraines, and persist between 15 minutes and three hours, several times a day. This continues for weeks, months, or even years. These headaches frequently occur during sleep, on only one side of the head. Researchers have dubbed cluster headaches "one of the worst pain syndromes known to mankind". Those experiencing one of these super-headaches enters into a disoriented state, with confusion, short-term memory loss, the inability to understand those around them, and unbearable pain.

Especially knowledgeable readers may notice that the above set of symptoms identically occurs with oxygen deprivation. Incidentally, a pure oxygen tank is one of the few things that stops these attacks. We have extensively researched this topic for the sake of those suffering from cluster headaches, and we have concluded that cluster headaches are the result of inadequate amounts of oxygen reaching the brain.

Throughout the Internet, people with these headaches are seeking illegal drugs to provide them with relief. The drugs effect the blood vessels leading to the brain, which could help to explain their benefits. Strangely, these drugs normally constrict blood vessels, which most people would expect to cause a reduced oxygen level. In actuality, the constriction of the vessels seems to increase the flow of blood, due to the increased blood pressure. Perhaps temporary vessel enlargement is responsible for an increased overall pressure on the brain, or the problem may be solely the oxygen starvation. Regardless, lower blood pressure means a slower movement of blood, and thereby, less overall movement of freshly oxygenated blood. Until much more research is performed, this mixture of facts and speculations is all that we have for diagnosis and treatment. Research concerning how medicines specifically effect cluster headaches is lacking, due to the current draconian drug laws against the only drugs that work. The inhumane drug war continues to stop people from accessing needed medicines, and it even prevents researchers from studying their effects.

> "The authors interviewed 53 cluster headache patients who had used psilocybin [hallucinogenic mushrooms] or lysergic acid diethylamide (LSD) to treat their condition. Twenty-two of 26 psilocybin users reported that psilocybin aborted attacks; 25 of 48 psilocybin users and 7 of 8 LSD users reported cluster period termination; 18 of 19 psilocybin users and 4 of 5 LSD users reported remission period extension."

> -- Harvard Medical School, *Neurology*, June 2006

Psilocybin mushrooms (commonly called "shrooms"), morning glory seeds, and L.S.D. have all been successfully used to mediate this condition. Dosages are much smaller than are used recreationally, with no hallucinogenic effects being noted in many cases. In addition to stopping the headaches, these drugs also seem to be able to prevent re-occurrences for several days. Considering the amount of pain that sufferers experience, it would be immoral for us to avoid mentioning these extremely effective remedies. However, we cannot officially recommend L.S.D., due to its extreme effects, length of "trip", and its unpredictable nature as a synthetic drug. Likewise, caution should be taken regarding the use of morning glory seeds, because retail seeds are often coated in chemicals to prevent this use, and the dangers of these chemicals are unknown. Anyone wishing to attempt medication with morning glory seeds should purchase only heirloom or organic seeds for safety.

Many cluster headache sufferers claim that their headaches are improved, or they have lower rates of occurrences when exposed to cooler air, or when exercising outside. All of these methods have a relationship with greater oxygen exposure and short-term increases in blood pressure.

Chlorophyll supplements have the fascinating property of allowing more oxygen to enter cells, while simultaneously protecting the cells from oxidation damage. It is the miraculous substance that is used by plants for photosynthesis (turning carbon dioxide and water into carbohydrates and oxygen). We strongly recommend that cluster headache sufferers purchase liquid chlorophyll concentrate, and place about ten drops directly onto their tongues several times a day, waiting for around 30 seconds, and then washing it down with a fluid. This will also provide the person with additional energy. Due to its copper content, it works best when combined with zinc.

Dr. Johanna Budwig pioneered what is now referred to as the Budwig Protocol (Reference the *Cancer* chapter). The protocol requires a special diet that is augmented with a mixture of flax seed oil and a source of sulfur proteins, such as goat cheese. Yogurt could be used instead of the cheese, but it is not as healthy, because it is made usually from homogenized milk. The Budwig Protocol was able to cure all types of cancers, reverse arthritis, and reverse some cases of heart disease. The protocol drives oxygen deeply into tissues, creating a healthier oxygen-rich environment, and an ideal alkaline body pH. For these reasons, it should be beneficial for cluster headache victims.

L-tryptophan can be quite helpful too. It likely has a dual effect upon the headaches. First, it increases serotonin levels, which causes brain blood vessels to constrict. Secondly, it elevates blood pressure as a powerful natural anti-depressant. This is because whenever people are depressed, their metabolisms slow and their blood pressure drops. People have experienced some relief from this supplement, and it is available at some health food stores. Tryptophan brings balance to the chemicals inside the brain, creating needed amounts of serotonin, melatonin, lactic acid, and niacin. It is therefore strongly recommended.

There have been many sufferers who have benefited from breathing exercises. Given the extreme nature of this condition, it would be prudent for people to attempt breathing exercises, such as those that are encouraged by the various traditional martial arts. Deep, proper breathing will allow more oxygen into the brain, thus helping during attacks. More information about breathing exercises can be found in the *Asthma* section of this chapter.

The principle of oxygenating the body will have some readers considering the use of hydrogen peroxide for treating this condition, either orally, or with an inhaled mist. Research shows it to be of little benefit.

Colds and Flu

Those who eat a balanced and wholesome diet should seldomly become ill. Healthy people are usually able to combat minor infections without showing any symptoms. However, even healthy people become sick when their exposure to pathogens is persistent or they become too lax in their diets. Emotional stress can weaken the immune system too.

Our usual recommendations about the avoidance of most sugars, and a diet featuring vegetables should be disregarded during sickness. While these healthy habits may be ideal for preventing illness, they can actually slow a body's recovery when an infection has taken hold. During sickness, normal digestion is essentially suspended, and it is very common for the intestinal yeast to overrun the beneficial bacteria that normally helps to digest the more challenging foods, like vegetables.

What the body needs most during routine illnesses are sugary, salty, and fatty foods. Most people crave junk foods when they are sick because the body needs the ingredients of these foods to repair and defend itself. Sugars are generally regarded as villains, but it is important to remember that sugar is what gives the body energy. When a body is busy fighting an infection, sugars will provide emergency energy that a body needs, and they help the patient to be more active. Foods that are high in fat allow the body to defend the nervous system from attack, and some of the fat will be used for energy production.

Most health-conscious people consume only small amounts of salt due to the categorical slander of salt by the medical establishment. As a result, health-conscious people are often deficient in salt, and the trace minerals that accompany sea salt. Salt helps to defend the body against invaders. Because of this, those who eat processed foods regularly are ironically better protected against routine illnesses than the health conscious are; but of course, those with healthier lifestyles fare much better against serious diseases. The white, minerally-stripped, and processed table salts have contributed to our modern epidemics by lacking the important minerals that salt is supposed to contain, so stick with sea salt if possible. Increasing salt intake during sickness would be a wise approach.

Some processed foods will actually be better for a person who is sick than what we normally consider to be healthy foods. The wisest approach during sickness is to obey any food cravings that arise, because the body knows exactly what it needs.

Some of the people who read this section will assume that our recommendations are terrible because the recommendations will produce an acidic body pH. This is true. However, it is impossible to maintain an alkaline body pH during times of infectious illness. The pattern is so recurring that the human body might actually be designed to become more acidic, as a means of creating an inhospitable environment for pathogenic invaders. We certainly know that attempts to maintain an alkaline pH during an infection are futile and counter-productive. Thus, a patient should try to work with whatever the body is doing, instead of against nature. When wellness is obtained again, all of the rules revert back to normal.

The following supplements are anti-viral and anti-bacterial. They will help the body to fight an infection. The dosages provided are just estimates, and minor changes will not be harmful.

The Anti-Virals

- Colloidal silver * (3 fluid ounces 2-4 times a day)
- Myrrh * (1.5 grams for an average adult)
- Neem * (500 mg. per 125 lbs. of body weight)
- Echinacea (400 mg. per 100 lbs. of body weight)
- St. John's Wort * (300 mg. per 150 lbs. of body weight)
- Yarrow (300 mg. per 150 lbs. of body weight)
- Goldenseal root (500 mg. per 120 lbs. of body weight)

- American ginseng (panax ginseng)
- Feverfew (250 mg. per 150 lbs. of body weight)
- Vitamin C (1 gram / 1,000 mg. twice a day for adults, and half for children)

> * Never take St. John's Wort or neem when pregnant, or while trying to become pregnant. Both are contraceptives, and St. John's Wort can induce abortions in early pregnancies. Myrrh is difficult to acquire, so we are listing our source as Monterey Bay Spice Company. Excessive doses of myrrh can lead to an upset stomach. Those with lung infections should also inhale colloidal silver through a nebulizer.

Astragalus (500 mg. per 100 lbs. of body weight) should be used if the lymph nodes are inflamed. It is particularly helpful against staph infections, and any infections targeting the lymphatic system. We do not recommend using these supplements preventively, because the body may develop a tolerance to them, and then they will lose their effectiveness. The exception is vitamin C, which a person should use daily in the same amount. Feverfew is especially helpful during headaches, or for reducing fevers.

There is public concern about the use of sulfide compounds as preservatives, but they are among the safest preservatives and natural antibiotics. Sulfides were the first antibiotics and they were among the original preservatives too. They have better safety records than any of our modern antibiotics, and they work well. Sulfide-based antibiotics were not abandoned because they had lost their usefulness. They were instead discarded because the associated patents had expired, so it was entirely about the money. Whenever people are sick, they can benefit from sulfur's antibacterial properties. One of the best sources of sulfur is wine. Sulfides are naturally produced during the fermentation process that transforms grape juice into wine. Additional sulfides are sometimes added to wines as preservatives. Another method for getting plenty of sulfur is to supplement with MSM (methylsulfonylmethane). It occurs naturally in some plants, and it is considered to be the most absorbable form of sulfur, because it the same form that is found in foods. Do not confuse MSM, a sulfur compound, with M.M.S., a chlorine-based toxin and health fraud that we discuss elsewhere.

Never attempt to diet, or perform any sort of cleanse while fighting an infection. Dieting will cause the sickness to last longer. Cleanses will place extra stress on the body, and the illness could become much worse. The degree to which the sickness is exacerbated will vary depending on the type of cleanse, but all cleanses should be avoided to allow the body to fully recover. Allow at least a week after all symptoms have passed before attempting a cleanse or resuming a diet.

Alcohol as Medicine

It has long been common for media companies to mock traditional therapies; even those which have had superior safety and efficacy. Perhaps the most memorable instance of this (for those of us who are old enough to remember) was "Tennessee Tranquilizer", or simply "the medicine", from the television show, *The Beverly Hillbillies*. This medicine was homemade liquor which was commonly referred to as "moonshine". The traditional use of alcohol as a medical therapy was a long-standing joke on the show. The joke took advantage of how indoctrinated Americans are about mainstream drugs being the only valid treatment option.

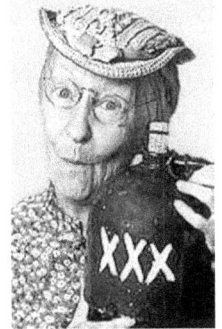

Alcohol has been used by the human race throughout most of its history as a method of boosting immunity, and for fighting active infections; as a truly natural antibiotic. Organic alcohol is one of the most effective and safe antibiotics ever discovered by man. It is a natural medicine and a gift from God. The only thing comparable in naturalness, safety, and effectiveness is colloidal silver. Alcohol's effectiveness is why doctors swab an area with alcohol before giving an injection. They choose alcohol instead of an antibiotic cream because most bacteria survives topical applications of antibiotics. In fact, we have written elsewhere about the frauds of antibacterial soaps and hand sanitizer products, and how they often have bacteria living inside them.

Alcohol is no longer recommended by doctors for the same reason that they do not recommend the use of marijuana (cannabis) or cocaine anymore. The use of natural products cannot be patented for monopolization, so the pharmaceutical industry will not allow them to be considered medicinal. The industry succeeded in banning all consumable alcohol in the United States during an infamous period of its history. If they are successful in their modern propaganda campaign, then readers will not be able to seriously consider alcohol as the safe and powerful medicine that it truly is. The truth is that about half of the viruses die faster in contact with alcohol than with any other substance on Earth. Prior to the advent of the germ theory, our grandparents already knew the truth about the benefits of alcohol, as did countless earlier generations.

It is our recommendation that vodka be chosen as the preferred medicine whenever alcohol is used as an internal therapy. This is because vodka is the purest source of consumable alcohol. Alternatives to vodka usually contain a variety of harmful impurities or yeasts, which further burden an immune system. Beer is absolutely the worst choice; due to its excessive yeast, unhealthy carbohydrates, and its low amount of alcohol per serving.

A therapeutic amount of alcohol will cause a patient to become tipsy, but drunkenness is not necessary. Human blood becomes somewhat toxic to both bacteria and viruses at only a slight degree of intoxication. It is often enough to rapidly give the patient's immune system an advantage. In the very least, this therapy will reliably eliminate much of the patient's suffering, without the long-term havoc that is caused by the residual fungal bio-toxins that are found inside today's 'real medicine'. The main negative consequence to drinking alcohol is that it is dehydrating, so plenty of other fluids should be consumed to forestall dehydration.

When to Avoid Medicinal Alcohol

The use of alcohol will be counterproductive during times of nausea or diarrhea. Alcohol may do more harm than good during times of kidney stress or kidney infection. On occasion, vodka may actually help during a kidney infection. In such cases, experiment in moderation, and use common sense. Tylenol (acetaminophen) should never be mixed with alcohol, because it can cause fatal liver toxicity. This is how many of the so-called "binge drinkers" have died on college campuses.

Colloidal Silver

Two thousand, three hundred years ago, Alexander The Great was surveying his battlefield and drinking water from silver urns. He knew nothing about bacteria, but he knew that silver containers have a seemingly miraculous way of keeping water fresh. Silver has been used for thousands of years in different forms for its health benefits. Throughout the middle ages, the wealthy gave their children silver spoons to suck upon to stave off illnesses. People have known about the benefits of silver for so long that it is incorporated into legends. Silver is the recommended agent for killing vampires, werewolves, and various forms of the so-called undead. According to ancient legend, a silver dagger was all that a knight needed to vanquish evil.

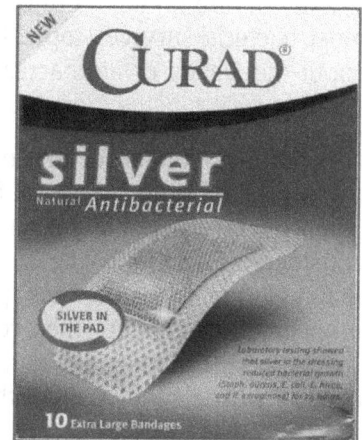

The new history of silver is a falsified history. Silver was once used extensively by all health care practitioners as an antibiotic, anti-viral, and as an anti-microbial. Nothing worked better then, and nothing does now. The F.D.A. began its crusade against silver products in the 1930's, because silver (as a natural substance) cannot be patented; but the organization's antibiotic and vaccine industry partners were able to patent their wares. Under the Food and Drug Administration's original name, The Bureau of Chemistry, its real mission was to legally protect the chemical industry by declaring toxic chemicals to be "generally recognized as safe", and to eliminate the chemical industry's competition through regulations. This history has likewise been obscured greatly in most modern historical texts, but the truth can be found in materials from its early period.

Silver medicine has been erased from the textbooks, and it is seldom given mention in medical literature. The official Pharmacopeia (physician's desk reference book) listed dozens of medicinal silver compounds prior to the mid-1930's; but thereafter, all mention of silver disappeared. Newer books report that it never really happened. Before the history was rewritten, silver was like the nuclear weapon of medicine. No human pathogen of any kind survived it. This was the gospel of medicine. Pure colloidal silver is still the most comprehensive and potent antibiotic and anti-viral known that is actually safe for human consumption, and it is absolutely safe for everyone in every condition. It is natural, has no side effects, and it was killing the worst viral diseases in the 1930's, long before it became impossible to kill viruses with medicine.

Over the past two centuries, silver has been used by both allopathic and alternative medicine. In addition to being used for routine ailments, silver has been used effectively against some of the most notoriously hard to kill illnesses, including tuberculosis and syphilis. It has been used as an anti-bacterial agent that was added to bandages and disinfectant sprays. It has been embedded into clothing to prevent bacteria from producing foul odors from sweat, and it has been merged into cloth that is used in burn centers. Attempts are still being made to lace hospital counter tops with silver, to prevent the growth of bacteria. Silver-lined containers are actively being used to disinfect water in third world countries.

Silver is remarkable because it is an extremely powerful natural anti-bacterial and anti-viral agent, yet it does not impair overall health like antibiotics do. It kills viruses, fungi, and parasites in cases where the parasites live in a symbiotic relationship with a bacterial agent. This is surprisingly common, especially in the case of blood-borne parasites, such as those of U.S. bio-weapons like Lyme disease. Because of the way that silver kills with an electrical charge, no pathogen can be found or engineered to be immune to it. No life can develop an immunity to electricity.

Since the late nineteenth century, colloidal silver has been the safest and most effective way to medicate with silver. Colloidal silver is manufactured by electrically combining silver with pure water. The colloidal manufacturing process uses no chemicals. While silver is now labeled as an alternative medicine, it was once used widely in hospitals as the premiere antiseptic and antibiotic. It is still used in hospital burn centers for its incredible ability to heal burns more rapidly than steroids. We were astounded when witnessing it eliminate a sunburn in the span of just an hour, and a burnt tongue within minutes.

Removing silver from the market was one of the first actions of the Food and Drug Administration when it changed its name in the 1930's. It has gradually changed its name from the Bureau of Chemistry to the more publicly palatable, Food and Drug Administration. In 1999, after a re-emergence of silver, the F.D.A. completely banned it in any form from being sold in over-the-counter health products, despite the fact that silver has safely been used as a medicine for millennia.

The devastation of the polio epidemic was largely caused by how the Food and Drug Administration suppressed silver to promote its new antibiotics and vaccine industries. By removing silver from the lists of approved medicines, it effectively removed the only treatment that reliably kills polio, which in-turn unleashed the full epidemic of polio. The F.D.A. later claimed a victory over polio in boasting that the new generation of vaccines had saved us. The agency cunningly waited until the epidemic was in its natural decline to release the vaccine, in order to ensure that people saw a connection between the vaccine's release date and the disappearance of the disease. The public, and quite a few doctors were distracted away from the fact that silver medications were a safe treatment, which effectively kills polio quickly, as well as virtually every other virus known. Prior to this entire smoke-and-mirrors routine, silver was recognized for doing what the establishment now claims is impossible. Had silver medicine not been stripped from the market, the polio epidemic would have never occurred. Today's huge vaccine and antibiotics markets would have never come into being. Silver had to go. Just to stack the dishonest vaccine marketing even more, the F.D.A. and the American Medical Association began promoting tonsillectomies for all children at the same time, while knowing that the tonsils are the only organ in the human body that produces polio antibodies.

The Food and Drug Administration now admits that antibiotic drugs are useless for most of the conditions that they have been prescribed throughout the last seven decades. The common cold, flu, and the most common type of pneumonia are all now believed to be caused by viruses for which antibiotics are useless against. However, silver is effective against viruses, so untold people have died as a result of silver being replaced with antibiotics.

Another suppression campaign against silver began around the time of the Second World War, when germ warfare agents were being increasingly studied as the new generation of warfare. Silver has the ability to neutralize almost every bio-weapon that has ever been created, because of how it attacks pathogens electrically. Silver will only be ineffective in cases wherein the bio-weapon is so toxic that it kills people too quickly for the silver to neutralize it, such as with ebola. Bio-weapons with that lethality are unlikely to be intentionally released, because they present too much of a risk for all parties. Silver's effectiveness against most bio-weapons is one of the primary reasons why silver has been suppressed and maligned so aggressively. There are groups within the U.S. Government that do not want anyone to be resistant to U.S. Military bio-weapons, so silver medications have been repressed throughout the world for the sake of a covert military weapons program that is forbidden by international laws. If silver medicine were still being distributed officially as the top tier of medicine, then the bio-weapons program would be rendered virtually impotent, because victims could simply use colloidal silver to recover from most germ warfare agents.

How Silver Medicine is Believed to Work

There are theories about how silver works. The leading hypothesis is that silver kills bacteria and viruses electrically, which would make it impossible for pathogens to become resistant to it. Indeed, it is true that there is no evidence of pathogens developing any resistance to colloidal silver. This hypothesis is impossible to prove (or disprove), because we cannot examine a single colloidal particle and its relation to a bacterium, or view the mechanism through which silver kills the latter. We can merely put colloidal silver and bacteria together, and see that all of the bacteria dies rapidly.

It is believed that each particle retains an electrical (ionic) charge, and that each particle of the same metal stores a charge of the same polarity. The charges ensure equal distribution of the particles throughout the solution. The theory is similar to that of magnetism, wherein the same poles of magnets are repelled by each other, and attracted only to their opposites.

There is evidence that silver interferes with copper and iron in the body, by binding with both electrically, to chemically form new metallic compounds. People who are using a large amount of colloidal silver regularly may begin to crave foods which are rich in iron, such as beef. It is wise to satisfy these cravings, since they are caused by a deficiency of an important nutrient. Copper can be safely supplemented through the use of chlorophyll, but virtually every other oral source of copper supplementation is dangerous, because it is so trivially easy to overdose with it and cause liver damage. Due to colloidal silver's ability to neutralize iron, men over the age of 30 will benefit from occasional colloidal silver supplementation. Iron accumulation in the bodies of men is believed to be one of the key reasons why women live longer than men do, and excessive iron is a major contributor to heart disease in men.

The Different Silver Products

There are many different types of silver solutions, including silver nitrates, ionic silvers, colloidal silvers, silver chlorides, and silver proteins. The only completely safe medicinal silver product, and the kind that we officially recommend, is colloidal silver.

Silver nitrate is produced by the pharmaceutical industry by combining silver with nitric acid. It can damage the liver and kidneys like most pharmaceutical drugs. It is the terrible side effects of silver nitrate that the establishment often uses to justify its attacks upon colloidal silver, in more slight-of-hand tactics. Pharmaceutical silver nitrate has a long history of turning patients' skin a bluish-gray color. Nitrates are the cancer-causing compounds that are added to meat products. In other words, the F.D.A. pushed the poisonous and carcinogenic nitrate compounds on the public again, and blamed the consequences on silver.

Ionic and colloidal silver are almost identically produced. The main difference between them is the size of the silver particles. In ionic silver, the particles are atomically small, to such a degree that even testing for their existence is difficult. It is possible that the particles in ionic silver are so small that the water itself becomes a different substance, because the silver particles are no longer completely autonomous. The particles in colloidal silver are microscopically small, but not as small as they are in ionic silver. Ionic silver can be made using very small voltages, over extended periods of time with silver plates. Higher voltages, or decreased resistance in the water produces colloidal silver. For true colloidal or ionic silver, the water must remain pure, so the only way to reduce the resistance of the water is to heat it, which most commercial manufacturers unwisely do.

Colloidal silver is much more likely to have a color, whereas ionic silver is always clear. This is because the larger particles in the colloidal silver provide a greater surface area. Ionic silver particles are so small that they are actually smaller than the wavelengths of visible light, making the silver invisible and colorless in even high concentrations. All colloidal silver solutions are mixtures of ionic and colloidal silver, but ionic solutions can be completely ionic. It is not possible to produce colloidal silver without also producing ionic silver. This is analogous to a construction worker who extracts materials from a brick wall. He might use a grinding tool that yielded only a fine powder, or he could bash the brick wall with a sledge hammer, which would yield a mixture of large chunks and fine powder. The use of higher voltages for colloidal extraction is like hammering the silver. The larger particles that are found in colloidal silver solutions are especially beneficial for external use, including the treatment of burns. Ionic silver is useless externally, and its internal effects have never been studied by independent third parties. Only colloidal silver and silver nitrate have been scientifically scrutinized for effectiveness, and only the colloidal variant is truly safe. Incredibly, colloidal silver is the only type which the pharmaceutical industry has never sold.

Another silver product is silver chloride. It is essentially made in the same manner as colloidal silver, but with the addition of table salt (sodium chloride). It is a cloudy liquid (often whitish) that is extremely photosensitive. Upon illumination or heating, the silver chloride solution separates into silver and chlorine. This instability makes it unsafe for human consumption. When ingested, silver chloride has a tendency to migrate to the outer tissues. Then, when the skin is exposed to sunlight, the silver chloride will break down into silver and chlorine. This causes the bluish-gray skin discoloration that has been heavily publicized as damning evidence against silver medicine. Victims of this phenomenon often claim that they drank colloidal silver, but the addition of salt transformed it into a very different substance that was chemically unstable. Conversely, true colloidal silver compounds are extremely non-reactive. Silver chloride has no benefits over colloidal silver, and it comes with risks. The salt is usually added to speed production time, but the same effect can be achieved with sodium bicarbonate (baking soda) in a much safer manner. The addition of sodium bicarbonate will yield especially large particles, which is unwise for internal use, but the resultant solution would nevertheless be ideal for external use. It would be excellent for burn treatments and infectious wound treatments.

Silver proteins contain much larger particles than either colloidal or ionic silver, and they should never be used internally. These were formerly approved of by the F.D.A., and they were preferred by the pharmaceutical industry. The silver particles in silver protein solutions are so large that they simply sink in the water, and the particles never stay evenly distributed without the aid of an added gelling agent. Due to the large size of the silver particles, and the silver's binding with proteins, there is a dramatically increased likelihood that silver will become trapped in the fatty tissues. Therefore, these thick solutions are likely to produce the infamous bluish discoloration of the skin too.

Dishonest Silver Companies

Misinformation is being spread by most sellers of colloidal silver. Most sellers boast about colloidal silver by showcasing its long history of safe usage, but they simultaneously claim to use a proprietary process that makes their silver superior to all other silver products. Their admitted usage of non-standard manufacturing processes means that they cannot sincerely use the safety history of colloidal silver as an example of their own product's safety, or honestly declare that their untested proprietary product is as effective. If a different manufacturing process is used, then the result cannot actually be colloidal silver. There is only one way to make colloidal silver, and any other manufacturing process will yield an entirely different product. Hence, the marketing for most colloidal silver is patently dishonest from start to end. This is not an indictment against colloidal silver itself, but its sellers tend to be morally bankrupt, and the products that they sell are potentially dangerous frauds. Every manufacturing short-cut has consequences.

We are aware from patent applications that some companies are producing silver solutions using fermenting bacteria combined with silver nitrates, instead of using electricity; but we do not know exactly which silver products are manufactured using this deplorable process. Whenever silver products are produced this way, they are inherently tainted with the dangerous nitrate compounds that the pharmaceutical silvers became infamous for. The effects of these toxic impurities can be much more severe than mere skin discolorations. Organ damage is a known consequence of using nitrate compounds, and cancers.

Most sellers of modern colloidal silver advertise that their product contains between 10 and 20 parts per million. They probably seek this concentration due to the research of Alfred Searle. He authored the book, *The Use of Colloids in Health and Disease,* in 1920. He is also the founder of Searle Pharmaceuticals. His company was respectable in its early history, and Searle was long dead before his company dishonored his memory by selling itself to Monsanto. In his book, Mr. Searle reported that a concentration of just 20 parts per million of silver was proven to be deadly to all known pathogenic life forms, including every known virus. However, these results do not equate to the 10-20 parts per million ratings that can be found on most silver products of today. The reason is that the methods of testing have changed dramatically.

Alfred Searle used a Tyndall meter to measure how many particles of silver were present in a solution. It is a device that uses light to test for hue and reflection, which are used to determine the particle count and their size. These devices use light wavelengths as the means of measurement. Most modern sellers of silver products instead purchase an electronic device that measures the conductivity of the finished product. The conductivity of different solutions will always vary greatly, so these meters cannot possibly do what they are advertised to do. For example, if salt were added to the water, then it would have a different effect on the conductivity than if copper were added, because of their differing electrical properties. Yet the sellers of these meters claim that they are able to get accurate results measuring particle counts regardless of a solution's ingredients. If salt or another electrolyte exists in the water, the conductivity of the water will increase dramatically, even whilst the number of particles will stay roughly the same. Particle size and the temperature of the solution also effect the conductivity, which the meter has no way of determining. Even a gust of wind will give a different reading, due to the electrostatic effect upon the surface of the solution. In the case of colloidal metals, electrically gauging the concentration is even more futile than it is for other types of solutions, because the metallic liquid is an electrolytic capacitor with a constantly changing capacitance. Electricity cannot be used to measure the amount of metal in a solution when the surface area of the metal cannot be verified, and when the capacitance of the solution is ever-changing. It is like trying to get a consistent light measurement from a fireworks display. The capacitive solution itself will produce its own tiny currents, and it will block currents from the meter, which makes electronic testing an exercise in absurdity. The only way to accurately measure concentration in a metallic colloidal fluid is using light. Thus, the parts per million rating given by most colloidal and ionic silver sellers is meaningless. Since colloidal silver changes the color of the water, clear colloidal solutions are frequently just expensive water, regardless of any measurement that sellers purportedly get. In the case of ionic silvers, it is impossible to measure the particle count, since the particles are too small to reflect light.

TDS Meter, the *de facto* manufacturer of the new testing equipment, even acknowledges the uselessness of its own meters on its website, in an amusing attempt at damage control:

> " ...temperature changes by a tenth of a degree may increase or decrease the conductivity. Additionally, the temperature coefficient (what the reading is multiplied by to adjust for temperature differences) changes slightly depending upon the range of ppm... Even a tiny air bubble that has adhered to one of the probes could potentially affect the conductivity, and thus the reading... Electrical charges off fingers, static eletricity off clothes, etc. on the meter and lingering electrical charges in the water will affect the conductivity of the water... Plastic cups retain lingering electrical charges more than glass. If the meter touches the side of the glass or plastic, it could pick up a slight charge. If the plastic is retaining a charge, it could also affect the water... The amount of water in the sample may affect the conductivity. Different volumes of the same water may have different levels of conductivity. Displacement may affect the conductivity as well... The depth and position of the probe in the water sample may also affect the conductivity. For example, if a meter is dipped into the water, removed and then dipped into the water again, but in a different spot, the reading may change... "

The expensive methods of testing colloidal solutions that are utilized by modern laboratories are likewise grossly flawed. Flame atomic absorption spectroscopy is one of the leading laboratory methods for analyzing colloidal solutions. It uses extreme temperatures to destroy a colloidal solution, and then observers rate the colors of the flames, in an attempt to visually gauge the metal concentration. Fire is impossible to control with the precision that is needed for a valid analysis; and of course, the test results are in the eyes of the beholder. These machines cost about $50,000 (U.S.), so it is unlikely that anyone outside of the chemical industry actually owns one. There are similar devices that utilize a beam of light that is projected through the flames during the analysis. These devices have the same inaccuracy issues, and they are even more expensive.

True Colloidal Silver

We have been unable to find any sellers of silver solutions whom we could fully trust, so this section is intended to assist people in producing their own colloidal silver. The silver solutions sold at retailers are essentially the homeopathic versions of colloidal and ionic silver products, which means that they are merely high-priced water. Some of the retail products that we examined had plenty of impurities (like iron that biologically neutralizes silver), but we found very little silver. Testing was impossible in the case of ionic silvers, which may be convenient for manufacturers. At many locations, the municipal water supply will contain more silver than the fraudulent retail products. The majority of retail products are fake, and these bogus products are the primary reason why so many people who are new to alternative medicine believe that silver is ineffective. The products that retail shoppers typically buy are usually no more effective than water, because they are water. People can either take their best guess in choosing the commercially-available products, or they can produce their own to ensure that it is real and of the best quality.

Manufacturing Colloidal Silver

The most important step in the production of colloidal silver is obtaining the right materials. Using distilled water is vital. Never use tap or spring water, because even minerals that would normally be beneficial can cause health problems once they are electro-chemically transformed through electrolysis. Ensure that the water has been distilled using steam distillation, which should be written on the container. Some "distilled" water containers have, "distilled through reverse osmosis" on the label, and these labels are entirely dishonest. True distillation uses steam to separate the water from its minerals and contaminants, whereas reverse osmosis is simply a type of pressurized filtration that does not render pure water. It is a much cheaper process, so some of the companies lie about their "distillation". Beware of Food Lion brand distilled water in particular, because our testing during the production of colloidal copper indicated that it is quite impure, even though it is labeled to have been distilled. Also be forewarned that the formation of black chunks and other strangely-colored precipitates during the electrolysis process is an indication of water impurities. Black is the most common color for these, because they are usually the charred carbon remnants of organic matter and bicarbonates. Some grayish chucks may form in the water. These particulates are actually safe and are produced by the silver. They are especially beneficial for burns and skin infections, but they should be filtered out of the solution for internal use. A coffee filter works exceptionally well for this, and the solution may be drained by gravity through a coffee maker. Silver particles which have not clumped remain in either a colloidal or an ionic state, and these will pass through any filter. In fact, the particles are so small that wooden spoons and plastic utensils will begin to develop a silvery appearance after several batches. Never use metal utensils. The only metals in the process should be the silver itself and the electrical connection wires.

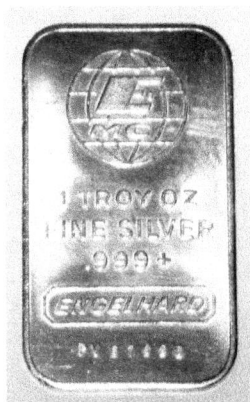

Using chlorinated tap water is especially dangerous, because when chlorine combines with other materials, it has a tendency to form dioxin compounds. It will also produce chlorine gas during electrolysis, which was used as a chemical warfare agent during World War I. Sodium chloride (salt) in the water will also release chlorine gas, so salt should never be added. As an important side note, tap water should never be used inside vaporizers for the same reason, because chlorine gas will be released into the air to actually worsen lung issues.

We strongly recommend that instead of obtaining silver wire, which is used for most colloidal silver manufacture, people instead use silver bullion bars (pictured). Most of the silver wire that is available comes from China, and it is simply not feasible to check every wire for impurities. Chinese wire should be assumed to be contaminated, since this is normal with Chinese products. When referencing the purity of their metals, companies use an obscure way of gauging it. Whenever a seller of a precious metal refers to it as having a purity of 925, it equates to 92.5 percent, so the given metal would be almost 10 percent impure. Most people will assume that a purity rating of 925 means that the metal contains only 0.925% impurities, and therefore that it would be over 99% pure. Be watchful of this gotcha. A large portion of the silver buyers seem to be ignorant of it. We recommend getting only 99.9% (written by sellers as 999) silver bullion bars.

However, modern buyers should beware even when buying "pure" silver bullion bars. It has come to our attention that the bullion market of the United States has been flooded with counterfeit bullion bars in recent years. Other countries are likely to be experiencing the same Chinese contamination problems. To minimize the risk of buying fakes, bullion bars should never be purchased from Craig's List, E-bay, or any other source that is not absolutely trustworthy, because the purity of the bullion is absolutely essential for health and safety reasons. We therefore recommend that our readers only purchase bullion bars from banks and other reputable institutions that service the financial market. In the not-so-distant past, bullion bars were an absolutely pure source of silver that were guaranteed to be safe, because they are regulated as an official currency. This once meant that any attempt to sell fake bullion bars would have risked a swift law-enforcement response for counterfeiting, and a plethora of additional charges that would have gotten a man imprisoned for the rest of his life; but alas that safety net has disappeared, for the Chinese have no fear of the law.

Coins contain a variety of metals that should not be consumed, so never use silver coins for colloidal silver manufacture. High purity is vital, because most metals are extremely detrimental to the health. Silver of such extreme purity typically only contains the impurities of copper and selenium, in trace amounts. Both of which are beneficial to health in these small quantities. In fact, both are vital nutrients. The selenium is actually used by the human body to chelate harmful metals.

To avoid any soap or chemical residues, the bullion bars should be soaked in a solution of white vinegar that is nearly saturated with salt for cleaning. They can also safely be cleaned with vodka. It is not absolutely necessary to clean the silver between uses, but we do. Be advised that the silver will never look new again, regardless of the cleaning method.

People may either use three 9V batteries that are interconnected in series, or a 30V DC power supply that has a rated output of at least 3 amps (3,000 mA), to power the electrolysis. A power supply does not have to be exactly 30 volts, but it is the ideal voltage. The range should be kept between 26 and 30 volts, which is also ideal for creating colloidal copper. Those who have no experience with electronics should opt for battery power, instead of using a DC power supply. Serious injury and fire can result from the improper use of a power supply. The electrical danger is elevated

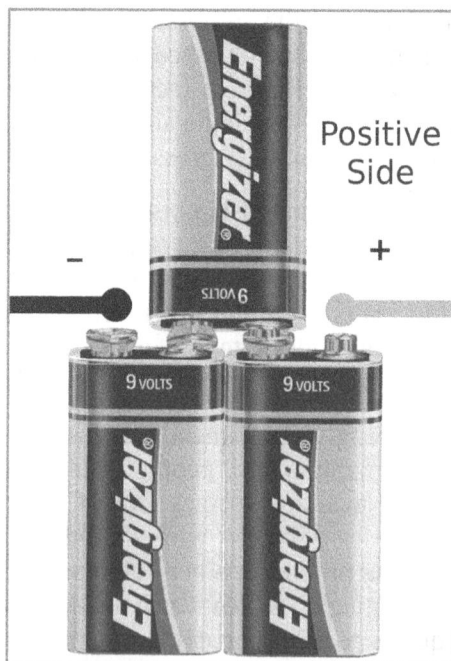

because water is being used. For liability reasons, we must officially recommend against using a power supply, and anyone using a power supply does so at his own risk. Batteries must be interconnected, so that the positive terminal of one battery is connected to the negative terminal of another battery. When properly connected, one battery should have an unused positive pole, and the opposite battery should have an unused negative pole. These two remaining terminals should be connected to the two pieces of silver. Most 9V batteries in the U.S. have terminals that can be used to interconnect with other 9V batteries, whereby connection wire is unnecessary for the battery to battery connections. Never use aluminum wire for any of the connections, and we strongly recommend the use of only copper wiring, for the sake of preventing unhealthy contaminants.

To make colloidal silver, fill a completely clean glass or plastic container with distilled water. We suggest cleaning the container with vodka immediately beforehand, to remove soap residues. Connect the batteries to the pieces of silver. Most people do this with alligator clips. We usually make our connections by inserting copper wires through tiny holes in the top of the silver bullion, and then we twist-tie the wires for maximum hold. Never solder the connection to the silver, and it is wise to even avoid soldering the wires to the alligator clips, for solder can leach lead or cadmium into the solution if the metal components become moist. Nobody should be supplementing with lead and cadmium.

The silver bars should be partially submerged in the water, and be about an inch apart. They should never touch, and the wire connections should never enter the water. If the connectors or silver are allowed to touch, the batteries or the power supply will have a dead short. This could cause overheating and an explosion. It could easily mean a quick death for the power supply. The electrical connections to the silver should be clearly above the water, else other metals will become infused into the solution. Nothing except for pure silver should be in contact with the water. We recommend that all other connectors and wires be maintained at least a quarter inch above the water's surface. We should offer one last reminder of the risks of using solder, which include the introduction of tin, lead, and cadmium into the product.

The time needed to produce colloidal silver will vary greatly depending on the purity of water that is used, and no commercially-available water is absolutely pure. One of the first indicators that silver is combining with the water can be seen with a flashlight in a dark room. Shining light through the water at certain angles will show what appears to be smoke coming from one of the silver plates. As time progresses, one of the silver plates will turn a flat gray color, and the other plate will blacken. Tiny bubbles may also form around the silver plates. Those producing a large batch over an extended period should gently stir the solution periodically, using a wooden or plastic spoon. Some people can produce a quart in twenty minutes, but our own experimentation in making 2 quarts required a duration of 4 hours to reach the acceptable strength and color. Due to the fact that silver is extremely non-reactive, a slower process indicates higher purity in both the silver and the water. Pure water and pure silver will both be very resistant to the electrolysis process. Readers may notice that many of the online manufacturing videos show colloidal silver being produced very rapidly, using silver wires that were obtained from China. The short manufacture time indicates the presence of other, more reactive metals, and perhaps impure water too. When producing our own colloidal silver by the gallon, we add about 10 fluid ounces of existing colloidal silver to speed the production time, without effecting the quality of the resultant product.

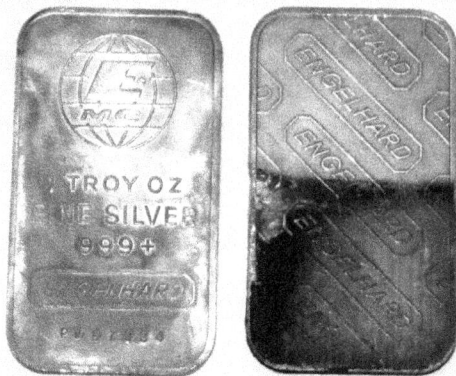

To make the silver bars last as long as possible, the polarity should be reversed each time. This means that the silver bar that is connected to the positive (red) wire in one batch should be switched so that it is connected to negative in the next batch. Otherwise, one of the bars will rapidly erode.

If a colloidal silver solution is black, brown, or purple, then it indicates that the silver particles are abnormally large. It may also reflect the presence of impurities. The huge particle size of these products makes it debatable if these solutions can truly be called colloidal. It is how most colloidal silvers from online sellers look. The ugly discolorations can also be caused by heating during production, or from the use of high voltages, which are common shortcuts taken by the commercial manufacturers. We recommend that such solutions be avoided, except as a last resort. These products are significantly less effective internally than properly-produced colloidal silver, and the abnormally large silver particles are more likely to get forever trapped in the tissues. Most commercial sellers have proprietary processes for production, which cannot be trusted, and there is no way to know what is really in their products. We do know from the color of their products that they are not selling true colloidal silver.

Properly Medicating with Colloidal Silver

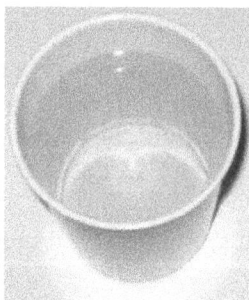

High quality colloidal silver, at an appropriate medicinal strength, usually looks slightly yellowish in a brilliant white container, under a fluorescent light. Some batches of colloidal silver will instead have a slight silvery tint. The two colors are an indication of a particle size difference, but there should essentially be no difference in effectiveness. Some batches turn yellow about a day after production. The strength of a colloidal silver solution can be judged by shining a laser pointer through the solution, whilst the silver is being infused. A red laser pointer is best, because it is least visible under normal conditions. As the silver solution gets stronger, it will become possible to see the red beam clearly through the water. As the solution becomes more concentrated, the laser beam will become more solid.

We recommend against making stronger concentrations for most uses, because silver appears to create iron deficiencies with extreme dosages. We do not truly know if the colloidal silver causes the increased excretion of iron, or if it simply neutralizes usable iron by bonding with it, or both. We believe that it is both. Either way, there are no real human toxicity issues, but the proper iron level should be nevertheless maintained for optimal health.

During times of sickness, we recommend using 3 fluid ounces of colloidal silver, twice a day. Best results can be achieved by holding the colloidal silver in the mouth for a minute before swallowing it. This technique allows some silver to penetrate through the walls of the mouth, and directly into the bloodstream. Expect for it to have a metallic aftertaste. Due to the wide variety of people who will read this book, we have made the recommended silver dosage very conservative, but some patients measure their dosages in cups.

Storage of Colloidal Silver

Colloidal silver may be stored in either plastic or glass. The ideal plastic is the type that is used to store milk. It is high-density polyethylene (HDPE), and it can be identified in the U.S. by a number "2" embossed into the bottom of the container. It is a very non-reactive plastic, but the microscopic silver particles may stain it.

Colloidal silver should be stored at room temperature, and never allowed to freeze. The silver will coagulate into visible chunks at the bottom when frozen, which will make the solution much less effective and create the possibility that it will cause argyria. Therefore, an interesting experiment to verify the presence of silver in the solution is to freeze a small amount of it, and then examine the clumped silver in the bottom of the container after thawing. If a choice must be made between storage in a hot or cold environment, the warmer environment should always be chosen.

Pure colloidal silver should not experience any of the serious breakdown problems that silver chloride solutions do whenever there is light exposure; but we nevertheless store our colloidal silver in a dark location, because darkness might somewhat help to keep it better preserved.

A good batch of colloidal silver should last for years, because the silver itself is a powerful preservative. In fact, we use it as a substitute for water in risky foods that use uncooked ingredients, such as raw eggs (for mayonnaise production). It is used to ensure that all of the bacteria is dead. A minute of blending with colloidal silver is enough to ensure that no bacteria survives.

Patients Experiencing the Blues

The medical establishment and the big media organizations have demonized colloidal silver by parading people who have developed a condition known as argyria. It is a bluish-gray discoloration of the skin that is reported to be permanent. However, every case that we investigated involved products that were not actually *colloidal* silver, and most cases were the result of pharmaceutical-industry silver products. Our exhaustive research could not find a single instance of argyria that was caused by pure colloidal silver. The pharmaceutical silver solutions are the most likely to cause it.

Regulators proclaim that the people who turned blue provide evidence of silver's toxicity, but the opposite is actually true. It proves that even after a person is so incredibly saturated with silver from 20+ years of misuse that he turns blue, he still does not suffer from any health problems. The blue patients are actually healthier than normal. Take for comparison: a patient who consumes enough aspirin to turn white. Actually, we cannot use this example, because within 20 minutes of such extreme aspirin consumption, the patient would be dead from internal bleeding -- long before he ever began changing color.

The National Institutes of Health documented one case of argyria that occurred when a man started producing his own silver solution and consumed 16 fluid ounces of it, three times each day, for a period of years. He measured his silver to contain a whopping 450 parts per million, which is 22 times stronger than is normal. This regimen gave his body the same concentration of silver as if he had consumed 1,056 fluid ounces of standard colloidal silver (8.25 gallons per day). The extreme concentration means that the silver had to be discolored and impure, and it almost certainly had salt added. Otherwise, it would have taken him days to manufacture each day's batch at such concentrations, so we can be certain that he was using silver chloride instead of colloidal silver. It is a reflection of the stupidity of turning to pharmaceutical manufacturing processes for the practice of alternative medicine, and then using the terrible results to prove that alternative medicine is bad. It is what we see most often in the politics of silver.

The most popularized case of argyria is that of Paul Karason, the so-called Smurf Man. He internally consumed large doses of a homemade silver solution for years, and then began also using silver externally on his face. He too made his silver solution using salt, which resulted in silver chloride. Despite it being a completely different substance, he refers to his solution as "colloidal silver", as does the media. We believe that after he noticed some slight skin discoloration, he actually increased his dosage, because he had found a way to become famous and profit from being a freak. He admits publicly to using excessive amounts of his silver chloride both internally and transdermally, daily for 14 years. He *still* continues to use it, despite his obvious saturation. He further admits that his face turned blue before the rest of his body; and yet he continued to use both silver products, despite the color change. Due to Karason's self-inflicted and intentional cosmetic alteration, the F.D.A. has used him in a public relations campaign that is intended to convince the public that colloidal silver is dangerous. We can only speculate about how much the media networks and the F.D.A. have paid him for his appearances.

Not one death or serious side effect has ever been recorded for pure colloidal silver, during the century of its existence. There are, however, plenty of horror stories from people who used the chemically-altered silvers that were made with various proteins, salts, or fermented bacteria.

Epilepsy

Epilepsy is a term that is used to encompass various types of seizure disorders that are believed to be caused by abnormal electrical signals in the brain. The standard therapies include anti-seizure pharmaceuticals, psychological counseling, and brain surgery.

Anti-epileptic medications are known for having horrific side effects, which include suicidal ideation, jaundice, kidney and liver failure, blurred vision, aplastic anemia (failure to produce blood cells), impaired cognitive function, bone loss, and more severe seizures. Doctors believe that these risks are acceptable, in exchange for an overall reduction of seizures. When the medical side effects manifest, doctors often fail to recognize that they were caused by the medication, and treat the side effects like spontaneously new disease conditions. The problems are caused by anything and everything -- *except for the pharmaceuticals*. This sometimes results in half a dozen absolutely unnecessary drugs being used, and worsening health problems from the untested combinations of pharmaceuticals. This is the standard of epileptic care.

There is no medical procedure which is more dangerous than brain surgery, yet this is seen as a viable option for some people who suffer from seizures. It is used by the medical establishment as a final shot (in the dark) at eliminating epilepsy.

Unless the seizures are triggered by stress, psychological therapy is not helpful for preventing seizures. However, seizures can be very traumatic for sufferers; especially when they include involuntary urination, so counseling can be helpful for some. We recommend seeking a Jungian Analytical Psychologist, when needed.

The Causes and Cures of Epilepsy

Epileptic seizures can be triggered by many additives that are in processed foods. Aspartame is known to induce seizures. Two main constituents of aspartame are phenylalanine and aspartic acid. Aspartic acid is an excitotoxin, which means that it over-excites nerves, causing them to literally burn-out and die. Phenylalanine is a known neurotoxin, so aspartame should be avoided by all individuals. Beware whenever you see "sugar-free" on a package.

Zinc deficiency has been shown to cause seizures. A study that was published in 1990, entitled, *Effects of dietary zinc status on seizure susceptibility and hippocampal zinc content in the El (epilepsy) mouse*, showed that zinc deficiency caused seizures, and this could be quickly corrected with adequate zinc supplementation. Many epilepsy sufferers have noted significant improvements in their condition with zinc intake.

Magnesium is a vital component of epilepsy recovery. Studies have verified a link between magnesium deficiency and epilepsy. Lots of people choose to supplement with magnesium using Epsom salt (magnesium sulphate). While this is an option, impurities may be present in Epsom salt, because it is not meant for oral consumption. Some companies are dedicated to selling completely pure, food-grade Epsom salt. We cannot attest to the integrity of any of these companies. If Epsom salt is used, then the ideal dosage is about 1/2 a teaspoon each morning. Otherwise, magnesium supplements are available from health food stores. Food sources of magnesium include almonds, cashews, peanuts, halibut fish, and spinach. Excessive supplementation with magnesium will cause other important minerals to flush out of the body to ironically cause even more nutritional deficiencies. So, the wisest approach is to fix the nutritional problems with diet, if possible.

The valerian herb is a very popular anti-spasmodic medication in Russia and Germany. In America, it is mostly known for its sedative effect, but it also has an anti-convulsant action that is beneficial for epileptic people. It has been additionally shown to aid concentration. Low doses are recommended to avoid its sedative effect.

Scullcap and Indian tobacco (lobelia inflata) have both been traditionally used for convulsions, seizures, and tremors. Although there have been few official studies concerning their effectiveness. Scullcap is believed to be calming, while Indian tobacco is believed to relax the muscles. Indian tobacco is technically not a tobacco, even though it is smoked. It is actually known for reversing the lung damage that is caused by smoking real tobaccos.

Vitamin B-1 and vitamin E have shown very positive results in helping people who are suffering with epilepsy. Epilepsy has been linked to a vitamin B-1 deficiency. Kava kava is a herb that contains nuciferine, an anti-spasmodic. Kava kava is relaxing, so it is best taken at night, before sleeping. Read about kava kava in the *Painkillers* section of this chapter.

Based on the aforementioned approaches, it is obvious that a good diet is essential for overcoming epilepsy. As always, we recommend avoidance of all "white" products, including white sugar, white flour, table salt, and white rice. It is especially important for an epileptic sufferer to avoid artificial sweeteners and additives. Drink spring water, and eat a balanced diet, which includes range-fed meats (preferably organic), whole grains, and organic fruits and vegetables. There are no healthy breads (not even whole wheat) in regular retailers anymore, so we recommend buying a bread maker.

People who suffer from this condition often benefit from a heavy metal cleanse, which can be purchased at health food stores or you can do it yourself using the approach in the *Cleansing* section of the *Wellness* chapter. Be sure to read the ingredients on these products before purchasing.

Radiation from sources such as the new generation of high-frequency televisions, energy efficient lights, microwaves, video game systems, radio towers, and cellular towers can trigger severe seizures.

Erectile Dysfunction

There are 30,000,000 men who experience erectile dysfunction in the United States alone. Most are over the age of forty. This is not being mirrored to the same degree in other countries, which affirms that E.D. is not simply a product of aging, or even a particular disease state. It is a product of an unhealthy lifestyle. Sexual stamina is usually the first thing to go whenever serious health problems begin to develop. This means that sexual problems, such as erectile dysfunction, are usually the first symptoms of other more serious health issues. Conversely, great drive and performance are among the best indicators of excellent health.

The Causes of Erectile Dysfunction and Loss of Libido

The American lifestyle is significantly unhealthier than that of any other industrialized country in the world. Even the water in the U.S.A. is laced with fluoride, chlorine, and various other toxic compounds, including pharmaceuticals, such as detectable levels of S.S.R.I. anti-depressants. All of these play a leading role in causing sexual difficulties.

Outside of the U.S.A., most processed American foods are considered unfit for human consumption and banned from store shelves. Some food producers actually have two recipes for the same product: one for the U.S.A. and another formulation for all the other countries not tolerating the mass-poisoning of their populations. One example is the case of Coca Cola having removed sodium benzoate from its Diet Coke throughout the United Kingdom, which was done to prevent a complete ban of the product. The ban was almost initiated because sodium benzoate causes cancers and destroys people's immune systems. In contrast, the regulators in the U.S. *work with the companies* to hide health effects from the public. It is sometimes shocking for Americans, who travel internationally for the first time, to notice the completely different recipes for exactly the same food items. Although, the two versions frequently come from the same food processing plant. In the long term, it actually costs these companies more money to maintain the dual production systems, so the mass poisoning of Americans is not done for financial reasons and it is not accidental.

Other nations do not tolerate water fluoridation, and we strongly encourage the use of non-fluoride toothpastes, due to fluoride's neutralization of iodine that is needed by the thyroid, and fluoride's overall destructive effects, including *causing* cavities. The astounding litany of poisonous effects are chronicled in the *Hidden Dangers of Tap Water* section of the *Poisoned World* chapter.

The worst chemicals seen in American-prepared foods were banned long ago in the U.K., and throughout most of Europe. There is no Food and Drug Administration elsewhere to categorically bless chemical contaminators by legally redefining dangerous chemicals as "generally recognized as safe". This is done solely to prevent legal recourse against the companies.

The bodies of average Americans are so incredibly toxic that a dead American's body will take 7 years longer to fully decompose than the dead of any other nationality, and this is not due to differences in embalming techniques. American bodies are actually embalmed long before they die by chemical preservatives that are present in foods.

It is not just the toxic chemical preservatives ruining our sex lives. Also contributing are petroleum derivatives, coal tar colorings, steroids, growth hormones, artificial fats, rancid omega oils, heavy metals, pharmaceuticals, artificial sweeteners, radiation, and now genetic engineering -- all of which are in American foods. Aggravating this is the fact that American foods are becoming devoid of all nutrition; for the vegetation that is used to feed American animals is as nutrient depleted from over-farming with chemically-engineered fertilizers as our produce is.

These things have helped the F.D.A. to make symptom management (standard medicine) the top money making industry in the U.S.A., and the leading cause of bankruptcies. Practically every adult American is taking a doctor-prescribed chemical to offset the damage that is being done by the other chemicals and the malnutrition. Americans have miniature pharmacies in their bathrooms and kitchens. Most international visitors to the U.S. are stunned when observing the chemicals in a typical American medicine cabinet.

If the previously mentioned factors were not enough, Americans have crippling degrees of stress that are unseen in other industrialized nations. Most Americans get about one quarter of the vacation (holiday) time that the rest of the industrialized world gets, and then there is the bankrupting medical system, which hardly needs further explanation. Americans are drowning in a perpetual enslaving sea of debt, even with both husbands and wives feverishly working in vain to escape their debt, and whilst getting very little rest. As long as this lifestyle is normal, new epidemics and diseases will manifest within our broken bodies and spirits.

The Mental, Emotional, and Cultural Aspects of a Healthy Sex Life

Many Americans have forgotten that they are the descendants of Puritans, and even those who are not directly related to the Puritans of yesteryear would still be the descendants of people who would be considered puritanistic by today's standards. This history still resonates throughout the American culture and within its churches.

Sex to the early Americans was in the domain of the Devil. Desire was considered impure and corrupting. Sex was only acceptable for the inducement of pregnancies amongst married couples. God had, after all, blessed both marriage and procreation. Sex was otherwise shunned by the Christian cultures of the past. It was demonized for hundreds of years by Christian peoples, and some groups still rebuke it. Indeed, sex can be sinful by Christian doctrine, whenever it is experienced at the wrong place, wrong time, or with the wrong person. The Puritans of the past took God's rules about sex to an extreme; including forbidding most sexual activities between husbands and wives. It was actually forbidden for sex to be enjoyable. They considered the enjoyment of sex to be a sinful expression of lust, even amongst married couples.

In the present, we are still suffering under the yoke of Puritan dogma. Our culture and churches sometimes still imply that sexual activities are "dirty" and ungodly, even if only indirectly. Despite our tendency to deny it, we are still so hysterical about sex that people have had their lives destroyed because someone found a picture of a naked child on a computer; and in most cases, these mentally ill individuals were given more prison time than real rapists were -- for thought crimes. So yes, Christian guilt is quite pervasive in American society, and it has impaired many married couples from experiencing one of God's greatest gifts. Sex is unquestionably one of God's greatest gifts, so he wants us to enjoy it; provided it occurs at the right time, place, and with the right person (e.g. your spouse).

Billions of dollars have been spent to foster the pop-a-pill mentality pervading society. This ongoing campaign by the pharmaceutical industry has caused Americans to forget how influential their mental attitudes are to their health and sex lives. Ask a typical American how E.D. is treated, and immediately a whole slew of pharmaceuticals will be mentioned by conditioned reflex. Pharmaceuticals are never the long-term answer to any of our problems. They only hide the symptoms, while actually aggravating the underlying conditions. Using drugs is making a deal with the Devil; for there is ultimately the *gotcha* at the end, which almost always entails slavishly needing even more pharmaceuticals. Please reference our side effects listing at the end of this section, before giving into the temptation to take the easy path.

Intimacy is a big part of sexual fulfillment, and there are always sexual problems whenever it is missing. Intimacy has become so rare for men that they rarely recognize it anymore, or notice its loss. The most romantic men (and practically all women) tell us that intimacy is sorely missing from our modern society. A little romance goes a long way toward making things work. Romance is like the foreplay of the foreplay. Skipping steps only leads to a frustrating journey. We know it is difficult to find the time, or the right state of mind in this era to be romantic, but it is so worth some extra effort. Many men assume that this does not apply to their E.D. issues, because it seems to them that only women feel a great need for romance, but this forgets a critical sexual aspect. It forgets that men are only half of the sexual equation at play, and if the woman involved seems less satisfied, then everything for the male is much more difficult. In other words, if a woman is completely aroused, then her partner becomes more capable, and he will get a tremendous psychological boost from her improved reactions.

To be romantically successful, find a time and place where you and your spouse can forget about everything else in the world. Spend that time together as if nothing else in the world matters. Both your relationship, and your sex lives are worth every minute of that invested time. Remember how you worked to impress and please one another whilst you dated? Surely that can be repeated for at least a couple of hours each week. Such time is an investment that always pays out more.

What the Allopathic Establishment Considers the Causes of E.D.

- Diabetes or pre-diabetes
- Poor circulation
- High blood pressure
- Heart disease
- Lack of exercise
- Drugs

You may notice from the list above that every one of these (except exercise) is caused by a combination of poor diet and pharmaceuticals.

Recommended Lifestyle Changes

The issues of diabetes really deserve a chapter of their own, so they are covered elsewhere. In the meantime, diabetics should know that they can reverse their condition through drastic changes in diet and lifestyle. Many pharmaceutical treatments, especially steroids and synthetic insulins, are known to cause full-blown diabetes.

Poor circulation will be encountered by anyone who has a poor diet, and it is therefore especially common in those who suffer with obesity. Remove artificial additives from the diet, along with processed sugar (use evaporated cane juice) and discontinue consuming bleached foods (e.g. white rice, white bread, white flour, white sugar). By doing so, you should be eliminating all processed foods. Remove all table salt and replace it with nourishing sea salt.

Excessively high blood pressure is something that almost never happens with a healthy and active person. Cayenne pepper is particularly helpful for blood pressure and heart issues. (It has been known to stop heart attacks.) Add it to your foods and drinks, or conveniently buy cayenne in capsule form at a health food store, to avoid the usual burning if you are especially sensitive.

Heart disease is neither genetic nor a natural product of aging. It is caused by a degenerative lifestyle for a period of many years, and the longer that this poor lifestyle continues, the worse it gets. This is why it is falsely considered to be a problem with aging, despite the fact that now even children are being diagnosed with heart disease -- telling us just how bad our diets and lifestyles have become.

In addition to blaming aging for heart disease, the medical establishment also blames cholesterol for cardiovascular problems. The whole anti-cholesterol industry and its science are frauds; and there has never actually been scientifically-valid proof that dietary cholesterol causes heart disease. Take for example that having elevated levels of cholesterol at the same time as heart disease is not necessarily evidence that one is the cause of the other; and in actuality, they are both just symptoms of the same underlying condition: namely inflammation.

Remedies for Erectile Dysfunction and Decreased Libido

- Maca root
- Fo-ti
- Horny goat weed
- Asian ginseng ("Panax" Ginseng)
- Ginkgo biloba
- Arginine (L-arginine) *
- Biotin
- Cayenne
- Vitamin E
- Minimize alcohol usage
- DHEA
- Perform a detox (cleansing) regimen
- A natural (hopefully organic) diet

> * Those with herpes may wish to avoid using arginine as a treatment, for it can trigger outbreaks. It should also be avoided during outbreaks of chicken pox or shingles, which are caused by a sister virus of herpes. Never use arginine in the months following a heart attack, because it increases the risk of another heart attack. However, it decreases the risk of heart attacks otherwise.

You may notice that the list above is for *treating* E.D. symptoms, but they cure nothing. We recommend correcting whatever underlying problem is causing the E.D., instead of just covering up the symptoms; since ignoring the root cause may lead to other serious long-term ailments.

The recommended supplements can help in the meantime. Gingko biloba is known for this, in particular. Vitamin E is known for helping with erectile dysfunction, because of its ability to boost the circulation. When buying vitamin E, read the label to ensure that it comes from a natural source. In a rather ironic twist, the best vitamin E supplements are extracted from soybean oil; which we normally recommend avoiding. Avoid all other sources of soy; especially if you are experiencing hormonal problems like E.D.

Erectile dysfunction is always a symptom of a much more serious health issue. There are herbs which can be used to treat the symptoms, like ginseng, but reckless usage can be dangerous. For instance, stimulants combined with excessively high blood pressure is a potentially deadly combination. Therefore, E.D. sufferers are advised to attack the root source of their problems, instead of merely seeking a quick fix.

The Known Consequences of Using Pharmaceuticals for Erectile Dysfunction

Viagra	headaches, flushing, abnormal or blurred vision, increased sensitivity to light, diarrhea, dizziness, shock, pain, chills, chest pain, angina pectoris, postural hypotension, cardiac arrest, heart failure, abnormal electrocardiogram, cardiomyopathy, vomiting, colitis, liver function tests abnormal, rectal hemorrhage, anemia, leukopenia, unstable diabetes, gout, hyperglycemic reaction, arthritis, tendon rupture, tenosynovitis, bone pain, myasthenia, synovitis, ataxia, hypertonia, neuralgia, neuropathy, paresthesia, tremor, vertigo, depression, insomnia, somnolence, abnormal dreams, reflexes decreased, hypesthesia, asthma, dyspnea, laryngitis, pharyngitis, sinusitis, bronchitis, sudden decrease or loss of hearing, mydriasis, conjunctivitis, photophobia, tinnitus, eye pain, ear pain, eye hemorrhage, cataract, dry eyes, seizures, anxiety
Levitra	anaphylactic reaction (including laryngeal edema), asthenia, face edema, pain, sudden decrease or loss of hearing, tinnitus, angina pectoris, chest pain, hypertension, hypotension, myocardial ischemia, myocardial infarction, palpitation, postural hypotension, syncope, tachycardia, abdominal pain, abnormal liver function tests, diarrhea, dry mouth, dysphagia, esophagitis, gastritis, gastroesophageal reflux, GGTP increased, vomiting, arthralgia, back pain, myalgia, neck pain, hypertonia, hypesthesia, insomnia, paresthesia, somnolence, vertigo, dyspnea, epistaxis, pharyngitis, photosensitivity reaction, pruritus, rash, sweating, abnormal vision, blurred vision, chromatopsia, changes in color vision, conjunctivitis (increased redness of the eye), dim vision, eye pain, glaucoma, photophobia, watery eyes, abnormal ejaculation, priapism
Cialis	asthenia, face edema, fatigue, pain, Nasopharyngitis, Dyspepsia, angina pectoris, chest pain, hypotension, myocardial infarction, postural hypotension, palpitations, syncope, tachycardia, abnormal liver function tests, dry mouth, dysphagia, esophagitis, gastritis, GGTP increased, loose stools, nausea, upper abdominal pain, vomiting, arthralgia, neck pain, dizziness, hypesthesia, insomnia, paresthesia, somnolence, vertigo, dyspnea, epistaxis, pruritus, rash, sweating pharyngitis, blurred vision, changes in color vision, conjunctivitis (including conjunctival hyperemia), eye pain, lacrimation increase, swelling of eyelids, sudden decrease or loss of hearing, tinnitus, spontaneous penile erection, hypersensitivity reactions including urticaria, Stevens-Johnson syndrome, and exfoliative dermatitis, migraine, seizure and seizure recurrence, transient global amnesia, visual field defect, retinal vein occlusion, retinal artery occlusion, Non-arteritic anterior ischemic optic neuropathy

The pattern is that each of these drugs in-turn generates more long-term business for the chemical companies and the doctors, and they slowly destroy the health of the patients. It is incredible that these are the drugs that are considered to be the most *safe and effective* by the F.D.A. There are men who were blinded by Viagra, and they would certainly disagree.

Female Hair Loss

Thirty million women suffer from hair loss in America alone, yet most people see hair loss as something that only effects men. It is usually a sign of poisoning. This problem is traumatic to the self-esteem of women, especially when they do not realize that their hair loss is caused by their supposedly "safe" medications. Contrary to what women are told, female hair loss is not hereditary, but a documented side effect of prescription drugs. A massive portion of pharmaceuticals cause hair loss, including antidepressants. This is a particularly disturbing finding, because those who are being treated for depression may suffer from this side-effect, and become further depressed by the hair loss. This combination is common for menopausal women. Beta blocker drugs that are used to treat angina, panic attacks, and social anxiety can also cause female hair loss. All hormone-effecting drugs are likely to cause hair loss, including anti-acne medications, and medications that are prescribed to increase a woman's libido. Birth control pills are especially bad for causing hair loss and other health problems that can last for years after they are discontinued. "The pill" is one of the most dangerous things that a woman can do to her body.

Doctors rarely inform women that the hair loss was caused by them. That would require ethics and taking responsibility. Doctors instead attempt to correct the condition with even more pills. There is only one prescription product that is F.D.A. approved for dealing with hair loss, which is minoxidil (brand name Rogaine). Minoxidil must be used consistently for 6 to 12 months before there are any signs of improvement, and the patient can never stop taking it without the hair loss resuming. In addition, minoxidil darkens the pigmentation of hair throughout the body in more than 80% of patients studied, and it produced heart attacks and cardiac lesions in animal test subjects.

Finasteride (brand name Propecia) is also being prescribed to some women "off-label" (without F.D.A. approval). It causes birth defects, and is therefore usually given to post-menopausal women. It is also known for causing dizziness, nausea, hypertension, and sexual frigidity.

Superior Treatments

The first thing that a woman should do if she is experiencing hair loss is look toward the medicine cabinet, and start throwing things in the trash. If the medications are anti-depressants, then be careful in discontinuing them. Most of these drugs cause severe withdrawal symptoms, because they were specifically designed to be addictive. Psychotic episodes are common withdrawal symptoms, as is the impulse to commit suicide.

Two of the most common causes of female hair loss, excluding pharmaceutical side effects, are iron deficiency and hypothyroidism. The root causes should always be dealt with instead of just utilizing symptom treatments, or else much more debilitating problems could eventually manifest. Vegetarians and vegans are the most likely groups to suffer from iron deficiencies. Eating organic, grass-fed beef will correct this condition. Certain pharmaceuticals deplete iron from the body too.

Many women experience hair loss due to extreme stress, such as from the loss of a loved one. Remember to take time out for yourself, and to do something that you love; especially physical activities. You may also wish to supplement with Saint John's Wort, a natural antidepressant. Do not take St. John's Wort whilst pregnant, or while trying to become pregnant; because it is an abortive and can cause pregnancy complications. See the *Depression* chapter for much more information.

Supplements

There are many people who use the following supplements to deal with hair thinning that is associated with aging. They can also be used to help in the re-growth of new hair, after the root cause of hair loss has been dealt with. We generally recommend vitamin E and green tea to everyone, regardless of their current health. Silica supplementation is recommended by quacks, but there is already ample silica in everyone's diets, and there is no credible evidence of it having any supplemental benefit whatsoever.

- Saw palmetto is a very popular remedy for hair loss. It is believed to work by balancing the hormone levels.

- Pumpkin seed oil stimulates hair growth, and it appears to block dihydrotestosterone in the liver, a major cause of hair loss.

- Vitamin E is used to strengthen hair, and stop the thinning of hair. Food sources of vitamin E include almonds and hazelnuts.

- Green tea is full of nutrients, and is great for the health. It is believed to help prevent hair thinning that is associated with aging, because it balances estrogen levels.

- Zinc is vital for normal hair growth. It thickens the hair, increases the speed of its growth, and prevents hair loss. Zinc is best utilized by a body when there is sufficient copper, so chlorophyll should be used as a safe copper supplement. Zinc should not be taken on an empty stomach.

- Iron deficiency causes hair loss. The safest way to increase iron is by eating beef, and beef's organic iron is considerably more effective than the iron of supplements. Lamb is an equally good source of nutritional iron.

The standard treatments for female hair loss are accurate demonstrations of the way in which the medical establishment operates. It creates the initial problem with its drugs, then it attempts to treat the new problems with even more drugs. If side effects were correctly identified, instead of being rationalized as new diseases, then less people would die each year as the result of this incredibly broken system.

Gallstones and Gallbladder Attacks

Gallstones are believed by the medical establishment to be formed inside the gallbladder: not the liver. They are thought to be few in number, instead of hundreds. Supposedly, gallstones are not linked to pains other than gallbladder attacks. Orthodox doctors believe these things, because whenever patients have acute gallbladder pain, some of the stones have already moved into the gallbladder, and they are big enough, and sufficiently calcified enough to view with x-rays. The stones inside the liver are rarely noticed. It is where gallstones actually originate.

Whenever the gallbladder is surgically removed, the acute gallbladder attacks disappear, but the bursitis, other miscellaneous pains, and digestive problems remain. Those who have had surgical removal of their gallbladders frequently continue to get bile-coated stones elsewhere that are identical to the supposed "gallstones" described by medical literature. Doctors virtually never mention this to patients beforehand, and dishonestly promote the surgeries as a permanent cure.

Gallbladder problems most often arise from poor dietary practices and lifestyles that are unhealthy. In most cases, this involves eating too much fat, whilst having few vegetables in a diet. Protein diets that minimize or eliminate vegetables are a recent fad, which easily causes gallstones, in addition to a myriad of other health problems from general malnutrition. Gallstones may also develop from rapid weight loss. Extreme weight loss usually results from the toxicity of pharmaceutical drugs, or a serious underlying health condition. Exercise reduces the likelihood of gallstones, although the mechanism through which this happens is not understood. Therefore, the story of obtaining a healthy gallbladder is a familiar one, for the rules are: get rest, get exercise, and eat your vegetables.

For the sake of long-term health, gallbladder surgery should be avoided, if at all possible. Therefore, it is actually unwise to go to a hospital for gallbladder issues, unless the problem becomes truly unbearable. We offer a pain relief solution that usually helps substantially. However, we do realize that there are occasional cases which require emergency intervention. In the worst cases, a person could use the remedy cited below before leaving for the hospital, or consume it during transit; and hopefully the problem will be resolved by the time that he arrives.

Fast Pain Relief from a Gallbladder Attack

Drink 1/4 a cup of apple cider vinegar (preferably stored in glass). If possible, also chase it with 8 ounces of apple juice (preferably organic), or mix both together. Most of the pain should disappear within 15 minutes. Do not attempt to perform the 2-day cleanse during an attack.

Prevention and Treatment of 'Gallstones'

The following natural protocol helps to correct liver dysfunction, in addition to helping combat gallstones (liver stones). It will holistically improve a person's overall health too. Several of the recommendations target cholesterol, because stones are often made of cholesterol.

- Reduce fat intake overall, especially unnatural and toxic fats like hydrogenated oils, soy, and canola. Natural fats (like butter) are better, but they should be used in moderation nonetheless.
- Ox bile can greatly ease the burden of the gallbladder, thereby giving it an opportunity to heal. It may be purchased in supplemental form, and it should be taken with fatty meals (e.g. meals which contain meat or lots of cheese). Ox bile also provides relief to individuals who have had their gallbladder removed, and who subsequently have difficulty in digesting food. Do not take ox bile on an empty stomach, because it can cause stomach disturbances.
- Omega-3 supplementation is recommended by way of flax seed oil capsules.
- Niacin (vitamin B-3) is helpful for people with cholesterol or skin problems.
- Red yeast rice reduces cholesterol, and its active compound is used to make pharmaceutical drugs for cholesterol. This has the benefits of the drugs, without the dangers, addictions, or expense. For years, the F.D.A. tried to block sales of unprocessed red yeast rice and supplemental extracts, because they compete with the patented drugs that are based on the same rice; so the all-natural rice was conveniently reclassified as a "drug". This has become a common trick ever since the U.S. Congress forbade the F.D.A. from regulating nutritional supplements, in lieu of its similar abusive behaviors.
- Sunlight exposure converts the excess cholesterol reserves stored inside skin into vitamin D-2, which is later used by the liver to make vitamin D-3. Therefore, sunlight helps in multiple ways. It dramatically boosts the immune system.
- Exercise. No explanation should be required.
- Milk thistle (available as a supplement) is a liver tonic.
- Dandelion root (available as a supplement) is another liver tonic.
- Avoid soy lecithin and all soy products. Soy products can have disastrous effects upon

hormone balance, and this is especially true for women. The phytoestrogens inside soy products attack the thyroid. The presence of gallstones has been shown to have a relationship with hormone imbalances. Also, be advised that all soy is now genetically engineered.

- Vitamin C makes cholesterol more water soluble, allowing a body to better eliminate excesses.

- Turmeric increases the solubility of bile.

- Consume apple cider vinegar, lemonade, or apple juice regularly. Supplementing with several tablespoons of apple cider vinegar per day is best.

- Castor oil transdermal packs neutralize inflammation. Reference the *Endometriosis* section of the *Women's Health* chapter for instructions on how to make and use one.

- Licorice is another liver tonic.

The 2-Day Gallbladder Cleanse Procedure

There are other, more thorough cleanses available, but these take a minimum of a week to implement. Anyone who is trying to rid himself of gallstones wants fast relief.

Ingredients

- 1/2 cup of cold-pressed, extra virgin olive oil
- 3 cups of fresh grapefruit juice or fresh apple juice
- Chamomile supplements
- 1 large grapefruit (or 2 small)
- 3 lemons (optional)
- 4 tablespoons of Epsom salt

Preparation

1. Test to see if you have a bad reaction to Epsom salt by holding about a 1/4 tsp. of it in your mouth for about half a minute, and then swallow it. If there are any problems, then this entire procedure should be aborted. The test is essential for safety, because an allergic reaction to the massive amounts used later could be fatal.

2. This is a 2-day procedure, so ensure that you have two days that are completely

free of obligations before beginning. Most people should begin on a Saturday.

3. Try chamomile tea to test for a ragweed allergy.

4. Discontinue all medicines, vitamins, pills, and herbs if possible.

Procedure

1. Eat a no-fat breakfast and lunch, such as cooked cereal with fruit, fruit juice, bread and preserves, bread with honey, baked potato, or vegetables that are salted only. Consume no butter, milk, or cheese. These fat-free meals allow bile to build up and develop increased pressure within the liver.

2. 2:00 P.M. -- Discontinue all food. No cheating! Breaking this rule can later cause illness and a failure of the flush. Prepare the Epsom salt solution by mixing 4 tablespoons with 3 cups (24 fluid ounces) of grapefruit juice or apple juice inside a large jar. This makes four servings of 3/4 a cup. Place the jar inside a refrigerator to get it cold (this is for convenience and improved taste). Both grapefruit and apple have properties that aid the cleanse, in addition to making the procedure more bearable.

3. 6:00 P.M. -- Drink one serving (3/4 of a cup) of the Epsom salt solution. You may add 1/8 tsp. of Vitamin C powder to improve the taste. You may also drink a few mouthfuls of water afterward, or rinse your mouth. Place the cold-pressed olive oil and grapefruit on the kitchen counter to warm up.

4. 8:00 P.M. -- Repeat by drinking another 3/4 cup of Epsom salt solution. Ready yourself for resting, because timing is important for success.

5. At 9:45 P.M. -- Pour 1/2 a cup of olive oil into the pint jar. Then squeeze out the grapefruit juice into the measuring cup. Remove the excessive pulp. You may add lemon juice to improve the flavor. Add the juice(s) to the olive oil. Seal the jar tightly and shake it vigorously. This should make at least 1/2 a cup (3/4 a cup is better) of this mixture, but do not drink it yet. Visit the bathroom, even if it makes you late for your ten o'clock drink. Do not be more than 15 minutes late, or you will expel fewer stones.

6. 10:00 P.M. -- Drink the olive oil solution. Take four 300 mg. chamomile capsules with the first sips to help you sleep through the night. Drinking through a large plastic straw helps it go down easier. You may use oil and vinegar salad dressing, or straight honey to chase it down between sips. Have these ready in a tablespoon on the kitchen counter. Make certain you drink it standing up. Get it swallowed within 5 minutes (fifteen minutes for very elderly or weak persons). Lie

down immediately afterward on your right side. The sooner that you lie down, the more stones you will get out. Be prepared for bed ahead of time. Do not bother with clean up, because timing is very important. Try to keep perfectly still for at least 20 minutes after laying. You may feel a train of stones traveling along the bile ducts like marbles. There should be no pain because the bile ducts are dilated to full size, due to the Epsom salt solution. Go to sleep.

7.   Next Morning -- Upon awakening, take your third dose of the Epsom salt solution. If you have indigestion or nausea at any point, treat it with ginger supplements, and wait until it has passed before drinking the Epsom salt solution. If you absolutely can not hold the ginger in the stomach, then hold the ginger powder in the mouth for direct blood absorption through your cheek tissues. You should return to bed after you have finally consumed the Epsom salt solution. Do not begin this step before 6:00 A.M.

8.   Two hours later -- Take your final dose of the Epsom salt solution and return to bed again.

9.   Two more hours -- You may finally eat again. Begin with only fruit juices. Half an hour later, eat fruit. After another thirty minutes, you may eat regular foods, but keep the meal light. By evening, you should feel recovered.

Conclusionary Remarks

Expect diarrhea during this procedure. It is normal, so do not be alarmed. This regimen does not brutalize an already weakened body, and leaves the person stronger in the long term. It is cheap, fast, effective, all natural, and generally very safe. Unlike modern medical treatments, these methods will usually cure the problem, instead of merely suppressing the symptoms until the problem becomes much worse.

Precautionary Statements

Disregard our entire cleansing procedure if you have allergies or other negative reactions to any of the ingredients used for it. If you are experiencing serious health issues unrelated to the gallbladder, then we recommend delaying this cleanse until the other issues have been resolved. Readers must use their own common sense to determine if they are having a health emergency, and to take appropriate action if so. Do not perform this cleanse during a gallbladder attack.

Hypothyroidism

Hypothyroidism occurs when the thyroid gland has been weakened by poor nutrition, thyroid toxicity, bad lifestyle, stress, and too much medical 'help'. A victim of hypothyroidism has a body that can no longer adequately produce vital hormones. The establishment considers it to be yet another "autoimmune disease"; unilaterally rejecting all legitimate causative factors. The immune system only attacks things that it detects as being toxic.

Symptoms of Hypothyroidism

- Mood swings
- Cold sensitivity
- Weight gain
- Depression
- Heavy or irregular menstrual periods
- Constipation
- Fatigue
- Dry skin
- Brittle hair, skin, or fingernails
- Hair loss

The thyroid gland is suppressed by the intake of soy; an ingredient in the great majority of processed foods, and even in most of the so-called healthy alternatives. Additionally, fluoride is extremely damaging to the thyroid. Until the 1970's, doctors prescribed fluoride to patients with hyperthyroidism (an over-active thyroid) in order to cripple it. It was shown to be effective at 2 mg. per day. People in the present are estimated to be consuming 2-10 mg. per day from tap water, non-stick cookware, toothpaste, pharmaceuticals, infant formula, processed cereals, and sodas. Hypothyroidism is also recognized to be caused by certain medications, such as lithium.

All S.S.R.I. anti-depressant drugs feature fluoride as a main ingredient, so these psychiatric drugs dramatically contribute to thyroid disorders, and they are the primary cause of hypothyroidism in some cases. S.S.R.I. drugs are notorious for causing nutritional deficiencies, due to their overall toxicity and because they dramatically disrupt the serotonin that is used for digestion. Contrary to the dishonest drug company marketing, only 10% of an individual's serotonin is used by his brain, while about 80% of it is used by his digestive system. Without the proper nutrients, hypothyroidism cannot be cured, because those nutrients are needed to balance the hormones and to strengthen the thyroid. S.S.R.I. drugs furthermore reduce usable calcium in the body, and thereby render magnesium unusable; since magnesium and calcium are interdependent. Magnesium deficiencies are rife in modern society because people do not eat enough green leafy vegetables. A severe magnesium deficiency can lead to sudden heart attacks, and lesser deficiencies cause heart attacks when monosodium glutamate (MSG) is consumed. People who have hypothyroidism are much more likely to have heart problems, because the hormones that are produced by a healthy thyroid help to strengthen heart contractions and regulate heart rhythm.

The medical establishment prescribes synthetic hormone pills to hypothyroidism patients, and patients must continue taking them for the rest of their lives. This is because these artificial hormones cause a body to stop producing its own thyroid hormones *permanently*; similar to what is experienced with diabetics taking synthetic insulins. In both cases, the result is perpetual customers who will forever after be reliant on the system, because the medications destroy the organ that they supposedly help. Be forewarned that there is no cure with orthodox therapies, and there may be no turning back.

The medical establishment's tests for hypothyroidism are unreliable, so multiple consecutive tests may produce differing results. As a result, some people are drugged for the rest of their lives for a disease that they did not actually have, until they began the drug regimen. Those who are given the pharmaceutical hormones develop hypothyroidism that is much more difficult to cure than those who did nothing at all, or those who turned to the alternatives immediately.

> *"Dessicated natural thyroid does not have FDA approval and its availability became quite limited in 2009. Many consumers complained to the ombudsman because of their preference for dessicated natural thyroid as thyroid replacement medication over the FDA approved synthetic versions"*

-- F.D.A.

In the 1890's, the original conventional medicine (what is now alternative medicine) began using all-natural hormones to treat hypothyroidism. These natural hormones were extracted from animal sources. In 1958, the chemical industry first began producing the completely synthetic versions of the hormones, which were marketed as being identical to the natural hormones that had been used for decades. Soon thereafter, the F.D.A. began playing a political game to suppress the use of the significantly safer, animal-based hormones for no other reason than increasing industry profits. Behind its corrupt shenanigans was the fact that chemical formulations can be patented, but natural hormones cannot. It avoided a political backlash by not *officially* banning the natural hormones, but it nevertheless accomplished the same goal by re-categorizing natural hormone treatments as "not approved" therapies. Thus, a doctor risks his medical license, and increases his lawsuit risk, if he prescribes the natural hormones. It is another example of the F.D.A. eliminating competition for its top pharmaceutical partners using cunning methods. Treating hypothyroidism has become much more expensive and dangerous as a result. The new synthetic hormones are addictive to the extreme, as only chemistry can provide. It follows the same addictive pattern seen with cholesterol medications, hypertension medications, diabetes medications, cancer treatments, anti-depressants, and pharmaceutical record-holders like Heroin (from Bayer). The chemical industry's synthetic hormones cause both heart disease and cancers, but they help to cover a doctor's assets.

How To Cure Hypothyroidism

In alternative medicine, there is very little difference in the curing of hypothyroidism and hyperthyroidism. This is because the treatments involve assisting the thyroid to heal, in either case. Those with hyperthyroidism should not use iodine, because it could overdrive the thyroid, worsening the condition.

Curing thyroid disease requires a long-term commitment for a period of at least a year. Creating this problem took years of self-poisoning, so fixing it is neither quick, nor easy. Hypothyroidism medications are addictive, and the body becomes reliant on them, which is why the mainstream establishment maintains that people must take them forever. Those who have been taking hypothyroidism medications for years must slowly wean themselves from the drugs. Abruptly stopping these medications will result in extreme fatigue, and additional thyroid problems.

Recommendations

- **Discard all non-stick cookware**

- **Eliminate soy:** Soy suppresses thyroid functions, imbalances hormones, and it has been shown to cause goiters (an enlargement of the thyroid gland) in previously healthy individuals, which shows that it disrupts iodine usage.

- **Adhere to an alkaline diet:** This is extremely helpful when curing any chronic disease. Reference the *Body pH and Disease* section of the *Wellness* chapter to guide you.

- **Balance estrogen levels (women):** Excess estrogen slows down the thyroid gland. This means eliminating birth control medications, increasing the fiber in the diet, and avoiding all non-organic meats. Reduce dairy intake, because milk often contains lots of estrogen.

- **Exercise:** Find a physical activity that is fun, and do it often. We believe that exercise could half the cure time in some cases, and curing is not possible without it.

- **Hemp fiber:** This is a broad-spectrum supplement and a mild laxative.

- **L-tyrosine:** Tyrosine is a natural amino acid which helps the body produce its own thyroid hormone. This is also known to help with the depressions that usually accompany hypothyroidism. Most naturopaths recommend that 500 mg. be taken 2-3 times daily.

- **L-arginine:** Arginine is known to stimulate the thyroid and its hormones. It also improves immune function, improves fertility, and alleviates erectile dysfunction.

- **Avoid all sources of fluoride:** As already mentioned, fluoride suppresses the thyroid, and is likely to be the leading cause of hypothyroidism. Drink spring water, avoid soft drinks, use fluoride-free toothpaste, use a shower filter, and throw away non-stick cookware.

- **Eat a natural diet:** To help the body heal itself, remove burdens on its immune system. This means that all processed foods, artificial flavors, colors, preservatives, white flour, white sugar, table salt, hydrogenated oils, aluminum, high fructose corn syrup, and etcetera should be eliminated from the diet. Organic food is the ideal. Do not trust marketing that reads "all natural", because this phrase is intentionally unregulated, so that anyone may use it for anything. Read labels carefully.

- **Iodine:** The thyroid needs iodine to function properly, and lots of people now suffer from iodine deficiencies. To test yourself, place some iodine (we use 2%) on your stomach. Make a dot the size of a silver dollar (or twice the size of a British 50p). If it disappears within 12 hours, then you are iodine deficient. Keep adding iodine in increasing amounts, until it no longer disappears in a 12-hour period. This works due to the fact that the body transdermally absorbs iodine at the rate that it is needed. Do not use povidone iodine and do **not** orally consume iodine. This is an especially important precaution for those with Hashimoto's thyroiditis. Red marine algae is the only means to safely orally supplement with iodine, but beware of other types of underwater vegetation. Baked fish is the safest and most natural way to consume iodine, but beware of bottom feeders, shell fish, krill, etc. Think kosher in regards to fish.

- **Chlorophyll:** Supplementing with chlorophyll provides essential copper, helps oxygenate the body, builds healthy red blood cells, and it overall assists with skin health. Chlorophyll is a safe method of orally supplementing with copper.

- **Pears and apples:** The ancient Chinese discovered that pears have a powerful tendency to balance hormones; especially in women. Pears help most when mixed with or juiced with apples. Try our pear juice recipe, and drink it regularly. It is titled *The Hormone Regulator* in the *Juicing* chapter.

- **Zinc and selenium:** Studies indicate that severe zinc or selenium deficiencies can cause decreased thyroid hormone levels. Never take zinc on an empty stomach. Brazil nuts are high in zinc and selenium.

- **Coconut oil:** Buy organic, cold-pressed coconut oil from a health food store. Take about 1 teaspoon of it daily. You can also use it to cook with, but be warned that it smokes at low cooking temperatures, so it should only be used for low-heat cooking. Coconut oil speeds the metabolism, encourages production of the thyroid hormone, and kills candida yeast.

- **Avoid canola oil:** Canola oil interferes with the production of thyroid hormones, amongst its many other dangers. Treat canola oil like the genetically-engineered abomination that it is.

Additional Notes

If depression becomes is a serious problem, then sufferers may wish to read the *Depression* chapter. Chronic constipation can be addressed by adding additional dietary fiber, such as psyllium or the superior hemp fiber. Sufferers will also want to take flax seed oil, and combine it with a food containing sulfur proteins; for example, goat cheese or eggs. This follows the Budwig Protocol's methodology, which decreases inflammation, increases oxygen intake, stimulates beneficial intestinal flora, and it provides a mild laxative effect.

Heavy metals and toxins can cause the thyroid to malfunction. This is particularly true in cases of Hashimoto's disease, wherein the thyroid is so poisoned that the immune system begins attacking it. Most people with thyroid disease will benefit from a heavy metal and liver cleanse, because thyroid impairment is generally the result of toxicity.

Hashimoto's Thyroiditis

There is a lot of conflicting information regarding the application of iodine to treat Hashimoto's thyroiditis, so it is prudent that we comment. Dosage is especially important in these cases, as an overdose of iodine can cause the thyroid to shut down completely. However, a small amount of iodine does help this condition. Problems usually occur for those who take potassium iodide supplements, and those who take internal iodine drops. However, there is no evidence of adverse effects for those who moderately apply iodine transdermally. Applying iodine to the skin allows the body to regulate the iodine's absorption rate.

Kidney Stones

Kidney stones are believed to be caused by mineral formations. They are frequently described by people as the most painful experience of their lifetimes. It is this intense pain that propels most sufferers to seek fast relief from doctors. Thereafter, drugs are prescribed that are intended to dissolve the stones, but if the stones are too large to pass, then surgery is conducted. Ironically, the surgeries can increase the risk of having further kidney stones; especially in overweight patients.

Mineral stones are the most common type of kidney stones. They can sometimes occur when people do not drink enough water, resulting in minerals and salts clumping together into "stones". It is believed that an excess of calcium causes kidney stones, but the stones are technically caused by a body lacking other minerals. The human body requires a diverse group of minerals, in order to be able to utilize calcium properly. If calcium cannot be properly combined with vitamin D-3 and magnesium, due to poor nutrition, then the resultant wasted calcium can bind with other materials to form into kidney stones, or the calcium may line the arterial walls to play a role in coronary artery disease, amongst a long list of problems. Various pharmaceuticals and artificial food additives, such as MSG, deplete minerals to make kidney stones, and a variety of other health problems much more likely. This mineral starvation is one reason why people with kidney problems will usually develop heart ailments too. The connection between the two was discovered about 3,000 years ago, by Traditional Chinese Medicine. Our modern doctors have not discovered it yet.

Prevention

To prevent kidney stones, people should drink enough water for the urine to run clear, and they should also have a diet that features fruits and vegetables. It is not possible to have completely clear urine in the hours following vitamin B supplementation, and excessive vitamin B-6 will cause neon-green urine. Magnesium is needed to properly utilize calcium. It is found in green leafy vegetables, cashews, almonds, and walnuts. Spinach is especially high in magnesium, and baby spinach is even more nutritious. We recommend against taking magnesium supplements, because excessive magnesium causes other important minerals to be flushed out of the body. Vitamin D is available in some foods and supplements. The vitamin D that is synthesized as a supplement has only partial effectiveness, and it is rejected by some bodies outright. The best food source of vitamin D is baked (not fried) seafood, but avoid fish that is farm raised or imported from God-forsaken countries. A body will also manufacture its own vitamin D with sunlight exposure, and the tanning process additionally helps a body to remove excess cholesterol.

Symptoms of Kidney Stones

- No symptoms will appear if the stones are extremely small, but the kidneys will not function optimally
- Sudden, severe pain that gets worse in waves. Stones may cause intense pain in the back, side, abdomen, groin, or genitals
- Nausea and vomiting
- Blood in the urine, or strange urine colors
- Inability to find a comfortable position
- Frequent and painful urination, which usually occurs when a stone lodges in a ureter, but it may also indicate a bladder infection that was caused by the stones

---

Eliminating Kidney Stones

Some people have managed to pass kidney stones by eating large amounts of watermelon. However, our research has concluded that the popular lemon juice and oil combination is the most effective method. Lemon juice breaks down the stones, while the oil provides lubrication to allow the stones to pass.

To perform a lemon and olive oil cleanse, blend 5 ounces of lemon juice with 5 ounces of olive oil. Extra-virgin olive oil is best because it is the healthiest, and it has a thicker consistency than most other food oils. People may wish to add a small amount of honey to improve the taste. Drink the solution as quickly as possible. Do this once in the morning, and once in the late afternoon. Continue this for several days, or until the stone passes. Drink plenty of water throughout this process, including extra lemon juice if possible.

Lyme Disease

For the sake of brevity, most of the research that we have compiled about Lyme disease is being omitted from this edition. The omissions include how Lyme disease is a U.S. Military bio-weapon that was accidentally released from the Plum Island facility, as was the West Nile Virus, bird flu, swine flu, and others. By the time that you read this, we may have a thorough report online, or an audio show at our site, HealthWyze.org. You may read about the illegal germ warfare program, which dates back to Operation Paperclip, in the book, *Lab 257*.

Finding useful and credible information about Lyme disease is exceedingly difficult, because those who have done research are usually afraid to talk about their findings. Our research causes us to conclude that weaponized Lyme disease employs a genetically-modified hybrid of syphilis, like the one that was used in the infamous Tuskegee Experiment. It lives in a symbiotic relationship with a microscopic parasite which it nourishes. This explains why the disease is so difficult to eradicate. Attacking only the virus without attacking the microscopic worm can enable the worm to flourish, reproduce, and to breed more of the viral component. Therefore, a two-pronged approach is needed to effectively cure Lyme disease. The virus and the worm should be attacked at the same time.

Jarisch-Herxheimer Reactions

Most commonly referred to as simply "herxes" or "Herxheimer reactions", this is when toxic die-off wastes result from the death of spirochetal pathogens. The name was given by Karl Herxheimer, who noticed this reaction when studying syphilis. When it dies, endotoxins are released. Whenever this occurs at a rate faster than a body can flush the wastes; fever, chills, rigor, muscle pain, hyperventilation, skin flushing, and a worsening of skin lesions can result. Due to these reactions, Lyme treatments can often make the symptoms worsen before they get better. It is important to differentiate this phenomena from a worsening of the actual condition. This reaction should be anticipated in any effective program.

The Health Wyze Lyme Disease Protocol

- **Astragalus** - The idea of using astragalus for a syphilis-like pathogen comes from Traditional Chinese Medicine, and this therapy was verified by American physicians in the early 20th Century (before the A.M.A. took over and eliminated natural therapies). It is known for strengthening the kidneys, liver, and heart. It also drives pathogens out of the lymph nodes, making it easier for the immune system to attack them. Some people who have had chronic Lyme for several years find that astragalus, even in small amounts, provokes too many symptoms, so they opt to forgo its use. However, this is unwise, and astragalus is one of the most important treatments. To understand the side effects, read about Herxheimer reactions above.

- **Parasite cleanse** - The topic of parasite cleanses is too large for us to adequately cover here, but a thorough and long-term parasite cleanse is of vital importance for killing Lyme disease. Read the *Parasites and Lupus* section of the *Alternative Medicine* chapter for detailed information about how to do it.

- **B vitamins** - The B vitamins, particularly B-6, B-9 (folic acid), and B-12 (methylcobalamin) are known for healing damaged nerves.

- **MSM** - MSM is a sulfur protein that helps with joint pain, and it assists in repairing nerve damage. A standard adult dosage is 1 gram daily (1,000 mg.). Do not confuse it with M.M.S., which is a dangerous fraud.

- **Food cravings** - It would be wise to satisfy specific food cravings, because the body likely knows what it needs. It is also important to remember that children may take advantage of this suggestion, and suddenly "crave" ice cream constantly.

- **Colloidal silver** - This is a natural and general purpose anti-fungal, anti-bacterial, and anti-viral. It works electrically instead of chemically, so pathogens cannot develop any resistance to it. A reasonable starting amount would be 1 fluid ounce that is taken twice a day. An ounce is equal to two U.S. tablespoons. For maximum effect in the bloodstream, it should be held in the mouth for a minute before swallowing. If the patient gets noticeably sicker, then you need to immediately decrease the daily amount. Later, you should increase the dosage, but you must not increase it too rapidly, due to the toxic die-off reactions. One method of determining the ideal therapeutic amount would be to increase the dosage every day until the patient gets slightly sicker, and then cut back to a dosage that is slightly lower than that amount. Then use this ideal dosage for a couple of weeks before trying an increase again. Read the *Colloidal Silver* section of the *Alternative Medicine* chapter to learn how to make your own, because bad colloidal silver is worse than none at all.

- **High salt diet** - Use unrefined natural sea salt in all meals. If it is bright white, and therefore stripped of minerals, then it should be avoided. Good salt can only be found in health food stores and online. The extra salt will make the body inhospitable to pathogens, and it will simultaneously give better penetration to the colloidal silver, making it more effective. Unrefined sea salt also contains trace minerals that will help to negate the negative effects of increased sodium. Extra salt has the benefit of making a patient drink more, and keeping fluids circulating. Having Lyme disease and a high salt diet will make high blood pressure very likely. Just be watchful that it does not become dangerously high.

- **High fat diet** - Healthy fats are necessary to protect against central nervous system damage, and to heal any existing nerve damage. A key component of the Budwig Protocol, which involves mixing flax seed oil with full-fat yogurt or cottage cheese, would be very beneficial.

- **Echinacea** - This is well known for its efficacy in removing venom from the body. It is a very common treatment by those who are fighting Lyme disease, for this reason. Do not begin taking echinacea until the correct colloidal silver dosage is determined, else it will be impossible to determine if the worsening symptoms are due to echinacea or silver. Echinacea is known for making people feel worse for a short time after taking it, followed by them feeling much better. Due to this, it should be taken only once each day. Break from using the echinacea after three weeks, because it will lose its effectiveness. Stop taking it for a week, before restarting for another three week period.

- **Chlorophyll** - This provides the body with better oxygen absorption, which will support the body overall. In addition, it provides a safe amount of copper, which will make the body more toxic to pathogens. It will also give the colloidal silver better penetration, because silver will electro-chemically bind with the copper that is inside the chlorophyll.

Optional

- **Niacin** - Otherwise known as vitamin B-3, niacin can increase the deep tissue penetration of the other treatments, especially colloidal silver. Niacin is an unusual supplement with unusual effects, so read the *Niacin* section of the *Supplements* chapter before using it. We recommend that people not use more than 100 mg. daily.

- **Gotu kola** - Historically, gotu kola was known for its toxicity to syphilis, so it can be assumed that it will help to kill Lyme pathogens. Gotu kola is typically supplemented using dosages of 500 mg. per day, but if it causes strong Herxheimer reactions, a lower dose is prudent.

- **Ginkgo biloba** - This is used to clear the mental fogginess that is a common symptom of Lyme disease. The standard dosage for an adult of average build is 120 mg. daily.

- **Bentonite clay** - Make a paste out of bentonite clay, and rub it over the spine every day. Lyme disease pathogens are known to congregate around the spinal column. Bentonite clay can somewhat penetrate the skin to cleanse venom and toxins out of the body, so it may be helpful in removing the die-off toxins.

Conclusionary Remarks

Lyme disease is a serious condition, and it is often permanent when it is treated with standard care. This is due in part to the fact that doctors usually deny the existence of chronic Lyme disease (most cases), and they categorically ignore the parasitic component. Symptoms which continue after two to three weeks of antibiotics are labeled as "Post-Lyme Syndrome", and victims are instructed to ignore future symptoms. Patients who do not comply in being silent are frequently accused of having mental illnesses, and they are then treated psychiatrically for the sake of medical political correctness, and to suppress meaningful investigation into what is really happening. It is the way that the U.S. Department of Defense wants to keep things. Curing Lyme disease is not easy, and it may require long-term dedication. To ensure success, the recommended protocol should be continued for three months after all symptoms subside. There has been some success in curing Lyme disease with standard therapy, for cases which were caught early enough, but only similar alternative therapies will work for well-established infections.

Migraine Headaches

Migraine headaches are caused by inflammation, and effort should be made to ascertain the cause, so that they can be prevented. The causes are almost always dietary, and the main aggravating factors are listed below.

Aggravating Inflammatory Factors

- Monosodium glutamate (MSG)
- Artificial sweeteners
- Magnesium deficiencies *
- Homogenized milk
- Unhealthy cooking oils
- Stress

   * Be careful not to over-supplement with magnesium, because it can cause other minerals to be stripped from the body. Magnesium is best obtained from a diet containing green, leafy vegetables, cashews, and walnuts. Sufferers should be aware that if their magnesium deficiencies are severe enough to cause migraine headaches, then they are at an elevated risk for heart attacks.

Migraines are most often related to gastrointestinal problems, and they occur frequently in those with irritable bowel syndrome and acid reflux disease. Most gastrointestinal problems are caused by an overgrowth of candida yeast in the digestive tract. Detailed information about this can be found in the *Allergies and Candida* section of the *Alternative Medicine* chapter.

Feverfew can prevent migraines if taken daily, and 90 mg. is ideal for the average adult. Feverfew should be used with caution in those who have ragweed allergies, due to the risk of an allergic reaction. Test with a small dosage, and increase if no reactions occur.

Stopping a Headache

Ginger can be helpful for when nausea accompanies a migraine. If the sufferer is too nauseous to take ginger capsules, then place ginger powder in the mouth for direct blood absorption through the cheeks. This may be necessary before pain-relieving methods can be attempted.

Butterbur is a herb that is effective in the prevention of headaches, and for stopping them when they occur. The recommended dosage is 100 mg. for an average adult. Ideally, butterbur would be taken immediately when any soreness is felt in the head. Waiting for the headache to manifest will result in diminished effectiveness.

Reflexology and pressure point techniques can help alleviate some of the pain from migraine headaches. This entails gently pinching and applying pressure to the tops of the first three toes of each foot in a massaging motion. The patient should notice unusually acute soreness in this part of the foot, and there may even be slight toe pain in the beginning. Begin with only slight pressure and eventually build to as much force as the patient can tolerate. Some temporary relief may also be obtained by applying pressure to the cheek bones, temples, or just above the eye sockets.

Migraines can be the result of spinal misalignment. This is most likely when the headache is accompanied by soreness in the neck or back of the head. These headaches can be typically cured by a chiropractor within minutes.

Blue lotus is a flowering lily. Its dried flowers may be smoked to relieve migraines and lesser headaches. The fact that it can be smoked is an advantage, because migraines cause nausea, which can make swallowing impossible.

Kava kava is a mild pain reliever and relaxant. Kava kava is an exceptional remedy when headaches are caused by stress and anxiety. Reference the following *Painkillers* section for more information about kava kava and blue lotus.

Smoking cannabis ("marijuana") is the most effective method for alleviating both nausea and the pain. It is the fastest method of obtaining relief, and it really ought to be recommended by doctors. It is wise to obtain it before it is needed, due to the fact that it cannot be purchased in stores. Some have reported success after smoking salvia divinorum during migraines, but research on the plant is very lacking. It is, however, much more readily available than cannabis.

Painkillers

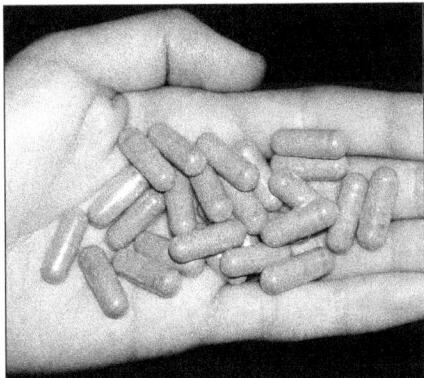

Information about these natural medicines has been sparsely distributed, but there is an underground movement of freedom fighters who are beginning to share it. This section is an attempt to unify critically important information, and to make it easily accessible for those needing serious pain relief.

We have personally tested some of these natural medicines, and we encourage our readers to not underestimate their power, or experiment with massive doses. They are strong medicines, and they should be wisely treated with respect. Consider the sap from opium poppy flowers as an example, for it was first used to make opiates, and then it was further chemically refined to make codeine, morphine, and Heroin. This simple flower is still the foundation of all pharmaceutical painkillers in one way or another.

We must not continue without an obligatory notice about caution. It is foolish to use any painkiller (natural or pharmaceutical) to merely mask pain in lieu of remedying its cause. Routinely doing so will lead to more suffering later, when more symptoms arise from the systemic problem that was ignored. Pain always indicates that something is wrong, so efforts should be made to uncover the cause and to correct it. Therefore, painkillers should only be used to temporarily mitigate a patient's suffering, while simultaneous efforts are made to eliminate the health issues that are causing pain.

Kratom (Mitragyna speciosa)

Kratom is used for severe pain, such as the pain that results from car accidents and botched surgeries. It is a very strong and capable painkiller, often replacing oxycodone (Oxycontin) and hydrocodone (Vicodin). It typically causes a feeling of euphoria, relaxation, and a bizarre tingling sensation in the frontal lobes. The tingling is usually brief. Kratom is also used for reducing addictions to the pharmaceutical derivatives of opium. Such addicts can use kratom instead of the addictive drugs to curb their withdrawals. After an extended period of this therapy, addicts can stop taking

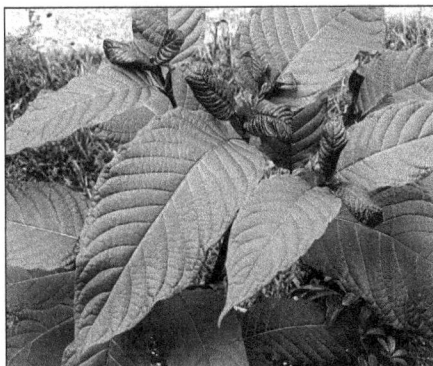

kratom without incident.

Our own experimentation with kratom has shown that it has a tendency to cause a user to serenely reflect upon his past experiences, including unpleasant experiences that would otherwise produce a traumatic effect. Therefore, it shows great promise for psychiatric use, in a very similar manner to the drug Ecstacy (3,4-methylenedioxy-methamphetamine). There are three varieties of kratom, and each has different properties. Although, all of the strains provide some pain relief.

The Three Types of Kratom

• **Red vein kratom** is the strongest variety for pain relief. It is also helpful for reducing stress and anxiety. Its mental effects are similar to cannabis (marijuana) in that it tends to make people much more relaxed and less worried. In other words, everything just feels right with the world, so contentment comes easy. This emotional affect helps in making it best for those in severe pain, because severely injured people should limit their activities, so that they can heal. Like cannabis, it may also cause a slight hunger whenever it activates. This phenomenon is commonly referred to by cannabis users as "the munchies", but it is much less intense with kratom. This variety is often sold as "Red Thai Kratom" or "Bali Kratom".

• **White vein kratom** is a stimulant, though it is different from pharmaceutical stimulants in that it tends to increase a person's drive, and his desire to accomplish; rather than just providing raw energy. It also acts as an anti-depressant. This herb would be an ideal aid for someone with attention deficit disorder, or anyone with energy and concentration problems. It is like an all-natural Ritalin. In this regard, it could be considered the opposite of the red vein kratom. Some people use white vein kratom in a tea, instead of having morning coffee. Although, it is alleged to have a disagreeable flavor. White vein kratom is often sold as "Maeng Da".

• **Green vein kratom** effects and affects its users like a blend of the other two strains, which is milder than either. It is a decent, general purpose pain reliever, and it provides some extra energy, but it does not provide the same motivational factor as the white vein kratom, nor does it blunt pain as effectively as the red vein type. It is frequently sold as "Green malay kratom".

Kratom Dosage Recommendations

For most people, the ideal kratom dosage is between 1 and 2 grams. However, starting at 0.5 grams is wise, because this is plenty for some people, especially those of lower body weights. Kratom capsules typically contain 0.5 grams each. Those who are using kratom for opiate addictions will need to use higher doses to offset their cravings. Some experimentation will be needed. Kratom must be swallowed to be effective. Smoking it provides no benefit. There will be variances in both the effect and the time that it takes to become active, because it is a natural herb that cannot be chemically standardized. In an empty stomach, its effects may begin within 10 minutes, but the time will be an hour in some cases. Once active, kratom has a very persistent effect that can last for 24 hours, or even more. High doses can cause nausea, which generally only happens to those who have taken extreme amounts in an attempt to get "high".

CBD Oil

CBD (cannabidiol) is useful for treating pain and anxiety. It is a compound that occurs naturally in the hemp and cannabis (marijuana) plants. It is the reason why cannabis has earned such an enduring reputation as a pain reliever. CBD has no known harmful effects, but it is known to come with a plethora of benefits. In fact, these medicinal benefits are the reasons behind the push for medical marijuana. Unfortunately, we cannot catalog those medicinal benefits, due to F.D.A. regulations which apply to product sellers, since we sell it in our store. People have known of its medicinal benefits for eons, including doctors who prescribed marijuana as an official medicine in past centuries, but it has only been in recent history that the specific CBD compound was identified and isolated. It has medicinal value only. There are no narcotic effects from CBD usage; so in other words, there is never a "high". In fact, CBD can be used to neutralize the "high" of cannabis, for those who take things a little too far. What a person instead gets is a state of normalcy. This normalcy can truly be heavenly for those who suffer from chronic pain or anxiety -- just being normal again. In some cases, CBD works better than kratom as a painkiller, which puts it on-par with the most powerful pharmaceutical painkillers. We have had reports that it can even alleviate much of the pain of neuropathy, which nothing else does. The beneficial effects of the CBD usually last 6-7 hours.

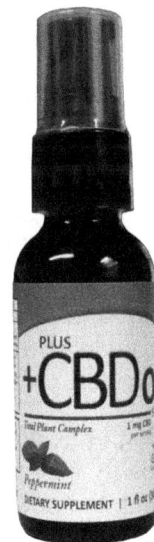

Wild Opium Lettuce (Lactuca serriola)

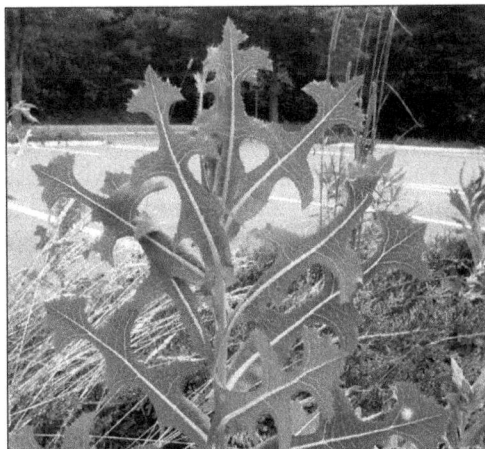

Opium lettuce grows throughout the world in various backyards and near roadsides. It loves to grow near asphalt. The plant is usually considered to be an invasive weed, and it certainly is the ugliest of the plants mentioned herein. When its leaves are scored, they release a milky sap. This sap mimics opium, hence its common name, "wild opium lettuce" or simply "opium lettuce". The plant's leaves are broken from the plant and scratched to release the sap. Then the sap is collected. It is a type of natural latex which is typically formed into pill-like balls. These can be directly consumed as pills, or smoked inside of a pipe. Opium lettuce is often reported to cause a numbing sensation that is felt spreading throughout the body. This feeling is particularly noticeable when the lettuce is smoked. It does not usually impart a euphoric or a "high" feeling.

There are few studies of opium lettuce in the Western world, but researchers in Iran have confirmed that opium lettuce was well known as a painkiller and sedative before the Victorian period. Thus, it is likely that it has been used for eons. In the paper, *Lettuce, lactuca sp. as a Medicinal Plant in Polish Publications of the 19th Century*, the Institute for the History of Science affirmed, "*The action of the substance was weaker than that of opium, but free of the side-effects, and medical practice showed that in some cases lactucarium produced better curative effects than opium*". Despite opium lettuce not containing opium, it has multiple characteristics that are similar to it. In addition to its pain-relieving properties, it is also known for assisting with coughs. It has even been used successfully in the mitigation of whooping cough (pertussis) symptoms.

The Servall Company published a catalog of medicinal plants in 1917, which was entitled *Health from Field and Forest*. It stated that opium lettuce was "*highly esteemed to quiet coughing and allay nervous irritation, a good safe remedy to produce sleep, to be used when opium and other narcotics are objectionable*". When it was written, codeine and opium were still widely available without a prescription. Both were considered to be safe and effective medicines, yet opium lettuce was known to be even safer.

Eating large doses of opium lettuce can cause nausea, vomiting, anxiety, and dizziness. So, it is probably best not to use it in a salad. The powdered leaves lack most of the effects of the sap, though the powder has a history of being used to remedy sunburns.

Opium Lettuce Dosage Recommendations

Approximately 1.5 grams of opium lettuce sap is typically infused in a tea. It is alleged to have a sweet taste. Only about 0.25 grams are smoked in a pipe. It is considerably more potent when smoked.

Blue Lotus (Nymphaea caerulea)

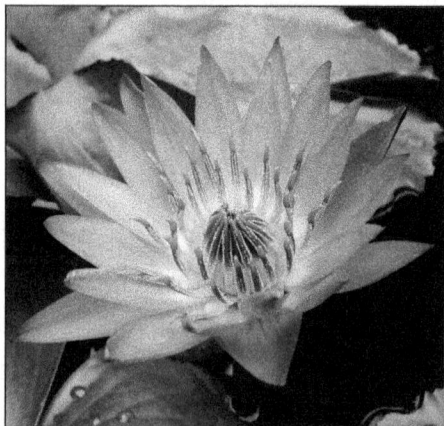

This flower can be used by both men and women as an aphrodisiac. It is a painkiller that is especially useful for relieving muscle spasms, migraines, and tinnitus (ringing in the ears). It can be smoked, which is especially beneficial for eliminating migraine headaches, since they usually accompany nausea. Blue lotus is reported to be "not as strong as codeine", but it is effective in remedying migraines, menstrual cramps, and various moderate pains. While it is weaker as a painkiller than the other herbs within this article, amongst the things that it does do, it does them best. Those who are researching this plant should be aware that it is commonly confused with the lotus (Nelumbo nucifera), but in fact, the "blue lotus" is a water lily. There are no blue members of the lotus family of plants. Blue lotus flowers are often used to make teas, wines, and martinis. The effects of the plant are amplified whenever it is combined with alcohol. There is very little of a mental effect from it, though it can produce a feeling of relaxation in high amounts. In large doses, it can produce a slight "high" feeling that is allegedly similar to that of cannabis. However, extreme dosages should not be necessary for medicinal use.

Blue Lotus Dosage Recommendations

Typical recipes involve soaking 10-20 grams of petals for up to three weeks in an alcohol solution. Blue lotus tea is prepared by boiling the flowers (the petals and flower heads) for 10-20 minutes. When it is smoked, the petals and the flower heads are combined inside a pipe.

Kava Kava (Piper methysticum)

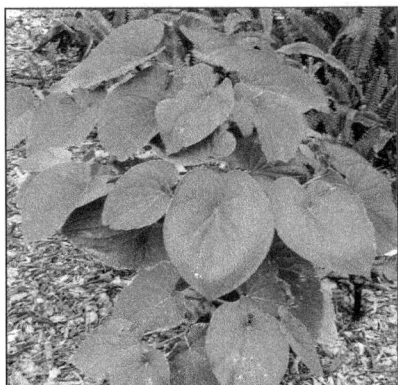

Kava kava (frequently referred to as just "kava") is used to relieve anxiety, or remedy the pain of sore muscles. It appears to have an ability to relax the muscles throughout the body. It imparts a euphoric state when it is consumed in large amounts. The euphoric feeling that is produced by kava has often been compared to alcoholic drunkenness. There are a few rumors of it having caused hallucinations on the Internet, though they all appear to have occurred from the use of strange mixtures that contained chemicals. It is known to be especially helpful for tension headache relief. Kava kava contains an anti-spasmotic called nuciferine, so it might be useful for both epilepsy and A.D.D. Note that attention deficit disorder is partly a seizure disorder, but this has been whitewashed by the psychiatric establishment throughout the last decade.

The University of Minnesota found that kava *"prevented the formation of 99 percent of tumors in a mouse lung tumorigenesis model that is routinely used in predicting lung cancer behavior in humans"*. In the same study, DNA damage resulting from cigarette carcinogens was reduced significantly with kava kava supplementation. Researchers noticed that despite similar smoking rates, the lung cancer rate in Fiji, where kava tea is a staple beverage, is approximately 1/20th of the rate for American smokers. Thus, we recommend it for everyone who smokes, alongside regular supplementation with L-taurine, and the use of self-rolled, organic cigarettes to prevent lung cancers.

Kava Kava Dosage Recommendations

The typical amount used in tea is about 3-5 flowers, which is about 5 grams. It may be drank in a tea form, or put into capsules and swallowed, or even smoked. The amount used for smoking varies greatly.

Additional Advice About Natural Painkiller Dosages

The dosage weights that are provided in this report are much smaller than what can be calculated by a normal scale. Scales that are designed for such small weights can be found in legal high stores ("head shops") and online. The typical cost is about $10.00 (U.S.D.). The type of scale needed is called a pocket scale.

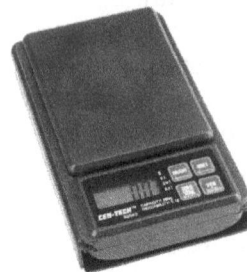

Obtaining Your Own Natural Painkillers

All the painkillers cited can be grown or purchased. For immediate help, these herbs are often found in local "legal high" stores, which are also called "head shops". These medicines tend to be very cheap, and yet very potent. Americans have the best chance of getting natural painkillers if they order from domestic sellers, since this will prevent the F.D.A. from intercepting the medicines at the border. Purchasing them online will almost certainly require using a credit card other than Mastercard. It is always best to keep painkillers available for whenever an accident occurs. Thus, purchasing beforehand is a wise decision, especially since some of these will likely need to be ordered online. Furthermore, the legality of these herbs could change rapidly, so ordering plenty would be a worthwhile investment.

Kratom is natively grown in Thailand, and it can be grown in warmer climates. It has been successfully grown in Florida, Hawaii, and parts of California. However, those in colder regions have had success with growing kratom indoors, near a window. Growing it indoors is problematic, because kratom is a tree that eventually grows to become quite large if it is not pruned regularly. Never use any fertilizer on kratom, except for natural manure. Chemical fertilizers always kill it. It is a mystery as to why this happens.

Opium lettuce grows like a weed. It does not need much care, and it will even die if pampered. It likes shade, and it does not like for soil to be too moist. Once cultivated outdoors, the plant should spread literally like a weed, so that opium lettuce plants will be found throughout the area. One only needs to loosen the soil, sprinkle the seeds atop the soil, and keep the soil slightly moist.

Given that blue lotus plants are water lilies, a pond is needed to grow them. However, the plants are usually sprouted indoors. To do so, add a layer of soil to the bottom of a small pot or pan, then fill to the brim with warm water. Once the soil has settled, attempt to level and compact it. Sprinkle the seeds as evenly as possible, and add a thin layer of white sand on top of the seeds. This helps to anchor them. Adding water after adding the seeds will bury them, and prevent them from growing. When leaves appear from the seeds, the baby plants can be gently moved to a permanent home, such as an outdoor pond.

Kava kava grows in tropical climates, and it favors Hawaii. It can be grown in cooler climates if it is taken indoors during the colder months, though it will need to be pruned to keep it manageable. It takes at least four years for kava kava to reach maturity. At four years of age, the lateral roots are then collected. These roots grow just under the surface of the earth. The plant will die if the roots are collected early, and the roots will not contain the active constituents.

Editorial: Defending Our Rights and Our Medicine

The existing research of kratom shows a fixation on the topics of whether kratom can induce addictions or cause harm, because all of the studies originate from an industry that is threatened by natural alternatives. In fact, most of the studies actually admitted that they were searching for unflattering results from the very beginning. We have not found a single study that was objectively searching for the true effects of kratom, or one that was seeking benefits. Most studies have concluded that kratom *must* be addictive, based on the gratuitous assertion that it effects the same area of the brain that painkilling drugs do. This is religiously recited throughout the studies, despite the fact that kratom usage tests have never shown any withdrawal symptoms whatsoever. Yet the detractors do not appear to be getting discouraged. Withdrawal symptoms were only observed in subjects who were using kratom to eliminate existing addictions that had been previously gained from pharmaceutical-style opiates. It means that the addictions that the system is blaming on kratom were actually from the system's own drugs. To make a long story short, the usual pattern was that the subjects were specifically chosen for already having addictions, and given kratom so that it could be falsely linked to the existing drug withdrawals. It is the sort of scientific slight-of-hand that our research has accustomed us to seeing. Whenever studies are manipulated to accomplish an agenda, then it is a perversion of science, of which we are prone to calling dirty politics.

To make the point about the politics that is involved, they are still trying to find a harmful effect for cannabis (marijuana), and they have not been able to document a single individual who has been harmed. They certainly scare us by decrying that the natural medicine might do this or that thing, but can they show us an actual individual with a verifiable injury in recorded history? Where are those millions of people who have been horribly hurt by "marijuana", if we do not count the ones whom the establishment has hurt and then imprisoned? Where did the victims disappear to? How many poor souls inside of the emergency wards are there because "pot" did them in, and how many are there because of the effects of "safe" pharmaceuticals? The only verifiable findings about cannabis' overall health impact are that it cures cancer, it improves lung capacity, and it boosts oxygen intake into the long term. Most people could easily learn to accept these things.

The U.S. Drug Enforcement Agency (D.E.A.) has described kratom as a "drug of concern", and pointed to a possible death to justify its aggressive posturing. Of course, kratom is not a "drug", but getting it considered to be a drug is another slight-of-hand trick that is used to manipulate the public into giving them the power to rob us of even more of our freedoms. In a case cited by the D.E.A., a coroner attributed a man's death to "*possible* Kratom toxicity", despite the man's history of Heroin abuse, and despite the fact that both a cold medicine and benzodiazepines were found in his body at the time of his death. Benzodiazepines are a family of tranquilizers, which includes Xanax and Valium. Xanax caused more than 150,000 emergency room visits in 2009 alone. Even if it were true that kratom had led to the death of this one individual, it could not compare with the 16,000 deaths that occur every year from what are considered to be the safest pharmaceuticals of all: Tylenol and aspirin. Unlike kratom,

Tylenol weakens the liver, and it can become a fatal poison whenever it is mixed with alcohol. The manufacturer leaves this pesky tidbit off of the labels, by the way. The Tylenol danger is one of the real reasons why so many "binge drinkers" die every year on college campuses, but we are not told the truth, because it would be disastrous for business. Pharmaceutical Tylenol (acetaminophen) has yet to be listed as a "drug of concern", despite its issues and the fact that it is actually a drug.

Considering the number of places in America that are now legalizing cannabis, Americans are simply not believing the lies anymore. They have begun to realize that there is an agenda to take away their freedoms for the sake of corporate and governmental interests. They are awaking to realize that it is not really the weed in their backyards which they should fear, but those who relish busting down our doors in the middle of night, shooting our pets, and shoving machine guns in our children's faces to supposedly 'protect' us.

The herb kava is already illegal in Australia, Canada, South Africa, and the United Kingdom. The strained justification was that some unethical suppliers were creating extracts from the plants using dangerous solvents. These poisoned products caused liver damage, and this was conveniently blamed upon the kava. Like the other natural medicines mentioned herein, organic kava has no known victims. Nonetheless, the psychiatric industry, acting alongside its governmental cronies, got an excuse to ban it in multiple countries. Like is the case for the other natural medicines mentioned, the real reason for the ban (the one that they never mention to the public) is because it is truly safe, effective, cheap, easily accessible, and non-addictive. This combination makes it a threat to the establishment.

The medical establishment does not want regular citizens to have access to safe and effective painkillers, because pain is the thing guaranteeing that the public will inevitably fall back to the system. Eventually, everyone gets injured in a way that requires pain relief. It is these instances which force even the most educated citizens to return to allopathic medicine for relief. If citizens had access to better and cheaper pain relievers that were outside of the system, then they could become completely independent and free. Prior to the last century, herbalists successfully competed with allopathic doctors, and the herbalists generally had much better results. This was partly due to the herbalists' easy access to painkillers, like opium and cannabis. These plants were also core medicines of the establishment as well, which had been doing poorly in the free and open medical market. The free market allowed people to choose their medicine based upon its true merits; instead of being controlled by legal requirements and regulations. Medicine was not our biggest killer in those days. It was the U.S. federal regulations combined with state licensure laws and forced changes in the university system that finally ended medical competition worldwide, as was shamelessly boasted about in public documents from the American Medical Association.

Strong pharmaceutical pain relievers are now only available by way of an official prescription. Most of these drugs are categorized as "controlled substances", which means that individuals can be criminally charged for just possessing them without permission. A free people never needs permission to treat their own pain, and free people are not required to officially report about it, replete with identity documents. The first thing asked is always something like, "Your papers please". At this time, doctors resist providing prescriptions for painkillers, due to their buying into the hysteria about painkiller addictions. Of course, some of the hysteria is merited, but it is mostly designed to ensure that patients literally keep coming back and begging for more.

In the U.S., the F.D.A. has been leading the charge to take painkillers away from the people for over a century. None of the natural painkillers that are cataloged in this report are illegal under federal law, but the F.D.A. has been illegally abusing its power to prevent people from getting access to these herbs. The *Federal Food, Drug, and Cosmetic Act* of 1994 gave the F.D.A. the power to intervene whenever a seller of a product makes "claims" that his product is helpful for treating or curing any *disease* without its official permission. Telling the truth about a competing medicine actually requires permission from the F.D.A., which it has never given for anything. Moreover, pain is not a disease, so the F.D.A. has been flagrantly violating the law by arbitrarily seizing pain relievers.

On September 25th of 2014, the F.D.A. seized 25,000 pounds of kratom from Rosefield Management in California, whilst claiming that it was because kratom is an "unapproved drug". For maximum intimidation, the F.D.A. sent armed Federal Marshals to perform the raid. Kratom is a plant. It is not a drug any more than a carrot is a horse. Following their usual modus operandi, they justified their criminal activity by stating that the seller's truthful claims about kratom's ability to greatly reduce pain and alleviate opiate addictions had somehow meant that it had been transformed into a drug, as if the seller's claims had some type of magical power. Even if that could be true, it does not account for the fact that neither pain nor addiction are diseases. However you examine the situation, they have been ignoring the law and making their own as they have seen fit. Such behavior is the hallmark of tyranny.

On November 7th of 2014, the F.D.A. issued an import alert on kratom, which effectively means that the F.D.A is attempting to seize all of the kratom that enters into the U.S.A. Kratom is not illegal at the federal level, nor is it illegal in the vast majority of states. When it issued its import alert, the F.D.A. claimed that kratom is a hallucinogen, which was a flagrant lie. Even if it were actually a hallucinogen, it would still not give them the authority to simply take whatever they want, whenever they want, in punitively stealing from the lawful citizens of whom they pretend to serve. This is the behavior of the Mafia, but not of an accountable regulatory agency. By confiscating kratom as it is being imported, in utter disregard of our laws, the F.D.A. is willfully sabotaging the basic human right of the people to heal themselves through God's natural medicine and our right to trade legal goods.

The reason why they are dishonestly claiming that kratom is a hallucinogen is because this belief would frighteningly differentiate it from the other "drugs" that are already legal and commonly used, like alcohol, nicotine, and caffeine. The agenda is to suppress kratom by saying and doing whatever is necessary, so that it can be stopped before the public begins demanding it. If herbs like kratom were to become controlled through transparent regulatory means, then we would have the power to effect changes in the policies, such as is already happening with cannabis legalization in state after state. So they plan to stop it before there is any public debate.

There have been no legal actions against opium lettuce, because the same compounds occur in farmed lettuce too, though to a lesser degree. Outlawing lettuce is simply not feasible for them, so they must ignore it while hoping that we do not notice. Taking action against lettuce would laughably expose the true agenda.

Lawmakers are usually quick to jump onto the bandwagon of banning various substances, to seem "tough on drugs". Most of the legislative bills that ban herbs are ironically intended to stop the dangerous synthetic drugs, yet within the fine print is usually found the alternative plants too. When contacted by concerned citizens, lawmakers were typically unaware that they had banned the natural substances. So perhaps our legislators should take the time to read what they vote for, and take into account the fact that corrupt agencies are manipulating our laws through trickery.

It is rumored that Mastercard has threatened and "fined" (electronically stolen from) companies which sell herbs like kratom. However, we have been unable to confirm this, and most of the sellers are too afraid to speak with us. The sellers are so embattled that they disingenuously tell their own buyers not to consume the herbs that they sell, as an attempt at appeasement by playing both sides. It truly expresses the degree of tyranny whenever the citizens are too afraid to openly speak about topics that are completely legal. It is reminiscent of how terrified people constantly swore that they were not Jewish in NAZI Germany. Kratom sellers normally display long disclaimers to make F.D.A. raids less likely. Here is one of those fear-driven disclaimers from a web site that is selling kratom:

> "...provides kratom to its consumers for ONLY aromatic or external applications. Our products are NOT MEANT FOR HUMAN CONSUMPTION. Our encapsulated products are NOT MEANT FOR HUMAN CONSUMPTION. All packaging will be clearly labelled with this disclaimer to ensure there is no mis-understanding. ...will not ship our products to any region where possession of kratom is prohibited. Please do not order if kratom is prohibited in your area."

In the routine fashion, the mainstream media is again kowtowing to its biggest sponsors and the regulators by openly attacking natural painkillers. Take for example that on September 22nd of 2012, Forbes magazine published an article that warned about kratom causing "vomiting, delusions and hallucinations". This was patently untrue, with the possible exception of vomiting, which can result from an overdose. This is actually a desirable trait from a safety standpoint. Would it not be wonderful if the doctor-prescribed medicines caused victims to vomit before the dosage became fatal?

The media circus has been claiming that kratom is addictive, and it has justified these reports by using the shoddy science that was referenced earlier. For example, they mention that mice repeatedly consume kratom whenever they are exposed to it, but this does not actually prove that kratom is addictive, but only that it is desirable. We could likewise argue that cheese and corn are addictive to mice using this same logic, since mice also choose to consume them again and again. Since human subjects can report that they have not suffered from any addiction withdrawals, the testing was moved onto animals, where the desired test results could not be disproven. This increasingly common type of scientific fraud is something that we call "data shopping", but most of society calls it "creative accounting". For now, we should all be afraid of corn, cheese, and of course, kratom addictions.

There are very few organizations that are fighting for our right to have access to natural medicines. The few organizations that exist are disorganized, and they typically only focus on a single herb. None are Christian, which is especially disturbing, for Christians should feel the call of duty. To be truly effective, a group needs to fight for our right to have access to all of the God-given medicines. This issue spans much wider than a single plant. It is about our basic right to use the much safer medicines that were provided by God.

It may help our American readers to put the tyrannical situation into perspective by learning that our Constitution and Bill of Rights were written on hemp paper (also outlawed), that Benjamin Franklin was the man who smuggled the national treasures of cannabis and hemp into the United States, and that Thomas Jefferson compassionately grew opium poppies on his plantation for those in need. Our Founding Fathers would have been hunted criminals by the F.D.A. and D.E.A., if these organizations had existed during their time. America's Founding Fathers would be deeply ashamed to witness what we have allowed to happen, and how we have apathetically squandered the greatest inheritance that any people ever had. Nevertheless, we believe that truth, liberty, and justice may once again rise, even in the United States.

It is crucial for people to be able to successfully treat their own pain. We should not be forced to endure pain unless we submit to the whims of our medical keepers and regulatory cronies. Moreover, the natural painkillers are always better than the pharmaceutical drugs, because they are never addictive, nor do they induce liver damage.

Parasites and Lupus

Parasitic infestations are an epidemic in the United States, with most sources estimating that a massive 85% of Americans have parasites. Because of this, we recommend a parasite cleanse every six months, care in choosing restaurants, and washing after exposure to animals.

Unfortunately, most doctors are not trained in the treatment of parasites. It is only when parasites are visually seen that American doctors will suspect them, which requires an especially terrible case. There are many symptoms of parasite infestation which people experience in daily life, believing that these issues are completely normal. While sickness has become somewhat normal in the modern lifestyle, it does not need to be. The amount of damage that can be caused by parasites is virtually limitless, because many types of them are small enough to travel anywhere in the body through the bloodstream. Parasites obtain sustenance by robbing the body of nutrients. They are the root cause of lupus, with all other issues being secondary to the parasitic infection. Therefore, lupus cannot be cured without a thorough parasite cleanse. Lupus is officially reported to be just another "incurable disease" and an "autoimmune disorder" by the establishment. Most parasites can be avoided by thoroughly cooking foods and by never drinking unfiltered water.

Identifying Common Parasites

- **Round worms:** Living in the stomach and intestines, these worms enter through undercooked and contaminated food. Remember that manure used in organic farming may be contaminated with worms. Therefore, this parasite is one reason to avoid raw produce diets. Always wash your hands after having contact with pets; especially if there has been any contact with their feces.

- **Heart worms:** It is extremely rare for heart worms to occur in humans. It usually occurred as a single worm in the lungs, instead of the heart, in the few cases that were reported. They cannot be spread from one animal (or human) to another, but must be spread through mosquitoes.

- **Tape worms:** These worms enter the body through undercooked beef, fish or pork. They live in the lower intestinal tract. Use gloves and wash thoroughly after preparing meat to prevent them.

- **Pin worms:** Living inside the intestinal tract and lungs, these small white worms come out at night to lay eggs around the anus. The eggs hatch, and then the young worms reenter through the anus. If the person scratches during his sleep, the eggs get under the fingernails, spreading to wherever the person touches. It is believed that they are small and lightweight enough to become airborne, leading people to inhale them. This is how they are purported to arrive inside the lungs.

- **Hook worms and thread worms:** These can be found in contaminated drinking water, or they can enter directly through the feet. They are tiny in size, and can enter through the soles of bare feet; even without open wounds. Always wear shoes when walking outside. These worms are unique because they have a lifespan of several years, and the eggs can incubate for up to 10 years.

Symptoms of Parasitic Infection

- Repeated diarrhea or constipation
- Chronic, unexplained nausea, often accompanied by vomiting
- Fatigue and weakness
- Intestinal cramping
- Unexplained dizziness
- Foul-smelling gas
- Indigestion

- Bloating
- Multiple food allergies
- Loss of appetite
- Itching around the anus, especially at night
- Difficulty sleeping
- Difficulty maintaining a healthy weight (over or underweight)
- Itching on the soles of the feet, often accompanied by a rash
- Itching or tingling sensations on the scalp
- Coughing blood (severe cases)
- Palpitations (hook worms)
- Anemia
- Facial swelling around the eyes (round worms)
- Wheezing and coughing, followed by vomiting, stomach pain and bloating (suggesting round worms or thread worms)

Allopathic Treatments

If a conventional doctor believes that you have parasites, he will prescribe an anti-parasitic pharmaceutical. These pharmaceuticals are always toxic, for it is their toxicity that kills the parasites. Thus, swelling of the lymph nodes, hands and feet are common with these drugs. Vision problems, lack of coordination, and convulsions can also occur. Diarrhea is typical.

Naturally Eliminating Parasites

- Black walnut hulls
- Wormwood
- Cloves
- Pumpkin seeds or pumpkin seed oil capsules
- Garlic
- Neem *
- Thyme
- Marshmallow root
- Diatomaceous earth

   * Do not take neem if you are pregnant or planning to become pregnant, because it can work as a contraceptive.

We do not recommend choosing any of the anti-parasite formulas that are available in retailers, for they are usually overpriced and formulated at very low concentrations.

Diatomaceous earth is probably the best natural anti-parasitic medication. It is a natural pesticide that does not harm humans or pets. It is believed to kill insects, worms and parasites by dehydrating them. When used on ants, it usually takes approximately 20 minutes before they are all dead. One tablespoon of diatomaceous earth taken by an adult, once a day for a week, is believed to be extremely effective for killing all parasites. When it is used on children, bear in mind that height is a better indicator of the size of their gastrointestinal tracts than their weights. Thus, a child who is 4 feet tall should take 2 teaspoons, and a child who is 2 feet tall should take 1 teaspoon.

If you take the diatomaceous earth route, then we advise you to only buy it food grade. Industrial diatomaceous earth is used for swimming pool filters, and it has been chemically treated, so this type is not safe to eat. Try to avoid rubbing it onto your hands, since it will have a drying effect upon the skin. Diatomaceous earth contains heavy metals as part of its mineral content, but it also contains selenium, which allows otherwise accumulative heavy metals to be safely flushed from the body. Therefore, it is not really a health concern despite the trace presence of aluminum and lead. We recommend taking selenium supplements for a week after discontinuing this treatment to ensure that the body thoroughly neutralizes the metals. Concerned individuals can follow the parasite cleanse with a metal cleanse. Our research indicates that diatomaceous earth is the best overall parasite treatment for humans, because it can kill blood-borne parasites as well. When using it, be sure to drink plenty of fluids, because it will dehydrate a person considerably.

Wormwood and black walnut hulls are known to kill adult worms, whilst cloves kill the eggs. Some people use this trio for treating parasites, instead of diatomaceous earth. It is recommended that you take 500 mg. of wormwood and black walnut hulls, whilst taking 1/2 teaspoon of cloves daily for about 14 days. The other herbs listed can be used to augment these two core protocols.

As parasites die, they release toxins through their excrement and from rotting. The most common parasites, the worm type, attempt to escape by burrowing deeper into the intestines, which can cause sharp cramps. Even when dead, the body is still burdened with the task of flushing them out. This whole process can make the person feel sicker than he was before he began the cleanse, but this is only temporary, and it is a sign that the cleanse is working. It is known as a Herxheimer reaction when people become sicker as a result of the toxins that are released by dying parasites. While fatigue and grogginess are to be expected, normal life may be continued, and diarrhea should not occur. Eat a good, wholesome diet throughout the cleanse to ensure that your immune system is at its strongest. After the cleanse, you should feel better, have more energy, and experience sickness less often.

Deworming Pets

A cat or dog is best treated with diatomaceous earth and pumpkin seed oil. Do not feed pets walnut hulls, wormwood, or any other supplement without first researching its effects upon animals. For instance, onion can kill dogs.

Animal Diatomaceous Earth Dosages

Animal	Amount To Use Daily
Kitten	1/2 teaspoon
Cat	1 teaspoon
Dogs up to 50 lb.	2 teaspoons
Dogs over 50 lb.	1 Tablespoon
Horses	1/2 - 1 cup (depending on size of horse)

Scabies

Scabies is a term that describes a parasitic skin infestation by the itch mite (*sarcoptes scabiei*). The name itch mite should give readers a clear indication of the effect of these little monsters. They burrow under the skin to lay their eggs, and they create bacterial infections in the process. The overall immune system is usually weakened. The itching only begins after 30 days of infection, and during this initial symptom-less period, victims may pass this condition on to all of their family members and friends. These highly contagious infestations can be transmitted whenever there is skin contact, or when there is shared contact with cloth fibers. Infestations have been known to run rampant in institutional settings.

Finding effective natural methods of eliminating such parasites can be a challenge for those who practice alternative medicine, because the methodology required is in opposition to normal procedures. Alternative medicine normally concentrates upon working with nature, to help it overcome whatever has caused an imbalanced state of dis-*ease*. In a sense, traditional methods can be thought of as a little too pro-life to be of any use. Poisons are the forté of our adversaries. The pharmaceutical industry poisons best, and they have literally transformed the poisoning of their own customers into a science. Allopathic medicine has plenty of poisonous chemicals that people can rub all over their skin, with their products often containing carcinogens such as benzene and formaldehyde.

Conversely, alternative medicine usually works by improving the health of the body, so that it may easily kill threatening bacteria or viruses. This left us in a research predicament, whereby we needed to find something that was both deadly to the insects, and yet safe for people.

Treating the Mites

Tea tree oil is one of the most popular remedies for eliminating scabies. It seems to be able to penetrate the skin and suffocate the insects. Be advised that nail polish will rarely eliminate scabies, because the mites will typically relocate before the nail polish dries. Tea tree oil treatments are applied directly to the bite areas with a cotton swab. The surrounding area and anywhere else with excessive itching is treated.

Neem oil is used by organic farmers as a natural insecticide. The E.P.A. reports that neem is "generally recognized as safe" for use in food products. This God-given "insecticide" is considered so safe for humans that they exempted their typical stipulations for maximum pesticide residues, so that unlimited amounts can be present in foods. Neem works differently to most pesticides, because it does not kill on contact. For some insects, it hormonally disrupts their life cycles and their desire to eat, whilst with others, it simply repels the insects by smell. Its smell is not strong to humans, however. In the case of scabies, neem oil prevents reproduction, a fact that is very pertinent due to their short life cycles. Neem seems to work by altering the hormones of insects (like soy), and in fact, neem is an all-natural contraceptive in humans too. It is a much safer contraceptive than "the pill". Most scabies sufferers stop getting bites after two days of neem treatments, but some adult mites are guaranteed to still be alive. If possible, rub neem oil all over the body with a cotton swab, and purchase neem soap to use in the bath or shower on a daily basis for two weeks (the life cycle).

Cayenne was described in the herbal book, *The Badanius Manuscript*, printed in 1552, for treating scabies. Topical applications of cayenne will quite literally burn the scabies, without causing any health problems for the host. Most people who use it place large amounts of cayenne into a warm bath and remain in it for an extended time (until the water becomes cold). You can purchase cheap packets of cayenne from the "Mexican" section of many grocery stores. Remember to protect your eyes while handling or bathing in cayenne. You should always keep an emergency eye wash solution in a dropper bottle containing colloidal silver and a pinch of sea salt.

Zinc can be used to help fight the secondary infections that occur under the skin and to prevent opportunistic fungal outbreaks. Grind zinc tablets into a powder, and add water until it makes a paste. Apply it to all irritated areas of the skin. Mixing turmeric with this can help to stop itching, and it has its own anti-parasitic qualities. This is also how to make a natural anti-dandruff cream. Zinc is the main anti-dandruff ingredient in commercial shampoos.

Our own colloidal copper lotion product will help to prevent secondary problems with bacteria and fungi.

Cleaning Your Environment

Mites can live in furniture, carpets, and clothing for several days. This can become a cause of constant re-infection. Thus, it is important to thoroughly clean the house to eradicate the pests. For regular vacuuming, we recommend using a vacuum with bags, and when finished, immediately remove the bags from indoors. If using a bagless vacuum, place a small amount of salt in the collection container before vacuuming to shred and dehydrate the mites. For optimal results, put borax powder into a steam cleaning mix, and steam clean the carpets. Try to limit direct skin contact and inhalation of borax. When you are vacuuming or spreading borax powder, we recommend that you use a high quality respirator mask like those used by painters, to protect your lungs from borax inhalation, at least until it has settled. These are available at most hardware stores.

Some people have successfully used diatomaceous earth to accomplish this task in a much less hazardous way. If this method is affordable, then we recommend it. However, diatomaceous earth is primarily silica, so a protective mask should still be worn to protect the lungs, whenever there is a chance of it becoming airborne.

Note that the cheap cloth-only masks that are sold in hardware stores will offer little to no protection. Get a real respirator mask. Read the included instructions about how to test if it allows any unfiltered air inside, before beginning the application process.

Shingles and Chicken Pox

Shingles (*herpes zoster*) is a secondary outbreak of the chicken pox virus. It can happen decades after the original infection. It is usually less severe the second time. It may strike people who have had either chicken pox or the chicken pox vaccination. It is often caused by the vaccine, and people who get the vaccine strain years after a vaccination get a much worse version of shingles. It is an opportunistic virus that will strike whenever the immune system is sufficiently impaired. Those who have never contracted chicken pox are at risk of contracting it from people with shingles. When it first occurs, shingles usually appears in circular patterns.

You Should Not Visit Your Doctor

Doctors will prescribe just about anything for these conditions, except for something that actually works. Some prescribe painkillers, anti-depressants, and petrochemical creams. The establishment's resultant help-to-harm ratio is rather disturbing. More often than not, standard treatments actually stress the immune system to make the outbreak last longer. Prescribing anti-depressants for a shingles outbreak is insanity, and places the patient at more risk than the original virus. All of the orthodox treatment options have risks, and are rarely effective. Chicken pox and shingles will eventually disappear without treatment, and the amount of time depends upon the strength of the immune system.

Natural Treatments

A natural, holistic approach takes into account that this virus is part of the herpes family. Whenever it is treated appropriately, the virus outbreak is short-lived. Herpes can only thrive in a body with a weakened immune system. The herpes family of viruses are particularly effected by a person's L-arginine to L-lysine ratio. These are natural amino acids that are found inside the human body, but they come from foods. There must be a greater level of arginine in the body for herpes viruses to thrive.

Lysine is found in proteins, dairy, and most vegetables. Arginine is found in nuts, chocolate, and tomatoes. Use the following chart to ensure that the diet is higher in lysine foods, until the outbreak passes.

Foods with Lysine (Encouraged)	Foods with Arginine (Avoid)
All meats	Tomatoes
Fish	Wheat Germ
Yogurt	Brussels sprouts
Cheese	Cashews
Milk	Grapes
Eggs	Pumpkin Seeds
Apples	Pecans
Pears	Blackberries
Apricots	Blueberries
Avocados	Peanuts
Pineapples	Chocolate
Green beans	Sugars
Asparagus	

It would be wise to temporarily supplement with large doses of lysine of up to 2,000 mg. per day (2 grams), until the outbreak is gone. However, this large dosage may cause health problems if it is continued for an extended period. A mere handful of peanuts is usually enough to unfavorably shift the balance in favor of arginine, so a carefully planned diet is absolutely critical for fast recovery. Oral doses of colloidal silver can be helpful too, because colloidal silver is harmful to viruses. Large doses of vitamin C are known for being helpful in reducing the recovery time. We intentionally neglected to list herbs as an option, because herbs have almost no effect on herpes, chickenpox, or shingles.

A chiropractor will generally be more helpful than a standard doctor. The virus dwells in the spinal column, where it may remain dormant for decades. Spinal misalignment is a strong contributing factor in outbreaks, and their duration. Therefore, chiropractic adjustments can dramatically speed the recovery process.

In order to reduce pain and stimulate recovery, soak a cloth rag in apple cider vinegar. Next, sprinkle cayenne pepper powder over the lesions, and cover them with the damp rag. Put a hot water bottle on top of the rag, or use some other safe source for heat. Be careful not to burn the skin. This procedure should dramatically reduce recovery time if repeated regularly. It will also provide much needed relief from the itching.

Weekend Headaches

For many people, headaches are a normal part of life, and are expected. Ironically, those who have stressful, and particularly thankless jobs will often experience headaches most often during the weekends, instead of during their work-weeks. As a result, stress factors are usually dismissed. There are many who spend months trying to track down the cause of their weekend headaches, to no avail. Readers who experience these headaches have likely tried multiple remedies, in an attempt to relieve them, but such trials in self-medication can be a perilous process.

For sufferers of weekend headaches, the sudden change from a state of stress to one of rest on the weekends causes the neurotransmitter chemicals of the brain to be massively discharged. It can create a painful headache (or even a migraine) that takes a particularly long time to fade.

The first thing that people need to do is learn relaxing techniques, for stressful periods. This can be challenging, and the process is different for each person, but relaxation (prayer/meditation) techniques are plentiful. If the place of employment is simply too horrible to ever relax in, then seeking employment elsewhere would be the best option. Those who have these routine headaches have an increased risk of strokes, so eliminating the headaches should be made a top priority. Even without having a stroke, the pattern of high stress will eventually take its toll upon the body in other ways. Of course, the effects of poor surroundings is partly determined by the individual. It really is a mind over matter issue. (If you don't mind, it doesn't matter.)

For those who need some extra help, L-tryptophan supplementation will be of immediate value. L-tryptophan is an amino acid that is naturally found in proteins, and has been traditionally used to treat depression. It can be found at some health food stores. Tryptophan is metabolized into several different neurotransmitters in a balance that is optimal for a body. This can bring emotional balance during the work week to eliminate the depression that results from poor environments. Many unhappy people are clinically depressed without realizing it; for instance in cases where a person uses anger to hide and suppress depression, even from himself.

While this type of headache has a very identifiable pattern, there are plenty of other causes of headaches. Common causes include excitotoxin exposure (MSG and artificial sweeteners), lack of oxygen (cluster headaches), magnesium or B vitamin deficiencies, bad eyeglass prescriptions, internal inflammation, mold exposure, and allergies.

Cancer

The Carnage

"If a patient with a tumor is receiving radiation or chemotherapy, the only question that is asked is, 'How is the tumor doing?' No one ever asks how the patient is doing. In my medical training, I remember well seeing patients who were getting radiation and/or chemotherapy. The tumor would get smaller and smaller, but the patient would get sicker and sicker. At autopsy we would hear, 'Isn't that marvelous! The tumor is gone!' Yes, it was, but so was the patient."

-- Dr. Philip Binzel

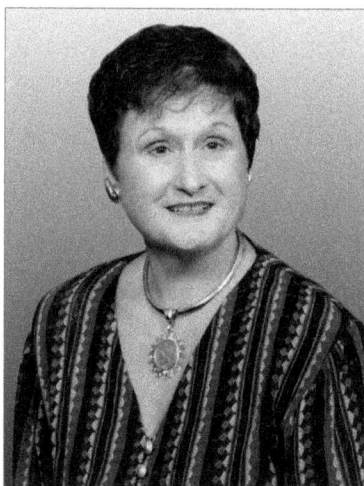

In late 2010, we released *The Cancer Report*, a documentary describing how cancer occurs, its causes, and the most effective alternative cures. It was especially aimed at those who have never been exposed to alternative therapies, and those who were unaware of the corruption of the cancer industry. The documentary was dedicated to Clara Corriher, who died of cancer treatments. After destroying her physically and mentally (e.g. "chemo-brain"), Clara's oncologist sent her away to a hospice, because he was unwilling to watch her die. She was removed from the hospital, even though more than half of the beds were free. The hospice staff put her into a drug-induced coma, so that Clara would not burden them. They killed her with complete starvation and dehydration. They re-drugged her whenever she awoke. Family and friends were told to ignore her gasping and gurgling sounds. The hospice staff pumped moisture into her lungs after she developed pneumonia from forced inactivity. Such treatment is considered normal, even noble, by those involved. Starving someone to death, while inducing pneumonia at a hospice passes for humane treatment, and it is always considered preferable to trying alternatives.

Cancer cells exist in every human body. They are a normal part of life. A healthy immune system eliminates cancer cells at roughly the same rate that they are created. Tiny outbreaks of symptomatic cancer have existed since ancient times. It was discovered in Roman and Egyptian remains having high levels of lead and other toxins. Before the 20th century, cancer was so uncommon that it was a medical oddity. By the early twentieth century, 1 in 25 people died of cancer. Now, about 1 in 4 people die of "cancer". These are almost always deaths by medicine. Forty-one percent of Americans will eventually be diagnosed with cancer, and virtually all Americans already have the pre-cancerous condition of acidosis.

After the industrial revolution of the early 20th century, humans were exposed to thousands of new toxins, including petrochemicals, fluoride, chlorine and radiation. Later, plastic compounds added to the assault, including plasticizing agents that are found in our foods and skin products. The onslaught to our immune systems was further compounded by a new generation of chemically-engineered fertilizers that depleted our soils of vital nutrients. Obesity has exploded because people are in a state of semi-starvation regardless of how much they eat, which in-turn stimulates poor eating habits, snowballing the nutritional problems further. Many people of the industrialized world, especially Americans, do not realize that they are chronically malnourished. Radiation exposure, malnutrition, and toxicity are the unholy trinity that combine to create a condition called acidosis. It is the fuse to the cancer bomb.

> *"The alarming fact is that foods (fruits, vegetables and grains), now being raised on millions of acres of land that no longer contain enough of certain minerals, are starving us - no matter how much of them we eat."*
>
> -- U.S. Senate Document No. 264

> *"Chlorine is the greatest crippler and killer of modern times. While it has prevented epidemics of one disease, it was creating another. Two decades ago, after the start of chlorinating our drinking water in 1904, the present epidemic of heart trouble, cancer and senility began."*
>
> -- Dr. Joseph M. Price, M.D.

> *"If* [fluoride] *gets out into the air, it's a pollutant; if it gets into the river, it's a pollutant; if it gets into the lake, it's a pollutant; but if it goes right into your drinking water system, it's not a pollutant. That's amazing..."*
>
> -- Dr. J. William Hirzy, E.P.A.

> *"According to the handbook, 'Toxicology of Commercial Products', fluoride is more poisonous than lead, and just slightly less poisonous than arsenic. It is a cumulative poison that accumulates in bones over the years... Epidemiology research in the mid 1970's by the late Dr. Dean Burk, head of the cytochemistry division of the National Cancer Institute, indicated that 10,000 or more fluoridation linked cancer deaths occur yearly in the United States. In 1989, the ability of fluoride to transform normal cells into cancer cells was confirmed by Argonne National Laboratories."*
>
> -- Dr. Michael Schachter, M.D.

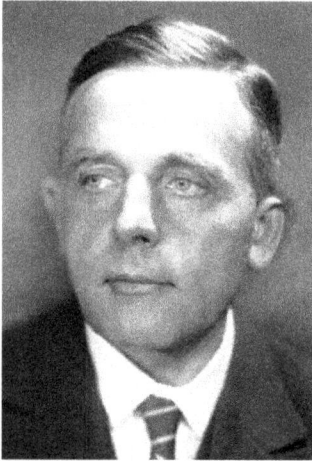

In 1931, Dr. Otto Warburg was awarded the Nobel Prize for medicine. Dr. Warburg discovered that cancer cells only thrive in the absence of oxygen, whereas normal cells require oxygen for respiration. He found that oxygen exposure actually has a poisoning effect upon cancer cells, and only cancer cells. He realized that mutated cancer cells do not derive their energy from respiration, but instead from a fermentation process that draws upon blood sugars. Warburg furthermore noticed that bodies with a low pH (acidic) were more cancerous, because having a low pH meant having a high resistance to oxygen absorption. When oxygen levels drop too low, and the cells start to suffocate, they must mutate into cells that can survive from fermentation, in order to prevent entire regions of the body from dying. Warburg's discoveries have since been suppressed by the medical establishment so successfully that only alternative medicine researchers ever learn of them, or of him. Medical students rarely learn of Warburg, despite him having made the greatest health discovery of the twentieth century, and despite his Nobel prize from an era when it meant something.

The number of American deaths from pharmaceuticals and cancer treatments every year outnumber the deaths for any war in U.S. history. On average, chemotherapy and radiation are effective 4-5% of the time for long-term recovery. They are always poisonous. The phrase "successful treatment" has been redefined by oncologists and the medical literature to mean having no tumors (without regard to cancers) for a mere 5 years, and they continue counting patients as "survivors", even when they die at 6 years; cooking the numbers about their cure rates. This is one of the ways that science is manipulated to render the 'right' statistics.

> *"My studies have proven conclusively that untreated cancer victims actually live up to four times longer than treated individuals. For a typical type of cancer, people who refused treatment lived for an average of 12-1/2 years. Those who accepted surgery or other kinds of treatment* [chemotherapy, radiation, cobalt] *lived an average of only three years."*

-- Dr. Hardin Jones, Physiology,
University of California, Berkeley

The medical establishment's attempts to correct cancer tend to worsen it, or cause it to appear in other areas. Mainstream attempts at prevention are just as dismal, because the diagnostic tests are almost always cancer-inducing. This includes radioactive mammograms.

"Children who are successfully treated for Hodgkin's disease are 18 times more likely to later develop secondary malignant tumors. The risks of leukemia increase markedly four years after the ending of successful treatments, and reached a plateau after 14 years, but the risk of developing solid tumors remained high and approached 30% at 30 years."

-- New England Journal of Medicine

These secondary cancers that are caused by the medical therapies are deadlier and much more horrific than the original cancers. All nuclear and chemotherapy treatments are known to cause and spread cancers. These are flippantly referred to as "side effects" by the medical industry in its own literature. Cancer screenings do the same, by likewise exposing victims to radiation and various industrial poisons. This is why breast cancer rates explode with expansive mammography testing. It is why early screenings catch so many cancers, because this year's cancer was caused by last year's radioactive screening.

Iatrogenic deaths (deaths caused by doctors) are the 3rd leading cause of death in the United States according to the medical establishment's own statistics from the Mortality Census. Death by doctor is so normal that they have actually coined a word for it: "iatrogenic".

Girls who undergo chemotherapy and radiation treatments face a 35% chance of developing breast cancer by the time that they are age 40, which is 75 times (7,500% increase) greater than average. Mammogram radiation likewise produces cancers, especially in the breast area. Statistics show that more tests equal more cancers.

"A study of over 10,000 patients shows clearly that chemo's supposedly strong track record with Hodgkin's Disease [lymphoma] is actually a lie. Patients who underwent chemo were 14 times more likely to develop leukemia and 6 times more likely to develop cancers of the bones, joints, and soft tissues than those patients who did not undergo chemotherapy."

-- Dr. John Diamond, M.D.

Getting chemotherapy means becoming permanently mentally challenged. They callously call it "chemo-brain", and conveniently have a multitude of drugs that we can purchase to "treat" and "manage" the new medically-caused mental handicaps forever after.

Dr. Ewan Cameron, and two-time Nobel Prize winner, Linus Pauling, did studies in Scotland (which were later duplicated by studies in Canada and Japan) comparing vitamin C therapy versus standard chemotherapy. Guess which group of patients lived longer on average, and by how much. The vitamin C patients lived an average of 6 times longer; and of course, they also had a substantially better quality of life. The difference was due to the fact that vitamin C strengthens the immune system, instead of damaging it further.

"As a chemist trained to interpret data, it is incomprehensible to me that physicians can ignore the clear evidence that chemotherapy does much, much more harm than good."

-- Alan Nixon, Ph.D., Past President
of The American Chemical Society.

Whenever a cancer patient dies of sepsis, it is virtually always because chemotherapy destroyed the patient's immune system, and thereby allowed sepsis to easily overwhelm the patient. These are usually counted as "sepsis deaths", instead of cancer deaths. It is another way whereby the medical community manipulates the statistics about the safety and effectiveness of chemotherapy and radiation. The same pro-industry chicanery is applied to explain fatal pneumonias, heart failures, and diabetes cases which were caused by cancer drugs and radiation.

The petrochemical industry, the medical community, and their regulatory partners in government have convinced us that sunlight is a carcinogen. Sunlight produces vitamin D in the skin from cholesterol, which removes excess cholesterol. A more important fact is that vitamin D (from sunlight) reduces the risk of getting over 70% of cancers, including skin cancer. People with greater sun exposure have higher rates of skin cancer because they are the group who uses the most sunscreen. Newer sunscreen formulations contain photo-reactive ingredients that become carcinogenic when exposed to light. Otherwise, the sunscreens contain persistent carcinogens, such as zinc oxide, titanium dioxide, and aluminum hydroxide.

The chemical companies created the problem, so they could sell us their solution. The real solution is simply not to expose oneself to the poisons. Their propaganda is so powerful that they now have us blaming our illnesses on the sun. Vitamin D deficiency is common, which proves that most of us do not get enough sun exposure. Skin cancer only became a major problem in the mid-twentieth century, after the advent of sunscreens, in much the same way that breast cancer became an epidemic only after the promotion of mammography. Breast feeding, not mammograms, is the surest way to prevent breast cancer. In fact, breast cancer was once known as "the nun's disease", because women who bore children (breast fed) appeared to be immune.

"It has been estimated that only 10 to 20 percent of all procedures currently used in medical practice have been shown to be efficacious by controlled trial."

-- Technology Assessment Health Program,
report to the U.S. Senate Committee, 1978.

The lifetime cure rate for cancers treated with standard therapies (not the mere 5 years of tumor remission that is used to cook the numbers) is about 4%. Therefore, with poisonous "conventional therapies", there is approximately a 96% chance that cancer will eventually kill the patient, or more likely, the side effects of the treatments will.

Cancer Industry Lies

First and foremost, cancer is not merely an outbreak of tumors. Although, the orthodox establishment apparently considers them to be the same. Endorsing perpetual treatments to create life-long customers is the overall agenda of policy makers, instead of curing. A dead patient is not profitable, nor is a healthy patient. The big money is made somewhere in the middle; in patients who are alive, but barely. The reason why they will never find a cure is because they are not actually looking for one. Curing would destroy the most profitable segment of the industry. Just the cancer segment of medicine alone is the 5th leading cause of bankruptcy in the United States. Any clinical researcher who announced a cure would quickly find himself looking for another career, or needing an undertaker. All of them know it. Cancer is the most profitable condition in medical history, and the establishment intends to keep it that way.

Cancer is essentially a modern, man-made epidemic from the food and chemical industries, which tend to be one in-the-same. There is some evidence that cancer existed in ancient history, but cancer was extremely rare in ancient times, except in cities with cases of mass heavy metal poisoning (again, man-made).

According to some statistics, cancer is expected to strike one person out of every three born, and this rate is rising rapidly. It is painfully obvious that there is something very corrupt about the industry, when cancer is treated by the three things that most reliably cause it: radiation, poison, and malnutrition. In fact, *properly prescribed* medicine is the 3rd leading cause of death in the United States according to the Mortality Census (not even counting the mistakes) and treatments are responsible for most deaths which are attributed to "cancer", which is the 2nd leading cause of death. Doctors never discuss the real statistics, because in 96% of cases, the treatments will greatly reduce a person's life, and most patients do not live longer than ten years. This data, which doctors keep private, is why surveys show that most oncologists would refuse some of their own therapies if they had cancer themselves. While well-meaning people continue to walk for the cure, the industry that they are supporting is still murdering their friends for profit.

The Unholy Trinity of Cancer

Toxins, radiation, and acidosis (from pharmaceuticals and malnutrition) are the unholy trinity of cancer. Acidosis is the first stage of this misunderstood condition. An astute reader will have noticed that these things are caused by the medical establishment itself, even in its supposedly valiant fight against cancer. When a person's body chemistry becomes acidic from the aforementioned factors or modern medicine, then his blood's ability to retain and carry oxygen is severely diminished. Healthy individuals have a blood oxygen level between 98 and 100 as measured by a pulse oximeter, but cancer patients routinely show only 60. Oxygen is replaced in a cancer patient's blood by wastes such as carbon dioxide. The oxygen starvation caused by acidosis leads to the formation of tumors as groups of cells which mutate to derive their energy from a fermentation process. Normal cells obtain their energy from cellular respiration, but oxygen-starved cells must mutate for survival, in order to utilize a type of direct sugar fermentation, which is the body's self-defense. This is not as biochemically clean as oxygen-based energy, and the waste products of fermentation build in the tissues causing even higher toxicities. This leads to even more acidosis and cellular oxygen starvation. Eventually, the entire immune system is debilitated by the process of cleaning the waste products, so that it can no longer cope with the removal of unhealthy cells. This allows the cancer cells to multiply even faster and to spread unchecked, creating the symptom of tumors, which happens in the latter stages of the cancer process.

The secret to beating cancer is that life-giving breath of God: oxygen. Technically, it is not so simple, but it is almost that simple. The real trick is getting oxygen into the deep tissue cells, and getting the cells to use it again. Dr. Johanna Budwig's regimen is just one of many for stimulating this. Most cancer cures (not treatments) involve adjusting the body's pH beyond neutral, and into an alkaline state. In the alkaline state, human blood is especially rich in oxygen, and this same oxygen is poisonous to mutated cancer cells. Oxygen is, of course, harmless to people who are eating a healthy diet that is full of anti-oxidants. Whilst mocked by the cancer industry, the alternative alkalizing protocols have superior degrees of effectiveness and merit further inspection.

The Budwig Lies

Most of the information that is found elsewhere about the Budwig Protocol is untrue. Dr. Budwig earned such a stellar reputation with her alternative therapy that a litany of con artists have sought to hijack her name to promote their bogus therapies. Her name is used throughout the Internet to promote ridiculous frauds that she never advocated. Some of the scoundrels have even manufactured quotes and attributed them to Johanna Budwig. The main reason for why we wrote this report was because it is so challenging to find truthful information about Dr. Budwig's work.

There is even a book that is falsely marketed to have been authored by Johanna. The book, *The Budwig Cancer & Coronary Heart Disease Prevention Diet*, was written by Dr. Budwig's opportunistic nephew, the dishonorable Armin Grunewald. Supposedly, Dr. Budwig wrote this book years after her death, which could be considered to be her most impressive accomplishment, if taken seriously. The dietary recommendations of this book do not even stay true to those of the Budwig Protocol, causing them to be of questionable safety to cancer patients.

We are citing another offender by name because the title of the clinic will deceive people into believing that the clinic is the handiwork of Dr. Budwig. In addition to that, The Budwig Center (budwigcenter.com) espouses a protocol that deviates from Dr. Budwig's, while pretending that it is the official protocol. The director of the Budwig Center (Lloyd Jenkins) has sent us threats, and filed an illegitimate D.M.C.A. take-down notice to suppress our reporting of his clinic. To be fair to the Budwig Center's director, he is no longer issuing threats, and he does appear to be slowly implementing changes to address the many concerns that we have had about his unique therapy.

As a general rule, we recommend that readers get information about the Budwig Protocol from Johanna Budwig's real books (listed herein), this report, or Lothar Hirneise, and that they assume that everything else is false. For some readers, it will mean the difference between life and death.

Dr. Johanna Budwig

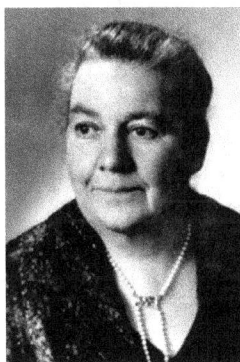

"I have the answer to cancer, but American doctors won't listen. They come here and observe my methods and are impressed. Then they want to make a special deal so they can take it home and make a lot of money. I won't do it, so I'm blackballed in every country."

-- Dr. Johanna Budwig

Dr. Johanna Budwig left us in 2003, at the age of 95, after being nominated six times for the Nobel Prize in medicine. She cured cancers in "terminally ill" patients in her homeland of Germany; even patients that the establishment had surrendered to fate, and claimed were "untreatable". She did not just cure specific or rare cancers. She cured all types of cancer, and she did it relatively quickly, cheaply, easily, and permanently; using only non-toxic ingredients, which had no adverse effects. Her medicine actually made her patients stronger. Her cure rate was over 90%, including the worst terminal cases. Dr. Budwig's success greatly contrasts the fact that the life-long cure rate of standard procedures averages less than 4%, and that the standard therapies are known to fuel future cancers and other diseases.

Dr. Budwig's weapons against cancer were quark cheese and flax seed oil. She quickly became an enemy to the pharmaceutical and nuclear industries. They have been so effective at suppressing her work, that for many of our readers, this will be their first instance of learning of the Budwig Protocol. Her bombshell findings were first published in the early 1950's. Yet they are still being institutionally ignored today.

Dr. Budwig found ways to oxygenate patients better and faster than other therapies. Her results catapulted past those of other alternative therapies by utilizing a solution made from common flax seed oil and quark cheese. She discovered that the low-fat diets were a huge part of the problem. Her regimen eliminated damaging fats and foods from the diet that cause cellular oxygen starvation, and replaced them with healing foods, such as life-saving essential fatty acids. Along with her special diet, she emphasized the benefits of sunlight, the natural source of the anti-cancer vitamin D-3, and the elimination of pervasive emotional issues.

"Without these fatty acids, the respiratory enzymes cannot function and the person suffocates, even when he is given oxygen-rich air. A deficiency in these highly unsaturated fatty-acids impairs many vital functions. First of all, it decreases the person's supply of available oxygen. We cannot survive without air and food; nor can we survive without these fatty acids. That has been proven long ago."

-- Dr. Johanna Budwig

The Budwig Protocol

There are two parts of the Budwig Protocol that are used concurrently. One of them is a natural medicine, which is a blend of something containing high amounts of sulfur proteins, and flax seed oil to provide safe omega-3 oils in the appropriate levels. Fish oil is avoided because there is a high risk of impurities, it is always rancid from heavy industrial processing, and it can dangerously upset the balance of the omega oils further. Dr. Budwig discovered that the body will synthesize omega-3 from flax seed oil in the exact quantity that it needs, and in the proper ratio with other omega oils. This medicine is normally taken orally, but in the most terminal cases, Dr. Budwig was also known to have given large doses of pure flax seed oil in enema form. The other phase of the Budwig Protocol is a special diet. Dramatic results are usually seen within 90 days, and sometimes within a week. Patients should continue the regimen for a minimum of 6 months, regardless of a disappearance of symptoms.

"...I investigated the high temperature treatment for fish oils, for the purpose of making them keep longer, and killing their fishy taste. I came to the conclusion that these oils do great harm to the entire internal glandular system, as well as to the liver and other organs and are therefore not suitable for human consumption."

-- Dr. Johanna Budwig, *Flax Oil as a True Aid Against Heart Infarction, Cancer and Other Diseases*

The Medicine

Dr. Johanna Budwig recommended the following meal, once a week for people of good health, as a cancer preventative. It was required for cancer patients as part of her protocol, wherein it was consumed at least once a day, though twice was preferred. This nutritional therapy is called the "Flax Seed Muesli", and it can be blended into a smoothie. Since genuine quark cheese is not available in most countries, see our later recommendations for alternatives to quark cheese.

Flax Seed Muesli

1. Add 1 teaspoon of honey and 2 tablespoons of freshly ground flax seeds to a bowl. Make certain to only use flax seeds that have been *freshly* ground.

2. Next, add a mixture of fresh organic fruits (any fruits that are in season, such as apples, berries, peaches, grapes etc.) Never use bananas, because Dr. Budwig felt that bananas quickly push the blood sugar level high in cancer patients.

3. Take 3 tablespoons of flax seed oil and mix it with 100 grams (about 7 tablespoons) of quark. Add about 3 tablespoons of unhomogenized ("creamline") milk to create a smooth mixture. It is best to blend it, in order to get it mixed most thoroughly. More flax seed oil may be used, depending upon personal taste, but if the quark does not fully absorb the oil, then more has been used than is needed. Add the resultant mixture to the bowl.

4. You may optionally improve the flavor by adding vanilla or cinnamon. The latter will help to regulate blood sugar.

5. Add some organic nuts on top. All organic nuts are fine, but peanuts are the least helpful.

Optional

- little garlic
- little cayenne pepper
- champagne (for the worst cases -- always given in the first couple of days)

In addition to this, Dr. Budwig incorporated flax seed oil or freshly ground flax seeds into her patients' diets every three hours. She often gave them Linomel. This is only available in Germany, but it is simply a combination of ground flax seeds and honey. She recommended 2 tablespoons of Linomel every three hours during the day, in addition to the muesli once or twice daily. Those who are seeking to grind flax seeds may use a coffee grinder to do so.

Those who do not have cancer, and are merely concerned with routine health maintenance, can simply combine 3 to 4 grams of flax seed oil with roughly 3 fluid ounces of sulfur proteins (e.g. quark, goat cheese, etc.), and consume this daily.

A cancer patient should not be concerned about getting too much flax. Dr. Budwig regularly created foods using flax seeds, but readers should beware of the flax that is used in modern foods. Flax should never be cooked, and it should not be stored after it has been ground, because its otherwise beneficial oils become rancid easily. This means that the flax found in retail foods is virtually always harmful, and it worsens cancers. What is truly despicable is that the companies selling it as a healthy ingredient must know this.

The Official Budwig Diet

- SUGAR IS ABSOLUTELY FORBIDDEN. Grape juice may be added to sweeten any other freshly-squeezed juices.

- Avoid pure animal fats, such as lard, fatback, dripping, etc.

- No commercial salad dressings or toppings.

- No commercial mayonnaise (bastardized, radioactive, genetically engineered, corn, canola and soy oils).

- No meats unless organic and preferably range fed.

- No butter, and especially no margarine or other artificial butters.

- Freshly squeezed vegetable juices are encouraged, especially carrot, celery, apple, and red beet. All-natural juice drinks are fine, with special preference to completely organic drinks.

- Three times daily a warm tea is essential. Good choices are peppermint, rose hips, or grape tea. Sweeten it only with honey. One cup of black tea before noon is fine.

- Avoid all artificial sweeteners (including high-fructose corn syrup).

- Entirely chemical-free diet.

- Avoid all processed foods.

- Avoid all soft drinks.

- Avoid tap water and bottled water, and use products free of fluoride.

- Eat all foods freshly prepared -- no reheating and no leftovers.

- Never use fish oil.

- Coconut oil is a source of omega-3 that is beneficial, and it was recommended by Dr. Budwig.

Our Suggestions

- Most patients will need to use an alternative to quark cheese, because it is unattainable in most areas. Non-homogenized yogurt is an acceptable option, and it is available in health food stores. Goat milk cheese is a better alternative. Most yogurt, cottage cheese, and other soft cheese products are less desirable, for they are made from homogenized milk. Such products should be assumed to be homogenized unless labels clearly state otherwise. They should only be used if goat cheese and non-homogenized yogurt are not available, or if they are unaffordable. It is important to supplement with vitamin C and folate if homogenized dairy products are used, in order to protect against inflammation and potentially irreversible arterial damage. The supplements do not provide complete protection against homogenized products, but they would be quite helpful.

- The flax seed (linseed) oil used in the protocol should be protected from air, heat, and light to prevent it from becoming harmfully rancid. It should always be cold pressed and preferably organic. Keep it refrigerated and sealed. Do not purchase flax seed oil in bottles unless each bottle will be used within 1 day after being opened. Discard opened bottles after 24 hours. If the oil develops any sort of rancid (fishy) smell before then, it should also be discarded. Unopened flax seed oil should be stored in a cold, dark place to prevent toxic breakdown. Those using the Budwig Protocol for routine health maintenance will use smaller amounts. They should instead purchase dark, light-resistant capsules of flax seed oil, puncture the capsules with a needle just before use, and squeeze out the oil. Avoid flax that is present in pre-made foods, such as flax cereals, flax flour, or flax-containing granola, because such flax is a rancid carcinogen from heat and processing. These precautions are necessary because of how reactive flax seed oil is with oxygen. There is breakdown of flax seed oil within 15 minutes of being exposed to heat, air, and light.

- Avoid non-flax sources of omega-3, except for baked fish and eggs. Avoid fried fish.

- Dr. Budwig never endorsed or used low-fat products, as many websites are now falsely claiming. Man-made and man-altered fats are the problem, and beneficial fats are part of the Budwig solution.

- We suggest either spring water or water filtered through a Berkey water filter that includes the optional fluoride filters.

- Green tea with honey and lemon juice. A pinch of cayenne may be helpful too.

- No microwaving food.

- Avoid hydrogenated oils.

- Attempt to wean off of all pharmaceuticals.

- Supplement with chlorophyll.

- Drink the Green Drink regularly to ensure proper nutrition. The recipe can be found in the *Nutrition* chapter.

- Eat an alkalizing diet. Reference the *Body pH and Disease* section of the *Wellness* chapter.

- Take a large dose of vitamin C daily. Do not take more than 5 grams per day, because massive doses will cause kidney stress. More than two grams could be problematic for patients with kidney or liver cancers.

- Avoid sunscreens, cosmetics, and the toxic lotions that are found at regular retailers.

- At least once a day, we suggest a lemon and pineapple drink, because of its ability to improve body pH rapidly.

- Avoid white bread, white rice, white sugar, white flour, and anything else that is overprocessed or bleached with chlorine compounds.

- Avoid table salt and use a high quality sea salt from a health food store.

- Delay detoxifying whenever a person is severely ill or unstable.

- Delay detoxifying if it is liver or kidney cancer.

- Get a high grade water filter for shower water with the priority of getting all chlorine removed.

- Do not use tap water in a vaporizer, because it will release chlorine gas.

- Find safer alternatives to common soaps, bleaches, and detergents.

- Eliminate candida, which should already happen with the Budwig Protocol.

- Avoid all vaccines.

- Avoid your doctor. *Seriously*. This could be the most important rule if you want to live.

- Avoid soy products and canola oil.

- Use iodine transdermally, but beware of povidone iodine. If a pill form is necessary, then supplement only with red marine algae capsules. Do not use any other type of oral supplementation for iodine.

- For deathly ill patients, see a specialist, such as a naturopathic doctor (N.D.) who can provide IV's, including safe hydrogen peroxide if necessary.

- Use vitamin B-17 for bad cases, but avoid for people with impaired livers.

- Do not use aluminum-based antiperspirants or deodorants, which is most of them.

Books by Johanna Budwig

Only three of Johanna's books have been translated into English. Six books are only available in German. The English books are listed below.

- *The Oil-Protein Cookbook (l-Eiwei-Kost)* Sensei Verlag (2000)

- *Cancer - The Problem and the Solution (Krebs. Das Problem und die Lsung)* Sensei Verlag (1999)

- *Flax Oil As A True Aid Against Arthritis, Heart Infarction, Cancer And Other Diseases (Fette als wahre Hilfe gegen Arteriosklerose, Herzinfarkt, Krebs)* 1972

Some of the information in this report was obtained from Lothar Hirneise, who was Johanna's student, even though he is too humble to call himself her apprentice. He is also the English translator of her books. We wish to express our gratitude to Lothar for preserving Dr. Johanna Budwig's memory, her honor, and her important work.

Additional Anti-Cancer Therapies

The Budwig Protocol is our recommended anti-cancer therapy, although there are other effective alternatives. We covered the best of them in detail in our documentary, *The Cancer Report*. What follows is a brief listing of the anti-cancer therapies that we consider to be the safest and most effective.

- Essiac Tea
- Vitamin B-17 (laetrile)
- Oxygen/ozone therapy (intravenous hydrogen peroxide)
- High-dose vitamin C therapy
- The Hoxsey Regimen
- Gerson Therapy

Most cancer patients react with panic upon learning of their diagnosis. This panicked reaction enables doctors to convince patients to do almost anything, including poisoning themselves with radiation. After years of brainwashing, many of the people seeking alternatives are tempted to try everything, because they have lingering doubts about the effectiveness of alternatives. This tendency to try them all is always a mistake. Combining a multitude of therapies together will usually put more stress upon a body, to ultimately be counterproductive. It is likely to worsen the cancer. For the panicked people who are insistent on "hitting it with everything", we recommend the following therapy combination. Begin with the Budwig Protocol, then augment it with Essiac Tea, vitamin B-17, and vitamin C. All of these should work together well, without producing more problems.

Important Precautionary Notes

Vitamin B-17 should never be used for liver or kidney cancers, or in cases wherein the individual has liver or kidney impairment. Chemotherapy will easily cause such impairment. Intravenous hydrogen peroxide should only be provided by someone who is knowledgeable enough to get the ratios correct, between it and saline. Administering or preparing an IV solution improperly can be fatal. Do not take more than 5 grams of vitamin C per day, because massive doses will cause kidney stress. More than two grams could be problematic for patients with kidney or liver cancers.

A.C.S. Admits Untreated Cancers Often Go Away

Naturally

While researching the use of alternative therapies that were utilized by Suzanne Somers, we came across doctors and media outlets who desperately tried to malign her reputation. Their responses were so hasty that they accidentally revealed statistics that are not normally shared with the public.

> *"We're finding that about 25 to 30 percent of some cancers stop growing at some point, that can make some treatments look good that aren't doing anything. Until doctors figure out how to identify which patients have cancers that won't progress, the only option is to treat everyone."*

-- Dr. Otis Brawley, American Cancer
Society's Chief Medical Officer

While some people might consider 25 to 30 percent to be a relatively low percentage, this is actually much higher than the success rate for chemotherapy. Since the life-long cure rate bounces between 2 and 4 percent for orthodox treatments, 30% suddenly becomes a very impressive figure with a gain of 10 times. Of course, this number speaks only for those who supposedly get no treatments at all. Alternative therapies get better life-long cure rates than 30%, but these numbers are not discussed publicly by medical officials, and rarely in private. Why aren't these figures ever given to patients who are diagnosed with cancer? Why are they instead told the lie that they will certainly die if they refuse chemotherapy and radiation when almost the opposite is true?

We have searched tirelessly for the success rates of those who decided to walk away from all treatments for years, but we only found it when the American Cancer Society stumbled in its attempts to defend its bruised reputation from meekly Suzanne Somers. Why didn't they publicly release those numbers before? The recovery of Suzanne Somers was obviously quite embarrassing for them, because not only is she one of many who has cured herself of cancer permanently (not just 5 years of survival), but she also went public about her experiences with alternative treatments. Had she religiously followed the orthodox therapies, she would have had a 96% chance of not being alive, and her protracted death would have been truly horrific.

The quotation cited earlier makes another interesting point. Doctors really have no clue which cancers will progress, and which ones will not. Therefore, we must ask if early testing is *really* a good idea. With early testing, not only do the tests actually stimulate cancers through radiation, cutting, and poisoning, but doctors frequently discover anomalies that would otherwise naturally disappear if left alone. They always treat those abnormalities, and the patients almost always die from the treatments. People nowadays die from the treatments instead of the cancers, and this is shown in the establishment's own statistics. Regardless of whether they existed initially; cancers will strike sooner or later whenever a body is exposed to chemotherapy. All chemotherapy drugs are carcinogenic, and they weaken all healthy cells. This is admitted in the official literature for adverse effects for all of the so-called anti-cancer medications, and massive cellular destruction is a part of standard treatments by design. They claim that their medicines attack the weaker cancer cells, but they actually do it by attacking all of the cells, and thereby the very immune system that is so critical for recovery.

> *"Call it the arrow of cancer. Like the arrow of time, it was supposed to point in one direction. Cancers grew and worsened. But as a paper in The Journal of the American Medical Association noted last week, data from more than two decades of screening for breast and prostate cancer call that view into question. Besides finding tumors that would be lethal if left untreated, screening appears to be finding many small tumors that would not be a problem if they were left alone, undiscovered by screening. They were destined to stop growing on their own or shrink, or even, at least in the case of some breast cancers, disappear."*
>
> -- Gina Kolata, The New York Times,
> October 26, 2009

The success rate of curing cancer is not going to rise much in orthodox medicine, because it is unwilling to consider any less profitable methodologies. Any rise in orthodox cancer treatment success rates would indicate that their methods of calculating cure rates have changed, not the actual survival rates. It is how the *science* of modern medicine is cooked. Barely surviving for 5 years is currently counted as a successful cure, but patients usually die between the 5 and 10 year mark. It is called "cooking the books" in accounting circles. Most people are shocked when they learn that those who die during drug trials are censored from the records, because the departed did not "complete the study". Getting killed in an experimental drug trial actually helps a drug company's chance of getting that drug approved, because those who get the sickest are not counted.

"Success of most chemotherapies is appalling... There is no scientific evidence for its ability to extend in any appreciable way the lives of patients suffering from the most common organic cancer... Chemotherapy for malignancies too advanced for surgery, which accounts for 80% of all cancers, is a scientific wasteland."

-- Dr. Uhlrich Abel

If the cancer industry were really concerned about scientific progress, then it would not hide its own statistics. Truth does not fear investigation. Instead, its numbers are repeatedly covered up, and the scientific community eliminates from its ranks anyone who refuses to accept the establishment's zealous dogma. It is not science. It is politics, and a very deadly form of it.

"Two to four percent of cancers respond to chemotherapy."

-- Ralph Moss, Ph.D

J.A.M.A. Admitted Chemotherapy Leads to Early Death

Reuters has reported some scientific findings that are not usually released to the public. The recent study *Clinical Ascertainment of Health Outcomes Among Adults Treated for Childhood Cancer* by Birmingham University (England) concluded that those who survive cancer treatments as children have extremely high chances of premature deaths. After monitoring 18,000 childhood cancer survivors, the university documented that these people tended to die early from a range of ailments including heart attacks, heart failure, heart disease, strokes, and additional cancers. Premature deaths were 11 times (1,100%) more likely than for the general population.

"Survivors experienced 11 times the number of deaths expected from the general population, and although this rate declined over the years, it was still three times higher than expected 45 years after their original diagnosis."

-- Reuters

Raoul Reulen, the lead researcher from Birmingham University, described recurrent cancers as a "recognized late *complication* of childhood cancer". How is that for spin? To the medical establishment, endlessly recurring cancers are considered to be just *complications*, instead of being hard evidence that their methods are not working and that the treatments are murderous.

"This is due largely to exposure to radiation during treatment, and to the side effects of some of the more toxic cancer drugs."

-- Raoul Reulen

Perhaps more shocking than the admission that these "complications" were caused by previous cancer treatments (rather than genetics) is that the study actually got published in the Journal of the American Medical Association.

Heart Disease

Broken Hearts and Ticking Time Bombs

No health topic is more important, more full of misinformation, and more complex than this one. This report tackles the four most common conditions associated with "heart disease": hypertension, stroke, coronary heart disease, and congestive heart failure. The information herein should be useful for all heart problems.

Heart disease is the number one killer in America, and yet it does not induce terror as cancer does. The reason for this is because people are horrified of the cancer treatments, not the disease itself. Alas, heart health is frequently ignored in lieu of cancer concerns, with breast cancer being an excellent example of this short sightedness. Case in point: For every woman who dies of breast cancer (cancer treatments), 11 more will die from coronary heart disease. About 60% of heart disease deaths happen suddenly in people who had no previous symptoms and normal cholesterol levels. These people simply collapsed unexpectedly. The real lesson to be learned, as you will see, is everything that we have been taught about heart disease is wrong. If the *experts* whom we have been listening to were right, then heart disease would not be the #1 failure of modern medicine.

Adhering to a critical holistic principle of alternative medicine, it is important that we never adopt the foolishness of a typical physician, who will obsessively focus on only the organ displaying obvious symptoms. It is wiser to treat the patient instead of an organ, which means correcting problems with both lifestyle and diet. As is the case for practically all other chronic diseases, a heart patient usually brings the disease upon himself with his irresponsible behavior for a period of many years, and only he can get himself out of the mess. Drugs can suppress symptoms for a while, like they always do, but real change comes only from real changes. Merely masking the symptoms with drugs is the health policy of fools. The time bomb is still ticking, even though the timer has been hidden from view.

Heart issues go beyond the physical, and merely physically treating heart conditions ultimately results in the failures that we all see around us in slowly dying friends and relatives. Numerous surveys have shown that asking people about their quality of life and happiness accurately reflects their heart health. Thus, we must not ignore the mental, and even the spiritual components of heart conditions. A healthy heart requires a healthy mind, body, and spirit. Emotional issues are commonly forsaken, despite their obvious importance. Throughout mythology, the human heart represents something greater than merely an organ to pump blood. It contains the soul of a person, including his memories and emotions. We frequently refer to emotional issues in modern life with phrases ranging from "heart-broken" to "faint-hearted".

In Traditional Chinese Medicine, the physical organs are correlated with emotional states. Such ancient science can seem ludicrous to modern readers, but one quickly learns of its persistent value when studying alternative medicine. Heart problems are indeed closely tied to depression, rage, nervousness, despair, insomnia, and restlessness. This has been repeatedly proven in studies of the Type A Personality and in studies of grieving patients. Therefore, people should look within themselves to deal with their own emotional issues as the first stage of healing their hearts. It is absolutely vital. Periodic meditation and prayer can save lives.

Heart Disease and Cholesterol

Everyone in modern society has heard about cholesterol, and how bad it is. Most do not understand why it exists, and simply see it as a menace that must be eliminated as quickly as possible. This misunderstanding is exactly what the pharmaceutical complex promotes, because it allows them to perpetually treat cholesterol with drugs. These drugs are prescribed for the remainder of a patient's lifetime, and when he eventually dies of a heart attack, family and friends will believe that the disaster was inevitable. The death will not be attributed to other health factors or to the drugs themselves, but to the "high cholesterol"; even though there are no known deaths from cholesterol in human history. It is all very convenient for the drug companies, so long as we do not examine what is up their other sleeve. We are reminded of restless leg syndrome, whereby the disease was 'discovered' immediately after the pharmaceutical for it was patented, as a reason to sell us that pharmaceutical. Now it has been upgraded to a "disease".

> *"Before 1920, coronary heart disease was rare in America -- so rare that when a young internist named Paul Dudley White introduced the German Electrocardiograph to his colleagues at Harvard University, they advised him to concentrate on a more profitable branch of medicine. The new machine revealed the presence of arterial blockages, thus permitting early diagnosis of coronary heart disease. But in those days, clogged arteries were a medical rarity, and White had to search for patients who could benefit from his new technology. During the next forty years, however, the incidence of coronary heart disease rose dramatically, so much so that by the mid 1950's, heart disease was the leading cause of death among Americans."*

-- Mary Enig, Ph.D.

The amount of cholesterol that you eat actually has very little relationship with the amount that you have in your blood. When you eat more cholesterol, your body produces less, and when you eat less cholesterol, your body produces more. A body usually produces between three and four times the cholesterol that one eats. The amount produced is generally related to how much is needed. Cholesterol is indeed needed and critical for optimal health. The purpose of so-called "bad cholesterol" is not to give us heart attacks, but to repair our damaged arteries. Whenever a poor diet and lifestyle lead to damaged arteries, a thick and sticky substance is required to patch them. That substance is known as LDL or "bad cholesterol". When this damaging behavior is continued, multiple patches are created, leading to what we know as "clogged arteries". The problem is not the cholesterol, which is doing its wonderful job of preventing our deaths from internal bleeding. The problem is the fact that the arteries are damaged enough to risk internal bleeding. Blocking a body's healthy countermeasures only leads to worse problems. It is the pharmaceutical standard of symptom suppression that is so much like hiding the timer of a time bomb, and then expecting it not to eventually go off. Thus, that "bad" cholesterol is not a bad thing to have, but it can be a warning sign of problems elsewhere.

Modern medicine spends a lot of time fighting this patch, instead of the actual causes of arterial damage. Thus, it is not surprising that cholesterol-lowering drugs cause heart disease and heart attacks. A massive portion of the elderly population is taking cholesterol-lowering drugs, even though research shows that the higher their cholesterol levels (especially HDL), the longer that they will live. Low cholesterol in the elderly is actually a sign that something is seriously wrong, and a heart attack may be imminent. Modern medicine has only recently come to accept that at least some cholesterol (HDL) is good.

Cholesterol is still suppressed with drugs, despite what science would make prudent. It also has been proven that these drugs cause high suicide rates. The drugs can lead to personality changes, in a manner similar to (but not as intense as) S.S.R.I. anti-depressants.

The anti-cholesterol hysteria began in the 1950's, when researcher Ancel Keys proposed the Lipid Hypothesis. It stated that cholesterol and saturated fats lead to heart disease. His beliefs were promoted heavily by the new hydrogenated oils industry, which spent obscene amounts of money to convince everyone of Keys' indisputable findings. This successful marketing campaign was on par with similar marketing for fluoride at about the same time. Studies which had oppositional findings to Keys' were ignored or maligned. As a result of his flawed scientific methodology (cherry picking results to match what he wanted to find) saturated fats like butter and eggs were used less, in exchange for the poisonous trans fats that are in hydrogenated oils. Heart disease rates have been rising exponentially since then.

The French eat more fats than any other group in the world, yet they have low rates of heart disease. There are plenty of countries with similar patterns. The French lifestyle especially counters Keys' hypothesis, and it also provides evidence that resveratrol (found in wines) improves heart health. Resveratrol has been shown to reverse atheriosclerosis (hardening of the arteries).

High cholesterol levels should be a warning to people that inflammation is present. It is a risk marker, and a symptom that can save your life, unless you follow your doctor's advice. Eliminating the cholesterol through drugs is the equivalent to eliminating the thermometer in a room that is too hot. It is illogical, and it does nothing to eliminate the dangerous cause.

Cholesterol levels naturally drop whenever the body's need for it does, and cholesterol should never be forced lower with drugs. Diet and lifestyle can reduce cholesterol, but it is never because of a lowered cholesterol intake. The natural drop in cholesterol happens only when a person stops eating toxic foods that attack the arteries, because healthy arteries do not need patching. Remember that a body typically produces 3-4 times the amount of cholesterol that is consumed. The fats that a person eats are therefore comparatively insignificant. Cholesterol will rise whenever the body's need for cholesterol rises, so trans fats and inflammatory substances are what need to be avoided. These attack the arteries, and a body will be required to do a great deal of patching as a consequence. References will be made to herbs that lower cholesterol levels later, but herbs do it by lowering a body's need for cholesterol, not by forcefully lowering it like pharmaceuticals do.

Studies on the link between cholesterol and heart health have been manipulated for decades. The first studies on eggs showed elevated cholesterol levels because they had used dehydrated eggs, and studies of coconut oil yielded similar results because they had used partially hydrogenated coconut oil to get the results that they wanted. Why will this billion dollar industry not test with organic, range fed eggs?

Why Allopathic Medicine Will Never Find the Cure

Allopathic medicine will not find the cure to any heart-related ills because they are not really looking for them. They are looking for new ways to *manage* diseases perpetually, and to keep their patients sick enough to require drugs. Thus, they are developing new drugs to help reduce cholesterol, eliminate renin (clotting agent), thin the blood, and other forms of symptom management. The utter insanity is shown by the fact that cholesterol is designed to prevent internal bleeding, so while doctors are giving anti-cholesterol drugs, which make internal bleeding much more likely, they are also simultaneously giving blood thinners to ensure that the bleeds are real gushers, and that the body will need *even more* cholesterol to save itself. They spend no time considering why the body creates cholesterol, the role of renin, and what causes thick, hypercoagulatory blood. The system is designed to ensure that heart disease is not curable.

A drug dealer will not help you to quit an addiction, unless he can give you another drug that is more expensive, and preferably more addictive. The medical establishment likewise relies on your sickness for its profit. They do not want you to die, because that is the end of their profit stream, but they do not want you to be independent either. When most people die, they have already fed most of their money into the system, and it is the leading cause of bankruptcy in the U.S.

Hypertension

Hypertension is bad, but hypertension drugs are worse. Blood pressure medications can cause heart failure with prolonged use. They all seem to have a pattern of side effects, which include heart and muscle damage, irregular or fast heart beat, restlessness, and light-headedness. Weaning off these drugs should be done slowly and cautiously, with frequent monitoring for dangerous spikes in blood pressure. Bear in mind that whenever weaning off of such drugs, one should expect sudden and temporary rises in blood pressure. This is temporary, and the instabilities should diminish in time. Dangerously excessive pressure will require emergency intervention at a hospital, so it is wise to decrease drug dosage gradually to avoid dangerous spikes in pressure.

People diagnosed with hypertension are often asked to undergo stress tests at routine intervals. There is actually very little science behind these. People have good days and bad days, and it has been repeatedly proven that the results of stress tests vary from one day to the next. Yet, when people do poorly on these tests, more expensive tests are always recommended, along with even more drugs. In addition to being useless, the stress tests themselves are prone to causing heart attacks. Sure, there are doctors on staff, but even minor heart attacks cause permanent damage to the heart, and some are deadly despite attempts at resuscitation. The heart attacks stimulated by the stress tests sometimes occur later, when the patient has returned to his home.

There is a much more effective way of determining if you are at risk for heart attacks, using a technique known as the ankle-brachial index test.

The Ankle-Brachial Index Test

A person begins this test by getting his blood pressure taken normally, and recording the result. Next, he lays on his back, and has his blood pressure taken at his ankle, just above the bone that juts out. This result should be recorded too. The index calculation is based upon the leg's systolic pressure divided by the arm's. Take for example, if the patient's first blood pressure measurement were 120 over 70, which is normally written as 120/70, and his blood pressure at his ankle were 110/68. We only need the first of these numbers in each set, the systolic measurements of 120 (arm) and 110 (ankle). For instance, $110/120 = 0.916$. A healthy index is 1.0 or greater.

The logic behind this test is sound. The arteries of the legs must exert more to assist with heart contractions than the arteries of the arms, so more pressure ought to be detected in the legs. Clotting disorders and signs of atheriosclerosis show up in the legs before anywhere else. These factors make this test a superior method of early detection. The sooner that a person notices heart disease, the easier it is to reverse damage.

There are plenty of medical industry tests surrounding hypertension, arterial plaque, and coronary heart disease, but there is very little purpose to them, other than to increase profits. For instance, a $3,000 test may tell a patient how severely clogged his arteries are, but modern medicine can do nothing to reverse it. They can create pretty pictures of the damage, but they are unable to actually do anything about it.

The following methods can eliminate hypertension. Many of these are explained in more detail later.

Natural Hypertension Remedies

- Weight loss must be done properly or the result will be further impaired health. For example, smaller and healthier meals should be consumed *more often*. Do not skip meals or use toxic diet products. Virtually all diet products are toxic and inflammatory. They exaggerate health issues (including heart disease) in the long term.

- Replace all table salt with unrefined sea salt, and avoid processed sodium sources, including monosodium glutamate.

- Follow the Budwig regimen of flax seed oil combined with goat cheese. Yogurt can be used in place of goat cheese, but it is not as healthy, because it is usually made from homogenized milk. If yogurt is used, also supplement with vitamin C and folate (or folic acid) to prevent inflammation and arterial damage.

- Do deep breathing exercises. Various martial art breathing techniques have had good success because of their emphasis on deep breathing exercises.

- American ginseng (panax quinquefolius) is sometimes used as a very mild stimulant, but it is weaker than the Korean varieties for this purpose. The American variant is most suited for heart patients, because it has been shown to improve heart health, reduce cholesterol levels (inflammation), and to normalize blood pressure.

- L-taurine is known for regulating the blood pressure, and bringing balance to the sodium and potassium levels in the blood. It also helps to regulate the pulse. It indirectly aids the heart by improving kidney function. Additionally, it can stop some heart attacks.

- L-arginine is used by the body in the production of nitric oxide, which makes blood vessels relax, increases blood flow, and improves blood vessel function. Do not take arginine following a heart attack. While arginine is good for prevention, it has been shown to have damaging effects immediately following a cardiac arrest.

- CoQ10 can be used to help people wean off of hypertension (blood pressure) medications faster and more safely and it is an overall heart tonic. It is especially useful for older people.

- Cayenne has the unique ability to regulate blood pressure as needed, either increasing or decreasing it, as is prudent. It is also useful for stopping a heart attack.

- Vitamin E thins the blood, and has been shown in studies to normalize blood pressure. Women should avoid blood thinners like vitamin E while menstruating, because they will cause heavier bleeding.

- Hawthorn is one of the best supplements for heart health, and it helps with blood pressure too.

Blood pressure instability or imbalance can be an indication of kidney damage. Additional symptoms of kidney impairment are fatigue, vision problems, muscle cramping, bleeding gums, swollen legs, excessive urination, and excessive thirst. Kidney stress can also result in imbalanced electrolyte salts, especially potassium, which will cause fluid retention or loss throughout the body. Kidney stress is commonly caused by excessive supplementation, a toxic diet, or pharmaceuticals. Doctors never blame the pharmaceuticals, because doing so would mean taking responsibility for damaging the patient's health. Kidney stress may also be caused by liver inflammation, which can be due to heavy metal toxicity, certain diseases, excessive alcohol usage, or pharmaceutical toxicity. The overall efficiency of the kidneys is also greatly effected by a person's emotional health, which ultimately effects the heart too. Therefore, the process of healing the kidneys could be very slow if the person has unresolved emotional issues, or if he continues harming himself.

The following list of supplements strengthen the kidneys. These dosages should not be exceeded, or else the supplements will ironically stress the kidneys further. When dealing with kidney stress, these should be the only supplements taken, and no pharmaceuticals should be used, if at all possible. During a period of kidney repair, it is important that a pristine diet be maintained, with preference being given to organic foods. As mentioned elsewhere in this report, special care should be exercised when weaning from blood pressure medications, because the discontinuation process may cause dangerous spikes in blood pressure. Discontinuing blood pressure medications should always be done gradually and with constant monitoring for dangerous spikes. Pressure spikes should be handled in a common sense manner, which may include increasing the dosage slightly, or visiting emergency medical personnel in the extreme cases.

For Kidney Support

- Dandelion (500 mg. for every 100 lbs. of body weight)
- Licorice (500 mg. for every 100 lbs. of body weight)
- Taurine (250 mg. per 50 lbs. of body weight)
- Vitamin E (133 I.U. per 100 lbs. of body weight)

- Cinnamon (500 mg. per 100 lbs. of body weight)
- Vitamin C (500 mg. for every 75 lbs. of body weight)
- Rhubarb
- Carrots

Congestive Heart Failure

Congestive heart failure is when the heart is too weak and damaged to properly oxygenate the blood, adequately circulate it, and clear the lungs. Blood cannot be circulated properly, and builds up in the heart, forcing it to beat faster. Fatigue and mental confusion are common, because not enough blood and oxygen reach the brain. As a result of this poor efficiency, fluids can then accumulate in the lungs, leaving the victim susceptible to pneumonia; which is one of the leading causes of death in the elderly population amongst those who have heart failure. Allopathic medicine claims that this condition has no known cause, because it ignores the findings of alternative medicine. Congestive heart failure is always caused by malnutrition over an extended period of time. This malnutrition is virtually always due to long-term pharmaceutical usage and toxic processed foods, which destroy a body's ability to retain and utilize critical nutrients. It can take many months, and a religious adherence to a nutritious diet to reverse congestive heart failure.

The B vitamins are crucial for reversing this condition. Vitamins B-1 (thiamine), B-3 (niacin), and B-6 (pyridoxine) are extremely beneficial. The essential vitamin B-4 is a name given to a specific group of amino acids found in some foods. It is strongly recommended that anyone with congestive heart failure does some thorough research for a B-complex supplement. When researching supplements, please be mindful that some companies are selling B vitamins that are made from liver, soy, and genetically-engineered yeasts, which we recommend avoiding.

The B vitamins are the main nutrient deficiency in the case of those with congestive heart failure. Proper supplementation can produce a massive improvement in health and well being. In addition to taking a B-complex supplement, heart patients should get plenty of vegetables. Patients should also drink cayenne tea or take a cayenne supplement (on a full stomach) daily. Cayenne's benefits are astounding to both heart health and blood pressure regulation. If cayenne supplementation causes burning in the stomach, simply eating some parmesan cheese should stop it.

Jiaogulan, otherwise known as "China's immortality herb" has been shown to increase the output of the heart without increasing the pulse or adversely effecting blood pressure. It can actually make the heart stronger. It may be used in conjunction with everything already stated.

See the *Reversing Heart Disease* section for information about CoQ10, because it has also been shown to be beneficial. Cases of congestive heart failure have been directly linked with a CoQ10 deficiency.

One of the hidden causes of congestive heart failure is an excess of iron. It is accumulative in the body, particularly for men, and an excess of iron causes an untold number of health problems. Patients can obtain a simple test to determine what their iron levels are (anything above 150 is considered dangerously high), or they can just begin treating it. Grown men practically always have excessive levels of iron inside their blood. Linus Pauling discovered that vitamin C and resveratrol help to remove excess iron. Resveratrol is present in red grapes, dark grape juice, and red wines. Its highest concentration is observed inside muscadine grapes. This is probably because these grapes have thicker skins, which is where resveratrol concentrates.

Vegetarian and vegan heart patients may actually harm their health further by removing iron, because they are likely to be deficient in iron, due to their self-imposed malnutrition. Iron is critical for the creation of oxygen-carrying, red blood cells. It is necessary to oxygenate a body properly. The stress placed upon the lungs from cellular oxygen starvation stems from a lack of red blood cells, which always equals an equivalent stress upon the cardiovascular system.

Strokes

Strokes are reported for 750,000 American people each year. A stroke occurs when the blood supply (oxygen) to the brain is impeded for an extended period. It is believed that hypercoagulability (excessive clotting) of blood causes 85% of strokes. This section will concentrate upon the minority 15% for which the cause is not hypercoagulability. The hypercoagulability group is discussed later in this report.

People who snore and have sleep apnea are at a much greater risk of having strokes. Sleep apnea can usually be detected by nearby people, who may notice that the person stops breathing for several seconds while sleeping. One remedy is a snore guard that can be obtained from a dentist, or a person may get one custom fitted from a variety of E-bay sellers. It is a device that is designed to maintain an unobstructed airway, which eliminates the primary danger of sleep apnea. These devices are obviously not a cure, but they will work to prevent any immediate risk that is posed by this condition. It is worth noting that those getting proper nutrition and exercise will rarely have sleep apnea.

Stroke patients unsurprisingly have a higher than normal level of fibrin in their blood. Fibrin is the blood-clotting factor. It is wise to supplement with vitamin E (400 - 800 IU) because it inhibits thrombin, the enzyme that converts fibrinogen to fibrin. This category of patients also has an increased level of infections in their blood, which will be discussed later as a cause of many additional heart problems.

The use of hyperbaric oxygen (pressurized oxygen chambers) has had tremendous success in helping those who have had strokes. It is now believed that parts of the brain may not simply die during a stroke, but that they may merely become dormant. All of the B vitamins should be provided to a stroke victim, because they are essential for good brain health and repairing the central nervous system. The oxygenating effects of Budwig therapy, taurine, chlorophyll, and NAC (N-acetyl-cysteine) are also very useful for stroke recovery.

Aspirin use increases the risk of aneurysms and internal bleeding, so it is not a wise preventative for strokes. Contrary to popular belief, it does not decrease the chances of having heart attacks. The studies which showed a reduced heart attack risk used Bufferin, an aspirin product that is buffered with magnesium. Magnesium can safely prevent some heart attacks, but aspirin without magnesium cannot. Heart disease patients do not suffer from aspirin deficiencies.

Causes of Heart Disease

While heart disease is a term used to describe all forms of circulatory problems, the most common circulatory ailment is coronary heart disease. It is a narrowing of the small blood vessels that supply blood and oxygen to the heart. Coronary heart disease is also referred to as coronary artery disease.

> *"The main cause of cardiovascular disease is the instability and dysfunction of the blood vessel wall caused by chronic vitamin deficiency. This leads to millions of small lesions and cracks in the artery wall, particularly in the coronary arteries. The coronary arteries are mechanically the most stressed arteries because they are squeezed flat from the pumping action of the heart more than 100,000 times per day, similar to a garden hose which is stepped upon."*
>
> -- Dr. Matthias Rath, *Why Animals Don't Get Heart Disease, But People Do.*

Dr. Matthias Rath worked closely with the late Dr. Linus Pauling. They discovered that cardiovascular disease is a slower, less-severe form of scurvy. In scurvy, cracks in the vessel walls are deeper, leading to massive internal bleeding. Dr. Linus Pauling labeled artheriosclerosis (hardening of the arteries) as a pre-scurvy condition.

It was discovered that the arteries actually pump blood too, which is common knowledge in medical circles. This phenomena is what makes it possible to test ones pulse with a finger pressure test. The pumping action of the arteries is stimulated by the heart. When the heart beats, arteries expand to create a negative, vacuum-like pressure to pull blood. When the heart relaxes, the arteries contract, exerting a force that is strong enough to aid in pushing the blood along. Neither alternative medicine nor orthodox medicine understands much about how this works. The big difference is that we admit that we do not fully understand, whereas typical doctors use medical buzz-words to disguise their ignorance.

Cracks in the arterial walls are repaired by the body using a sticky protein known as APO(a) and a lipoprotein called LP(a). Then LDL, the "bad" cholesterol comes along to help them form the finished repair patch. Due to deficiencies of the anti-oxidant vitamin C, these fats may oxidize, leading to a hardening of the arteries. Oxidation, which is unchecked by vitamins, leads to the calcification of the cells. "Plaque deposits" is the phrase given to the calcification of fats lining the arterial walls, which is the end result of malnutrition-induced oxidation damage.

The coronary arteries are the most stressed; and hence, they need the most repair. Plaque forms as the inner walls of the arteries oxidize. When the interior of arteries become narrow, due to plaque formation, dislodged pieces of plaque can lead to blockages. Blockages may also be caused by traveling blood clots, whenever they become wedged inside thick plaque deposits. These blockages are commonly called myocardial infarctions by medical professionals, and heart attacks by the rest of us.

Within five years of diagnosis of coronary heart disease, 50% of American patients die from it or the long-term effects of medical treatments. Diuretics, for example, are the most common medications given for the worst heart problems, but they flush out the B vitamins that a patient's heart desperately needs, along with flushing potassium (a deficiency of which may lead to sudden heart failure). To highlight just how moronic this approach is: diuretics stress the kidneys (and the rest of the body) by chemically forcing a body to purge itself of fluids. In other words, the most popular treatment for severe heart problems is forced chemical dehydration, and attacking the kidneys, which have a direct effect upon heart health.

Our modern lifestyle has paved the way for the epidemic of heart disease. Most municipal water is contaminated with pharmaceutical drugs, fluoride, BPA, and chlorine. Chlorine-tainted water changes the preferred HDL cholesterol into LDL cholesterol, creates free radicals inside the body that require more anti-oxidant vitamins to neutralize, and it destroys fatty acids that are needed by the heart. According to the book, *Coronaries Cholesterol Chlorine* by Dr. Joseph M. Price, chlorination was first suspected of causing heart disease during the Korean War, because the men who had canteens with the highest amounts of chlorine also had the greatest damage to their arteries. Physically fit soldiers in their twenties had arteries reminiscent of their seventy-year-old grandfathers.

> *"Chlorine is the greatest crippler and killer of modern times. While it prevented epidemics of one disease, it was creating another. Two decades ago, after the start of chlorinating our drinking water in 1904, the present epidemic of heart trouble, cancer and senility began."*

-- Dr. Joseph M. Price

A massive amount of chlorine is inhaled and absorbed during a typical shower, and thus a shower filter is strongly recommended. We recommend drinking spring water, or getting a Berkey water filter with the optional fluoride-removing add-ons. Be aware of filters which only remove the taste of chlorine, and instead get one that removes all impurities.

Most cooking oils are already oxidized (rancid) before they are even bottled, because of the processing. Even otherwise healthy oils become slightly toxic and carcinogenic when they are rancid. It is vital to get cold-pressed oils for this reason. Chemical deodorizers are sometimes added to hide the unpleasant scent of rancidity. Rancid (oxidized) fats are chemically unstable and provide damaging free radicals. Trans fats cause inflammation that may induce arterial patching. Beware of both trans fats and healthy oils that have been made rancid. Use cold-pressed, extra-virgin olive oil for most cooking, and peanut oil for high-heat applications. Cold-pressed, extra-virgin coconut oil is easily the healthiest oil of all for cold recipes, but it breaks down rapidly in heat to become rancid. Pristine coconut oil is an extremely healthy dietary supplement that will help to protect the arteries, like other healthy saturated fats will. Trans fats are industrially-produced artificial foods. They commonly contain aluminum, lead, and cobalt residues, as a result of their manufacturing processes.

The same biotechnology industry that brought us trans fats has more recently created genetically-engineered soy and canola. Both soy and canola oils are used as pesticides. Soy causes drastic hormone imbalances, which has resulted in the epidemics of hypothyroidism and endometriosis. Soy is toxic in even its organic state, and it has to undergo a fermentation process just to make it safe for human consumption, with very mixed results. As a general rule, soy should be considered unsafe for human consumption. The canola plant has no organic variety, because the first canola plant was born in a test tube in the 1970's. The nuclear industry assisted in genetically engineering it. Canola is the Frankenstein spawn of the deadly rapeseed plant. Rapeseed oil was banned in foods for causing heart tumors. Rapeseed's bastard child, canola, is being deceptively marketed as being free of trans fats. The lie is based upon the fact that they only use the test results from before the oil is heated, and flagrantly ignore the test results of heated canola oil. Then, they market canola as the healthiest cooking oil, using cherry-picked test results from only uncooked oil. The biotechnology companies forget to mention that canola oil becomes a trans fat as soon as it is heated. However, they never forget to place the FDA-approved "heart healthy" label on every bottle of canola oil. Canola oil is also marketed as being high in omega-3, but all of the omega-3 becomes rancid and carcinogenic as soon as it is heated. Studies have shown that canola oil can produce heart lesions, particularly when accompanied by a diet that is low in protective saturated fats. It also produces high levels of benzene and formaldehyde when it is heated. The biotech industry brought us trans fats to ironically save us from heart disease, and it is now bringing us genetically-engineered canola and soy, whilst promoting the very same con-job.

Heavy metals inside the body accumulate, leading to immune system suppression and inflammation in increasing amounts with age. Heavy metal toxicity leads to obesity, which in-turn leads to even more inflammation and heart stress. Thus, metal extraction through chelation therapy is immensely beneficial for reversing heart disease. All heavy metal cleansing should first begin with a liver cleanse. The liver will need to be at maximum efficiency for additional cleansing to be effective.

Allopathic medicine is beginning to believe that renin (the clotting agent in the blood) is the main cause of heart disease. It is trivial to pharmaceutically-lower renin levels, just as drugs may reduce cholesterol levels. Both are typically expected to be life-long treatments, but neither is advisable. The presence of either renin or cholesterol in elevated amounts is a warning that the real problem elsewhere should be dealt with properly. The standard procedures of merely suppressing the symptoms has led to the huge mortality rate, because patient bodies have been prevented from defending themselves.

Symptom suppression as heart medicine is a dangerous strategy, but it is nonetheless typical. For instance, cardiac arrhythmia is often caused by severely imbalanced hormones, and it is frequently the result of birth control drug usage. Treating the arrhythmia with more pills can be a deadly cocktail, and masking the symptom could shortly result in a heart attack, because the real cause was never addressed: namely the other medication. Unfortunately, allopathic medicine tends to negate the significance of symptoms, as if they were just a menace to be suppressed with chemical warfare; but symptoms should always be traced to their root causes, in order to map courses toward life-saving interventions.

Homogenized milk is one reason why heart disease is the number one killer in America, and we suspect that it could actually be the main culprit. Homogenization causes the fat in milk to be broken into such tiny particles that milk does not separate from its cream. These fat particles are so unnaturally small that they are absorbed directly into the bloodstream without proper digestion. These undigested fat particles stress the immune system greatly and cause extreme inflammation. There is an enzyme in cow's milk that becomes dangerous whenever milk is homogenized. It is called "xanthine oxidase" or simply "XO". This enzyme is used by young calves to aid with digestion, but it causes cardiovascular disease in humans whenever it is unbound from the fat by homogenization. With raw, or even pasteurized milk (creamline milk), this toxic substance is not absorbed into the blood. Prior to homogenization, this offensive enzyme was always chemically bound inside milk fats, which were too large to enter into the human bloodstream undigested. The natural particle size of fat inside unadulterated cow's milk acts as a shield to protect humans from the milk's xanthine oxidase. Homogenized milk should always be avoided, but if complete avoidance is not an option, then some of its negative effects can be neutralized with folate or folic acid supplements combined with vitamin C. Folic acid is inferior to folate for supplementation purposes. Be advised that the homogenized fats will still be damaging to the heart, even if the arteries are somewhat shielded from the xanthine oxidase. We recommend whole creamline (non-homogenized) milk, which can be found at many health food stores. In some cases, heavy cream can be used as a perfect substitute to milk, and it is unhomogenized. There is no significant benefit to using raw milk over pasteurized milk, so our recommendation is to simply stay with sterile milk.

"Bovine milk xanthine oxidase (BMXO) may be absorbed and may enter the cardiovascular system. People with clinical signs of atherosclerosis have greater quantities of BMXO antibodies. BMXO antibodies are found in greater quantities in those patients who consume the largest volumes of homogenized milk and milk products."

-- *The XO Factor*, by Kurt Oster,
M.D. and Donald Ross, Ph.D.

Most soft dairy products are made with homogenized milk. Although they are rarely labeled as being so. Some people eat yogurt in an attempt to become healthier, and it is something that we have recommended many times in the past. Overall, yogurt usually helps more than it harms, but due to homogenization, it is not as healthy as most people believe. Most soft dairy products will cause inflammation and arterial damage, because of homogenization. Those who eat homogenized products should compensate somewhat with vitamin C and folate (or folic acid), in order to shield the body. Hard cheeses and butter are currently not being made with homogenized milk, so they are safe. Goat milk and products made from it are safe, because goat milk is never homogenized.

No person, especially a heart patient, should ever consume high fructose corn syrup. It is one of the most damaging ingredients that a person can consume. It is present in a wide variety of processed foods and all major brands of soft drinks. It has long been implicated in causing heart disease and obesity. More recently, it has been tied to diabetes, dementia, and metabolic disorders. High fructose corn syrup is frequently made from genetically-engineered corn, and the resultant chemically and genetically-engineered fructose produces scarring inside the arteries. In contrast, natural fructose that is metabolized by the body, such as fructose derived from fruits, does not have any known harmful effects. The arterial scarring caused by high fructose corn syrup becomes a permanent hindrance to the cardiovascular system. It is vital for anyone with any health problem (particularly heart disease, cancer, or diabetes) to avoid high fructose corn syrup completely.

Refined sugars cause inflammation in the body. The harmful sugars are those which have been bleached white, or which have gone through intensive industrial processing, such as high fructose corn syrup, and bleached sugar (also known as table sugar). These sugars cause inflammation, which damages the arterial walls, requiring the body to produce cholesterol to repair them. These sugars cause both inflammation and oxygen starvation at the cellular level. This makes a person much more likely to acquire diabetes and cancer. Refined sugars also disrupt intestinal flora, which is a beneficial bacteria that is necessary for the proper absorption of nutrients from foods. When flora is damaged by toxic sugars, people become malnourished because they can no longer properly absorb nutrients, even from nutrient-dense foods. The same problems come from processed carbohydrates, which convert into sugars inside the body. As is the case with sugars, what makes carbohydrates especially dangerous is being over-processed and bleached. Thus, whole grain carbohydrates are significantly healthier, and significantly less inflammatory. This rule also applies to rice, so whole grain rice is much preferred over bleached, processed white rice. We would like to include a special warning about purchasing whole wheat breads, because we have found that the chemical ingredients in commercial whole grain breads tend to be significantly worse than those of white breads. Therefore, the only safe bread is homemade bread, which is preferably whole wheat. Healthy sugars, such as those found naturally in fruits, honey, and evaporated cane juice do not contribute to inflammation, and they do not damage the intestinal flora. If a powdered sugar is needed for cooking, choose one whose only ingredient is "evaporated cane juice". It should have a beige to brown color, as any natural sugar will.

As shown, there are many causes for heart disease, but it always comes back to what we eat and drink. Congenital heart failure is present at birth, but it too can always be traced back to a malnourished mother, pharmaceuticals taken during pregnancy, or nutrient-depleting toxins inside the mother.

Heart Attacks Which Strike the Healthy

Some heart attacks occur without warning signs, within people having normal cholesterol levels and blood pressure. Here is how that usually happens. Infections routinely occur in the blood, and a healthy immune system eliminates them without displaying any symptoms. However, if a blood infection is not dealt with rapidly, then the infection becomes more prominent. In such cases, extreme inflammation may be created by the viral wastes or by direct arterial attacks, and then the "bad cholesterol" must provide protective patches over the resulting scarred tissues. Then the cholesterol patch is covered by a fibrous cap. Macrophage cells then come along, whose job it is to assimilate things that are causing problems, like cholesterol. Eventually, they become too full to function, at which point scientists call them "foam cells". These foam cells can die underneath the fibrous cap, forming into something like a boil. Eventually, the boil will burst, and when it does, the body must clean up these bits. The blood cells in the area then join together to form a patch. A poor diet and lifestyle results in excess fibrin in the blood (the clotting factor) which means that it is already thick, sticky, and ready to clot. This, in turn, may cause the patch to become much bigger than it should be, allowing it to be dislodged easily from pressure and contractions. When it is dislodged, it floats through the blood supply to possibly arrive at the brain to cause a stroke, or to the heart causing a heart attack. People experiencing these things may have had no prior symptoms of heart disease. For these victims, the combined effects of their poor lifestyle suddenly come together at once like an avalanche, with no warnings, and the game is over.

Reversing Heart Disease

The longer that a person has had heart disease and hardening of the arteries, the more challenging it is to reverse. In some cases, the damage will be too severe to completely eliminate, but stopping the progression and reversing it partially is possible in even the worst cases.

Hawthorn has been proven to help those with congestive heart failure, pulse irregularities, and angina. It is the most recommended supplement for heart health, in both alternative and mainstream medicine. Hawthorn is considered to be the swiss army knife of heart supplements. According to the University of Maryland Medical Center, hawthorn has been used since the 1st century as a remedy for heart and respiratory ailments. In Germany, it is regularly prescribed by mainstream doctors to those with heart failure or hypertension. Hawthorn also reduces the likelihood of blood clots, and has a strong anti-inflammatory effect. The research study, *Alternative Therapies: Part II. Congestive Heart Failure and Hypercholesterolemia*, aggregated the results of 50 clinical trials. It was performed by the Louisiana State University School of Medicine. It concluded that a "clear improvement in the subjects receiving hawthorn was observed". The standard dosage in the studies was 500 mg. per 100 lbs. of body weight.

Perform a heavy metal cleanse. Those with heart disease generally have a history of heavy metal toxicity, and the difference that a heavy metal cleanse makes can be dramatic. As noted earlier, always begin with a thorough liver cleanse. When heavy metals are removed, the body can properly create nitric oxide. Nitric oxide allows vessels to expand and contract efficiently, and it allows greater oxygen into cells.

Toxic iron accumulation inside the blood is a problem specific to men. Therefore, adult males should never use supplements containing iron. Men develop an excess of iron in their bodies because of male hormones, and because the male body will not remove excess iron without proper nutritional augmentation. The typical resultant iron excess in males is believed to be one of the main reasons why men die younger than women. The bodies of females of child-bearing age flush excess iron through their menstrual process, which acts as a natural blood-letting. A woman's remaining iron reserves are then used to produce replacement blood. Donating blood is the quickest way for a man to reduce his iron levels, and it may therefore save two lives. The study, *A Historical Cohort Study of the Effect of Lowering Body Iron Through Blood Donation on Incident Cardiac Events*, has shown that men who give blood have a 30% reduced risk of heart disease. An unusual but potentially effective option is to occasionally supplement with colloidal silver, for silver is able to neutralize iron in the body. Please read our *Colloidal Silver* section of the *Alternative Medicine* chapter before using colloidal silver, because bad colloidal silver is always worse than none at all.

Dr. Linus Pauling discovered that resveratrol, found in grape skins, aids in the removal of iron. Resveratrol can also directly reverse plaque deposits. A study by the University of Wisconsin found that when people with coronary artery disease drank 20 fluid ounces of purple grape juice for just two weeks, their blood vessels became noticeably more elastic, and both platelet aggregation and LDL oxidation decreased. Due to its resveratrol content, wine consumption has been identified as one of the primary reasons for France's low rate of heart disease.

In perhaps the greatest irony herein, salt is needed to reverse heart disease. Natural salts are needed because of the trace minerals that they contain, which are not attainable by any other means. We recommend that readers replace all table salt with mineral-rich sea salt. Do not buy the fake sea salts from regular grocery stores, because they are just as refined as the table salts, and are thereby counterproductive. True sea salt should never be a bright white color. Always avoid salts that are. Use unrefined, non-adulterated, mineral-rich sea salt that can be purchased online or from a health food store. Small amounts of natural sea salt should be added to home-cooked meals as a healthy and flavor-enhancing supplement. Be cautious about adding it to foods that are already salted, however.

The human body can create new arteries whenever its old arteries become clogged, but it needs copper to accomplish this. Oral supplementation with copper is dangerous, because it quickly becomes toxic with an overdose, and it takes only a tiny amount to overdose. Excessive amounts are known to cause severe organ damage; especially to the kidneys and liver. Therefore, we discourage people from orally consuming any man-made copper solutions, such as colloidal copper or copper hydroxide. For the sake of safety, copper should only be supplemented by way of the following nutritional methods. Natural sea salts contain safe amounts of natural copper and important trace minerals. Another option is chlorophyll extract, which will have the additional benefits of increasing the number of red blood cells, increasing blood oxygenation, protecting against radiation, and neutralizing benzene compounds. It contains much more copper than sea salt. It is a recommended supplement for all heart disease patients. Chlorophyll safely gets large amounts of copper into the human body.

Avoid all processed foods. They contain excessive amounts of sodium from dangerous sources, such as monosodium glutamate. MSG is especially dangerous to the heart, because it neutralizes taurine, which is necessary for pulse regulation. Monosodium glutamate intake in combination with deficiencies of both magnesium and taurine can make MSG deadly. This combination is the cause of many unexplained heart attacks in otherwise healthy people; including young athletes in their prime years, whose only mistake was that last meal at K.F.C. (Kentucky Fried Chicken).

Two-time Nobel Prize winner Linus Pauling recommended 2 grams daily of vitamin C for everyone, and 5-6 grams for those suffering from any kind of heart problems, or for those who are at high risk. He also recommended 2-5 grams of L-lysine.

Dr. Matthias Rath, M.D., who has continued much of Dr. Pauling's work, explained that the first step in reversing coronary heart disease is nutrition, and people with coronary heart disease are deficient in trace minerals. In particular, vitamin C supplementation is essential. In his book, *Why Animals Don't Get Heart Disease, But People Do*, Rath explained that the only other species to get heart disease is the guinea pig, and it is also the only other species that does not internally produce its own vitamin C. Hardening of the arteries is a pre-scurvy condition, and it will occur if not enough vitamin C is available. The two doctors proved that vitamin C also bonds with iron, allowing excess iron to be removed, it suppresses cholesterol oxidation, and it shields the body against so-called "free radicals".

Niacin (vitamin B-3) and pantothenate (vitamin B-5) work in conjunction with vitamin C. Niacin protects the arteries, and is metabolized in the body from L-tryptophan. L-tryptophan naturally occurs in eggs and meats, but can also be obtained through supplementation. It is recommended that people avoid time-released niacin, because too many people have had bad experiences, including blackouts and hallucinations from the chemical impurities. Both niacin and L-tryptophan are effective for treating depression, and this again reinforces the connection between emotional and heart health. Vitamin B-5 (sold as "pantothenic acid") works with vitamin C to protect against arterial damage, thus reducing a body's overall need to produce cholesterol. Vitamin B-5 can be found naturally in eggs, peanuts, legumes, and meats.

In the 1950's, Dr. Johanna Budwig was reversing heart disease with what is now known as the Budwig Protocol. However, this alternative protocol is much more famous for reversing cancers, and there is a strong connection between the two inflammatory disease states, but that connection is too complex to explain in this report. At the core of Dr. Budwig's protocol is a combination of flax seed oil and a food item that is rich in sulfur proteins. Johanna discovered that maximum absorption of omega-3 into cells required it to be mixed with sulfur proteins. Whenever properly combined, this solution is best able to penetrate into the deep tissues and through cellular membranes. Flax seed oil supplies the building blocks for cellular repair, helps dissolve excess cholesterol inside the arteries, balances the high omega-6 concentrations that are found in trans fats and processed foods, increases cellular energy, increases the efficiency of respiration, and it is an overall tonic to general cellular functions. The heart benefits of flax seed oil (omega-3 supplementation) are now well recognized, even by orthodox medicine. Whenever flax seed oil is heated or exposed to air, it rapidly becomes rancid, and thereby harmful. People should avoid products which contain heated or exposed flax seed. This often includes cereals, breads, and flour. The companies that sell these products deceptively promote them as being healthier, but ironically, most of the omega oils have been destroyed by the processing, and any remaining oils have become inflammatory and carcinogenic.

The medical establishment has sabotaged alternative medicine's otherwise beneficial Budwig Protocol into being something harmful. Instead of following the original protocol that uses only flax seed oil as the source for omega-3 supplementation, the medical establishment prescribes fish oil to heart disease patients, which has been industrially processed by the pharmaceutical industry with high-heat and poisonous chemical solvents to extract the oil from fish livers. The livers of fish are where the PCB's, heavy metals, and pesticides are stored; because such substances are too toxic for their digestive and immune systems to excrete normally. A liver is a body's toxic waste dump, in other words. The high heat and extreme processing that is used to chemically extract the omega oil from fish livers means that the derived oil is always rancid by the time that it reaches the patients; and therefore, this doctor-prescribed 'medicine' *actually causes* heart disease and cancers. Most of the fish that are used to pharmaceutically produce omega oil have high amounts of the inflammatory omega-6 and very low amounts of omega-3, because the pharmaceutical industry's fish are farm-raised in unhealthy conditions in Chinese fish farms. Adding an even greater insult to the injury, American patients are charged hundreds of dollars for this impure and carcinogenic version of omega-3 by the medical industry, while the safe and more effective equivalent (flax seed oil) can be found cheaply at any health food store. Health food stores also sell fish oil, but it too should be avoided in lieu of the superior flax option.

Co-enzyme Q10 is absolutely essential for recovery from heart disease and heart failure. It can be found in some foods (particularly meats and fish) and it is produced by the body during exercise. While studies have shown great benefits through intravenous supplementation, oral supplements are unfortunately not absorbed well. Thus, it is best obtained through dietary sources and exercise. CoQ10 is essential for the emulsification of fats. It lowers the blood pressure and provides an increased chance of survival following cardiac arrest. Research has also found that those with gingivitis have a deficiency of CoQ10. Vegetarians may attempt supplementation, even though absorption will be very low. Nevertheless, even a small amount will be helpful.

Japan currently has the lowest rate of heart disease in the world, so it is logical to examine their dietary and medicinal practices, in order to adopt them into our own society. The Japanese eat lots of fish, and thereby get large amounts of vitamin D, omega-3, and safe iodine. In addition to that, whenever heart disease is diagnosed, L-taurine is a common recommendation by Japanese doctors. Taurine is a natural nutrient, which makes it unpatentable (unprofitable), so it is "not approved" for medical use in the United States. It can stabilize the heart rate, neutralize MSG, and it helps the body to better regulate potassium, calcium, and sodium in the body. It is known for its ability to protect the kidneys from damage.

Taurine supplementation has also been shown to reverse some of the damage caused by smoking, even amongst smokers who continued smoking during the clinical trials. A 2003 study by the Royal College of Surgeons found that damage caused by chronic smoking can be reversed in as little as five days with a dosage of 1.5 grams of taurine. The inner lining of the blood vessels and the diameter of blood vessels returned to normal in the study.

It is wise to take anti-inflammatories when attempting to reverse heart disease. As already stated, inflammation is the first step in arterial plaque. Effective natural anti-inflammatories include devil's claw, vitamin C, MSM, cherry concentrate, and resveratrol. Curcumin, a component of the turmeric spice, is also an anti-inflammatory and it has the added benefit of reversing some arterial plaque. Never underestimate the benefits of culinary spices, which are sometimes known as herbal medicine.

We have already written an entire section (*Supplements* chapter) about the benefits of cayenne pepper, but it is absolutely vital for people with heart problems. It aids circulation, stabilizes blood pressure, and it can actually stop a heart attack in its tracks. *Seriously*. Remember this, because cayenne pepper can save a life. This is especially true whenever it is mixed with taurine. The suffering patient may need to hold them in his mouth for fastest results. During a heart attack, nobody ever complains that something tastes too spicy. Cayenne pepper is even good for painless weight loss. It can be conveniently supplemented in a pill form that is available from health food stores. We recommend that everyone with heart problems supplement with cayenne, or put it into a tea daily. Dr. David Christopher has been labeled "Dr. Cayenne" for his endless promotion of this spice.

Another reason for calcification inside the arterial walls is an excess of blood-borne calcium, which is typical in Western nations. Vitamin D and magnesium are critically needed for a body to make proper use of its calcium, so that it does not simply get dumped onto the artery inner walls. A large portion of people are not able to properly assimilate vitamin D supplements, so it is best obtained through sunlight and fish. When purchasing fish, bottom-feeders should be avoided because of their heavy metal content. Farm raised fish have the wrong omega ratio along with various other toxicities from chemicals, hormones, and antibiotics. Americans should carefully read the packaging for fish, because much of America's fish is coming from China now. Fish will typically cause more harm than good if they are not wild-caught. With the exception of bottom feeders, most wild-caught fish will contain enough selenium to counteract any metals found within them. Eat fish that has been baked, not fried. Magnesium is vital to prevent calcium waste, but supplementing with it can be risky. Too much magnesium will cause other nutrients to be flushed out of the body. Thus, magnesium is best obtained from green leafy vegetables. Magnesium steadies the blood pressure, and aids in the absorption of potassium, which likewise regulates the heart rhythm. Migraine headaches are a common symptom of people who are deficient in magnesium too.

It is important that you reduce or eliminate nicotine in cases of severe heart problems. Nicotine, along with alcohol, caffeine, and a host of pharmaceuticals, interferes with the absorption of key nutrients, which are vital for recovery. If you must smoke, ensure that you are making your own cigarettes with organic tobaccos and a rolling machine, or else you will be inhaling a host of chemicals including (but not limited to) carpet glue. Modern cigarettes have been made much more harmful than they need to be by the chemical industry, and they are fertilized with radioactive fertilizers. Indian tobacco can help eliminate a large number of addictions, including nicotine, and it can also help to clean the lungs.

Nuts lower the heart disease risk because they contain alpha-linolenic acid (LNA). It is an omega-3 fatty acid. Countries with the most LNA in their diets also have the lowest risk of heart disease. Walnuts and cashews are the most nutritious nuts available. Peanuts contain the least amount of nutrients and are likely to have pesticide residues.

Ginkgo biloba improves circulation, and it reduces cholesterol concentrations in the arterial walls. It also enables the arteries and veins to more fully relax between pumping cycles. The National Institutes of Health reported that ginkgo is very useful for alleviating leg pain that is attributed to blocked arteries.

Exercise is essential for preventing heart disease or recovering from it. Not only does exercise allow the body to create its own CoQ10, but it also creates nitric oxide and L-carnitine. As already stated, nitric oxide aids the vessels to expand and contract more efficiently, and L-carnitine can improve the heart's function. We recommend finding an exercise that you can enjoy, and if possible, do it with others. Try to remember how enjoyable exercise was when you were a child, and attempt to make it that way again. Let us not forget that positive emotions are vital to heart health. Jogging on a treadmill is a chore, and it can even be a humiliating, demeaning experience.

Grapefruit pectin is available in supplement form. It reverses arterial plaque, reduces cholesterol, and widens the arteries. While it is not a standard supplement, we would nevertheless recommend it to anyone with chronic heart problems.

Due to the importance of nutrition, we recommend that people try a juice fast for about two weeks when they are strong enough. Juicing is the process of mixing fruits and vegetables together in a blender or juicer, and then using the extracted juices as a food source. A juice fast is a means of flooding a body with nutrients that it is normally lacking in due to our modern diets. The first few days may be difficult, but the long-term benefits can be dramatic. We recognize that many people will require a source of pure protein each day (such as organic eggs) to be able to continue with their normal lives uninterrupted. The fasting procedure should vary, depending on each individual's needs, so a little bit of common sense is required.

The Prognosis

Throughout this report, we resisted the temptation to rant about the sorry state of cardiac medicine, if it can indeed be reasonably called medicine. We began by citing that the medical industry's own statistics prove that standard medicine for cardiac issues is the single biggest failure of orthodox medicine. Now we end this report with an honest commentary about our well-earned biases against the status quo.

Sometimes emergency medical personnel save lives with emergency medicine, but this is the best that orthodox medicine can do. They fail at everything else, and this is partly because effective therapies are illegal. All approved therapies must be drug-based, which means that all of the successful nutritional therapies (to what is a very nutritional problem) are forbidden to all doctors who wish to remain licensed to practice medicine. The consequence is that it is actually illegal for any licensed doctor to cure or to successfully mitigate heart disease, since successful and natural therapies are not approved by medical regulators. If you receive the standard treatments (chemical symptom suppression) for heart conditions, or the establishment's supposedly preventative treatments, which usually do the opposite of what they are presented to do, then you will either die of heart disease, or the treatments themselves. It is equally likely that you will die of complications caused by the medications, such as the development of a cancer, or liver failure, or diabetes. They call it "progress".

Heart disease is not truly normal or natural, and it is not genetic. The only thing that is genetic about our cardiac catastrophe is that lifestyles, family doctors, and eating habits are inherited. At the core of the problems are ignorance and irresponsibility that span generations. In this sense, there are genetic components to heart disease, but the problem was never God's engineering.

Heart disease takes lots of work to reverse, but it is more-or-less curable in most cases, regardless of what a doctor tells you. Remember that it took years to get yourself into this state of ill-health, and it may take a long time to get yourself out of it. Do not disregard the importance of emotional and spiritual health, because these things have a major impact upon the heart, and a full recovery may not be possible otherwise. Whenever we use the term "spiritual health", we are referring to real spirituality, such as forming a personal relationship with our Creator, not the type of empty ritualism like that which is practiced by yoga practitioners, or the paganistic Earth worship that has become prevalent in the alternative health movement.

Symptoms of a Heart Attack

- Discomfort, pressure, heaviness, or pain in the left arm or chest
- Discomfort radiating to the back, jaw, throat, or arm
- Fullness, indigestion, or choking feeling (may feel like heartburn)
- Sweating
- Nausea
- Dizziness
- Extreme weakness
- Anxiety
- Shortness of breath
- Rapid or irregular heartbeat

Emergency Treatment for Heart Attacks

In the event of a heart attack, do not forgo calling for an ambulance. The establishment's forté is emergency medicine, and the risk is too great to delay calling for help. While waiting for the ambulance to arrive, small amounts of these supplements should be placed into the mouth of the victim, and allowed to absorb through the walls of his cheeks:

- L-taurine
- Cayenne
- Magnesium

Please have these supplements available beforehand. Get them now. They could save your life, or the life of someone you love, and there is no time for shopping when a heart attack strikes. Being able to respond within minutes could mean the difference between life and death. Try to get the patient laying on his back, taking slow deep breaths, if at all possible. It is also important to keep the patient calm and reassured. Keep the patient warm if he appears to be entering into shock.

Americans need not be concerned with legalities when trying to employ these methods. Every American state has a Good Samaritan law, which provides special legal protection to those who make a good faith effort to save a life.

Diabetes

A Medical Quagmire

Chronic diseases such as diabetes are becoming more prevalent. Diabetes diagnoses are increasing at a steady rate of 5% annually in the U.S., and there is no sign of either a cure or a preventative from the medical establishment. The total cost of treating diabetes was approximately $245,000,000,000.00 ($245 billion) in the United States alone for the year 2012, according to the American Diabetes Association. Until very recently, type 2 diabetes did not occur in children, so it was formerly known as "adult onset" diabetes. Now, type 2 diabetes occurs in children as young as two years old. Meanwhile, the medical establishment refuses to acknowledge that diseases could be caused by artificial food ingredients that are manufactured by the chemical industry, its own drugs, and by overall toxicity. Therefore, the victims will continue to get younger.

The average American consumes 100 to 160 pounds of toxic, inflammatory, chlorine bleached, chemically-refined sugars every year, and this is one of the primary reasons for diseases such as diabetes, heart disease, and cancer. Additionally, a large percentage of American foods are artificial. The chemical industry has entered the kitchen, and every processed food now contains a variety of chemical compounds. Just like prescription pharmaceuticals, these foods have serious side effects, and they include all of the modern epidemics. The Big 3 chronic diseases were once rare, but they are now a routine part of modern life; thanks to the capitulation of governments, the food industry, the chemical industry, and now, the nuclear industry.

The massive amount of refined sugars that we eat each year destructively inflames the pancreas, kidneys, and liver. When these organs finally become dysfunctional from such abuse, people develop a condition known as carbohydrate intolerance. Carbohydrate intolerance is a condition in which a body can no longer properly metabolize carbohydrates and sugars. Most Americans somewhat already have this pre-diabetes condition, and this is why the carbohydrate-free diets seem to work so well, for a human body places compounds that it cannot process into fat storage to shield itself. This explains both the effectiveness of carbohydrate-free diets, and why diabetics tend to have such terrible weight management problems. The dramatic loss of weight that some diabetics experience stems from a completely different cause that is related to kidney stress. Carbohydrate intolerance is a precursor to diabetes, but most people remain undiagnosed until full-blown diabetes begins disrupting their lives.

The Top 15 Symptoms of Diabetes

- Frequent or excessive urination
- Unusual thirst
- Extreme hunger (usually type 1)
- Unusual weight loss (usually type 1)
- Unexplained weight gain (type 2)
- Extreme fatigue and irritability
- Frequent infections
- Blurred vision
- Cuts and bruises that are slow to heal
- Tingling and numbness in the hands or feet
- Recurring skin, gum, or bladder infections
- Swollen, tender or bleeding gums
- Intense cravings for sweets
- Impotency
- Kidney pain

Manufacturing Diabetics

The medical industry is known for producing full-blown diabetics out of pre-diabetics by prescribing synthetic insulin. Synthetic insulin poisons the pancreas, which eventually stops producing its own insulin. The pharmaceutical itself creates diabetics, who will conveniently be dependent upon the system thereafter. This is by design. The F.D.A. now refuses to provide approval for natural animal insulins, which are cheap, unpatentable, non-addictive, and do not cause full-blown diabetes to develop.

The best natural insulin available in previous times was a mixture of beef and pork insulins. Less of the natural insulin was needed to achieve optimal blood sugar. It was absorbed slower, which led to greater stability in blood sugar levels. Its U.S. production halted in 1998, when Eli Lilly suddenly stopped producing it; without providing an explanation. The company was ready with its patented "insulin" that could be produced in its chemical factory for much less cost, and yet it is sold at a much higher price. The F.D.A. soon after declared that there were no longer any approved animal insulins, and it officially banned them from entering into the United States, unless a doctor officially petitions the F.D.A. in writing for permission, and then only on the basis of the animal insulin being "essential for treatment". Of course, doctors who wish to keep practicing medicine in the U.S. do not write such letters; so the F.D.A. had politically maneuvered to ban the animal insulin without *officially* banning it. Due to the patent of the only legal synthetic insulin, and the corroboration of F.D.A. cronies, Eli Lilly has been exclusively given a lucrative medical monopoly in diabetes treatments. There were no scientific reasons for it, for the natural insulin was safer, more effective, and cheaper. It was about money, power, destroying natural alternatives, and ensuring addiction. To maintain a facade that the diabetes market is open and full of competition, the F.D.A. allows Eli Lilly to market its insulin under a variety of different names, in order to convince the American public that it has multiple products to choose from.

Type 2 Diabetes

Insulin is a hormone that is designed to pull sugar into cells. "Insulin resistance" and "type 2 diabetes" are actually the same condition. It is believed that the aggravated cells of a person who is suffering with type 2 diabetes resist insulin, whereby his body rejects its own natural insulin to cause an excess of blood sugar. A vicious chain reaction begins when the pancreas creates too much insulin to compensate for the low insulin absorption of the cells, which in-turn causes even more cellular inflammation, which then causes the cells to become even more resistant to insulin.

The pancreas will continue to produce excessive insulin, because very little sugar gets into the cells to provide energy. When the amount of insulin becomes excessive enough, it will sometimes completely overrun the cellular resistance, causing unnaturally rapid absorption of sugars into the cells, which then creates hypoglycemia (low blood sugar). This stimulates the production of additional hormones, especially from the adrenal glands, as a body will try to right itself with emergency energy reserves. These hormones increase the blood sugar level temporarily, but over time, this process stresses the adrenal glands. When the standard sugar-laden diet is continued, the adrenal glands eventually start malfunctioning, resulting in overall imbalanced hormones. In the most extreme cases, a person experiences adrenal failure, adding yet another diseased state to his already full platter. Regardless of whether full adrenal failure happens, the constant flood of otherwise unnecessary hormones, and the over-driven adrenals can eventually lead to vision loss, kidney failure, and such poor circulation that amputation of the feet or legs may be required.

Type 1 Diabetes

Type 1 diabetes occurs when there is a failure of the pancreas, whereby it loses its ability to produce insulin. The body cannot properly utilize sugars as a result. The subsequent excess sugar in the blood can cause damage to the nervous system, leading to a variety of other disease states. The medical system has no explanation for type 1 diabetes, so it rationalizes its ignorance by predictably reporting that diabetes must be genetic, and therefore not preventable.

It has also periodically reported that type 1 diabetes may be caused by a mysterious virus, or that it is an autoimmune disease (caused by a malfunctioning immune system). At no point do they ever suggest that the malfunctioning immune system might be due to dietary issues, lifestyle, environmental factors, and above all, they never mention that their own pharmaceuticals often have diabetes listed as a known side effect. They also refuse to acknowledge that this man-made disease was a rare condition throughout most of history. The human race did not suddenly adopt a new type of DNA beginning with the industrial revolution of the twentieth century, when chemical fertilizers, chemically-laced tap water, and pharmaceuticals became the norm. Ignoring these facts, while gratuitously placing the guilt upon genes is the epitome of bad science, so often expressing itself in the politics of promoting biotechnology that is supposedly needed to fix the 'bad genes'. They are actually correct in their statements about diabetes constellating amongst certain families, but so does lifestyle, family doctors, and environmental factors. These things do cause diabetes. The often ignored evidence shows that type 1 diabetes is caused by an onslaught of chemicals, usually at an early age, followed by a poor diet. Some parents will notice diabetic symptoms shortly following vaccinations.

Curing Diabetes

When we consider that 85% of Americans suffer from parasitic infections, it is easy to conclude that a diabetic almost certainly has parasites, due to his less-than-ideal diet and lifestyle. Poor diets are equally conductive to parasitic invaders. Therefore, we strongly recommend a parasite cleanse for all who suffer from diabetes or pre-diabetes. Some readers will ponder why a candida flush is not being suggested, but it should not be necessary with the diet being recommended.

Juice fasting is an extremely important step to curing diabetes. Juicing is a quick and tasty way to consume large amounts of fruits and vegetables each day. Two weeks should be long enough for most people. It is generally wise to also eat one small, pure protein meal each day (e.g. organic white meat or organic eggs). While a blender is the only necessary appliance for juicing, an actual juicer will remove excess pulp. For those who can tolerate pulp, it provides plenty of helpful fiber. While a raw produce diet can cure diabetes, we feel that getting some protein, especially from white meat, is important for the adrenal glands, which are already stressed in the body of a diabetic. Eating only raw (uncooked) plant-based foods will generally be impossible for those who have to attend the workplace or conduct everyday activities.

Moderate exercise is recommended during the juice fasting period and beyond. Exercise is not being recommended for weight loss, even though weight loss may be a welcome side effect. Most diabetics will nevertheless begin losing weight after adjusting their diets, with or without exercise. In the process of curing diabetes, exercise has a benefit of much greater importance. Exercise helps toxins to get expelled through the sweat glands. So exercise is vitally important, especially for anyone with the life-long habits of using aluminum-containing antiperspirants, metal-laden cosmetics, processed foods, or pharmaceuticals. Otherwise, toxins that are stored inside fat cells will simply get re-released into the blood during the period of weight loss, where they will again exacerbate health problems. Exercising is a wise choice that will lead to greater long-term health, and exercise is the only way that toxins are removed from the lymph nodes.

Sweet cravings occur often in those with diabetes. It is possible to eliminate these cravings without turning to something unhealthy. On many occasions, fruits and fruit juices will eliminate sugar cravings, but always remember moderation. At other times, a patient may supplement with a small amount of organic evaporated cane juice crystals. It is truly organic sugar that has usually been sun dried. It is sugar before it has been bleached and chemically refined, and amazingly; it will actually help to cure diabetes if periodically taken in tiny amounts. We recommend holding one teaspoon of it in the mouth for about 15 seconds, and then swallow. Use as needed throughout the day. Sugar, in the way that God made it, is not usually harmful in moderation. If you have full-blown diabetes (either type) then of course, monitor your blood sugar levels for dangerous spikes. Be aware that the effects of this sugar intake will vary greatly as your health improves, and the sugar must be exactly the type specified: organic evaporated cane juice. Products with similar names, such as "evaporated sugar" are not the same thing. People with especially bad cases of diabetes may need to instead use only small amounts of all-natural (100% pure) fruit juices in the beginning. The process will be different for every individual, and results will vary. Beware of juice cocktails, and juices from concentrates, because they are always impure and contain processed sweeteners. Begin the process slowly and on a small scale, and monitor with appropriate safety precautions; like having a partner in the beginning, and being sure that he is ready to intervene with insulin in the event that things go too fast. This process literally retrains a person's body to accept that natural sugars are not toxic. The consumption of poisonous sugars has typically done just the opposite over a period of many years, in exactly the same way that vaccines train a body to overreact to certain substances. In fact, vaccines are a primary reason for infantile diabetes. Sugar is the energy of life, so this retraining process is absolutely vital for curing diabetes.

Dietary and Supplemental Suggestions

Alpha lipoic acid is the most effective supplement for helping to remedy diabetic neuropathy. Diabetic neuropathy is a painful condition, whereby nerves are damaged by excessive sugar in the blood (hyperglycemia). The condition typically manifests with sudden pains that are intensely sharp; like electric shocks. It also produces random tingling sensations, numbness, and on rare occasions, the feeling that bugs are crawling upon one's skin. Alpha lipoic acid can reverse nerve damage, thus eradicating or reducing neuropathy. The typical dosage is 300 mg., which is spread throughout the day, but it has been studied at dosages of 600 mg. with no ill effects. People may need to experiment to get the ideal dosage for their needs. Take care to not confuse alpha lipoic acid with alpha linolinic acid, which is also abbreviated as A.L.A.

Diabetics virtually always have a dysfunctional pancreas, which is the organ that is responsible for insulin production, and other important hormones. Digestive enzymes, sometimes known as "pancreatic enzymes", are supplements that contain many of the compounds that are made by the pancreas. These enzymes help in the digestion of foods, especially meats and fats, which are the most difficult foods for a body to digest. Taking digestive enzymes alongside meals will alleviate much of the pancreas' burden, allowing it to perform its other tasks more efficiently, and give it an opportunity to heal. A diabetic cannot be cured until his pancreas is repaired, and the damage to his pancreas is most often the primary cause of his diabetes. Whenever a pancreas is malfunctioning, it prevents a body from being able to properly digest its food, so diabetic patients subsequently become malnourished, which slowly causes other failures throughout a body over time. This explains how diabetes seems to be able to attack anything and everything, and why digestive enzymes are such a critical therapy.

Evidence suggests that a lack of vitamin E provides an increased risk for developing type 2 diabetes. Studies have demonstrated a benefit from vitamin E for blood flow into the kidneys, and for repairing kidney dysfunction; both of which are known issues for type 2 diabetics. Most importantly, vitamin E helps to correct insulin and glucose tolerance.

Cinnamon should be added to foods whenever possible, and one may even wish to take it in a convenient capsule form that is available. Cinnamon is remarkably effective at lowering the blood sugar, and many diabetics are starting to use it as a replacement for metformin, the most common diabetic pharmaceutical.

Supplementation with B vitamins is practically essential for recovery. Many diabetics suffer from vitamin B-12 deficiencies, in particular. This is exacerbated by the fact that metformin, a drug commonly used for the treatment of diabetes, is known to destroy B-12. Vitamin B-12 has been shown to be very helpful in the treatment of diabetic neuropathy. Vitamin B-12 should always be purchased in the form of methylcobalamin, instead of cyanocobalamin.

Vitamin B-6 (pyridoxine) is also used for diabetes. While there is lots of B-6 found naturally in grains, the process of modern milling removes it, by eliminating the shells. A vitamin B-6 deficiency has been associated with type 1 and type 2 diabetes, as well as gestational diabetes (diabetes which starts during pregnancy). Vitamin B-6 is known to normalize the blood sugar, to help prevent diabetic neuropathy. The use of oral contraceptives will increase the need for vitamin B-6.

The Linus Pauling Institute recommends biotin for both types of diabetes. Biotin is a B vitamin which has been shown in studies to lower the blood glucose levels by gently stimulating insulin, and it has also been shown to prevent diabetic neuropathy.

Chromium supplements can decrease glucose tolerance in people with both type 1 and type 2 diabetes, by increasing sensitivity to insulin. Chromium works best in conjunction with small amounts of niacin (vitamin B-3). Diabetics should not exceed 100 mg. of niacin daily, because high doses of niacin can make the blood sugar level unstable.

Diabetics almost always suffer from a deficiency in magnesium, a critical nutrient. Many in the medical profession believe that a deficiency in magnesium both decreases the production of insulin and increases insulin resistance of the cells. Magnesium absorption is hindered by caffeine and nicotine, so limit these whilst trying to cure diabetes. The best food sources of magnesium are: almonds, cashews, and spinach. Despite the bad reputation of spinach's flavor, the vegetable is flavorless until it is cooked, so it can be added to a salad or a juice easily, without any unpleasant taste. Organic baby spinach is even more nutrient dense than regular spinach is. We *strongly* recommend making custom salad dressings, due to the toxic ingredients found in virtually all commercial salad dressings. The hormone-disrupting properties of the soy and canola oils, which are the main ingredients of most commercial salad dressings, are enough to make recovery impossible.

Synthetic insulin reduces the amount of potassium in the body, and potassium is needed by the body to reduce insulin resistance. Potassium can be found in oranges, lemons, tomatoes, and bananas. Readers may be surprised to learn that an 8 ounce glass of orange juice has more potassium than a banana. There are other sources of potassium. For example, salt substitutes are often made with potassium chloride instead of sodium chloride. These can be used as a potassium supplement, but carefully check the labels for impurities. Also remember the rule of moderation in all things. Excessive potassium can lead to blood clots, especially for women who are taking birth control medications.

We strongly recommend stopping all hormone-effecting medications during the diabetes curing process, such as birth control pills. Patients may continue these pharmaceuticals at their own risk, but we warn about them being dangerous during this process, and they greatly impede progress.

Natural insulin is stored inside a zinc crystal that resides in the pancreas. Thus, zinc plays a critical role in insulin delivery. The staff of the Linus Pauling Institute believes that a deficiency in zinc could be one of the initial causes for diabetes, and zinc supplementation could definitely help to reduce the epidemic. This position has been supported by other studies. Always take zinc on a full stomach. The preferred type of zinc for supplementation is zinc orotate. Healthy food sources for zinc are: cashews, almonds, kidney beans, flounder, and eggs.

L-Taurine is an amino acid which is depleted in people with diabetes. This deficiency is believed to be one of the key reasons for kidney failure and liver problems. It can be found in all protein-rich foods, and it can be purchased as a dietary supplement. Taurine helps to stabilize the blood sugar and the pulse rate. Sometimes it can even save a person from a heart attack, especially when it is combined with cayenne pepper and magnesium. A rarely known benefit of taurine is that it neutralizes MSG. We recommend purchasing a supplement to obtain higher concentrations of taurine.

Studies have shown that diabetics have very low vitamin C levels. Vitamin C lowers sorbitol, a type of sugar that is known to accumulate in type 1 diabetics to damage the eyes, nerves, and kidneys. Recommended supplementation varies from 1,000 mg. to 3,000 mg. (1-3 grams) based upon the body weight of the individual. Sorbitol is a sugar that is made in the body, but it is not properly metabolized because of the adjuvant reaction of the vaccines containing it, causing a hyperimmune response to the sugar that can last for a lifetime. This is another link between diabetes and vaccines.

Diabetics should decrease their intake of carbohydrates (bread, cereal, rice, and potatoes). If a juice fast is undertaken, then simple carbohydrates should be completely avoided during the duration of the fast. Only whole wheat, whole grains, and unprocessed carbohydrates should be consumed. Acceptable carbohydrates include: whole wheat bread, brown rice, organic potatoes, and perhaps evaporated cane juice for when sugar is needed. Other truly natural sweeteners are fine, such as fruit juices and honey. Modern molasses is not natural or healthy.

The single most important aspect of a diabetic cure plan is diet. Diabetes cannot be cured without a change of diet to natural, wholesome foods. Diabetes is purely a disorder of malnutrition and poisoning. Juicing is a stupendous start for curing it, but then the individual must transition to a long-term diet of healthier foods when the juice fast finishes. Nutritious foods (especially organic) taste much better, and they are much healthier too. We would never recommend a permanent vegetarian diet, and we wish to make it clear that a long-term vegetarian lifestyle is foolishly unhealthy. A diabetic should eliminate all processed foods, white foods (white bread, white flour, white sugar, white rice), artificial sweeteners, tap water, artificial additives, and begin to cook wholesome foods for himself. He should replace table salt with sea salt. When people begin to cook real food, using real ingredients; they have more energy, feel better, and they even look better. The tastier home-cooked meals eventually become addictive. We recommend drinking spring water, or using a Berkey water filter. Americans should get the anti-fluoride attachments with Berkey filtration systems.

Kidney Stress

Both diabetes and excessive supplementation can weaken the kidneys, and thereby cause health consequences. Indications of kidney stress include fatigue, muscle cramping (particularly in the calves), vision problems, bleeding gums, leg problems that are caused by swelling, excessive urination, and thirst. Kidney stress can result in imbalanced electrolyte salts, especially potassium, which will cause fluid retention or loss throughout the body. While strengthening the kidneys, the use of other supplements and pharmaceuticals should be limited as much as possible. The following strengthen the kidneys.

- Dandelion (500 mg. for every 100 lbs. of body weight)
- Licorice (500 mg. for every 100 lbs. of body weight)
- Taurine (250 mg. per 50 lbs. of body weight)
- Vitamin E (133 I.U. per 100 lbs. of body weight)
- Cinnamon (500 mg. per 100 lbs. of body weight)
- Vitamin C (500 mg. for every 75 lbs. of body weight)
- Rhubarb
- Carrots

What To Expect

When first starting this plan, many people will feel low in energy. If the body is especially toxic or effected by candida, then there may even be some minor flu-like symptoms indicating that toxins are being moved (flushed), and that there is new stress upon the immune system. This is completely normal when the body is healing itself. Energy eventually returns, and the skin becomes visibly healthier. Those who are on diabetes medications, or insulin, should monitor their blood sugar throughout the program, and they should be able to gradually remove those medications. It is recommended that diabetics ask their loved ones to help monitor them, in case the withdrawal is done too quickly.

Both types of diabetes have been cured many times, but the media refuses to cover these politically-incorrect stories. An entire industry has been developed to ensure that people are never free of the pharmaceutical cartel, but real freedom exists for the taking.

Wellness

Fraudulent Health Products

Typical retailer shelves are full of products that are marketed as having health benefits, despite the fact that most of them are more damaging to us than the unhealthy products that they replace. As a general rule, you should beware whenever you see labels such as: "diet", "sugar free", "fat free", "no trans fats", "with flax", or "with omega 3". These are usually tricks to hurt you at someone else's profit. The U.S. Food and Drug Administration uniquely redefines common words to protect a chemical industry that is happily poisoning us. Some of the label terms listed herein mean something entirely different from what any reasonable person would expect. These word games will be explained.

Sugar Free Products

The phrase "sugar free" commonly means that normal food sugars have been replaced with chemically-extracted sugar alcohols, such as sorbitol, mannitol, and maltitol. These "diabetic safe" sugar compounds tend to increase a person's blood sugar levels more than real sugar does, and they cause *even more* inflammation than the standard processed sugars do. "Sugar free" frequently means being more sugary and more dangerous. These alcohol sugars are especially common in chewing gums.

Diet Products

Weight loss is a $35 billion industry. If diet products actually worked, then the industry would not allow them to remain that way for long. Effectiveness equals losing repeat customers. It is like how the medical industry cures nothing, because health freedom is bad for business. Just as pharmaceuticals make people sicker in the long term, diet products make people fatter. The wonders of chemistry indeed.

Diet products frequently contain monosodium glutamate, artificial sweeteners, and aluminum compounds. All of these cause victims to gain weight. Aluminum is a heavy metal that accumulates in the body forever. Fat tissues are produced as a defense mechanism against it, for a body utilizes fat cells to isolate toxins that it cannot expel; in much the same way that an oyster protects itself with a pearl. Most Americans (64%) believe that the government requires warnings about side effects on weight loss products, and 54% believe that diet products are approved for safety by the F.D.A. Neither is true.

Another example of industry deceit is how the artificial sweeteners in most diet products *cause* obesity at a *faster* rate than normal sugars and carbohydrates do. A typical "zero calorie" drink will stimulate fat build-up in two ways, and both involve destroying a victim's overall health. Firstly, all the artificial sweeteners are either inherently toxic or they metabolize into toxic compounds within the body. Take for example that the artificial sweetener, aspartame, is an excitotoxin (neurotoxin) in its normal state, like MSG is. During metabolisis, aspartame is broken down into various poisons inside the body, such as formaldehyde and aspartic acid, which are then circulated by the blood. This generates extreme inflammation and an over-driven immune system; as if the person were poisoned, because he really was poisoned. Most artificial sugars are excitotoxins, which means that they directly attack the nervous system; causing terminal brain cancer, fibromyalgia, cardiac arrhythmia, diabetes, obesity, and a whole host of other severe, life-destroying neurological disorders. Secondly, artificial sweeteners produce artificial sugar crashes that produce extreme cravings for sugars and carbohydrates. You may have found yourself irresistibly tearing into a loaf of bread or a bowl of pasta after consuming one of these "healthy" diet colas, all-the-while trying to understand why you could not stop yourself. Now you know, and perhaps you finally know how evil these companies are. If you wish to lose weight, then you should stop buying diet products.

If you are a diet cola drinker, you should feel especially cheated and betrayed. For they likewise forget to mention that the sodium benzoate from these drinks is not really the safe salt that we are supposed to believe it is; but a benzene derivative. Benzene is one of the most carcinogenic substances on Earth. It literally is paint stripper.

With Added Omega-3 or Flax

Flax seed oil is a major source of omega-3 supplementation, so food manufacturers have been cashing-in on what they see as the flax craze. Flax seed oil is a supplement that we recommend whenever it is cold-pressed, properly distributed in light resistant capsules, and protected from temperature extremes. All of this is necessary to keep the flax oil stable. If these precautions are not taken, then flax oil quickly becomes a nutritionally-useless, rancid, and carcinogenic oil. It is better to get no flax seed oil supplementation than to get oil that has been mishandled.

Always beware of "omega-3" labels, for it is impossible for any processed omega-3 to still be omega-3. It is one of the fastest oils to break down, and its extreme oxygen reactivity is what normally helps it to be so beneficial to the human body; provided that it is consumed in its natural and pristine form. The omega-3 found in the overwhelming majority of products is not only useless, but it is dangerous too; if those variants can even be called omega-3. Most of the finished products will not test positive for omega-3, because it is utterly destroyed by the time it reaches retail shelves. The processed products usually test positive for high levels of omega-6 and omega-9, which exaggerate the problems of omega-3 deficiencies. Our recommendation is to not only avoid such foods, but to boycott the manufacturers as well. These "flax added" products are currently being sold at Whole Food's Market, despicably alongside canola oil and soy products.

Decaffeinated Products

Decaffeinated products have a long history of being removed from the market because of toxicity issues. First, the industry used benzene and chloroform to remove caffeine, but these ingredients were later "discovered" to be highly toxic (as if they didn't already know). Next, dichloromethane became popular in the 1970's. It was claimed to be less dangerous, but it was eventually proven to be carcinogenic too. Of course, this also totally surprised all the regulators too. Most of whom have chemistry degrees, but they somehow never realized that these chemical warfare agents might be harmful to health. This is the selective amnesia of F.D.A. science.

Nowadays, coffee beans are usually soaked in solvents, which include methylene chloride and ethyl acetate (nail polish remover). Sure, only trace amounts remain in the coffee beans as is claimed, but a person nevertheless risks cancers and other diseases for avoiding a relatively harmless and naturally-occurring substance: caffeine.

Turkey Bacon

People choose turkey bacon as a healthy alternative. They rarely read the ingredients, and tend to be unaware that turkey bacon usually contains more additives. It is not uncommon for turkey bacon to contain both MSG and canola oil. These are completely unnecessary ingredients, which are not present in regular bacon. Truly healthy turkey bacon can be purchased at some health food stores, but always make certain to read the ingredients. The celery-derived nitrates in some healthier products are safe, unlike the chemical industry nitrates.

Fruit Juice

Fruits are healthy. This apparently still needs to be said, since certain news sources have been reporting about the purported dangers of sugary fruits. None of the studies purporting to show a connection between childhood obesity and juice used pure organic fruit juice, so the tests actually proved the connection between childhood obesity and high fructose corn syrup. There are no risks in consuming completely organic fruit juices. Freshly squeezed juice is always the ideal.

The only people who may suffer adverse effects from truly organic fruit juices are those whose bodies have been destroyed by the chronic use of synthetic insulin. Natural fruit juices can only be made dangerous with help from the 'miracles' of modern chemistry. *Natural* sugars do not have the same effects as refined sugars, or the chemically-extracted sugars that are perverted beyond all recognition. Pure, organic, chemically unprocessed, and natural sugars, like those from evaporated cane juice, fruits, and honey are actually beneficial to the health, and that goes for most diabetics too. In fact, natural sugar is an absolute requirement for curing diabetes.

The food industry has amazingly managed to make some fruit juices unhealthy. When drinks are made from concentrate, they are frequently re-hydrated with tap water. So drinking these juices is just as harmful as drinking municipal water that is fluoridated and chlorinated. Some companies additionally add high fructose corn syrup to their juice products, or they add regular processed and bleached sugar. The residual chloride from food processing and municipal water supplies can produce dioxin compounds, similar to those found in DDT. For a thorough explanation of the major problems caused by high fructose corn syrup, we recommend watching the documentary, *King Corn*. The list of consequences includes the Big 3: heart disease, diabetes, and cancer.

Natural sugars are perfect for the human body. It knows how to properly process them, and how to transform them into almost pure energy without harmful byproducts. The human body can metabolize natural sugar without any appreciable inflammation. The amount of natural sugars required to cause excessive weight gain would be so high as to be nearly humanly impossible to consume. One would have to drink so much fruit juice that his kidneys would begin failing before his belly ever grew.

Aluminum Pans

Aluminum is a cumulative heavy metal toxin, and particles of it may become part of the foods being cooked, due to mechanical friction with the utensils being used. Never use metal utensils in aluminum cookware, since scraping can dislodge metal particles. The ideal for most cooking is old-fashioned cast iron, but stainless steel is a reasonable second best.

Margarine

Margarine was first marketed to prevent heart disease. It and other butter substitutes are a main reason why heart disease is the #1 killer of Americans today. The hysteria surrounding butter was created in order to make way for a new industry of artificial hydrogenated oils that were patented by the chemical industry. The public was deceived, and too many people still believe that margarine is the answer to obesity and heart disease. Instead, margarine is a major cause of them. Read the *God's Nutrition* section of the *Nutrition* chapter for an explanation of the bad science behind the lipid hypothesis, which is the disproven belief that saturated fats and cholesterol lead to heart disease. Like in the case of diet items, chemically-engineered fats perpetuate the very diseases which we were told they would prevent. The multitude of studies disproving the lipid hypothesis over a period of decades have been greatly overshadowed by the original one (from the 1950's); which by the way, is *still* used by the A.M.A. to prove that a body metabolizes the new chemically-engineered fats better than natural, organic, food-based fats. Heart disease was a medical rarity when butter was a staple of the diet, but now it is the #1 killer.

Condoms for S.T.D. Protection

The belief that condoms will prevent sexually transmitted diseases is being passed throughout school systems, as if it were an indisputable fact. However, condoms cannot reliably prevent most of the common S.T.D.'s, including genital herpes (H.S.V.), human papillomavirus, chlamydia, syphilis, chanchroid, and trichomonas. Condoms are only partially effective for the H.I.V. virus, which is hardly the assurance that most people seek. The unreliability of condoms has been known since a 2001 investigation by the U.S. National Institutes of Health. A problem with quality control occurs when manufacturers transport condoms in extreme temperatures, as this causes the latex to expand, leading to larger pores. Many diseases can readily pass through the holes in condoms that easily pass standard quality tests.

Salads

One of the first things that most people do when they begin eating well and becoming healthier is start consuming salads. However, lettuce actually has very little nutrition; and moreover, the commercial dressings that people buy are toxic. Almost every commercial dressing contains soybean oil or canola oil as its base, and they are full of chemical additives. This includes the so-called "healthy" options that are found in health food stores. Some dressings are cold-pasteurized, which means that they have been 'treated' with radiation, and they are likely to still be radioactive when they reach store shelves. Such irradiation of foods causes benzene to be produced inside the proteins, alongside super-poisonous radiolytic compounds, which are likewise carcinogenic. Mayonnaise is also cold-pasteurized, which is the industry euphemism for a food being made radioactive. The process of making the food toxic and radioactive allows for an extended shelf life, despite the presence of raw eggs. Salads *can* be healthy, but they are not usually. We recommend salads that feature organic baby spinach, and be aware that the bad flavor for which spinach has become infamous only occurs whenever it is cooked. Uncooked spinach has very little taste. It is similar to lettuce. Always make your own dressings. They are easy to make with some recipe searching. We have some salad dressing recipes already available. You may read our online article, *Why Salads Are Not Usually Healthy* at our healthwyze.org site, for more detailed information.

Calcium Enriched Products

Be wary of foods which advertise added calcium. Excess calcium is a leading cause of the illnesses that we are experiencing today. Contrary to what you may have been told, very few people actually need more calcium, with the usual exceptions of young children and pregnant women. For the proper utilization of calcium in a body, a body needs enough vitamin D (sunlight), and an adequate amount of magnesium. Calcium is useless and detrimental in anyone without enough vitamin D and magnesium. The synthetic types of vitamin D, like those which are added to milk, are useless for about half of the population. Nobody knows why this is, but it is obvious that natural vitamin D cannot be identically produced in a laboratory.

Fish is a good source of vitamin D for those who can neither utilize the supplement version nor get enough sunlight. Diseases which are falsely blamed upon calcium deficiencies, such as osteoporosis and brittle bone disease, are usually caused by fluoride that neutralizes calcium, pharmaceuticals that cause malnutrition, sunlight deficiencies, or MSG depleting magnesium.

Read product ingredients to avoid "calcium phosphate" and "tricalcium phosphate". These are made from ground-up bones, and companies do not disclose where they get those bones from. We do know that these compounds are usually imported from China; so for all we know, they could be from the bones of Chinese political dissidents. Monocalcium phosphate is a naturally-occurring mineral that is completely safe, but it is not an adequate substitute for the minerals obtained from vegetable sources.

Mouthwash

Mouthwash is completely useless for cleaning the teeth. Instead, it kills all of the bacteria in the mouth, including the beneficial bacteria. As a result of its extermination of the beneficial flora (bacteria), yeast will multiply faster to make a person far more vulnerable to bad breath, sore throats, and cavities. Many brands of mouthwash contain excessive amounts of fluoride, which sinks through the walls of the mouth and into the blood to produce disastrous health effects. A healthy person does not have yeast overgrowth in his body, and therefore, he does not have bad breath. For more information about this, read the section about *Allergies* in the *Alternative Medicine* chapter.

Anti-Bacterial Soaps, Hand Sanitizers, and Baby Wipes

Anti-bacterial soaps, hand sanitizers, and anti-bacterial baby wipes should be avoided. They contain triclosan, an antibiotic which produces chloroform whenever it comes into contact with chlorine (another common ingredient). Chloroform is a known carcinogen. Triclosan does not actually kill the bacteria that is responsible for causing common colds or other routine illnesses; so it has very little value in consumer products. There have been numerous recalls in recent years due to bacteria colonies growing inside antibiotic products, which clearly demonstrates the safety and effectiveness of these products.

If any of these products were at all useful, then surgeons would use them instead of spending 15 minutes washing. In studies that compared these products with regular soap, it was shown that regular soap is more effective at killing bacteria than these "anti-bacterial" products are. The chemical industry has made fools of us again.

Hand sanitizers and anti-bacterial baby wipes are especially unhealthy, because these products are not washed off. The poisons remain on the skin for extended periods, so that much of it invariably sinks through the skin to further burden the person's immune system. The end result is that people who are exposed to these products become sick *more often* than people who never use them.

Most of the public elementary schools in the U.S. now use commercial hand sanitizer products on the hands of young children, without washing their hands at all. This means that the children have a bacteria-laden poison rubbed on their hands, which is applied just before they eat; so they ingest it too. This is ironically done in the name of health.

Even the effective antibiotics have the long-term effect of weakening the immune system overall, since they are all made from toxic, allergy-inducing mold compounds. It is a common misconception that only penicillin was manufactured from mold; but in fact, all antibiotics are made from molds. They are usually genetically engineered nowadays. Antibiotics are routinely found to contain fluoride and heavy metals. They are known to decimate intestinal flora (helpful digestive bacteria) for years, making malnutrition chronic for most Americans, and making both illnesses and allergies worse.

The true purpose behind these anti-bacterial products is to drive lagging antibiotic sales, and to promote a belief that we are totally dependent upon the pharmaceutical industry for our health.

Fluoride

Consumer fluoride is literally a toxic waste product from the aluminum, nuclear, and fertilizer industries; and this industrial waste product is what is added to municipal water supplies. There is no special high-purity pharmaceutical fluoride for U.S. water supplies. The material used is literally an industrial waste product. It is the main ingredient of most rat poisons, and U.S. Governmental statistics show that oral ingestion of fluoride from municipal water supplies *causes* cavities, along with a variety of other diseases. In some cases, fluoride is also radioactive because it is derived from radioactive materials. It is common for it to contain lead and aluminum impurities.

Fluorine gas from a super volcano is widely believed to have wiped out the dinosaurs world-wide, in just a matter of days. Those with pure water virtually always have lower rates of cavities and other dental problems. We found these statistics on a governmental website, but strangely enough, the American Dental Association persistently does not seem to find such studies. Fluoride weakens the immune system, kills the beneficial bacteria of the mouth, and neutralizes the calcium needed for maintaining the teeth. Fluoride does not make teeth strong. It makes them brittle, which is almost the opposite of strong. So it practically guarantees expensive dental work for everyone eventually. It can also directly induce cavities by causing pitting in the enamel, which is a known (but rarely reported) side effect. Fluoride can stain the teeth permanently (fluorosis) and it damages the bones (brittle bone disease). Of course, there is that cancer thing too.

Other ways in which the chemical industry has tricked us into buying its toxic waste is the radioactive component (americium-241) that is used in smoke detectors, and the radioactive (high phosphate) fertilizers that are used on tobacco fields, which is one of the main reasons why modern tobacco is so dangerous. Modern tobacco literally produces radioactive smoke, thanks to more 'miracles' of chemistry.

Body pH and Disease

The origin of the word "disease" is dis-*ease*: to not be at ease and harmony. Most medical practitioners have forgotten this, and they merely participate in what is essentially chemical warfare against the symptoms of bodies that are in a state of dis-ease.

Times have changed much over the eons to create dis-ease. Nowadays our diet hardly mimics the flora of Eden. Even when we try to eat well, our foods are saturated with insecticides, growth hormones, raised in deficient soils, have so-called "flavor enhancer" chemicals, and are genetically modified -- usually without any warning labels. Regulations have even been rewritten to redefine what can be presented as "all natural" on food labeling, so that the term "natural" is now routinely used to hide chemically-engineered ingredients that would be far from what any reasonable human being would call "natural". Take for instance, how certain genetically-engineered yeast products are made in unsupervised Chinese factories and are often labeled as "natural ingredients".

The goal of the involved powers-that-be is to engineer cheap, mass-producible foods, that are highly addictive; and to keep us ignorant of it. These foods line the aisles of typical grocery stores. Even colorings have been altered from being natural, and they are petroleum-based in some cases.

In the tap water, we have chlorine and fluoride, in addition to hundreds of other toxins. Some of these are poisonous heavy metals and they are never naturally flushed by the body. Even when not consumed orally, these still enter our bodies through absorption into our skin and lungs via the water mist of showers -- both direct paths into the blood.

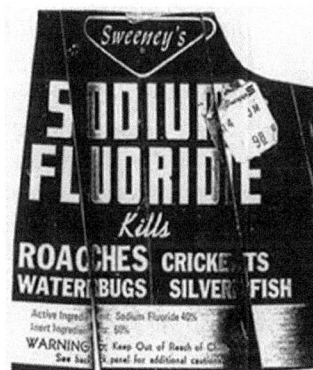

The end result of our accumulated toxicity and everything mentioned previously is that our body chemistry has been altered to become acidic. The relationship between an acidic body and illness has long been established, and the medical term for this condition is "acidosis". It ironically leads to an acid deficiency in the only organ requiring acid: the stomach. There is an inverse relationship between the pH of the stomach and the rest of the body, so whenever a stomach is not as acidic as it ought to be, then the rest of the body is acidic. The toxicity of the majority of foods in a typical diet causes the body to become more acidic during digestion, and this includes most tap water. An acidic body (most bodies nowadays) destroys its own cells, has a weakened immune system, ages rapidly, experiences skin and hair problems, has metabolic and weight regulation problems, is disease prone, is prone to allergies, cannot effectively absorb nutrients, cannot effectively flush toxins, cannot properly cope with cholesterol, cannot properly regulate minerals such as calcium, and most importantly, cannot maintain high levels of oxygen.

The opposite of being acidic is being alkaline. Chemicals (and blood) which are alkaline readily absorb oxygen. Most pathogens and cancers cannot survive in an oxygen-rich, alkaline environment. For instance, oxygenated water (hydrogen peroxide) is an effective infection killer, because harmful microorganisms consistently die in the presence of anything highly oxygenated.

Our typically acidic bodies cannot retain enough oxygen to function properly or fight infections well. When a body reaches a pH level of 7.4 (alkaline), cancers become dormant, and at 7.6, all cancers die rapidly, along with almost every type of invader.

> "Drugs, medications and toxic chemicals have the effect of lowering the pH of the body, that is the reason why there are side effects to drugs and none of them effect a cure. When body pH drops below 6.4, enzymes are deactivated, digestion does not work properly, vitamins, minerals and food supplements cannot effectively assimilate. Acid decreases energy production in the cells, the ability to repair damaged cells, the ability to detoxify heavy metals, and makes the body more susceptible to fatigue and illness. Your body pH affects everything. Research has proven that disease cannot survive in an alkaline state, and that, viruses, bacteria, yeast, mold, fungus, candida and cancer cells thrive in an acidic, low oxygen, low pH environment. An acidic pH can result from an acid forming diet, emotional stress, toxic overload, and immune reactions or any process that deprives the cells of oxygen and other nutrients. The body will try to compensate for acid by utilizing alkaline mineral reserves, like sodium from the stomach, and calcium from the bones. This is a primary cause of osteoporosis and a number of other diseases. If there are not enough minerals in the diet to compensate, acid build-up in the cells will occur, resulting in symptoms like pain, arthritis, fibromyalgia, MS, and lupus. Cancer is not compatible in a healthy pH environment full of oxygen. For example, cancer of the heart doesn't exist. This is because blood flowing from the lungs into the heart are at the highest pH and oxygen levels within the entire body. As the blood travels through the lungs, acidic toxins are thrown out of the system leaving it rich with oxygen and a high blood pH. In the absence of oxygen, glucose undergoes fermentation to lactic acid. This causes the pH of the cell to drop even lower. Urine and saliva pH of terminal cancer patients almost always runs between 4.0 and 5.5. When the cancer goes into metastases the pH drops even lower.

> "In 1964, only 1 person in 214 contracted cancer. Today it is 1 in 3 females and 1 in 2 males. The determining factor between health and disease is pH. It is not uncommon for the average American to test between 4 pH and 5 pH."

> -- Keiichi Morishita, *Hidden Truth of Cancer*

Potential hydrogen (pH) is the measurement of hydrogen ion concentration in any solution. The higher the pH reading, the more alkaline it is, and the more oxygen rich the fluid may become. A lower pH reading indicates that a solution is more acidic and oxygen resistant. The pH scale is from 0 to 14 with 7.0 being neutral. Anything above 7.0 is considered to be alkaline, and anything below 7.0 is acidic. For curing cancer, that $1.23 bottle of liquidized oxygen (hydrogen peroxide) is considerably safer and more effective than the $300,000.00 chemotherapy regimen that a doctor would recommend.

Dr. Otto Warburg (pictured) was awarded the Nobel Prize for medicine in 1931, but his discoveries have been suppressed by the medical establishment so successfully that only alternative medicine researchers ever learn of them, or of him. The Nobel Foundation explained why it awarded Dr. Warburg the Nobel Prize by writing, *"For his discovery of the nature and mode of action of the respiratory enzyme, the Nobel Prize has been awarded to him in 1931. This discovery has opened up new ways in the fields of cellular metabolism and cellular respiration. He has shown, among other things, that cancerous cells can live and develop, even in the absence of oxygen"*.

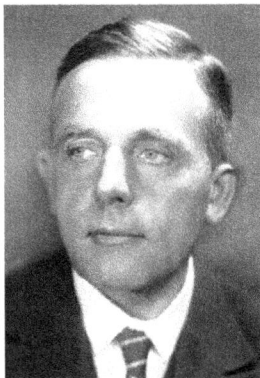

Dr. Warburg discovered that cancer cells are not fueled by oxygen as normal cells are. The high levels of oxygen that are found in healthy, alkaline bodies are toxic to cancers. He found that cancers get their energy from sugars and a process of fermentation in acidic environments. He proved empirically the relationship between cancers, acidic body pH, and cellular oxygen starvation. His findings demonstrated that cancers are merely a symptom of acidosis, and therefore it is impossible to truly cure any cancer without first curing the underlying acidosis.

Standard cancer care now means almost certainly dying from either the cancer, or more likely, the treatments. Cancer deaths usually result from the toxic effects of mainstream cancer treatments. These increase a body's acidity, virtually guaranteeing that cancer symptoms will return elsewhere, even if the initial tumors are destroyed. Thus, the dismal lifetime failure rate of standard cancer medicine is a jaw-dropping 96%. They call it "medicine" and claim that it is scientifically validated, but the *science* only works 4% of the time. Doing nothing is a more effective treatment for cancers than standard therapies. To manipulate the statistics, any patient who does not die within 5 years is reported to have had a successful treatment. The treatments stimulate the acidic conditions that originally caused the cancers. They damage the same immune system that is needed to fight cancer cells, and the treatments randomly damage the organs throughout a body. Therefore, cancers tend to spread rapidly (metastasize) following 'conventional' treatments of modern, experimental medicine.

Medical Quotations

"But nobody today can say that one does not know what cancer and its prime cause be. On the contrary, there is no disease whose prime cause is better known, so that today ignorance is no longer an excuse that one cannot do more about prevention. That prevention of cancer will come there is no doubt, for man wishes to survive. But how long prevention will be avoided depends on how long the prophets of agnosticism will succeed in inhibiting the application of scientific knowledge in the cancer field. In the meantime, millions of men must die of cancer unnecessarily."

-- Dr. Otto Warburg, medical Nobel Prize winner

"Everyone should know that the war on cancer is largely a fraud."

-- Dr. Linus Pauling, two time winner of the Nobel Prize

"To the cancer establishment, a cancer patient is a profit center. The actual clinical and scientific evidence does not support the claims of the cancer industry. Conventional cancer treatments are in place as the law of the land because they pay, not heal, the best. Decades of the politics-of-cancer-as-usual have kept you from knowing this, and will continue to do so unless you wake up to their reality."

-- John Diamond, M.D., Lee Cowden, M.D.

"Chemotherapy is an incredibly lucrative business for doctors, hospitals, and pharmaceutical companies. The medical establishment wants everyone to follow the same exact protocol. They don't want to see the chemotherapy industry go under, and that's the number one obstacle to any progress in oncology."

-- Glen Warner, M.D.

"You wouldn't believe how many FDA officials or relatives or acquaintances of FDA officials come to see me as patients in Hanover. You wouldn't believe this, or directors of the AMA, or ACA, or the presidents of orthodox cancer institutes."

-- Hans Nieper, M.D., alternative medicine practitioner

"When Dr. Hamer was arrested in 1997 for having given three people medical advice without a medical license, the police confiscated his patients' files and had them analyzed. Subsequently, one public prosecutor was forced to admit during the trial that, after five years, 6,000 out of 6,500 patients with mostly 'terminal cancer' were still alive. With conventional treatment the figures are generally just the reverse."

-- Dr. Caroline Markolin, Ph.D.

"As a chemist trained to interpret data, it is incomprehensible to me that physicians can ignore the clear evidence that chemotherapy does much, much more harm than good."

-- Alan Nixon, Ph.D., Past President of the American Chemical Society

"Two to 4% of cancers respond to chemotherapy."

-- Ralph Moss, Ph.D

"The FDA protects the big drug companies, and is subsequently rewarded, and using the government's police powers, they attack those who threaten the big drug companies. The thing that bugs me is that the people think the FDA is protecting them. It isn't. What the FDA is doing, and what the public thinks it is doing are as different as night and day."

-- Dr. Herbert Ley, former Commissioner of the F.D.A.

"In point of fact, fluoride causes more human cancer deaths, and causes it faster, than any other chemical."

-- Dean Burke, Former Chief Chemist Emeritus, U.S. National Cancer Institute

"Most cancer patients in this country die of chemotherapy. Chemotherapy does not eliminate breast, colon or lung cancers. This fact has been documented for over a decade. Yet doctors still use chemotherapy for these tumors. Women with breast cancer are likely to die faster with chemo than without it."

-- Alan Levin, M.D.

"When a patient is found to have a tumor, the only thing the doctor discusses with that patient is what he intends to do about the tumor. If a patient with a tumor is receiving radiation or chemotherapy, the only question that is asked is, 'How is the tumor doing'? No one ever asks how the patient is doing. In my medical training, I remember well seeing patients who were getting radiation and/or chemotherapy. The tumor would get smaller and smaller, but the patient would be getting sicker and sicker. At autopsy we would hear, 'Isn't that marvelous! The tumor is gone!' Yes, it was, but so was the patient. How many millions of times are we going to have to repeat these scenarios before we realize that we are treating the wrong thing?"

-- Dr. Philip Binzel

Cancer Cells are Normal -- Acidosis Is Not

Every person who takes breath on this Earth has cancer. Cancer cells are a normal part of existence. A healthy body with a healthy immune system will eliminate these cancer cells at roughly the same rate that they are spawned. The human body eliminates thousands, and perhaps millions of cancer cells every day, to ensure that it is clean of these mutated cells. It is how things are supposed to work. As tissues and cells die, such as those of killed cancer cells, the decaying tissues ferment to make the body somewhat more acidic and toxic. With the very active participation of the liver and kidneys, the body's regulatory and immune systems simultaneously trigger the chemical reactions to shift the blood from being slightly acidic back to alkaline by harnessing key minerals. This is how a healthy body cures itself of cancer every day.

If a body is made too acidic by diet, toxins, or a suppressed immune system, then things no longer work as they are supposed to. Excessive acidity impairs the immune system, which is the core of life itself. When the immune system is compromised, the body loses its ability to alkalize itself, and then the body loses its ability to absorb oxygen effectively.

With the low amounts of oxygen that are seen with extreme acidosis, cells must use fermentation for energy, and this transforms healthy cells into cancer cells. The transition into cells that live from energy that is derived from fermentation is actually part of a survival response. Whenever there is oxygen depletion, there may be an excess of cancer cells that may form into tumors. This "cancer" is no disease in itself, but merely a troubling symptom that the body's immune system can no longer regulate itself, because external forces have overwhelmed it. The cause may be vitamin and mineral depletion, illnesses, extreme stress, chemical carcinogens, unhealthy (chemically altered) fats and oils, pharmaceuticals, or a lack of omega-3. Diet usually plays a huge role in making a person acidic, and therefore oxygen depleted; especially the synthesized food products that are ironically marketed as "healthy alternatives" to natural fats and oils.

352

Acidosis is a byproduct of an over-taxed immune system, for it is known that the human body is always acidic during sickness. The orthodox establishment considers acidosis to be a symptom of whatever disease happens to be present, instead of considering that acidosis could be the root cause of multiple disease states. The establishment's utter lack of success in curing cancers is largely due to a fundamental misunderstanding of these relationships.

Cancer is one of the many symptoms of acidosis: albeit one of the worst. Therefore, tumors are not really a symptom of cancers, but of acidosis. Cancer cells are normal in even healthy bodies, after all. To the orthodox schools, the tumors are treated like they are the disease, and this mysterious disease is believed to be caused by another mysterious force called "cancer". It does not require 12 years of intensive college study to immediately see glaring flaws in the logic. One only needs to holistically look at the big picture to see it. Given that acidosis is known to appear at the onset of most serious diseases, including cancers, and all general infections, it is apparent that acidosis is not merely a coincidental symptom of hundreds of unrelated diseases. It is a core cause of disease.

Cancers have been cured countless times with alternative therapies designed to adjust patients' pH (and thereby oxygen intake). People have been literally saved with food-grade hydrogen peroxide. Of course, there are much better methods available, and virtually all alternative therapies are more reliable, safer, quicker, and cheaper than standard treatments. Remember that orthodox cancer doctors can only boast of a 4% lifetime cure rate, and "survival" has been redefined to mean just 5 years of life after diagnosis -- to cook their own statistics. A "cancer survivor" is likely to die between the five and ten year mark after diagnosis, if he undertakes standard therapies. We would do very little bragging if 96% of our patients died from our treatments in less than 10 years. The orthodox cancer industry is nothing short of a system of genocide.

According to the official statistics published by the German Research Centre On Cancer in Heidelberg, 98% of patients treated with chemo die within 7 years, and 95% within 5 years. With Germanische Neue Medizin (alternative medicine) however, 98% of those patients who did not previously receive treatments with chemo and morphine survived.

Due to space constraints, specific dietary recommendations were not cited here, but there is a pH food chart at our website (healthwyze.org).

Sudden Infant Death Syndrome

In 1774, it was discovered that sudden infant death syndrome, which is closely linked to acute infantile scurvy, is preventable in nearly all cases. Dr. James Lind, a Scottish physician of the British Navy, conducted experiments concluding that citrus fruits cured scurvy. He wrote the following about scurvy (vitamin C deficiency):

> *"Persons that appear to be but slightly scorbutic are apt to be suddenly and unexpectedly seized with some of its worst symptoms. Their dropping down dead upon an exertion of their strength or change of air is not easily foretold."*

The resemblance between these symptoms and S.I.D.S. is not merely coincidental. While the name, sudden infant death syndrome is relatively new; this identifiable pattern of sudden death has been around for a long time, and the methods of preventing it were known centuries ago.

Dr. Archie Kalokerinos volunteered to undertake the mission of reducing the rate of S.I.D.S. amongst aboriginal people in the opal mining region of Australia. At the time, approximately 50% of all aboriginal infants died of sudden infant death syndrome. He found that almost all of them were terribly deficient in vitamin C, so he provided them with supplementation. None of the infants died from S.I.D.S following the supplementation. He later wrote about it in the book, *Every Second Child*, with co-author and the Nobel Prize winner, Linus Pauling. He noticed that during his work with the aboriginal people, the pharmaceutical companies had been using the aborigines for mass vaccine experimentation, in what he felt was a campaign of genocide. He also reported that vaccines in Africa contained H.I.V., and this whistleblowing is why the medical establishment began maligning his reputation.

The good doctor went on tour with other doctors throughout the United States, in an attempt to spread the word about the main cause of sudden infant death syndrome. Kalokerinos and his peers were ignored by the medical establishment, because his findings were not politically correct medicine. The doctor was preaching that the cure was nutritional instead of pharmaceutical. Additionally, he proved that there was a direct link between unexpected child deaths and vaccines that had caused deficiencies of vitamin C. What other doctors heard was that modern medicine was actually *the problem*. To them, it made Dr. Kalokerinos the problem. As a result of this cover-up, approximately 2,600 babies die each year from sudden infant death syndrome in the U.S. alone.

All deceased S.I.D.S. victims who are tested for vitamin C deficiency show only trace amounts of this vital nutrient, without exception.

Dr. Kalokerinos wrote that many of the aboriginal babies died immediately after receiving vaccines. He blamed this on the amount of extra sodium ascorbate (vitamin C) that their bodies needed to counteract the toxic effects of the vaccines. He recognized that massive amounts of vitamin C are utilized whenever someone is sick, or when his immune system is otherwise aggravated. Vaccines are designed specifically to force a hyper-immune response, and this is done by the use of poisonous adjuvants.

Babies need vitamin C for development in the womb, and prenatal vitamin C helps to prevent the future onset of S.I.D.S. Even after birth, most infants desperately need the natural vitamins found in breast milk. Nutritional deficiencies place infants at risk of developmental problems and infantile death. The commercial infant formulas are not a healthy option. The inability of manufacturers to properly mimic human breast milk and vitamins is shown in the reduced immune systems of children who are fed infant formulas. Statistics show that the nutritional deficiencies caused by infant formulas vastly increase the likelihood of childhood health disasters, such as S.I.D.S.

Many scientists, especially those from New Zealand, have partially blamed mattresses for the modern epidemic of "cot deaths". Since the 1950's, mattresses have been doused with arsenic, phosphorus, and antimony to make them flame retardant. A fungus that grows inside mattresses (scopulariopsis brevicaulis) can cause these poisons to become airborne by way of fungal gas emissions, resulting in sudden halts to the central nervous systems of infants. It is a sound hypothesis considering the constant drooling of infants, combined with their tendency to place everything in their mouths, and their overall exaggerated vulnerability to toxins.

New Zealand manufacturers created specially formulated mattresses for infants to sleep on, which eliminate the risks of fungus and chemical poisons. No infant has ever died from S.I.D.S. whilst sleeping on these mattresses. Of course, New Zealand has not adopted the ridiculous vaccination regimen that the U.S.A. has either, nor are its foods so depleted of nutrients, nor laden with chemically-engineered artificial ingredients: all of which the body needs vitamin C to cope with.

Mattresses can obviously play a large role in producing S.I.D.S., but S.I.D.S. has been around since well before the 1950's. Nutrition should be the first concern for parents. Organic materials should certainly be used for everything that children are exposed to; but above all, remember the nutrition. Also remember that there is no acceptable substitute for breast feeding. For the sake of your child, remember that regardless of the billions that are spent in research, we cannot out-engineer God, and there is a high price for the arrogance of trying.

Shaken Baby Syndrome

Shaken baby syndrome has been increasingly diagnosed over the past 50 years, but the evidence is all anecdotal. The evidence mainly consists of individual case reports that were written by doctors who detailed their post-mortem observations and presumptions.

Medical literature reports that the symptoms of shaken baby syndrome include extreme irritability, decreased appetite, no vocalization, poor sucking or swallowing, rigidity, difficulty breathing, seizures, inability for the eyes to track movement, swollen head or a soft spot on the head which appears to be bulging.

When a child is taken to the hospital with these symptoms, physicians often perform a brain scan to find signs of hemorrhaging and swelling. Parents are often charged with child abuse when these symptoms are discovered, and they are virtually always accused of murder whenever the child dies. There is rarely any investigation into other possible causes. The medical establishment is galvanized in asserting that shaking a child is the only way for such injuries to occur, while studies on animals have already shown that this is not the case. In mice, brain swelling that is identical to the swelling that supposedly occurs from shaken baby syndrome is caused by the pertussis (whooping cough) vaccine.

An analysis of available shaken baby syndrome cases reveals two distinct patterns:

- The infant was usually delivered prematurely, or there were other complications during pregnancy, and the delivery supposedly required "medical intervention".

- The symptoms almost always appear within 15 days of vaccinations, and the overwhelming majority of cases happened within 10 days of vaccinations. A surprisingly high percentage of shaken baby cases were within 2 days of a vaccination.

The Vaccine Connection

Shaken baby syndrome usually occurs when an infant has had lots of *help* from the medical establishment and he remains too weak to survive the toxic onslaught from vaccines. The horrible aftermath of all that *help* is used as proof that the parents must have been abusive, since the over-medicated child was always so sickly. The vaccine reactions are always presented to be indicative of abuse whenever an infant is taken to a hospital with mysterious brain swelling and brain bleeding issues. Shaken baby syndrome deaths should more rightly be labeled as "iatrogenic deaths", because these are deaths that are caused by allopathic medicine.

The U.S. Centers for Disease Control admitted in its DTaP (diphtheria, tetanus and pertussis) vaccine information sheet that the vaccine may cause seizures and brain damage. These are considered acceptable risks for other people's children, for these risks are rarely mentioned to parents. In the same C.D.C. vaccine document, they ironically reported that the DTaP vaccine is much safer than the original DTP vaccine that it replaced in 1997; but they conveniently neglected to mention that its manufacturer (Wyeth Pharmaceuticals) was sued so often that the National Childhood Vaccine Injury Act of 1986 was created specifically to shield Wyeth from lawsuits and to prevent constitutionally-guaranteed jury trials against them. That law makes it illegal to sue *any* vaccine manufacturer in the United States *for any reason*. Lawmakers and industry lawyers felt that convulsing children have a tendency to generate sympathy amongst jurists, and attorneys actually mentioned this in their justifications. Despite its known risks, the DTP vaccine was sold for use on infants and children for 48 years before the "safer" DTaP formulation was marketed. Wyeth (now Pfizer) blamed the F.D.A. for having an approval process that is too slow, but it was more likely due to the fact that DTP is more profitable than DTaP. The newer DTaP vaccine *still* causes the same brain swelling reaction (encephalitis) that is blamed upon shaken baby syndrome. The biggest change is that it has become illegal to sue vaccine manufacturers, which is an unconstitutional privilege that is shared with no other industry.

The C.D.C. reported that yet another consequence of the DTP/DTaP vaccine is a fever exceeding 105 degrees. Such high temperatures are another cause of severe brain damage. Brain-related side effects are admitted for most childhood vaccines; so the categorical relationship between brain damage and vaccinations has already been demonstrated and documented in the medical literature. Parents are virtually never told; and in fact, they are told the lie that vaccines are completely safe and backed by incontrovertible science.

Evidence of a Lie

In most cases of supposed shaken baby syndrome, there are no indications of abuse or any history thereof. Even proponents of the current shaken baby syndrome theory acknowledge that signs of abuse, such as bruising and grab marks, are extremely rare. Parents who are accused of shaken baby syndrome were typically viewed by others as caring, and they invariably have no history of violence. Yet, according to the prevailing opinion, parents who have been nurturing their children may suddenly start violently shaking them to death, without any cause or explanation. In real cases involving abusive personalities, the abusers become progressively more violent toward their victims over time. This mental illness had never occurred in history until the 1980's, when the vaccine schedules were increased.

> *"Human shaking may cause lethal brain stem and cervical spine injuries in a 0-to 2-year-old child, as the forces necessary for these injuries are well below the level needed for fatal brain injuries and are consistent with the forces that can be produced in shaking."*

> -- Chris Van Ee, Ph.D., Injury Biomechanics Researcher

There is strong evidence that it is impossible to induce the type of brain injury that is found in cases of shaken baby syndrome without first causing extreme neck and spinal injuries.

However, spinal injuries are virtually never seen in these cases of alleged abuse.

Some parents actually confess to shaking their child, because upon finding their child unconscious, their natural reaction is to attempt to wake him by shaking him. It was never the shaking that caused these children to become comatose, but parents nevertheless confess to shaking their children, due to the intense pressure stemming from both their loss and the incessant interrogations. Such confessions are then used as evidence that the parents murdered their child. They are condemned in the courts and the press regardless of their emotional state. Strong emotional reactions are proclaimed to be expressions of guilt, whereas parents who show no emotions are said to be obviously unremorseful and sociopathic. Either way, the parents lose.

Real research into the causes of shaken baby syndrome is lacking, because there can be no controlled studies. Such studies would involve killing infants, or at least exposing them to a very high risk of harm. Nevertheless, lives and families are being destroyed on the basis of fraudulent scientific evidence. The parents of vaccinated children who suffer with encephalitis find themselves being tried for murder; lest the doctors and hospitals be held accountable. The manufacturers have already been legally immune since 1986. It is business as usual.

Cleansing and Detoxifying

We have received an enormous volume of questions about cleansing. This chapter attempts to answer the fundamental questions. Cleanses should never be attempted during illness. During most cleanses, the toxins that begin flowing throughout the blood (prior to being flushed) can cause hormone irregularities that lead to mood swings. Loved ones should be warned to expect this before a cleanse is begun.

Gallbladder Cleanse

We have a comprehensive gallbladder cleanse in the *Gallstones and Gallbladder Attacks* section of the *Alternative Medicine* chapter. Please reference that section for more information about cleansing the gallbladder, because there is too much information to include here. A gallbladder cleanse is only necessary if there are ongoing problems that are specific to the gallbladder, such as gallstones. Gallbladder cleanses are stressful on a body, and should not be utilized as routine preventative care.

Liver Cleanse

Always begin a cleansing regimen by cleaning the liver. Never bypass the initial liver cleanse. A body will not function optimally whenever a liver becomes burdened, but there is an even greater reason for cleaning the liver first. Until the liver is cleansed, its toxic load will prevent a body from coping best with new toxins and flushing them out. This is why a liver cleanse is so vital, because no other cleanse will work effectively until the liver is functioning well. Cleansing any other part of the body while the liver is partially dysfunctional is like cleaning a floor with a filthy mop and filthy water.

The liver works in close partnership with the kidneys to clean the blood. Toxins can get stored inside the liver whenever a body becomes too toxic to excrete them, or whenever materials are too toxic for the kidneys to expel. In a sense, a liver will self-sacrifice to defend the rest of the body when all else fails against antibiotics, heavy metals, chemicals, etc. Thus, many people have extremely impaired livers as a result. The worst toxins accumulate in the liver, and tend to remain permanently, unless there is intervention. The eventual result of years of chemical onslaught against the liver is a crippled liver that is too impaired to efficiently eliminate future toxins. This is the genesis of many chronic diseases; and in the worst cases, death by liver failure. Extreme liver toxicity can cause an avalanche effect, whereby the more toxic the liver becomes, the less a body is able to prevent the accumulation of further toxins, so it must therefore store even more of them in the liver. This is surprisingly common for people of the Western world, and it partially explains why Western societies are constantly becoming more sensitive to chemicals and allergens.

There is a wide variety of herbal liver cleanses available that are prepackaged to make the process easy, and there are reasons to choose commercial formulas. There is a complex array of herbs and supplements that must be properly combined and properly administered to effectively flush the impurities from a toxic liver. Such formulations are exceptionally difficult for any individual to create. The research alone takes weeks for a skilled researcher. It is even considerably more expensive to purchase all of the ingredients separately. Eventually, we determined that doing-it-yourself for liver cleanses is unwise, so we purchased Nature's Way's Thisilyn Daily Cleanse for ourselves. As always, we recommend reading the ingredients before purchasing any product to ensure that it does not contain any toxic additives. The ingredients for Thisilyn Daily Cleanse may have changed by the time that you read this, so buyer beware and examine the ingredients carefully for any product that you consider using.

As an example of the problem with reformulations, we previously recommended Perfect Cleanse brand, but the ingredients changed to include chlorella, since the use of chlorella has become a dangerous fad. Chlorella and other underwater plants are likely to increase toxicity and damage the liver, so we cannot recommend Perfect Cleanse anymore in good conscience. Please take the time to read and learn about the ingredients in whichever product you use. We have historically seen that products by Nature's Way have been amongst the best in virtually every category, but this could change at any time.

Liver Tonics

- Licorice
- Dandelion
- Milk thistle
- St. John's Wort *
- Nettle
- Fennel
- Peppermint
- Fenugreek
- Burdock root
- Wild yam

    * Do not use Saint John's Wort if you are pregnant or if you are attempting to get pregnant. It can cause pregnancy complications or abortions.

The above supplements will help with a weakened liver and various liver problems, but they will not necessarily provide the level of cleansing needed. If taken in excess, they can stress the liver more, so use common sense.

Heavy Metal Cleanse

For a healthy person with limited candida albicans (yeast) growth, we would recommend a heavy metal cleanse after a liver cleanse. Heavy metals are toxic to almost all living things, including candida. Metals constantly keep candida in the body suppressed, so removing the metal can result in an immediate candida overgrowth. The aftermath is general sickness, lethargy, yeast infections, confusion, and mental fogginess.

The wise approach is to first starve the sugar-loving candida colonies by eating a good diet for one to two weeks. Avoid processed carbohydrates and all sugars (except honey), get plenty of fruits, vegetables, and organic meats. Honey actually helps the process. Alongside this good diet, get some plain unsweetened yogurt (preferably organic) and eat some each day. The beneficial bacteria in yogurt will attack the candida inside the intestinal tract. Commercial yogurts are homogenized, so supplement with vitamin C and folate (or the inferior folic acid) to protect against inflammation and arterial damage. It would be wise to mix the yogurt with flax seed oil for extra health benefits. Read about the Budwig Protocol (cancer chapter) for a full explanation of this combination.

A general heavy metal cleanse can be done simply using cilantro supplements combined with selenium, although it would be wise to include apple pectin too. Combining just these three supplements should result in a metal cleanse that is remarkably effective, whilst being relatively gentle on the body. A cleanse employing all of the supplements listed below is only recommended in the most extreme and time-sensitive cases, such as for those with Alzheimer's disease or autism. Heavy metal cleanses should be followed for 10 days.

- Cilantro (supplement 100 mg. per 50 lbs. of weight)
- NAC (N-Acetyl-Cysteine)
- Selenium (100 mcg. per 100 lbs. of weight) *
- B complex vitamin
- Alpha lipoic acid
- 5-HTP
- Garlic
- Exercise
- MSM (Methylsulfonylmethane) (optional)
- DMSA (optional)

> * It is dangerous to exceed 400 mcg. of selenium.

With all heavy metal cleanses, selenium should be used constantly, because it neutralizes the metals in the blood from a toxicity standpoint. DMSA is used in alternative medicine to cure autism. Sweating further helps to expel some toxins, and exercise is the only way that the lymph nodes expel toxins. EDTA also chelates metals, including mercury and lead. It is used by hospitals for metal poisonings, but it should be reserved for emergencies.

Apple pectin is a food-based cleansing agent that is much more gentle than most. Yet, it is surprisingly effective. It should be used by individuals who need a long-term constant cleanse, such as those with mercury (so-called "silver") dental fillings. It has been studied for its ability to remove lead, mercury and cadmium. It performs the dual task of dislodging toxic compounds from the tissues, and it assists the body in discarding them through the stools. It can also remove radioactive particles from the body, and it was used by victims of the Chernobyl nuclear disaster. The standard dose for heavy metal removal is 500 mg. per 100 pounds of body weight. The dosage increases to 800 mg. per 100 lbs. when treating radiation poisoning.

"Silver" Dental Fillings

Silver dental fillings are not really silver, and they are largely made of mercury. Mercury is one of the most toxic substances on Earth. Cilantro is able to remove mercury from the body. Japanese physician, Dr. Yoshiaki Omura, demonstrated this by using cilantro (chinese parsley) to remove the mercury that had leached into patients' bodies during amalgam filling removal operations. The mercury concentrations that had been observed in the patients were so great that they resulted in abnormal heart rhythms. Doctor Omura successfully chelated mercury out of patients using 100 mg. capsules of cilantro extract, four times a day, for two weeks.

People who have mercury fillings removed should cleanse the mercury from their bodies, regardless of the precautions that are taken during the operation. Those who have mercury dental fillings are constantly exposed to mercury, so it would be wise for them to regularly supplement with cilantro and selenium. Mercury exposure causes routine mental disturbances, lowered intelligence, confusion, weakened immunity, and potentially Alzheimer's disease.

Iron Issues

We highly recommend the regular intake of grapes, raisins, grape juice, or red wine for adult males. Resveratrol is a compound in these foods that men require. It can be obtained in supplement form too, but the supplements are quite expensive. Without regular resveratrol intake, an adult male will accumulate toxic levels of iron in his blood. It happens to practically all adult men who lack grape products in their diets. The only men who are not at risk of having excessive iron are those who have been life-long vegetarians, and it can sometimes happen to them too. Resveratrol is critical for men because typical heavy metal cleanses do not remove iron from the blood. Without regular resveratrol intake, a man's iron level tends to grow constantly throughout his life. The fastest way for a man to rid himself of excessive iron is to donate blood, so that his body must create pure blood to replace what is lost. His body otherwise recycles the iron endlessly. The toxicity of iron overload in adult males is a huge component of heart disease. Alongside truly toxic metals, iron is likewise involved in the development of Alzheimer's disease. Excessive iron can also cause strokes. It can be an issue for post-menopausal women too. The avoidance of beef is not a wise solution. Beef or lamb are a critical part of a healthy diet. These "red" meats provide nutrients that are not found elsewhere, and the best type of vitamin A (retinol).

Metal Cleanse Completion

The procedures outlined above (liver cleanse followed by candida cleanse and then a metal cleanse) should remove most of the stress from cleansing, so that life can continue relatively uneffected. Nevertheless, even with the best protocol, it will not happen entirely without incident. In the very least, the patient should expect to become moody and to suffer from bouts of fatigue. These are normal signs that the cleanse is working. These symptoms are a result of the stagnant toxins migrating through the body again, which triggers the immune system to activate, as if the body were being invaded. The result is what some people refer to as a "healing crisis". Initially experiencing mild flu-like symptoms means that the immune system is working like it is supposed to, so the patient should be emotionally supported to maintain a positive attitude throughout the process.

Kidney Cleanse

Having a combination of bad body pH and tiny undetected kidney stones are the most common reasons for kidney dysfunction, alongside infections and toxicity. Hormone imbalances often cause kidney problems too. Everyone knows about using cranberry juice, but it causes acidic body chemistry, so it should always be used in conjunction with lemon juice, pineapple juice, or something else that has a significant alkalizing effect. The following will cleanse the kidneys if used for a week, 2-3 times a day.

- Homemade Lemonade (sweetened with honey)
- Cranberry Juice
- Lots of healthy (e.g. spring) water

Lung Cleanse

If you have ever been a smoker, then your lungs could probably benefit from a good cleanse. This is also true for most asthma sufferers. One way to cleanse the lungs is with harmless and non-addictive Indian tobacco. If you smoke commercially-made cigarettes in the U.S., then you are in more danger than you know, because carpet glue is being added to every U.S. brand. Taurine supplementation has been shown to reverse some of the damage caused by smoking, even when smokers continue to smoke during treatment. Reference the *Indian Tobacco* section of the *Supplements* chapter for more information. A 2003 study by the Royal College of Surgeons found that most of the damage caused by chronic smoking can be reversed in as little as five days with a dosage of 1.5 grams of taurine. The inner lining of the blood vessels and the diameter of blood vessels returned to normal in the study.

Colon Cleanse

A colon cleanse should not be necessary for anyone having a high fiber diet. In other words, people who eat plenty of fruits and vegetables should never need a colon cleanse. A lifetime of poor diet may merit a colon cleanse, but prevention is always preferred. There are natural do-it-yourself colon cleanse protocols, but we do not recommend them. They generally entail living on top of a toilet, for days, in a manner reminiscent to having salmonella. The do-it-yourself solutions are insanity, and such cleanses give the allopathic doctors justification to laugh at our community. If you feel that you need a colon cleanse, then we recommend using a commercially-formulated product from a reputable health or herbal store. These products are often the result of years of research, and they have been perfected. Most of the products are "gentle" cleansers, which means that you will not be spending a week on a toilet. Unfortunately, we cannot recommend any specific brands.

Activated charcoal is an old do-it-yourself method, but be advised that it can cause malnutrition, constipation, and it neutralizes virtually everything (including medications).

Reference the *Activated Carbon* section of the *Emergency Medicine* chapter to learn more about using it for poison emergencies.

Extra Cleansing Aids

Chlorophyll has been shown to flush a wide variety of substances out of the body. It removes dioxins, benzene, and aflatoxin. All of which are extremely carcinogenic. It has the rare property of aiding a body in excreting such chemicals, while simultaneously drawing beneficial nutrients into cells, due to its special effects upon cell membranes. We get a tiny bit of it every time we eat green vegetables. It is the source of green coloring in plants.

Niacin (vitamin B-3) is well known for its ability to flush the body of various toxins. We recommend reading the *Niacin* section of the *Supplements* chapter before supplementing with it, because of its strange effects.

Throughout alternative medicine, there is a drink that many believe cleanses the blood. We call it "The Blood Cleanser", and it can be found in our *Juicing* chapter. Current scientific understanding tells us that the resveratrol present in grape juice removes excess iron and copper from the blood, and this drink seems to have unique properties in detoxifying after immediate exposure to unhealthy ingredients. It is *extremely* invigorating, and it can keep a person awake all night if taken too late in the day. We recommend that it be used alongside heavy metal cleanses.

Cooking Oil Safety

People tend to thoughtfully consider the nutritional value of the cooking oils that they choose, but the rancidity of oils is actually of greater importance. Whenever an oil is heated enough, it undergoes a chemical breakdown, which leads to it becoming rancid. The heat-induced process transforms healthy oils into dangerous oils. This happens regardless of the original nutrient content.

Every oil has a smoke point. This is the temperature at which the nutritional content of an oil begins rapidly degrading. The smoke point is when oils become harmful, and it is when they begin actually emitting smoke, which is often more toxic than the destroyed oil. Every time an oil is reused, its smoke point temperature is lowered, because it has already undergone some breakdown from previous uses. The reuse of oils is one of the main reasons why eating at restaurants is discouraged, because the oils will be bad even in restaurants that purchase healthy oils. Although, it is not often that they do.

Canola oil is always the worst choice, because it becomes toxic long before it reaches its smoke point. This is information that has been somewhat obscured from public view. We are outraged about the situation with canola, and its wide-scale promotion by Whole Food's Market, which also promotes hormone-destroying soy as well. The high rates of lung cancer in China are largely due to the use of canola oil and rapeseed oil, despite the country's low cigarette smoking rate. "Vegetable oil" once referred to corn oil, but now it usually refers to soybean and canola oil; so beware whenever you see "vegetable oil" on a label.

The low smoke point of flax seed oil is the reason why we recommend avoiding most of the so-called "healthy" foods that include flax. Flax oil becomes rancid much faster than other oils whenever it is exposed to heat, light, or oxygen. Thus, those 'healthy' flax-enriched foods are likely to destroy the arteries faster than anything else, and to eventually cause cancer. We still recommend flax oil supplements, but only when the oil has been properly cold-pressed, and packaged to protect it from heat, light, and oxygen. The same rancidity issues are also true for other oils that are high in omega-3. Omega oils are very unstable, so baked goods that boast about containing omega-3 are always rancid and should be avoided.

We recommend peanut oil for high-heat cooking, and olive oil for everything else. By high heat, we mean such temperatures that may be obtained from cooking in a wok or a deep fryer. Both olive oil and coconut oil are known for their health benefits and nutritional value, but both need lower temperatures. Coconut oil should only be used in low heat or no heat recipes.

If you are searching for something like butter, then simply use butter. Butter is actually a healthy substance that is full of fat-soluble vitamins and minerals, which are difficult to obtain from other sources. The best type of butter is organic, unsalted, yellow butter, which is more nutrient dense than standard butter. Natural butter, in moderation, will do much more good than harm; contrary to what your doctor may have told you. Butter can be used whenever extreme heat is not required. Never use margarine or other artificial fats. Margarine is a butter imitation that was created by the chemical industry, and it is largely responsible for the soaring rates of heart disease, which natural saturated fats like butter have been blamed for.

Please note that the oils marked as "refined" in the following table are the standard versions that are sold in most grocery stores, and these tend to have lower nutritional values. The inclusion of an oil in the list is not a recommendation from us. We would never promote the use of canola or soy, for example. We generally recommend against corn oil too, in part because it is genetically engineered, like soy and canola.

Type of Oil	Smoke Point in Degrees Fahrenheit
Canola oil (refined retail variety)	470
Extra-light olive oil	468
Canola oil (expeller pressed)	464
Pomace olive oil	460
Palm oil	455
Coconut oil (refined retail variety)	450
Corn oil (refined retail variety)	450
Peanut oil (refined retail variety)	450
Safflower oil (refined retail variety)	450
Soybean Oil (refined retail variety)	450
Sunflower Oil (refined retail variety)	450
Hazelnut oil	430
Virgin olive oil	420
Low acidity extra virgin olive oil	405
Walnut oil (refined retail variety)	400
Extra virgin olive oil	375
Coconut oil (unrefined)	350
Hemp oil	330
Peanut oil (unrefined)	320
Walnut oil (unrefined)	320
Flax seed oil	225
Safflower oil (unrefined)	225
Sunflower Oil (unrefined)	225

Sea Salt Versus Table Salt

The mainstream media villainizes salt at the behest of the misguided medical establishment. Society is constantly told that salt can raise the blood pressure, cause cardiac failure, damage the kidneys, aggravate asthma, and cause kidney stones. The establishment makes no distinctions between the different types of salt.

Sea Salt

Unrefined and unadulterated sea salt is not harmful in moderate amounts. Its benefits over table salt contrast the immense differences between God's engineering and man's. The human body requires a certain amount of sodium for optimum health, and we could not live without it. Healthy sea salts make a body a hostile environment for pathogens, such as bacteria and parasites. Its specific toxicity to pathogenic life forms is why salt is such an excellent preservative, awhile leaving the nutritional value of foods completely intact. Even mainstream medical doctors will admit these things when probed, but their institutionalized attacks upon salt continue unabated.

Sea salt naturally contains selenium, which helps to chelate toxic heavy metals from the body. It also contains boron which helps prevent osteoporosis, and chromium which regulates blood sugar levels. Sea salt is one of the few sources for safe copper ingestion, and copper helps the body to form new arteries whenever the main arteries become too clogged. Small quantities of sea salt will actually *lower* the blood pressure of most individuals, because it provides the trace minerals that aid with blood pressure regulation. It can only stabilize the blood pressure when the industry-depleted salts are removed from the diet. Mineral deficiencies are partly responsible for the rising obesity epidemic. Obese people are invariably malnourished, and their bodies are starving, because regardless of how much they eat, they are not getting the minerals and nutrients that they need. Processed table salts and conventionally grown produce are a big part of the problems.

Table Salt

The more common "refined" table salts have been been stripped of their minerals during processing, which manufacturers then sell to supplement companies. It makes the unmistakable point that the producers of table salts are stripping what they know to be the most nutritious part of the salt, and actually increasing profits by malnourishing their own customers.

Table salt has all of its minerals removed, which would otherwise help to balance the blood pressure. Consequently, table salt causes gross blood pressure fluctuations, instead of stabilizing it. This well-known danger has created an entire industry of "low sodium" foods.

Processed foods are very high in sodium, but it is always in the form of table salt, artificial flavors, or flavor enhancers. In the ultimate heart-health irony, low sodium products often contain monosodium glutamate, a sodium-based excitotoxin that causes heart attacks in people who do not have enough magnesium (from organic vegetables and sea salt). It is probably the most common reason for mysterious heart failures in young athletes, who simply fall-over dead at sporting events. The profuse sweating imbalances their electrolytes even further, to become the final straw on the camel's back.

Contrary to popular belief, table salt is not just sodium chloride. It also contains additives that are designed to make it more free-flowing. Ferrocyanide, talc, and silica aluminate are commonly included. Aluminum intake leads to neurological disorders, particularly when no selenium is provided to help the body to chelate it. Aluminum bio-accumulates inside the body, causing further degeneration over time. Talc is a known carcinogen, though its effects upon ingestion have not been heavily studied. While it was once used in baby powders, the majority of such products now use cornstarch instead of talc, because of the known health risks. The F.D.A. has a special provision to allow talc in table salt, even whilst it is prohibited in all other foods, due to toxicity issues. Current U.S. regulations allow table salt to be up to 2% talc.

Fake Sea Salts

Some companies sell bright white salts that are labeled as "sea salt", but they have had all of their minerals removed, just like table salt. It is the minerals that give real sea salt an off-white color. Depending on where it originates, real sea salt will be either gray or slightly pink. Salt that contains saltwater minerals is never bright white. Most of the sea salt that is available at major retailers is just as mineral depleted as table salt. These alleged sea salts sometimes contain anti-caking agents too, because they are produced by the same despicable companies that produce table salt. The reputable sea salt companies that we have investigated do not use any anti-caking agents or other impurities.

Iodine and Iodide

The potassium iodide that is added to table salt is not adequate to compensate for most iodine deficiencies. It is usually sufficient to stop goitrous boils from swelling in the neck, which are caused by an extreme deficiency. However, not enough iodine can be obtained from table salt to maintain optimal health, unless a dangerous amount of sodium is consumed. Naturally-occurring iodine is present in unadulterated sea salt with complimentary minerals, but even the vastly superior and healthier sea salt may not be enough for a tiny fraction of people who have extreme iodine deficiencies, which are frequently caused by fluoride toxicity and other mitigating factors.

F.D.A. Deception About Sea Salt's Iodine

The F.D.A. mandates that any salt, which does not have iodine added (at a chemical plant) must bear a warning label. It must state, "This salt does not supply iodide, a necessary nutrient". As a result, sea salt distributors are required to lie on their labeling. Unadulterated sea salt usually contains *more iodide* than iodized table salt does. Iodide is iodine that is mixed with a salt. In fact, iodide really ought to be called either "potassium iodine" or "sodium iodine", depending on which salt it has been added to. The naturally-occurring iodine in sea salt is maligned by false labeling to favor the chemical industry's bastardized products and profits. Moreover, the inorganic iodide in table salt is less healthy, because it is lacking the trace minerals that work with it, which are only found in natural sea salts. Sea salt distributors are not allowed to put any of this truthful information on their labels.

Dishonest Labeling

Consumer groups have been battling with regulators for consistent labeling for almost two decades, and yet current labeling has been largely defined by lawsuits, instead of meaningful regulatory guidelines. In the case of "all natural", the F.D.A. has intentionally left the phrase completely undefined for the benefit of its corporate partners. In 1993, the F.D.A. did not recommend any definition of the term in its Nutrition Labeling and Education Act, "because of resource limitations and other agency priorities". The Food and Drug Administration's thousands of employees were too busy to type the word "natural" during the year leading up to the Bill's passage. *They were so hard-working.*

Geraldine June from the F.D.A. spoke with the Food Navigator web site, and admitted that they are aware of the many misleading "all natural" labels out there. However, that supposedly did not merit an F.D.A. remedy.

> *"Even if people interpret it in different ways, it doesn't mean there is confusion out there. If there was, then we would definitely raise it as a priority".*

> -- Geraldine June, F.D.A. Food
> Labeling and Standards Department

A Typical "All Natural" Example

The non-profit Center for Science in the Public Interest (C.S.P.I.) threatened to sue 7-Up in 2006 after its advertising claimed that the soft drink was "all natural", whilst leaving high fructose corn syrup (H.F.C.S.) in the ingredients (made with sulfuric acid amongst other things). High fructose corn syrup may have once started as corn, but it is not something that is produced naturally or simply, and the result is not even chemically similar to its predecessor. As a result of the potential lawsuit, 7-Up changed its labeling to read, "100% natural flavors" (not ingredients). Of course, this was just another lie, because high fructose corn syrup is a sweetener, and sweetness is a flavor.

"High fructose corn syrup isn't something you could cook up from a bushel of corn in your kitchen, unless you happen to be equipped with centrifuges, hydroclones, ion-exchange columns, and buckets of enzymes."

-- Michael Jacobson, C.S.P.I. Executive Director

It is relatively well known amongst the health conscious that the phrase "all natural" has no real meaning on packaging. Although, most of us believe that the term "organic" is clearly defined. When looking at a product which holds a "USDA-certified Organic" label, most people have no idea that it may not be entirely organic.

What Do the Organic Labels *Really* Mean?

- **100% Organic:** This is what you should be purchasing, but this label is rarely seen. This product contains all organic ingredients. By law, no synthetic ingredients are allowed. Additionally, the production process must meet federal organic standards and it must have been independently verified by accredited inspectors. This is the gold standard of wholesome and healthy food. Foods under this category may bear the U.S.D.A. Organic label.

- **Organic:** This is where it gets deceptive. Ninety-Five percent of the ingredients need to be organically produced. The remainder can be non-organic or synthetic ingredients. Foods under this category may also bear the U.S.D.A. Organic label. While 95% organic may sound good enough, be advised that these foods can contain 5% toxic chemical additives.

- **Made with Organic Ingredients:** Products in this category contain at least 70 percent organic ingredients. They are not allowed to bear the U.S.D.A. seal. Consider the damage that could be caused by 30% synthetic ingredients. This ratio is normal for processed foods, which means that practically anything could bear this label.

The deceptions of modern labeling are not accidental, for an informed consumer is dangerous to the chemical industry. For instance, if ingredients lists replaced "gelatin" with the more honest "de-haired pig skins and flesh remnants melted in an acid bath", then what would happen to the sales of Jello and gummy bears? Always read food ingredients carefully, despite any marketing or special industry seals which appear on the packages. Study the chemicals that you and your family consume, and make the decision to become healthy in spite of their efforts. Remember that remaining healthy is much cheaper than health insurance, and it is long past the time to stop rewarding the people who are poisoning us.

Aspirin and Heart Attacks

For years, we have been told that an aspirin a day keeps heart attacks away. The science behind this belief is seriously flawed. Nevertheless, Bayer pharmaceuticals has had a heyday in marketing aspirin to doctors and the public for preventative cardiac medicine. As a result of this marketing, which twisted the results of otherwise valid studies, virtually every orthodox doctor in the United States now recommends aspirin to customers who have experienced heart problems. Millions of people ridiculously believe that heart attacks are caused by an aspirin deficiency.

The original studies from 1974 through 1988 showed that aspirin was not helpful for cardiovascular diseases. Then in 1989, another study was done, which tested aspirin that was buffered with magnesium (Bufferin brand). This type of aspirin acted as a magnesium supplement, and thusly reduced heart attacks by 44%. Since then, aspirin (not magnesium) has been recommended for those who have an increased risk of heart attacks. The magnesium content of the buffered aspirin from the paradigm-shifting study was completely ignored; since after all, only a pharmaceutical could benefit health. Magnesium was institutionally ignored, even though it was the only differing ingredient in the aspirin that actually worked.

While some heart attacks can be prevented by the magnesium in buffered aspirin, the number of aneurysms and other internal bleeding issues rise proportionally because of the aspirin itself, to make the overall death rate about the same as those not 'supplementing' with aspirin. In other words, by recommending aspirin instead of magnesium, the establishment kills about as many people as they save; because they are going to great lengths to avoid promoting competing nutritional medicine.

A serving of organic spinach would be significantly more effective and safer than an aspirin a day. Magnesium is necessary for healthy heart function, and it is lacking in Western diets. Multiple studies have shown that magnesium reduces the risk of coronary heart disease and balances the heart rhythm.

Aspirin is probably the safest pharmaceutical in existence, largely because it is based on natural and alternative medicine. It was first created from the bark of white willow trees by the American Indians for mild pain relief. This fact seems to never get mentioned, since natural medicine is, of course, "quackery". About 75% of the drugs in use were borrowed from our quackery, just like aspirin was. In this modern age, aspirin is "enhanced" with chemical engineering and it is made synthetically like all of the other "real medicines". Unlike the original pain reliever, the *improved* version is now fatal in large quantities.

The New York Times reported that pain relievers are being linked to gastrointestinal bleeding and ulcers, especially when taken on a long-term basis. When we combine this with the fact that ordinary aspirin does not actually prevent heart attacks, then we see the product of corporately manipulated science. The so-called "baby aspirin" that is most often recommended by doctors is not buffered with magnesium. It does absolutely nothing for heart health. Although buffered aspirin can be purchased as a substandard magnesium supplement.

Best Natural Sources of Magnesium

- Halibut fish
- Almonds
- Cashews
- Spinach
- Peanuts

Some people supplement with magnesium through small amounts of Epsom salt, but readers should be aware that it may contain impurities, because it is not manufactured for consumption. Furthermore, excessive magnesium will cause a body to flush other important minerals, so it is wisest to get it from foods.

The above list of foods are very nutritious, and we strongly recommend them to anyone who is wishing to improve his health. Regular supplementation of magnesium through good nutrition is the single best way to prevent heart attacks, and it comes without the risks which accompany pharmaceuticals. We also recommend supplementing with cayenne and taurine for heart health, as we have written about elsewhere, as well as the avoidance of homogenized milk. Cayenne can actually stop a heart attack in-progress, in many cases. So can taurine.

People who sell and distribute magnesium cannot make such "medical claims", even though the benefits are proven by the establishment's own studies. We would have to be silent about magnesium too, if we sold magnesium supplements. This is why the labels for most supplements only cite vague descriptions of their effect, because we are not supposed to know. The agenda is to keep us sick enough to remain drug dependent upon the system.

Heirloom Seeds and Tainted Varieties

Growing your own food makes a lot of sense, given the rising costs of healthy foods, the increased nutrition that will be gained from your own organic produce, and the sunlight that you will get in the process. However, most people do not know which seeds they should be buying. There are multiple brands selling what seem to be exactly the same seed products, and the companies use industry lingo that is misunderstood by the general public.

If a seed packet does not specify what type of seeds it contains, then you should assume the worst. The seeds will be clearly labeled if they are organic or heirloom.

Seed Types

Heirloom, Heritage	You cannot find these seeds in most stores, because these seeds are not very profitable. You can buy them online, or at some farmers' markets. These seeds have been saved by farmers for generations to preserve their genetic integrity. They have strong, full flavors, and are virtually always organic. They are generally easier to grow than most seeds. They are never genetically modified, but they unfortunately cost about three times more than regular seeds. They are worth the price.
Organic	The parent plant was not genetically modified, grown with synthetic pesticides, or fertilizers. These are usually a good option if heirloom seeds are not available. Try to buy from a small company if possible, because larger companies generally produce organic varieties that are less nutritious. This is because their soils are so depleted by synthetic fertilizers from previous years. There is also an elevated risk of cross-pollination contamination with the larger companies.
Open Pollinated	These seeds can be dried out, and saved over winter, to be grown the next year. There are no guarantees about the use of pesticides or fertilizers in the parent plant, and there may be some chemical residue on the seeds themselves. It is unlikely that they are genetically modified, because genetic modifications usually hinder fertility.
Hybrid	These seeds have been cross-pollinated to yield produce that does not bruise as easily and ripens much faster. They have the drawback of having a diluted taste, significantly lower nutrition, and if the seeds do germinate the next year; they could have different characteristics. Often, these can not be saved for the next year. Most supermarket varieties are hybrids. The chance of these seeds being genetically modified is still fairly low, as groups like Monsanto, the leading provider of G.M.O. seeds, prefer to market to large scale farmers. It is not easy to convince the general public to grow genetically modified foods, and Monsanto wants to monitor those who do, in order to ensure that their customers do not save patented seeds. Just remember that hybrids are never a desirable crop.

Nutrition and Diet

The Green Drink

This turbo-charged drink seems to do miraculous things within 8 to 12 hours, including improving eyesight, and the results can last for days. People with fast metabolisms may feel the results within a couple of hours.

Ingredients

- 4 carrots
- 1 celery stalk
- 1 box of baby spinach (5 oz.)
- 1 bunch parsley
- 2 Granny Smith apples (4 if not organic)
- 1 cup of pineapple juice
- Water (to thin)

It is strongly recommended that organic fruits and vegetables be used to make this drink, for being organic really does make a tremendous difference in improved taste and potency. It is an acquired taste for some, which is difficult to describe. However, the taste is far from bad, and the effects of this drink make it so worth acquiring its taste. This drink is so nutritious, in the extreme, that it has been known to suppress hunger for as much as 24 hours. Having a large glass of this stuff every 2-3 days keeps us healthy, energized, and feeling great. Armor yourself with this drink during the flu season, and we promise that you will have no regrets.

A juicer is required to properly extract this drink. Before being placed in the juicer, the vegetables are blended on a liquefy setting with water inside a blender. After that, all the ingredients can be poured into the juicer for finishing. The drink is technically healthier when the juicer part is skipped, so that it retains all of its fibrous pulp. It is a matter of weighing all of the taste and nutritional considerations. Everyone finds the drink tastier when it has been thoroughly chilled.

If the drink tastes terrible, then it probably indicates that your body is acidic. Try decreasing simple carbohydrates, processed foods, sweets, red meats, and drinking only pure pineapple juice for about 12 hours, and then taste it again. You could easily find yourself shocked at the difference in taste. If this test works on you, then you should begin learning about how to adjust your acidic body pH, before serious health problems occur.

Some people cannot drink this formulation, due to an aversion to the taste of celery. It is okay to remove it; but of course, the benefits of this secret weapon will be lessened.

Please note that if you make it organic, then you will only have about 48 hours to consume it before it starts becoming rotten. Keep it refrigerated, or drink it immediately. You should label its creation date, and religiously trash it after 2 days. If you dare drink this stuff three or more days after its creation, then it is going to *really* ruin your day. This is because bacteria finds this drink to be just as nutritious and stimulating. You should immediately clean the juicer and blender too, in order to avoid mold and fungus.

Do not store the green drink in an air-tight container, because if it is not able to release its gasses, then it will become putrid rapidly.

Homemade Bread

One of the most unhealthy items in the average household is bread. Commercial breads are atrocious, despite all of the marketing claims about its nutritional qualities and high fiber. The modern breads that are sold in retailers always contain soybean oil, and they usually contain aluminum too. The days of false marketing about the health benefits of soy are almost over. Aluminum is a toxic heavy metal that builds up in the human body to cause neurological problems over time, and numerous disease states.

It would be healthiest to simply eliminate bread from our diets altogether, but this is not feasible for most households. Commercial whole wheat bread is not actually a safe alternative, as most health conscious people would assume. This is because the ingredients added to commercial whole wheat breads make them even unhealthier than the commercial white breads. If you must use retail breads, then the white breads are usually the lesser evil, because so many altered food additives are added to whole wheat breads in an attempt to make them more flavorful.

Bread-eating families should start making their own, because the breads that are found in retailers are so lacking in nutrition and so harmful to the health. Making bread by hand is known to be a very time-consuming task, but breads and crusts are easy with a bread maker. Bread makers knead the dough, allow it to rise, and then they cook the bread without any assistance. The only work is adding the ingredients into the machine and activating it. Your entire family will be much healthier as a result of making your own breads, especially if you choose to use whole grain flours and sweeten with honey. The taste is so worth the little effort involved. Once you taste your own homemade bread, you will never be able to go back to store-bought bread. Homemade bread is cheaper too, so a bread maker will eventually pay for itself.

If a recipe calls for baking powder, always purchase an aluminum-free powder. We also recommend avoiding chlorine-bleached flours, and "enriched" flours that are laced with synthetic vitamins, which often do little more than strain the liver, kidneys, and immune system. It is possible to purchase unbleached white flour, which is safely bleached with hydrogen peroxide (oxygen) in most cases.

Non-Stick Coating Issues

The baking areas inside bread makers are coated with non-stick Teflon. Non-stick cookware is normally to be avoided, but there should be no safety issues for bread makers. The heating elements in bread makers are almost in direct contact with the dough, unlike ovens which have large open spaces separating the heating elements from the food. This means that bread makers cook breads at much lower temperatures than is possible with ovens. It is believed that non-stick coatings must reach about 500° F before the food is tainted by Teflon breakdown. Thus, it is very unlikely to get contamination from the non-stick coatings inside bread makers.

Dieting Right

Obesity has become an epidemic in the U.S., along with most other countries throughout the civilized world. The Western world has adopted an unhealthy approach to eating, which would have been considered gluttonous in the not-so-distant past. We pay little attention to the amount that we eat, and we hypnotically stare at entertainment throughout our meals; neglecting meaningful interaction with others. As such, an industry was born to cater to the obese. Weight loss is estimated to be a $40 billion industry, whose executives would be most unhappy if people really did lose weight. If their diet plans worked, then we would surely have a population of fit, healthy, and slim people. The industry would be self-terminating. It would have served its purpose. Instead, we have two and six week diet plans that help customers to lose a tiny amount of weight (usually less than 10 pounds) to soon regain it with even more. This is actually part of the business plan, because this industry profits most from people who remain unhealthy and miserable. Keeping people in a perpetual state of highly-profitable managed disease care is a familiar story. Diet products fail because that is part of their design, just as the medical industry has no cures for its cash cows, and policy makers will make certain that it never does. There is no money to be made from healthy people. Meanwhile, surgery-enhanced celebrities create an air-brushed, two-dimensional facade of how people should look; to the delight of the diet industry.

The great irony of it all is that we are overweight because we are starving for nutrition. We are deficient in magnesium, the B vitamins, vitamin D, and almost every trace mineral, due to our synthetic fertilizers having depleted the soils and our chemically "enhanced" foods. Our foods are so nutritionally deficient that the more we eat, the hungrier that we tend to become, because our bodies must exert ever-increasing work to make use of the empty calories. It is like the case of some early American colonists, who lived on diets of corn throughout the winter months. A huge portion of those settlers died of starvation and illness, whilst nonetheless becoming incredibly obese. Corn has very little nutrition, so those poor souls could not eat enough of it to stay satisfied for long.

Mental and Emotional Barriers

Most of our failures throughout life are due to our own internal self-sabotaging tendencies. For instance, many people remain overweight because they have such a low self esteem that they unconsciously feel unworthy of looking better. This secret desire is a manifestation of a self-destructive tendency, and it is often part of a deeply-repressed suicide wish. Every day in continued self-destructive behaviors, the individual slowly edges closer to obtaining that goal of self annihilation. Learning to respect and love oneself is usually the first step before other successful steps can be taken. Thus, letting go of a lifetime of pain and rejections can be the very trial by fire that is necessary for the required spiritual rebirth. The key is forgiving oneself and others.

Some of us were taught as children that food is a comfort to life's tough problems, and this training still resonates unconsciously through us into adulthood. Some of us were taught that food is something that we should reward ourselves with whenever we have accomplished a goal, as is the case with celebration dinners and birthday parties. Food is our sustenance, and we bear massive psychological problems whenever we perceive food as either a punishment or a reward. Unfortunately, almost all of us have fallen into these traps, and it happens purely unconsciously.

Winning the victory over one's own mind is the most important step to success. For it is certain that you will fail, if you already believe that you will. Your issues and beliefs determine your future reality, because you will unconsciously transform them into self-fulfilling prophesies. You will unconsciously work to prove your pessimisms right without ever realizing that it was you causing the problems -- that your failures were caused by a long chain of self-sabotaging actions. If you begin impeded by your own internal demoralizations, then the war can be lost before it begins.

For these reasons, we recommend that people with serious weight problems first see a hypnotist to uncover and deal with any unconscious barriers to successful dieting, as well as get themselves reprogrammed to be positive about managing their health. Hypnosis works powerfully, and it is probably the wisest first step that a person can take before beginning such a serious life transformation. Permanently improving one's well-being requires nothing less than a life transformation. It is safest to be hypnotized by someone who can be completely trusted, such as a close relative. It is not a difficult skill to acquire. The process is explained in detail in episode 34 of our audio shows.

The Truth About Beef

Eating non-organic meat while trying to lose weight is a mistake. The greediness of large food corporations has destroyed the traditional farm, and transformed our healthy foods, such as beef, into things that are sickening. The great majority of meat in the United States is fed on an unnatural and deficient diet of genetically-engineered corn products, instead of grass. This was exposed in the hard-hitting documentary, *King Corn*. Corn causes animals to become fat quickly, but the quality of meat produced is grossly inferior when compared to meat produced by traditional methods.

Despite all of this beef gloom, it is nevertheless so nutritionally beneficial that we still recommend it in moderation for every diet, and we strongly encourage our readers to seek organic meat whenever possible. Beef is actually an extremely healthy food in its organic form. Beef is not the health-destroying monstrosity that most health conscious people believe it to be, until it is *helped* by the chemical industry, pharmaceutical industry, and the biotechnology industry. A red meat, such as beef or lamb, is occasionally needed to maintain optimal health. Range fed beef is always superior to factory-farmed beef, but truly organic beef with 15% or less of it being fat is the ideal. Lamb is a more nutritious option, but it is unavailable in certain regions. More information about finding safe, nutritious beef is available in the *Beef* section of the *Poisoned World* chapter.

The Chopstick Diet

The Chopstick Diet now exists to force people to pay attention to how much they eat and pace themselves. It has been a resounding success, unlike most diets. While it may be fairly impractical for most people, it does point out that there are many paths to weight loss that are free of chemical aids. Many of the modern diet plans involve taking pharmaceuticals to drop the pounds.

As a society, we are forever searching for miracle cures for obesity, diabetes, cancer and heart disease. While we acknowledge that such advancements would be wonderful; these are nevertheless unattainable dreams. We should break out of our delusion that there is a quick and easy fix for our problems in the form of a pill.

Alli is a Typical Diet Product

Alli has become one of the most popular diet pills, due to its ability to limit the absorption of fats. It has been marketed as a "miracle", which is the standard hype for diet products and drugs. Alli promises to allow dieters to eat all that they wish, and yet lose weight. It was approved by the F.D.A., despite its deplorable set of ingredients and a rather unique set of negative side effects.

Around 50% of Alli users experience extremely loose or oily stools, gas, oily spotting on the underwear, or incontinence. Taking Alli gives you a 7% chance of needing adult diapers; and eventually, some serious counseling. This chance increases with the length of time that this *miracle* is used. Incontinence (explosively uncontrollable diarrhea) has a huge impact on the

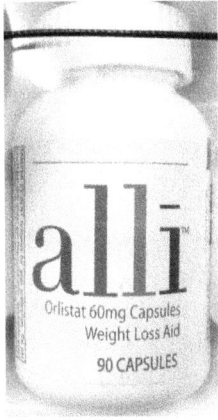

confidence, career, and social life of a person. It can be especially traumatizing to dieters, since most dieters already experience self-esteem issues. This is usually their main motivation for losing weight, and the reason for the extra weight in the first place.

Alli contains ingredients that we have never before seen in products that are intended for internal consumption. The active ingredient, sodium lauryl sulfate, is used as an industrial engine degreaser, floor cleaner, and as the oil stripper of most shampoos. Alongside it is talc. Talc was discovered to cause cancer with just skin contact; so now corn starch is recommended for infant diapers. In 1971, a group of researchers found that particles of talc were embedded in 75% of the ovarian tumors studied. What possible purpose could two such dangerous chemicals have in a product that is marketed to improve health, and what unique version of *science* was used to prove them safe for human consumption? Alli is actually typical of diet products instead of being an exception.

MSG and Friends

Many of the weight loss plans are not merely regimens, but they also provide their own patented, proprietary formulas that marketers promise will yield miraculous effects. The ingredients in these formulas are appalling. Diet foods are the most unhealthy foods that a person could ever eat, yet the deceptive marketing on these products leads dieters to believe that they are eating healthy snacks containing everything that their bodies need.

Artificial sweeteners are frequently used alongside the infamous monosodium glutamate (MSG). It is an excitotoxin that directly *causes* weight gain, Alzheimer's, heart disease, juvenile asthma, and cancerous tumors. Public pressure urging removal of this ingredient has caused companies to start disguising MSG under the names: yeast extract, sodium caseinate, hydrolyzed protein, autolyzed yeast, glutamic acid, calcium caseinate, hydrolyzed vegetable protein (HVP), textured protein, monopotassium glutamate, hydrolyzed plant protein (HPP), sodium glutamate, glutamate, autolyzed plant protein, yeast food, yeast nutrient, glutamic acid, sodium caseinate, vegetable protein extract, soy protein, hydrolyzed corn gluten, natural flavor, artificial flavor, and spice. Learn to spot these and boycott the guilty companies. MSG has the capability to conceal the rancid flavors of processed foods. Without the MSG, the processed foods would rightly be detected by the tongue as unfit for human consumption, so MSG is marketed as a "flavor enhancer". More accurately, it is a rottenness concealer. One only needs to examine this to understand why disease and obesity are so rampant. It is how the food industry maintains record profits every year, at the expense of our nutrition. Throughout most of history, our taste helped us to differentiate the good foods from the bad, but this is intentionally being prevented through chemistry.

Diet foods usually contain sodium aluminum phosphate or titanium dioxide. It is ironic to consume these foods whilst trying to lose weight, because heavy metals like these are stored inside the fat cells of the body, which makes losing weight immensely more difficult. The human body attempts to store toxic heavy metals inside of fat cells as a matter of self defense, in much the same way that an oyster will wrap an impurity inside of a pearl to protect itself. This is why a heavy metal detoxification (heavy metal cleanse) should be a part of every diet plan. Titanium dioxide is so cancerous that it can produce cancers merely from skin contact, and aluminum is a factor in every neurodegenerative disease known.

"Sugar Free" Means Extremely Fattening

Sugar is usually removed from diet products, under the guise of helping dieters to lose weight. The sugar is replaced with artificial sweeteners such as aspartame (Nutrasweet or Equal), saccharin, or sucralose (Splenda). All of these sweeteners have been proven to actually *cause* weight gain by stimulating carbohydrate cravings. It is believed that these sweeteners successfully trick a body into detecting that these products contain glucose, so a person experiences an artificially-induced sugar crash -- only the crash is worse because there was never any real sugar for the insulin to handle. Call it nature's revenge, if you like. Before artificially-enhanced foods and drinks, there was no sweet taste without calories, and a body does not understand how to regulate these artificially sweet substances. The proponents of these artificial sweeteners pretend that their chemicals do not effect insulin, but the carbohydrate cravings prove that they must, and a body really needs carbohydrates or sugar to compensate for the insulin imbalances that are caused by these products. These sweeteners are the primary reason why both dieters and diabetics have such difficulty overcoming their problems, which coincidentally benefits the industry.

Created by chlorinating (bleaching) some of the molecules in sugar, sucralose has been proven to worsen diabetes (which many overweight people suffer with), abort pregnancies, and enlarge the liver and kidneys. All of these are unmistakable signs that sucralose is a very toxic substance, but it is the least-studied artificial sweetener. Aspartame and saccharin are even worse.

> *"It's only been relatively recently that foods have been introduced that violate those kind of relationships, such as something very sweet that has no calories."*

-- Susan Swithers, PhD., Purdue University

The "Natural" Diet Aids

All-natural weight loss aids can seem like a desirable alternative, but these typically-deceptive products are most often created by the drug companies, not naturopaths. Fortunately, it is possible to attain long-lasting weight loss without commercial products. Be sure to only use diet aids alongside your regular dieting and exercise plans. Do not rely upon dieting aids, or anyone else to manage your health for you. Above all, buyer beware, even when labels proclaim that products are all natural.

Many herbal formulas were among the list of weight loss aids recalled by the Food and Drug Administration in December of 2008. These products were discovered to be laced with pharmaceutical drugs. One of which is known to cause anxiety, suicidal thoughts, and aggression. This is yet another reminder that we must check the integrity of the companies that we buy from. Trust only companies that are dedicated to delivering natural products. In other words, don't trust GlaxoSmithKline for your echinacea. The following statement was posted on the F.D.A.'s website:

> *"An FDA analysis found that the undeclared active pharmaceutical ingredients in some of these products include sibutramine (a controlled substance), rimonabant (a drug not approved for marketing in the United States), phenytoin (an antiseizure medication), phenolphthalein (a solution used in chemical experiments and a suspected cancer causing agent) and bumetanide (a diuretic)."*

Dieting Wisely

Effectively losing weight cannot be done in a two week program, but it can be done. Holistic health advocates look for the root causes of health-related issues; but with excessive weight, there are many possible causes. For some, a toxic diet in childhood is to blame (chemicals, heavy metals, bad sugars, processed carbohydrates, processed foods, liver, or undercooked meat), so they have consequently been overweight from a young age. Others eat excessively due to depression, and some people have hypothyroidism (the thyroid does not produce enough hormones and causes a slow metabolism). Hypothyroidism is now epidemic, so readers should check themselves for it. Be advised that the official tests are notoriously inaccurate and mainstream treatments should be avoided to prevent a lifetime of suffering.

As mentioned earlier, most dieters have problems losing weight because fat is their bodies' storage place for the toxins. While we would like to immediately recommend a heavy metal cleanse, it can be counter-productive for people who have yeast overgrowth in their gastrointestinal tract; which is actually most of the population. The heavy metals suppress bacteria, parasites, and fungus that are inside a person. In theory, that would seem to be a good thing; but the metals are also toxic to the brain, kidneys, liver, almost every other organ, and they hinder weight loss efforts. An unintended consequence of cleansing could be that the harmful candida yeast and existing parasites will breed unchecked, as never before.

Dieters should note that big changes in eating habits should be implemented to suppress candida, before any detoxification is done. The extent of these changes will depend upon the dieter's existing diet. If you are not prepared to commit to this, then successful dieting is just not for you. Successful weight loss takes commitment and some tasty sacrifices. While what follows next is only the first step of the program, you are likely to lose weight the entire way through.

Stage I: Destroy Intestinal Yeast / Candida

(Two Weeks)

- Eliminate all sources of refined ("white") products like white flour, white sugar, white rice, and table salt.

- Use a small amount of sea salt with every meal, unless the food is already salty. The sea salt is fake if it is bright white and it looks completely pure. Sea salt impurities are also known as "trace minerals", and lacking them is part of the problem.

- Limit carbohydrates, especially simple and processed carbohydrates. Avoid any that are not whole grain.

- Eat 2 tablespoons of organic plain yogurt 2-3 times daily. Since yogurt is usually homogenized, supplement with vitamin C and folate (or the inferior folic acid) to protect against inflammation and arterial damage. Unhomogenized yogurt can often be found at health food stores.

- Avoid all soft drinks, including the so-called "diet" drinks.

- Incorporate daily fruits and vegetables into your diet.

- Drink plenty of mineral-rich spring water, well water, or water filtered by a Berkey system with fluoride filters.

- Avoid yeast by avoiding mushrooms and alcoholic beverages.

- Buy organic foods whenever possible (More nutrients, but less antibiotics, pesticides, growth hormones, fertilizers).

- Eat small meals *more often* instead of the typical 2-3 large meals. Five small meals is usually ideal.

- Consume 1/2 teaspoon of cold-pressed coconut oil daily.

- Do not use anti-bacterial products, including colloidal silver. These will kill the beneficial intestinal flora that you are trying to stimulate. You must not do anything that would hinder the good bacteria, and therefore, pharmaceuticals can be a show-stopper.

- Sweeten with only honey.

- Avoid antacids, and use apple cider vinegar instead.

- Limit fruit juice, but it can be had a couple of times a day if it is 100% pure, and it is not from concentrate. Always avoid fruit juices from China, because they are likely to be tainted, and the distributor will try to hide the country of origin -- often near the cap and far away from the ingredients list. We recommend boycotting such companies, which often put flags on the products that are designed to deceive.

Read the ingredients on all of the foods that you eat. As a general rule, every unrecognizable ingredient should be avoided. These are the ingredients that have been designed in a chemist's laboratory. They are preludes to cancer, diabetes, and all the other epidemics -- including obesity. Do not be fooled, these diseases are not normal or natural. They are the result of malnutrition and chemical poisoning through our food and water supplies. Remember that it is harmful if it was not made by God. Do not be afraid to drink lots of water. Follow the water advice in the list above, and note that water from most plastic bottles absorbs hormone disruptors that will make things more difficult. The same problems exist with most metal bottles, because they secretly have an inner lining of clear plastic, so they are plastic bottles in disguise. Natural water will not make you fat, and it is needed to flush out toxins. Do not worry about water weight, for it is lost just as quickly, and it helps in the long term.

Light exercise is strongly recommended during the first month, and exercise should be increased as the dieter gradually gets stronger. Exercise is a crucial aspect of improving overall health so that weight loss can occur. Exercise is also the only way to clear the lymph nodes of toxins, such as carcinogenic aluminum compounds that were accumulated from antiperspirant absorption.

A Short-Term Juice Fast

(Ten Days -- Optional)

After following the stage I protocol for a couple of weeks, a short juice fast could be helpful before beginning stage II. A juice fast should last for no more than 10 days. Purchasing a juicer or blender would prove to be a great investment, for these make the intake of lots of fruits and vegetables easy, give you the option of great dietary variety, and there are hundreds of free juicing recipes all over the Internet.

The first few days may leave the dieter feeling fatigued, as candida fights to stay alive by scavenging all of the sugars that it can. Do not get disillusioned, for this is only temporary, and it is a sign that the diet plan is working to kill the pathogenic yeast. You will soon feel better than you have in a long time. Fortunately, the initial fatigue will only be severe for those who suffer from particularly bad cases of yeast overgrowth. For most dieters, it will be necessary to include a daily source of protein. Eggs are ideal for providing this, and a small amount of beneficial saturated fat. Butter is helpful too. This is not cheating. It is balancing.

Stage II: Cleansing Time

After a dedicated two weeks of Stage 1, or four weeks that included the optional juice fast, it will finally be time to remove the heavy metals that have accumulated throughout your life. Your body cannot successfully eliminate certain heavy metals without aid, so depending on the quality of your old eating habits and whether you have silver dental fillings, there could be massive amounts of heavy metals stored in your excess fat. This stage of the plan will permanently make losing weight much easier.

The following may be used together for approximately 10 days to detox from metals:

- Cilantro supplementation (100 mg. per 50 lbs. of weight)
- Apple pectin
- NAC amino acid supplement (N-Acetyl-Cysteine)
- Selenium (100 mcg. per 100 lbs. of weight) *
- B complex vitamin

- 5-HTP
- Regular Exercise

  * It is dangerous to exceed 400 mcg. of selenium.

Cilantro may need to be used several times a month forever after, if the dieter has mercury ("silver") dental fillings. Always use it with selenium to neutralize the moving metals. It is difficult to find multi-vitamins that are both safe and usable by the human body. Be wary of so-called "food-based" vitamins, because they are usually genetically engineered using pathogenic yeasts, and most are manufactured in unaccountable facilities in China. There is usually little to no food in the "food-based" vitamins, and many of these products are health-destroying scams from the biotechnology industry. The totally synthetic vitamins are therefore safer, but they often act to simply place more strain on the body, because they are likewise not identical to vitamins from natural foods. The cilantro supplement was cited because it will be difficult to get enough to have a major impact from diet.

According to the Linus Pauling Institute, these are the best food sources of the B vitamins:

Food Sources for the B Vitamins

- Vitamin B-1 (thiamin) -- pecans, cantaloupe, peas, spinach, and sunflower seeds
- Vitamin B-2 (riboflavin) -- almonds, turkey, chicken, eggs, fish and legumes
- Vitamin B-3 (niacin) -- chicken, fish, beef, and turkey
- Vitamin B-5 (pantothenic acid) -- cod, tuna, chicken, and eggs
- Vitamin B-6 (pyridoxine) -- potatoes (especially the skin), fish, chicken, and bananas
- Folate -- pickles, spinach, orange juice, and asparagus
- Vitamin B-12 -- beef, salmon, and eggs
- Biotin -- eggs, salmon, tuna, and avocados

Health food stores have ready-made heavy metal cleansing kits available, if that approach is more desirable. Please read the ingredients of those kits carefully, instead of trusting their cover marketing, because every company wants to sell a product. While going through a heavy metal detox, it is likely that you will experience some behavioral changes, as metals begin migrating through your bloodstream again. Therefore, a firm warning to your loved ones may be in order. Warn them to expect some flaky behavior and abrupt mood swings. These side effects are especially noticeable for people who have A.D.D./A.D.H.D., since these are conditions that are primarily caused by toxic and allergic overload. There may also be some mild flu-like symptoms for the first couple of days, showing that your immune system has detected the presence of threatening materials freely flowing in your body. Make sure to drink plenty of fluids to help the body flush them.

Stage III: The Diet

This is the easy part. Be sure to consume some apple cider vinegar each day with food. Those who have had a bad diet usually have reduced acidity in their stomachs, making it more difficult to absorb the nutrients that they need. Taking apple cider vinegar helps to ensure proper nutrient absorption, so that less food is needed.

- Add plenty of lean proteins to your diet. Along with regular exercise, they will help to replace lost fat with firm muscle. This includes eggs, chicken, fish, beef and nuts. Always avoid pork.

- Supplement with selenium to neutralize metals from diet, pharmaceuticals, and dental fillings.

- Supplement with biotin, because it helps the body to burn off carbohydrates and regulate dietary fats.

- Eat plenty of fruits and vegetables or juice them. They will provide energy and vital nutrients.

- Healthy fats are essential, and people who attempt to live without them will be hungry often. Real butter and nuts contain healthy fats that maintain health and curb the appetite. The same is true for coconut oil. Avoid all manufactured and homogenized fats.

- Do not consume energy drinks, even if "natural ingredients" are mentioned in the marketing. The natural thing is usually a lie.

- Avoid all artificial additives (colors, preservatives, sweeteners, and etcetera).

- Avoid "white" processed foods (e.g. white rice, white bread, white sugar, and table salt).

- Use sea salt.

- Avoid "enhanced" fruit juices containing sugars or high fructose corn syrup. Avoid all juice "cocktails" and juice "from concentrate". Juice is healthy if it is 100% pure and hopefully organic. Freshly-squeezed juice is best.

- Eat many tiny meals instead of a few large ones. Five small meals are the daily recommendation.

- Drink plenty of pure water and organic green tea with honey and lemon (that you brew yourself).

- Nuts have natural properties to curb appetite, so use them as snacks. Cashews and walnuts are the best. They provide incredible nutritional benefits too.

Following our recommendations will make you look and feel dramatically better, regardless of whatever the scales read. It is likely to get you off the pharmaceutical treadmill as well, to finally realize good health. Stop hopping on the scale each morning, and stop torturing yourself over meaningless numerical values. If you really need to torture yourself about something numerical, then count how many fruits and vegetables you eat each day. Any perceived lack of success on the scale only leads to depression, which contributes to real failure. As you transform fats into muscle tissues, you are likely to actually *gain weight* -- but look better and be much healthier. Muscle weighs about 3 times more than the equivalent amount of fat, so weighing on a scale is totally self-sabotaging for almost everyone. Our advice is to throw your scale into the trash and completely ignore the weight charts that are used by the medical establishment.

There are lots of natural supplements available to assist you, but they will be ineffective if you do not make the effort in other areas. Feel free to pick and choose from these lists. Combining herbs together will not produce negative effects.

Appetite Suppressants:

- Chickweed
- Cumin
- Evening primrose oil
- Chamomile
- Hoodia
- Cashew Nuts
- Various fruit and vegetable snacks

Metabolism Boosters:

- DHEA *
- Nettle
- Dandelion
- Cayenne
- Korean ginseng
- L-tyrosine
- Gotu Kola
- Guarana
- Coconut oil

> * Avoid DHEA if you are suffering with adrenal fatigue, hypothyroidism, heart problems, or male pattern hair loss. This is because it stimulates the adrenal glands and the production of male hormones.

Coconut oil should be cold pressed and preferably organic. Kola nuts are a natural stimulant, appetite suppressant, and they enhance mental and physical performance. Drinking herbal teas will also help you to lose weight. They are very popular throughout alternative medicine, and in particular, we recommend yerba mate, red raspberry leaf, and especially green tea. They are natural appetite suppressants and metabolism boosters.

Green tea is always encouraged. The ready-made green teas found in most retailers are horrible. You must brew your own for it not to be a chemical-industry monstrosity that does more damage than good. The health fad of green tea has become another opportunity to poison us for some very evil corporations. Take for instance the diet green tea from Lipton. It contains the following.

> "sodium hexametaphosphate, natural flavor, phosphoric acid, potassium sorbate and potassium benzoate, sucralose, pectin, acesulfame potassium, calcium disodium edta"

Yes, that's benzene (the paint thinner). Never mind that this "healthy" diet product is therefore a carcinogen more risky than cigarettes. "Natural flavor" means, as the F.D.A. officially allows -- that this is an ingredient that will never be disclosed, and it is almost certainly not natural by any reasonable definition. Oftentimes, we have discovered that "natural flavor" hides MSG, which was made from genetically-engineered bacteria. Companies like Lipton have worked tirelessly to ensure that such poisonous G.M.O. ingredients never get labeled, as they did in influencing the vote for California's Proposition 37 referendum.

Due to the problem in finding high quality green teas from trustworthy companies, we are making an exception to our normal rule about not mentioning specific brands. At the time of this writing, we officially recommend the Kirkland brand of green tea. Its quality and the company's ethics may change in time, so do your own research and buyer beware.

Good Dieting is a Journey -- Not a Destination

Diet products are usually scams advocating the continuation of a bad diet, but they may initially cause some weight loss through chemically-induced starvation. Gaining weight all over again is inevitable, because whenever real food is introduced into the diet again, the body will immediately store it as fat, because starvation will have tricked the body into believing that there has been an emergency state of famine. Emergency starvation hormones such as leptin and adiponectin get released, and this can last for years afterward. Storing fat is the body's emergency response mechanism, and most diets trigger it. This is one of the reasons why we advocate many small meals, instead of fewer meals. The starvation hormones must be switched off.

Many diet plans insist on regular exercise throughout the program, which makes it impossible to credit lost weight to the proprietary foods that were eaten, since it is most likely that exercise is what deserved credit. This is good news for the natural dieter, for it means that real weight loss is achieved without the help of chemicals. Losing weight using natural methods helps people to keep it off, since they attack obesity at its root cause -- a poor and toxic lifestyle.

The motivation for weight loss should be much deeper than the desire for a better appearance. True health goes beyond the cosmetic. We live in a society that is sinking into a sea of disease and sickness. We all know somebody who is fighting cancer, or diabetes, or heart disease, and maybe even Alzheimer's. Obesity is just a symptom that identifies a person as a future victim. All of it is due to toxic lifestyles.

Depression goes with weight problems like a hand in a glove. For success, you should read the *Depression* chapter too.

The Perverted U.S.D.A. Food Pyramid

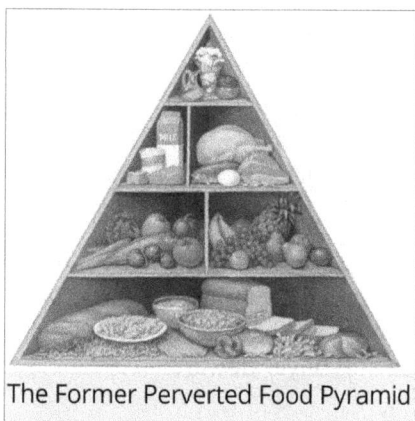
The Former Perverted Food Pyramid

The U.S. Department of Agriculture's food pyramid once contained four food groups: fruits and vegetables, meat, grains, and dairy. The fruit and vegetable category made up the base of the pyramid, to show that they were the most important component of the diet. Unfortunately, this superior food pyramid from yesteryear is long gone. It was replaced with a grotesquely-bastardized version (pictured left) that contains five food groups; one of which is comprised of sugars and fats. Perhaps even worse is the fact that carbohydrates were made to be the base of the revisionist pyramid. It was supposed to be a guideline that explained how our foods should be proportioned, but it instead came to identify what we were already eating as a society.

Luise Light, Ed.D, a former U.S.D.A. nutritionist, wrote extensively about the food pyramid, long after she was asked to help revise it. Since leaving the U.S.D.A., she has written the book, *A Fatally Flawed Food Guide*, which chronicles her experience. It explains how the food pyramid was not redesigned in the interest of health, but on behalf of those in the processed foods industry.

"Where we, the USDA nutritionists, called for a base of 5-9 servings of fresh fruits and vegetables a day, it was replaced with a paltry 2-3 servings (changed to 5-7 servings a couple of years later because an anti-cancer campaign by another government agency, the National Cancer Institute, forced the USDA to adopt the higher standard). Our recommendation of 3-4 daily servings of whole-grain breads and cereals was changed to a whopping 6-11 servings forming the base of the Food Pyramid as a concession to the processed wheat and corn industries. Moreover, my nutritionist group had placed baked goods made with white flour -- including crackers, sweets and other low-nutrient foods laden with sugars and fats -- at the peak of the pyramid, recommending that they be eaten sparingly. To our alarm, in the 'revised' Food Guide, they were now made part of the Pyramid's base. And, in yet one more assault on dietary logic, changes were made to the wording of the dietary guidelines from 'eat less' to 'avoid too much', giving a nod

to the processed-food industry interests by not limiting highly profitable 'fun foods' (junk foods by any other name) that might affect the bottom line of food companies.

"But even this neutralized wording of the revised Guidelines created a firestorm of angry responses from the food industry and their congressional allies who believed that the farmers' department (U.S.D.A.) should not be telling the public to eat less of anything.

"I vehemently protested that the changes, if followed, could lead to an epidemic of obesity and diabetes -- and couldn't be justified on either health or nutritional grounds. To my amazement, I was a lone voice on this issue, as my colleagues appeared to accept the 'policy level' decision. Over my objections, the Food Guide Pyramid was finalized, although it only saw the light of day 12 years later, in 1992. Yet it appears my warning has come to pass."

The new food guide was influenced by the processed foods industry, as other health guides are usually written by the pharmaceutical industry. How convenient it all is. Perhaps this is why Jello (gelatin) is a staple of the diet inside American hospitals. For readers outside of the United States, we are completely serious.

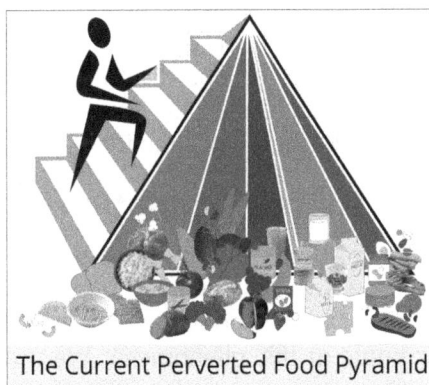

The Current Perverted Food Pyramid

In recent times, the pyramid was changed yet again, so that it no longer gives any clear recommendations whatsoever. It is fairly open to artistic interpretation. This is the goal. There is no legitimate health reason for having carbohydrates as the most important food group. That is, unless the agenda is to make people fat and diseased.

God's Nutrition: From the Big Guy Himself

"If you will listen carefully to the Lord your God and do what he considers right, if you pay attention to his commands and obey all his laws, I will never make you suffer any of the diseases I made the Egyptians suffer, because I am the Lord who heals you."

-- Exodus 15:26

The Good Book

The Bible is the best selling book in history, and it is also the most debated of all books. Some believers think of the Bible as a tool, while others consider it to be a history book, and another category of believers considers the Bible to be a guidebook for life. For eons, people have practiced its dietary edicts and in particular, it has been the Jewish people who followed the Bible's instructions most rigorously about which foods are acceptable. The foods Biblically blessed for human consumption are commonly called kosher foods. Modern Christians tend to ignore the kosher rules of the Old Testament section, using several quotes from The New Testament as justification. There is no place in the Bible where the Christ actually gave us permission to defy God. It was only Paul, who is falsely believed to have been one of the disciples. He is believed to have been one of the chosen twelve, despite his murderous history, and having never met the Christ. For more information about this topic, see *The Unapostle Paul* article at our site, healthwyze.org. Christian views about discarding Kosher law reflect how Paul successfully corrupted the church from within.

God's laws of good nutrition are still relevant today, and our refusal to obey them has resulted in almost all of our diseases. This chapter proves that God was always wiser, and more knowledgeable than us. It also explains scientifically the reasons for his nutrition rules, and how his kosher diet is the ideal diet.

The Science Revolution

Science and technology have progressed at a dizzying rate in recent history. They have become so pervasive that people are now more likely to use science than the Bible to discriminate between what is good and what is bad for their families. Food consumption is probably the best example of this phenomena. We now have scientific agricultural organizations, the science of biology, and various distribution organizations which inform us about what is best for us to eat regularly, in addition to the government.

God is no longer in the equation, with the exception of farmers, who occasionally pray for desirable weather. Now the equation is scientific. Science has produced an impressive array of information about our foods, including their calories, glucose content, vitamins, minerals, and how all of these effect our bodies. Science has also provided us with the knowledge of which foods are the most beneficial and which ones promote diseases.

For the first time in history, we actually have the scientific capabilities to test if God was right. Was it possible for him to understand nutrition 6,000 years ago, without the aid of science?

Forbidden Fruits: Scientifically Testing the Biblical Laws of Nutrition

> "And God said, *'Behold, I have given you every herb bearing seed, which is upon the face of all the earth, and every tree, in the which is the fruit of a tree yielding seed; to you it shall be for food.'"*

-- Genesis 1:29

The food granted to man in the above passage was vegetation. Vegetation was acceptable so long as it originated above the Earth's surface, and so long as it produced seeds. Thus, it is quite clear that God originally had no qualms with vegetarian diets.

Despite the encouragement of underwater plant and algae consumption by certain rogue health food gurus, these are not healthy. They are forbidden by God's diet. Science has proven that seaweed and kelp are excellent bottom-feeding water cleaners. They are sometimes utilized in alternative medicine, due to their phenomenal ability to absorb toxins; especially heavy metals. They absorb lead, arsenic, mercury, uranium, boron, fluoride, chlorine, molybdenum, aluminum, cadmium, and nickel from the oceans. The same is true for most algae. By consuming such underwater plants, one also ingests these toxins. Undoubtedly, repeated ingestion of seaweed, kelp, and other underwater plants results in severe long-term disease consequences from toxicity, which would be impossible to trace back to the original cause. Mercury alone is a cumulative heavy metal poison that is known to cause permanent damage to the brain, kidneys, and the immune system. The National Institutes of Health warns that contaminated algae products cause liver damage, and even certified algae is potentially contaminated. This is because algae can only be accurately tested whenever the testing laboratory already knows what contaminants to test for. It is impossible to test for random unexpected contaminants, and these are found in sea water. With most algae supplementation, the infused ocean pollutants will accumulate inside the liver, doing cascading organ damage over time. When the symptoms of a dysfunctional liver become severe enough to get noticed, the unchecked damage is usually quite serious. Health Canada reported that almost all of the blue-green algae supplements that they tested contained organ toxins, and they strongly cautioned against their usage. God was right about underwater plants.

Not every plant bears seed, and not every tree bears fruit. This eliminates some plants as kosher (acceptable) food sources. Examples are mushrooms, ferns, lichens, molds, and mosses. Science tells us that mushrooms are the fungal spore-spreading vampires of the plant world. They bottom-feed off of the corpses of dead plants and animals instead of getting nutrients from the soil, and they often die in the presence of sunlight. Only experts can determine which mushrooms are safe, and even experts have died gruesome deaths from accidental mushroom poisonings. The risks are so great that commercial mushrooms are grown indoors with specially-treated soil to prevent infestations of poisonous varieties. Even non-poisonous mushrooms feed candida, the harmful yeast that resides in the intestinal system and causes cavities. Candida stimulates hyperactive allergies and it compromises the immune system -- overwhelming the body with its toxic waste products. The side-effects of candida are seldom attributed to the foods being consumed, because we have been convinced by the broken health care system that random allergies and random illnesses are a normal and common part of life. When in actuality, everything happens for a reason. We were not designed to be routinely sick.

Ferns produce illness-inflicting spores just as mushrooms do, and like mushrooms, about half of the species are poisonous. A large portion of lichens are poisonous too. Some American Indian tribes used wolf lichen to create poisoned arrowheads. Ground lichen was the cause of death for 300 elk in Wyoming in 2004. Visiting elk from Colorado ate this lichen, which caused tissue decay and eventual death. The native elk were not effected, because their immune systems had developed a tolerance to the toxins. We shall skip the topics of molds and mosses, but most readers should already know. God was correct about mushrooms, ferns, lichens, molds, mosses, and all fungal life forms.

> *"Just as I gave you the green plants, I now give you everything. But you must not eat meat that has its lifeblood still in it."*

-- Genesis 9:3-5

Bloody meat is undercooked meat. Eating uncooked or undercooked meats exposes a person to e. coli, almost every type of bacteria imaginable, and dozens of parasite varieties. Many people choose to eat "rare" steak, but would never consider engaging in drinking an animal's blood, even though they are doing so with their undercooked steaks. It is a very risky behavior. Most people experience occasional parasites, but this group is especially likely to have them in massive numbers, and the routine sicknesses that follow.

> *"Never eat any fat from cattle, sheep, or goats."*

-- Leviticus 7:23

Both animals and humans store toxins inside of fat cells to isolate them from internal organs. These are the substances that are so toxic that a body is unable to excrete them. By consuming the fat of an animal, a person is ingesting something that has calories but no nutrition, and toxins but no benefits. A diet with any appreciable flesh fat therefore impairs overall health, is a known cause of cancer, and a major component of heart disease. The process of storing toxins inside fat partially explains why diet programs are so prone to failing. It is because without detoxification, a body simply cannot let go of its toxin-storing fat as a matter of self-defense, and most commercial diet programs increase the amount of toxins.

> *"Do not cook a young goat in its mother's milk."*

-- Exodus 23:19

Milk interferes with the absorption of meat-iron and proteins which are important for muscle growth and general health; especially in children. For this reason, you should never consume milk with meat. Some Jewish people go so far as to not drink milk for six hours after consuming meat, but the Bible does not make a statement based on time.

> *"The rabbit, though it chews the cud, does not have a split hoof. It is unclean for you. And the pig, though it has a split hoof completely divided, does not chew the cud. It is unclean for you. You must not eat their meat or touch their carcasses. They are unclean for you... You must distinguish between the unclean and the clean, between living creatures that may be eaten* [cloven hoofed and cud chewing] *and those that may not be eaten."*

-- Leviticus 11:6-8, 11:4-7

Distinguishing between clean and unclean foods has been largely ignored for centuries. Eating fats has become common, along with huge amounts of chemicals. We were granted surface vegetation and lean meat, but never something that was not previously alive. Chemicals in foods express the forbidden art of sorcery, for what is sorcery other than mixing concoctions together to defy the laws of nature?

The animals that are deemed clean (fit for consumption) are herbivores, while the unclean animals are either carnivores or scavengers. Pigs, for instance, are scavengers who will happily eat almost anything, which includes engaging in cannibalism and consuming their own wastes. They are notorious for being infested with parasites like tapeworms, because they roll around in feces and mud for most of their lives. Pigs also carry a parasite called trichinellosis. The U.S. Centers For Disease Control explained:

> "Trichinellosis, also called trichinosis, is caused by eating raw or undercooked meat of animals infected with the larvae of a species of worm called trichinella. Infection occurs commonly in certain wild carnivorous (meat-eating) animals, but may also occur in domestic pigs. Nausea, diarrhea, vomiting, fatigue, fever, and abdominal discomfort are the first symptoms of trichinellosis. Headaches, fevers, chills, cough, eye swelling, aching joints and muscle pains, itchy skin, diarrhea, or constipation follow. If the infection is heavy, patients may experience difficulty coordinating movements, and have heart and breathing problems. In severe cases, death can occur. For mild to moderate infections, most symptoms subside within a few months. Fatigue, weakness, and diarrhea may last for months."

Rabbits, despite being remarkably clean animals, also eat their own waste and often carry a bacteria called tularemia (rabbit fever). Those who eat and handle rabbits are susceptible to contracting this sometimes fatal disease. Tularemia was documented in the early 1900's during an outbreak in California, when the ailment became frequent with hunters, cooks, and agricultural workers.

> "Of all the creatures living in the water of the seas and the streams, you may eat any that have fins and scales... Anything living in the water that does not have fins and scales is to be detestable to you."

> -- Leviticus 11:9-12

Fish which do not have fins and scales are bottom feeders and scavengers. They collect wastes and toxins from the bottoms of the oceans. They are the cleanup crew of the environmental world. Scientists have discovered that fish with scales and fins are equipped with a digestive system that prevents the absorption of toxins into their flesh.

While the majority of fish have both fins and scales, many of the popular options, including shrimp, crab, lobster, mussels and squid are fin or scale-free, and thus they are forbidden. These bottom-feeders are full of toxins, and they are the only fish with LDL cholesterol. God was even correct about fish. He knew about cholesterol 6,000 years ago, without the aid of science.

> *"Therefore the Lord Himself shall give you a sign; Behold, a young woman shall conceive, and bear a son, and shall call his name Immanuel* [Christ]. *Butter and honey shall he eat, that he may know to refuse the evil, and choose the good."*

-- Isaiah 7:14-7:15

Perhaps science will finally prove God wrong on this point, after all, he was promoting butter -- a saturated fat. The medical establishment has warned us for decades about the dangers of using saturated fats, such as butter. It has been very convenient for the corporations who make butter substitutes, and profits are soaring for cardiac medicine as never before. Their statements about saturated fats are false for all but exceptional cases.

Butter's Nutrition

- It is rich in selenium, a powerful anti-oxidant that neutralizes toxic heavy metals.
- It contains iodine, which is a very common deficiency.
- It is a rich source of easily absorbed vitamin A, which is needed for a wide range of functions, from maintaining good vision to keeping the endocrine system in good shape.
- Butter contains all of the fat-soluble vitamins (E, K and D).
- It is rich in butyric acid, which is used by the colon as an energy source, and it has been identified as an anti-carcinogen.
- Lauric acid from butter is a potent anti-microbial and anti-fungal substance (kills candida and boosts immune system).
- Butter provides conjugated linoleic acid (CLA) which provides even more protection against cancer.
- Butter contains glycospingolipids which protect against gastrointestinal infections, especially in the very young and elderly.

Only naturally-occurring vitamins like those in butter can be readily absorbed into the body. Your body knows the difference between natural vitamins and the synthetic ones, even when chemists do not. Synthetic vitamins added to "enrich" many foods (like artificial butters) are not only practically useless, but they actually stress the body, since the body correctly identifies them as unnatural, potentially toxic substances, which should be flushed. In choosing the foods for his child (butter and honey), God was sure to point out the best.

Honey is composed primarily of carbohydrates and water. It also contains an important array of vitamins and minerals, including niacin, riboflavin, pantothenic acid, calcium, copper, iron, magnesium, phosphorus, potassium, and zinc. Honey contains a variety of flavonoids and phenolic acids that act as anti-oxidants: scavenging and eliminating free radicals. The carbohydrate blend in honey is well-suited to sustain ideal blood sugar concentrations after strenuous physical activity. The potent anti-bacterial activity of honey has been used to keep wounds free from infection, while its anti-inflammatory attributes reduce pain and improve circulation; hastening healing processes. Honey stimulates the growth of tissue involved in healing. It boosts the immune system, while decreasing allergic reactions with its naturally-occurring antihistamines. It does not cause dramatic spikes in the blood sugar of diabetics as most other sweeteners do.

About Listening to 'The Experts'

Mary G. Enig, PhD., from the Weston Price Foundation, reported:

"Fats from animal and vegetable sources provide a concentrated source of energy in the diet. They also provide the building blocks for cell membranes and a variety of hormones and hormone-like substances. Fats [e.g. butter and cheese] as part of a meal slow down absorption so that we can go longer without feeling hungry. In addition, they act as carriers for important fat-soluble vitamins A, D, E, and K. Dietary fats are needed for the conversion of carotene to vitamin A, for mineral absorption and for a host of other processes. Politically Correct Nutrition is based on the assumption that we should reduce our intake of fats, particularly saturated fats from animal sources. Fats from animal sources also contain cholesterol, presented as the twin villain of the civilized diet. The lipid hypothesis (which began the butter and cholesterol hysteria) states that there is a direct relationship between the amount of saturated fat and cholesterol in the diet and the incidence of coronary heart disease. It was proposed by a researcher named Ancel Keys in the late 1950's. Numerous subsequent studies have disputed his data and its resultant conclusions.

"Nevertheless, Keys' articles have received far more publicity that those presenting alternate views. The reason behind this is the usual one: money. The vegetable oil and food processing industries, who are the main beneficiaries of research which found fault with competing traditional foods, promoted and funded vast research designed to support the lipid hypothesis, which in turn supported their new hydrogenated oils industry. They paid for the 'scientific' results they got, and the medical establishment ran with them. There are many 'experts' who still assure us that the lipid hypothesis is backed by incontrovertible scientific proof, including the American Heart Association. Most people would be surprised to learn that there is, in fact, very little evidence to support the contention that a diet low in cholesterol and saturated fat actually reduces death from heart disease or in any way increases one's life span.

"Consider the following: Before 1920, coronary heart disease was rare in America -- so rare that when a young internist named Paul Dudley White introduced the German Electrocardiograph to his colleagues at Harvard University, they advised him to concentrate on a more profitable branch of medicine. The new machine revealed the presence of arterial blockages, thus permitting early diagnosis of coronary heart disease. But in those days, clogged arteries were a medical rarity, and White had to search for patients who could benefit from his new technology. During the next forty years, however, the incidence of coronary heart disease rose dramatically, so much so that by the mid 1950's, heart disease was the leading cause of death among Americans.

"Today, heart disease causes at least 40% of all U.S. deaths. If, as we have been told, heart disease results from the consumption of saturated fats, one would expect to find a corresponding increase in animal fat in the American diet. Actually, the reverse is true, and most people have been following the advice of their physicians and the American Heart Association. During the sixty-year period from 1910 to 1970, the proportion of traditional animal fat in the American diet declined from 83% to 62%, and butter consumption plummeted from eighteen pounds per person per year to four. During the past eighty years, dietary cholesterol intake has increased only 1%. During the same period, the percentage of dietary vegetable oils in the form of margarine, shortening and refined oils increased about 400% while the consumption of sugar and processed foods increased about 60%. Again, heart disease now causes at least 40% of all U.S. deaths, yet it was practically a freak occurrence when butter was a staple of the American diet. Americans are dying from heart disease in record numbers from chemically manipulated hydrogenated oils -- the very ones they promised were going to save us.

"Hydrogenated oils are artificially processed oils that never appear in nature. They are created by food producers for the convenience of food producers -- primarily to add shelf life and consistency to foods, so that those foods can sit on the shelf for months at a time without going bad -- a clear indicator of their toxicity. Hydrogenated oils (chemically perverted oils and butter substitutes) are the number one cause of heart disease, and a major contributor to neurological disorders around the world. Hydrogenated oils are poison to the human body. They accelerate the buildup of plague in the arteries by causing inflammation, thus stimulating the body to patch the inflamed artery regions with calcium deposits. The human body simply cannot process these unnatural oils. As a result, they bring on heart disease far more quickly than could ever happen naturally."

Switching to olive oil and butter may be among the best ways to fend off not only heart disease, but cancer as well -- another well-known side effect of the man-made oils and fats. Most modern studies confirm this, but you will have to dig to find them, because the food industry and the medical establishment ignores them. It is difficult to know how much of this behavior is influenced by professional arrogance, years of brainwashing, and how much of it is just old-fashioned greed.

"For the Lord your God is bringing you into a good land, a land of brooks of water, of fountains and springs, that flow out of valleys and hills; a land of wheat and barley, of vines and fig trees and pomegranates, a land of olive oil and honey."

-- Deuteronomy 8:7-8

Olive oil was once scorned by the orthodox medical establishment, but it has recently become a recommendation. Olive oil contains cancer-fighting properties and its consumption leads to more efficient cardiac contractions. It contains large amounts of omega-3 and anti-oxidants. Spanish research shows that olive oil will prevent colon cancer. Coconut oil is the only food oil that matches olive oil for health benefits, but coconut oil quickly becomes rancid whenever it is heated.

Conclusionary Remarks

If we ate all of our foods as God commanded in the Bible, then we would undoubtedly be much healthier and happier. It has probably been noticed whilst reading this article that the forbidden foods tend to be scavengers, who spend their lives consuming toxic materials and wastes. Whether it be seaweed, pigs, or shrimp; God knew well before we did that these were not good for our health. Repeatedly reassuring his love throughout the Bible, he set unerring rules that we must follow to avoid self-injury.

God did not create these rules just to give us something to follow, but because he had good reasons for everything. Some of the reasons were outlined here. Perhaps you will think twice before eating one of the forbidden foods whenever you find yourself tempted, and be assured that there will eventually be a price to pay if you ignore the rules, and it may result in meeting God long before you planned.

Medical Victims

Shane Geiger

Spraining an ankle should never be a death sentence, and historically it was not cause for funeral arrangements. It now sometimes is, alongside heart disease, high blood pressure, diabetes, and the long montage of other medically-aggravated conditions. Spraining an ankle was a death sentence for Shane Geiger. We were not given much opportunity to get close to him before his life was lost. Shane was an up-and-coming member of our Sarah's elite Web Team (network engineering) for Architects and Engineers for 9/11 Truth, during the period when she worked for them. He was previously an honorary staff member of Prison Planet, and his pointed questions at a governmental press conference about the Trade Center attacks left one cronie almost running to escape. We watched the video wherein Shane left a N.I.S.T. representative stuttering and making a rapid departure. We were proud to call him an ally. He was known for being a little bit paranoid, but in light of his bizarre death, his paranoia may have been justified.

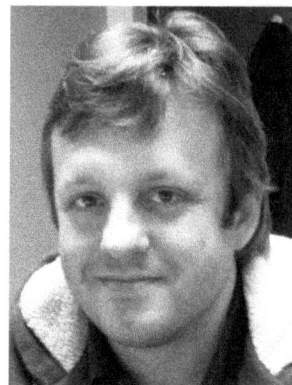

The biggest mistake that Shane ever made was visiting a doctor about a sprained ankle. Most people would not expect for such a visit to become a fatal encounter. We are certain that Shane never expected to die from it. The whole fiasco began in July of 2011, while walking his dog. We do not know if the dog or Shane was more to blame, but on that fateful walk, Shane's ankle got sprained. For about a month, Shane waited for his ankle to heal itself, and for the swelling to subside. Shane was not satisfied with the slowness of progress during that month: meaning that he likely had a damaged nerve or there was another secondary injury at play. So he did something that is becoming increasingly dangerous in this era. He visited (or revisited) a doctor. After getting medical care, his sprained ankle suddenly turned into "blood clots". They will never admit what really happened.

The most astounding aspect is that his close family and friends never questioned any of this insanity. Society's level of brainwashing is staggering. What if *we* had given him a drug, and suddenly he died of "blood clots"? We'd be in prison now, and Shane would have undergone a thorough autopsy for evidence of manslaughter or murder. The doctors are legally immune, and you can be sure that no investigation will ever take place. This is normal! This is routine! A healthy, thirty-something man is dead, and everybody is too afraid of looking crazy to question what *really is* crazy. Blood clots are not caused by sprained ankles, and they never have been. They are caused by the potassium-altering diuretic medications that are routinely given by doctors, and they were almost certainly giving him these drugs to reduce swelling. This class of drugs is documented to cause heart failure, but it is called "blood clots" upon death; to make it the victim's fault. That way, the doctors remain 'heroes'. You can't argue when you're dead, after all.

We are disturbed by the fact that we could have helped him, if only he had asked. With the right combination of anti-inflammatory herbs, healthy fats, joint-supporting supplementation, and nerve-supporting supplementation, we could have had him back to normal in a matter of days. Instead, he made the mistake of opting for 'real medicine', and the results speak for themselves. How many times does it have to be said before everyone realizes that the emperor has no clothes? We can promise that some of those who witnessed his burial soon thereafter mindlessly spewed platitudes about "the miracles" of modern medicine, before the dirt even settled. It is sickening, and it is disrespectful to those who have been killed thusly. There is little hope of history teaching us anything with the masses being so brainwashed that they cannot even see what is unfolding before their eyes.

Remember Shane Geiger, the next time that you are tempted to visit a doctor. Rest in peace our fallen comrade. We salute you.

Michael J. Fox

Certain celebrities have been associated with specific diseases. For instance, Patrick Swayze will be associated with pancreatic cancer indefinitely. Michael J. Fox represents Parkinson's disease, and the Marlborough Men ironically came to represent lung cancer. For those who do not remember, the Marlborough Men were the smoking cowboys who attempted to make filtered cigarettes seem more masculine. The commercials were a huge success, until all of the actors began dying from lung cancer. The demise of the Marlboro Men was publicized heavily by the mainstream media, because it has long been open season against tobacco products; ever since it became illegal for tobacco companies to fund news shows.

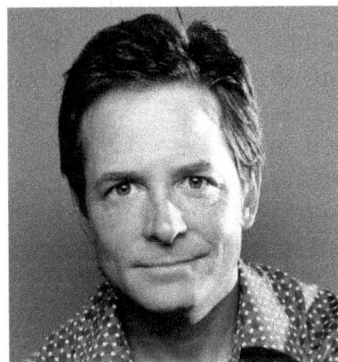

The cause of Michael Fox's Parkinson's disease is always side-stepped by the media, similar to the dishonest tobacco precedent of former times. Readers may notice there has never been a peep about the cause; and moreover, the talk has been singularly about finding the supposedly elusive cure. The cause of Fox's disease is not yet politically correct to attack. It would get most reporters fired.

Throughout the 1980's, Michael did commercials for Pepsico, and he promoted Diet Pepsi cola exclusively in the latter years of his contract. It is believed that he became an ardent consumer of Diet Pepsi throughout this period (even off-set). Then, in 1991, Michael was diagnosed with young-onset Parkinson's disease. It would be seven years before he told the public about his diagnosis, so the link has been missed by most people.

In 2000, Michael founded the Michael J. Fox Foundation, which was supposed to help discover the cause and cure for Parkinson's disease. Various groups have sent information to the foundation about the link between aspartame (found in diet colas) and Parkinson's disease, but they have been ignored. The foundation instead donated $175,000,000 to researchers of Parkinson's disease, while wholly ignoring the existing information about aspartame, just as most researchers have. The foundation is yet another organization which apparently believes that funneling even more money into the petrochemical cartel will help to find an elusive cure, for something that would require an admission of guilt to cure, and the loss of a billion dollar diet drinks industry. The chemical industry is *the problem*, not the solution. Their profits from treatment regimens soar higher with every new Michael that they create. Meanwhile, they continue promoting super-toxic diet drinks as the healthy alternative, because sugars, after all, are bad.

The mainstream medical establishment apparently does not know the cause of Parkinson's disease, but it has been linked with heavy metal exposure and excitotoxins. N-methyl-D-aspartate (NMDA) receptors in the brain are responsible for the excitotoxicity associated with Parkinson's disease. Aspartate is one of the main components that is released when aspartame is metabolized, and it directly effects the NMDA receptors. Regular intake of aspartame damages those receptors, and can eventually lead to Parkinson's disease.

It is known that Parkinson's disease occurs whenever the dopamine-related nerve cells inside the brain are decimated. With dramatically decreased dopamine, the nerve cells in the effected part of the brain cannot properly transmit messages. In studies, aspartame has been shown to decrease dopamine levels in the brain, inducing the unmistakable neurological decline that is seen in Parkinson's patients. A troubling study from the Norwegian University of Science, verified aspartame as an excitotoxin, and as a neurotoxin that is particularly dangerous to children. None of this is ever mentioned by either the Michael J. Fox Foundation, nor any mainstream media outlets, who carefully avoid the topic of aspartame.

Aspartame will cause the death of brain cells and damage to the brain neurons without any other implicating factors. It is a pure poison that is sometimes used to kill ants, and it is known to be the surest way to cause brain tumors in laboratory rats. Some cancer studies have used aspartame to induce cancers in laboratory rats, for the purpose of later testing anti-cancer drugs. Aspartame is chosen because it is so reliable at producing cancers in high dosages. In addition to its ability to cause Parkinson's disease, it also causes multiple sclerosis, diabetes, fibromyalgia, heart arrhythmias, reduced intelligence, obesity, asthma, muscle spasms, and a total of 92 symptoms that even the F.D.A. was forced to confess. There is a great irony that obesity is one of the side effects of aspartame, considering that it is used exclusively in diet products. The same chemical industry that produces this poison is the industry that sells even more lucrative treatments for the aftermath, so it is a case of one hand washing the other. Therefore, the cure will not be found anytime soon.

Perhaps Michael J. Fox will someday realize what caused his disease, and if he does, we hope that he will use his celebrity influence to inform others about aspartame. There are very few people who drink Diet Pepsi as frequently as Michael did, particularly at such a young age. Thus, Parkinson's disease rarely occurs in people so young. Finding the cause of these events is not difficult, except for people who are intentionally avoiding the obvious. Most of the organizations pretending to seek a cure, do ignore the obvious as official policy. They prefer genetic explanations, since these mean that nobody is to blame, and there will never be reason for the funding to stop. Genetic explanations mean that they are certain to never find that cure, and that's money in the bank.

If the mainstream media were to spend as much time attacking excitotoxins like aspartame and MSG as they did tobacco, then it would not be long before many of the major diseases, including Parkinson's disease, became a thing of the past. The closely-linked disease of fibromyalgia would disappear completely.

The Politics of Aspartame and Why It is Still Legal

In January of 1980, the F.D.A. advisory board banned aspartame, because their research showed that it caused brain tumors. This decision could only be overturned by the commissioner. Then, in November of 1980, Donald Rumsfeld was hired as part of the transition team for President Ronald Reagan, prior to which, he had been the President of Searle (the company that created aspartame). On the first day of the new administration, the previous F.D.A. commissioner's authority was suspended, and Rumsfeld assigned Dr. Arthur Hayes as the new head of the F.D.A. Hayes was previously just a defense contractor, but he had a close relationship to Rumsfeld, because they had worked together under the Nixon Administration in close contact with the President of Pepsico. Hayes' first decision was to approve aspartame for dry foods, and by the end of 1983, he had approved aspartame for soft drinks too. He was later forced to leave the agency, due to media pressure for his acceptance of corporate "gifts". The defense contractor then went to the Searle public relations firm as its "Senior Medical Adviser". Shortly thereafter, Monsanto purchased Searle. Rumsfeld received a $12 million "bonus" for his help in ram-rodding the F.D.A. into unbanning aspartame.

Patrick Swayze

In March 2008, the actor Patrick Swayze was diagnosed with pancreatic cancer. Standard medicine has deplorable success rates in suppressing pancreatic cancers, and most of its patients die within two years of diagnosis. The mainstream media publicized Swayze's case heavily. The devastating effects of the treatments became very apparent from photographs of him. Patrick Swayze died two years following his diagnosis, following the usual pattern. His quality of life by that time had been completely eroded. Patrick's doctors publicly boasted of Swayze's treatments, as if they represented the gold standard of medical care. An "excellent response" as described by Swayze's doctors is shown in the images below. You have probably already learned the ultimate conclusion of that "excellent response" from other media outlets. Swayze died on September 14th, 2009, of medicide. The establishment calls these "iatrogenic deaths", because outsiders do not know what the term means.

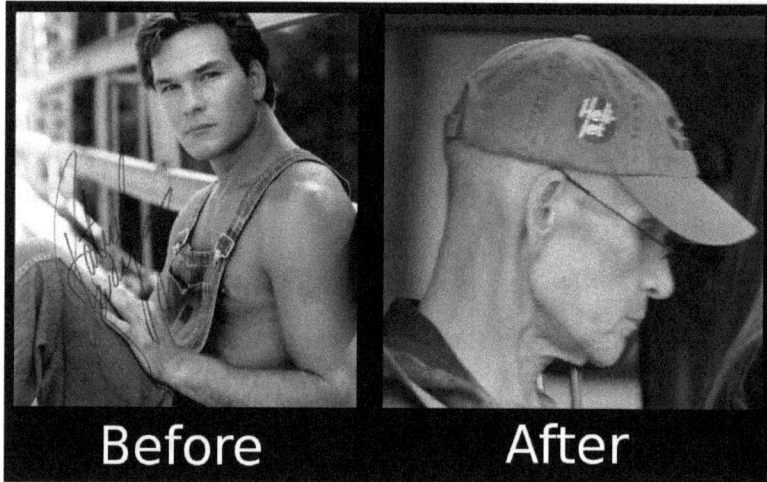

Before   After

If *our medicine* had this effect on someone, we could not possibly boast about it to the press. Dr. George Fisher, Swayze's oncologist, had plenty of proud remarks concerning his handiwork and the type of medicine he practices.

> *"Because of his excellent response, he* [Swayze] *will continue the same therapy at Stanford."*

How about this?

> *"Less than 25 percent of patients with pancreatic cancer that has spread survive a year after diagnosis, and yet Swayze is proof that it is possible."*

Let's not forget:

> *"Patrick has a very limited amount of disease and he appears to be responding well to treatment thus far."*

The problem (and usual slight-of-hand trick here) is that the death rate soars *only after diagnosis*, which means that patients start dying rapidly *only after* they begin standard treatments. It was not cancer that killed Patrick. The people who killed him are still patting themselves on the backs and cashing their checks. Untreated patients live better, and live longer than those who are given "conventional" medicine, which is actually new and experimental medicine. The results are always better with alternative (non-poisonous) remedies -- the ones that actually work to permanently cure more than the pathetic 4% that the allopathic establishment gets. It is worth noting that the most common reasons for cancers to "spread" are chemotherapy, surgery, and radiation -- the very treatments themselves, and these are officially known as side effects in the medical literature. Swayze would have lived longer and better if he had treated his cancer with cigarettes. Anything would have yielded better results than poisoning him to death.

Swayze made the common mistake of seeking poisonous *treatments* from allopathic doctors, when he should have been seeking *cures* from alternative medicine. Ultimately, Swayze made a leap of faith -- or more aptly -- a leap of very misguided faith. He paid dearly for his mistake, and millions of people will do the same; all the way to their graves.

Phil Collins

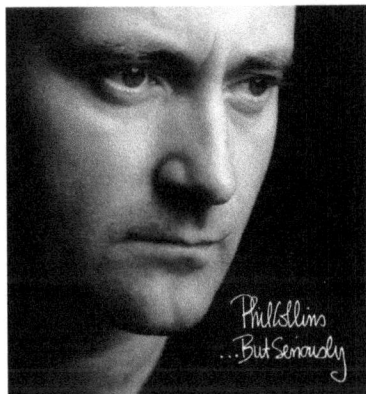

Young people need heroes, and today's young generation sadly lacks them. One of my heroes from the 1980's was Phil Collins. I admired Collins not just for his musical gifts, but also because he was a member of the rock and roll elites who managed to hold onto his soul. Even in the 1980's, this was no small feat for a successful musician. Phil was on par with the best of the best, and yet he did it without becoming a drug addict, was never into Satanic stuff, and he never gyrated on the stage half-clothed. I know of no other successful entertainer of equal talent with comparable character. These things made him a giant amongst his peers.

Collins' stellar career began meekly as a drummer for multiple gigs and groups, but Collins realized that he was on the brink of greatness when he joined a group of musical gods, known as Genesis. Within five years, Collins would graduate from being the drummer, who was known for providing the group's creativity, to being its lead singer. He replaced the esteemed Peter Gabriel. Some people feel that Collins was a better Peter Gabriel than Peter Gabriel. Every person exposed to the new Genesis under Phil's leadership could see it, and they could definitely hear it: big things were about to happen for Genesis. The world of rock music laid before them for the taking, and they took it.

Collins still exudes class and character in everything that he does. We desperately need more people like Phil Collins in the world. He was born as an Englishman, but he managed to overtake American music like a typhoon during the Reaganesque, *Miami Vice* era. One of the things that touches me about Phil Collins is, of course, his music; but it goes beyond that.

Collins crafted some of the most sincere, moral messages ever to be penned, and then blended them into some of the most beautiful music ever created. He used his music as a tool for changing people for the better. The following lyrics below provide an excellent example of Collins' moral fortitude.

Excerpted lyrics from *Tell Me Why*, by Genesis

Mothers cryin' in the street. Children dyin' at their feet. Tell me why, ooh, tell me why? People starvin' everywhere. There's too much food, But there's none to spare. Tell me why, oh, tell me why?

If there's a God, is he watchin'? Can he give a ray of hope? So much pain and so much sorrow. Tell me, what does he see? When he looks at you? When he looks at me? What would he say? 'Cos it seems there's no one listenin'.

Who would think it still could happen? Even in this time and place? Politicians, they may save themselves. Oh, but they won't save their face. So hope against hope, It's not too late.

You say there's nothing you can do. Is there one rule for them and one for you? Tell me why, just tell me why?

The Medical Downfall of Phil Collins

In 2009, Phil began to suffer from serious pain in his neck, resulting from a dislocated vertebrae. He went to see a regular doctor, and this was likely to have been the biggest mistake of his life. One surgery later and Phil had lost control over his priceless drumming hands. Not only is this elite musician completely unable to drum, but he cannot let go of a spoon, or even open his car door unassisted. The surgeons accidentally cut the nerves to his hands, and short of a miracle, he will never drum again. He will not be able to hold a microphone again, or let it go if he actually manages to hang onto it.

Collins told Rolling Stone Magazine:

> *"My vertebrae has been crushing my spinal cord because of the position I drum in. It comes from years of playing. I can't even hold the sticks properly without it being painful... The first time I picked up the drumsticks after my neck surgery, they flew across the room because I couldn't grip them. When I play, I've had to tape the sticks to my hand... I'm having an operation soon and there's a good chance of it improving over time."*

We are not so optimistic about Collins' prognosis. What Phil should really expect, if he could accurately appraise the situation, is dozens of surgeries over the next 10 years. At no point is there going to be any substantial improvement until he steps off the treadmill of allopathic medicine, and never looks back. It is his only hope.

The frustrating part of such situations for us is knowing how avoidable they are. Let's take for example the very worst case of spinal aggravation and misalignment, as if Phil's spine had been pulverized in an automotive accident. A competent chiropractor could have healed (permanently cured) Phil's back in a matter of months, or perhaps a year for this extreme example; with considerably less pain, risk, money, and time. Instead, Collins submitted to being butchered, and his butchers cut the wrong thing. If he had been wiser, he would have applied a chiropractic approach and combined it with strength training exercises to support his weak back areas, and perhaps undertook a diet that would have helped him to resist such aging issues. He could have cured his problem relatively cheaply and easily, and perhaps reversed 20 years of aging in the process.

That is not how it happened. We scoured the 'Net searching for any reference of Collins seeking alternative therapies, but it was as we suspected. Did Phil ever stop to reflect on just how patently stupid it was? It hardly requires 12 years of intensive medical training to see something is terribly wrong with an approach of slicing and dicing an already injured area of the body, and his severed nerves stand in silent testament to it. We have to wonder what the surgeons hope to accomplish with additional surgeries. Consider the following: The problem with Phil's hands is that his nerves were cut, and according to the medical establishment, cut nerves do not heal. So what could possibly be the goal of cutting into Collins' back even more? Finishing the job? Get his feet the next time?

Using naturopathic techniques, it is sometimes possible to heal nerve damage, even severed ones. The orthodox doctors will tell Collins that it is impossible, but history should prove to him that they cannot be trusted. I believe in miracles, and I hope that by fate or divine intervention that Phil Collins will someday stumble across this. If he does, I hope it will inspire him to take control of the situation, and to save himself. As he so poetically said himself: *"So hope against hope. It's not too late"*.

In June of 2012, Phil Collins announced that he felt it was necessary to retire from the music industry forever, because he would never again be able to perform as he once had.

Fraudulent Alternative Medicine

Just Like Magic

The truth is usually stranger than fiction, and we have been studying alternative medicine long enough to know the truth. There are two main categories of frauds in alternative medicine. One category consists of illegitimate therapies that are emulations of poisonous orthodox medicine, such as the use of radiation.

The other category of alternative medicine frauds is much more disturbing. This latter category is heavily influenced by dark religions. Due to the religious undertones, many of the involved lost refer to themselves as being "spiritual". They are pagans (witches), who are following the wicked religions of the ancient Egyptians, from before the time of God's wrath. Many Americans will immediately laugh at suggestions that witches exist, but there are modern-day witches with their own churches (covens), and their own set of "sacred" books. They have infiltrated all American institutions, managed to convince the American people that witches do not exist, and rewritten history to show that the witch trials were conducted against innocent victims of the bad Christians. The greatest trick that the Devil ever pulled was convincing people that he does not exist. In much the same way that Christians worship "The Father", these people worship the "Great Mother", who is also known as "Mother Earth", "Mother Nature", and "Gaia". They flaunt their religion; whilst hiding it from us in plain sight. It is one of the methods wherein they mock the better people. Upon inspection, the breadth of corruption that they have had upon our society should become obvious. They ironically worship nature, despite the fact that nature is God's handiwork. Following their satanic tendencies, they put all of nature in dominion over man, in opposition to God's earliest commandment that humans rightfully have dominion over all of nature. So witches play a big role in the environmentalism movement, and they started that work in 1970, when pagan groups manipulated the U.S. Government into creating Earth Day. The commands of God specifically forbid such idolatry.

Every part of the pagan religions is meant to mock God. Instead of prayer, they have spells and magic. Instead of teaching the virtues of celibacy before marriage, they have demonically-inspired naked rituals in the woods that we really should not describe here. For the upper level and old-school covens, these rituals sometimes involve child molestation and child rapes using their own children. That's part of their "religion" too, once a person has obtained enough "priesthood" to have these "religious mysteries" revealed. Their infiltration of churches is the reason for the child molestation cases, in order to malign the church, like they have done with their new version of history. It is why our forefathers burned and tortured these people to death, because no earthly punishment could be bad enough. The end game of the so-called "mystery religions" is to eventually migrate lower-to-mid level witches into full-blown Satanists. It goes without saying that none of these people can be trusted to even the slightest degree. They are everywhere, and their greatest power is in their manipulative ability to blend in, and to make us believe that they do not exist. They are in control of our laws and institutions. You will find them in the leadership of every major church, in fact.

Where they enter into alternative medicine most directly is in their promotion of magic. They no longer in public call it magic -- anymore than they call themselves witches ("Wiccan" etc.). The terms "witch" and "magic" tend to be very bad marketing for them, because both are truthful descriptions. They delude themselves that they have magic-energy healing therapies and "faith healing" that is entirely absent of the faith component. Their "spiritual healing" is an attempt to seduce us away from God and into their fold.

They sometimes begin by first attempting to pull Christians into alternative religions, because a more frontal attack against God would meet with too much resistance. The "spiritual" promotion of Yoga for instance, is one of their methods of pulling the faithful toward the Hindu religion. Once an individual is taken by this and lost, it is much easier to begin a conversion process. If even they fail, they still win, because the most important thing -- defiance of the one true God -- has been accomplished. Corruption is the goal, but they call it "spiritualism". Like with all of the other lies, it is actually the very opposite of being spiritual.

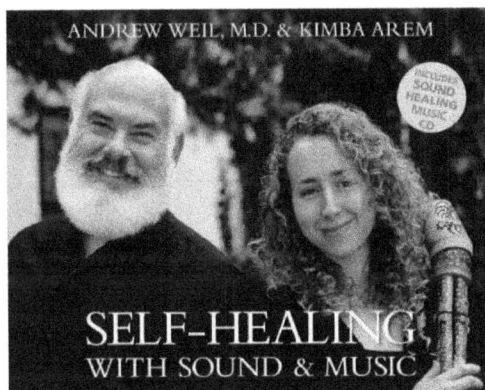

ANDREW WEIL, M.D. & KIMBA AREM

SELF-HEALING
WITH SOUND & MUSIC

REVITALIZE YOUR BODY & MIND WITH
PROVEN SOUND HEALING TOOLS

Attempting to alter nature through the use of special sounds is otherwise known as spell casting. The "self" part of these dark religions is significant too, because they promote selfishness instead of selflessness. The message is to help yourself, but not others, in other words.

The witchcraft is usually disguised under a variety of other names, such as "Reiki", "remote healing energies", "life force healing", and "spiritual energy healing". The common factor is that they promise power from an invisible mystical force. There is only one source for such forces outside of God.

Urine Therapy

Urine therapy is the process of drinking one's own urine, and slowly increasing the amount that is consumed each day, whilst ignoring the obvious health effects. People are told by online 'experts' that the nausea, vomiting, and sicknesses experienced are indications of ongoing detoxification. There are niché groups who are obsessed with urine, and they are always seeking new uses for it. They are tied with the pagan religions mentioned earlier. Urine was originally used as a magical medicine by the ancient Egyptians, who were notorious for their plagues.

Dr. Stanilaw Burzynski

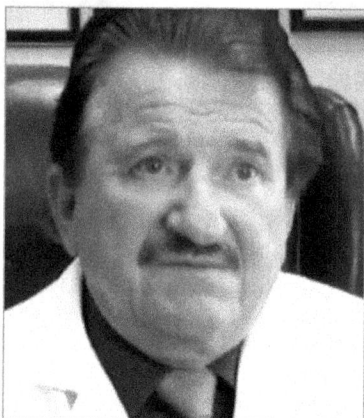

One of the offshoots of the urine therapy insanity is Dr. Stanilaw Burzynski's "antineoplaston therapy". Dr. Burzynski is a Polish-educated doctor, though his Ph.D. is of questionable origin. He operates in the United States, treating American cancer patients by injecting synthetic versions of human urine into them. The urine is chemically copied, which allows it to be patented; since natural substances like urine are normally unpatentable. Dr. Burzynski claims that his treatment is "normally free from serious side-effects", but the Office of Technology Assessment to the U.S. Congress revealed that platelet and white blood cell counts become so high after treatment that they could cause blood clotting. Furthermore, 65% of his patients develop hypernatremia, a life-threatening condition, which is associated with high levels of sodium in the body. Deaths have been reported as a result of the therapy. In order to improve the statistics of his treatment, Burzynski fraudulently claims "complete remission" from cases wherein the cancers were already in remission before his treatments. Even with such tactics, his own statistics still show a 75% failure rate, which is worse than the death rate of patients who receive no cancer treatments at all, within the same time frame. The F.D.A. has been actively involved in legitimizing Burzynski's "alternative therapy", by feigning impotent legal actions against him in a very public way. This has conned a flock of very vocal followers, who speak out against and protest his supposed persecution. Part of the slight-of-hand is that his 'treatment' has actually been approved by the F.D.A. for him to practice, and he was allowed to patent his 'therapy'. He has been negotiating partnerships with pharmaceutical companies for years, so he seems to be playing everyone. For a comprehensive report about Dr. Stanilaw Burzynski and his 'alternative therapy', you may listen to our audio report, *Dr. Burzynski and Other Evil People* (episode 25), in our audio archive at our site, healthwyze.org.

414

Borax

Borax is sold as a laundry detergent. It is a toxic bleaching agent. Small amounts of it can be fatal. Some fringe groups advocate its consumption for a never-ending litany of conditions, and even as a preventative medicine. Borax seems to prevent the initial onset of many routine illnesses, because it poisons the body to such a degree that it acts as an immunosuppressant. A thusly crippled immune system may be unable to manifest noticeable symptoms. This actually fosters more severe illnesses that are more difficult to overcome. Masking illness symptoms through poisoning is the very epitome of stupidity, of which the medical establishment is infamous for doing.

When the organs fail to such an extent that symptoms are finally visible, it will likely be too late to reverse the damage. Borax can cause liver and kidney failure, or irreversible damage to these vital organs. Ignorant people sometimes kill themselves with borax to merely suppress a case of sniffles.

Borax is promoted most amongst quacks and scoundrels for its ability to treat arthritis. Borax will kill viruses, because it is so toxic. This is how it helps certain arthritis patients. For arthritis is sometimes caused by a virus. There are much safer agents to be used instead, such as colloidal silver. There is never a legitimate reason to consume borax, because there are always non-toxic alternatives that work better. It is a medicine of fools, which closely mimics chemotherapy.

Sun Gazing

Sun gazing is the practice of looking directly at the sun, without any protection, with the supposed benefit of aiding the eyes, or even "getting vitamin D in the eyes". Staring at the sun is known to damage the eyes, and can lead to blindness. It should be avoided even when wearing sunglasses. Vitamin D cannot actually be made using the eyes. Vitamin D-3 is produced in the liver after sunlight converts cholesterol in the skin to vitamin D-2. Staring at the sun presents no known benefits.

Electromagnetic Therapy

Using radiation in place of medicine is dangerous and patently stupid. In some cases, such as when a virus is active within the body, using radiation devices will provide some relief. The relief, in the form of symptom remission, is mostly the immunosuppressant effect of damaging the entire body. The true underlying condition will actually worsen in most cases. Radiation is always damaging to the human body, and exposure greatly increases the chance of cancer. The most famous device in this category is known as the Rife Machine. Any electrical device that is said to cure chronic diseases should be viewed with great skepticism. There are some specific conditions, such as Bell's palsy, wherein the application of a tiny electric current through the nerves can help to sterilize them. However, such conditions are rare, and radiation is entirely different.

Homeopathy

There are two main variants of homeopathy. There is the modern, and the original homeopathy. Both are steeped in fraudulent medicine. The original homeopaths believed that "like cures like". They professed that a substance which causes a particular condition is also needed to cure it. It was the fighting fire with fire approach. The influence of this homeopathic idiocy is partly responsible for why the medical establishment is so broken. For example, radiation and chemotherapy are both causes of cancer in healthy people, yet they are used in vain attempts to cure cancers, with very dismal results. Similarly, in homeopathy, known allergens were given to patients who were experiencing symptoms like wheezing, sneezing, and coughing. What is now allopathic medicine (orthodox medicine) is largely the result of homeopathic influence. As the competitor of the original homeopathic establishment, the American Medical Association destroyed the original homeopathic industry though licensing laws. Nevertheless, likes are still treating likes, as in the case of pancreas-destroying diabetes drugs, heart attack causing cholesterol drugs, and psychiatric drugs that induce mental illness. Doctors who practice homeopathic medicine are at every hospital.

Modern homeopaths rely entirely on the placebo effect, so their 'medicine' is much safer. Using deception, they found a way to bypass the licensing laws by not really providing or prescribing medicine. Modern homeopathic preparations contain no traceable amount of the substance that is claimed to be active in them. These water-only formulations are alleged to work based upon the notion of "water memory". Modern homeopaths attest that water has a special ability to "remember" the "metabolic structure" of any compound that it has previously contacted, so long as the water is properly shaken while it is still in contact with that compound. Shaking imparts water's special property, they claim. There is absolutely no evidence of water having any "memory" capabilities, and the dilution that is used for homeopathic remedies is approximately that of 1 drop added to a swimming pool, or less. The active ingredient is undetectable, and so, such remedies are useless. We should be thankful that homeopathic remedies do not contain the substances that are claimed, because it is not unusual for potent poisons to be recommended, such as antimony. That too was once a "drug" of the competing orthodox establishment, which essentially hijacked everything homeopathic before killing the competition.

Readers may notice that "homeopathic medicines" are sold unopposed by the F.D.A., in various retail locations, regardless of the incredible claims that its sellers make. These products are allowed specifically *because they are frauds*, so that alternatives will be unilaterally maligned. The homeopathic wares will normally be found close to the equally fraudulent "energy healing" bracelets, and "healing magnets".

Homeopathic medicine is neither a legitimate alternative medicine nor a natural medicine, and it is not even medicine at all. Although, enough of the modern homeopathic medicine could be used to successfully cure dehydration.

Anti-Radiation Devices

Hundreds of fraudulent products are marketed as being able to suppress radiation inside buildings. Most of them are electronic, which ironically means that they increase the amount of radiation. All anti-radiation and anti-EMF devices are frauds. There is no way to electronically absorb radiation, or neutralize it via electronics. Harmful radiation can be compared to light (light technically is a type of radiation). For instance, there is no such thing as an anti-light device, whereby a switch can be thrown to suck all of the light from an area. Like other types of radiation, light must instead be stopped at its source or blocked with shielding. There is however, no such thing as an anti-light vacuum, anymore than there is anti-radiation, unless we count black holes.

Those who have purchased the radiation-neutralizing products can be absolutely certain that their devices are frauds if their cell phones and wireless devices continue to function, because the devices communicate via radiation.

It is technically possible to line a building's walls with metal to block most radiation from entering a building, which some companies provide; but doing so requires major expense. It risks turning the building into an oversized lightning rod, and the occupants will have to forgo cellular phone service indoors.

Some of the anti-radiation systems are special food plates or crystals that are marketed to neutralize all forms of harmful radiation. Some of these are promoted to have magical powers that counteract the radiation.

Sacred Geometry

The origin of sacred geometry was in the design of Christian churches, wherein architects designed structures to include symbolism. An example is how the spire or steeple of a church is designed to point up toward God. The term "sacred geometry" has since been mockingly hijacked by pagans, and its redefinition is far from sacred. These heathens create objects that feature various crystalline patterns, which are supposed to have special properties. The claims vary from the elimination of radiation to unlimited health benefits, or even ironically, a "cleaner soul". The claims are all bogus, and no honesty can be expected from such deluded people.

Krill Oil

Krill is widely being marketed as a superior source of omega-3, primarily by the companies that are selling it. The arguments in favor of krill oil supplementation are nonsensical and self-defeating. For example, one of the arguments is that fish oil contains contaminants from the oceans, and therefore, fish oil is inferior. Krill is a type of fish, so krill oil is fish oil too. Moreover, krill is a bottom-feeding fish, so it will contain *more* contaminants than most fish. Proponents also demonize fish oil because of the extreme processing necessary to extract supplemental oil, and it is true. What they cleverly neglect to mention is that the processing for krill oil is identical. Krill is shell fish that primarily eats algae. It is therefore worse than most fish, because algae is virtually always contaminated with heavy metals, PCB's, and other ocean contaminants. It is the job of algae to clean the oceans of these things. Some algae even produces its own bacterial toxins.

Each year, hundreds of people get sick from seafood that was contaminated by algae-related bacterial toxins. When they visit hospitals, physicians base their antidote upon the revelation that the patients recently ate seafood. The new krill supplements will undoubtedly lead to very sick people, who do not equate their sickly condition with the supplements that were used, and thus unknowing doctors will be unable to help them. There are no tests for all of the bacterial toxins from algae.

Neither krill oil nor fish oil should be used for supplementation. Even when contamination is not present, the processing of these oils is extreme, and solvent byproducts often remain in the oils as remnants of the manufacturing process. The resultant oils are always rancid by the time that they reach retail shelves, and rancid oils are carcinogenic. The best way to get omega-3 is from cold-pressed flax seed oil, in light-resistant capsules.

Shark Cartilage

The hoopla regarding shark cartilage first began as an Internet rumor that was promulgated under the contention that "sharks don't get cancer". The intellectually challenged and the unscrupulous are claiming that shark cartilage is a "miracle cure" for everything. The gratuitous and disrespectful use of the word "miracle" usually indicates that someone is working for the other side. The truth is that no fish or animals get cancers when they eat their natural diets and live in their natural habitats. Cancers appear only in captivity, due to exposure to the same things that cause cancers in humans; like the compounds from genetically engineered and commercially-processed foods.

Shark cartilage has been promoted for every condition that is known to plague man. It is primarily imported from China, so the purity of such products is always dubious. Regardless of origin, shark cartilage is very unlikely to have any positive health benefits, and there is a high probability of contamination, due to the unethical nature of the companies who promote it.

Nutritional Yeast and Brewer's Yeast

Yeast products are now being promoted as nutritional supplements. They do contain certain nutrients, but they are also very damaging to the body. Yeast is never a wise supplementation strategy. Due to the fact that it feeds the harmful yeast in the gastrointestinal tract, it will lead to gastrointestinal problems, such as irritable bowel disease. It will also cause malabsorption of foods, and the subsequent plethora of diseases which arise from malnutrition. Be forewarned that most allegedly food-based supplements are now made using genetically-engineered yeasts instead of food. Be forewarned that most of the supplements being marketed to the health conscious, and those found in most health food stores, are made with yeast and genetically-engineered bacteria. Reference the *General Recommendations* section of the *Supplements* chapter for more information about yeast-based vitamins.

Mushrooms

Mushrooms are fungi, and they too aid the candida yeast in the body. They act like algae, in that they absorb the contaminants that they are exposed to. They are known as the vampires of the plant world for absorbing the putrid wastes and toxic compounds in soil. Mushrooms often contain varying levels of heavy metals. There has been a plethora of health scams involving mushrooms, most of which are proclaimed as "miracle" cures from Asian countries. The most frequent claim is that they can cure cancer. Cancer is caused by a type of fermentation, so mushrooms will always worsen cancer, instead of helping. They should never be considered a health food. Most varieties of mushrooms are poisonous, so it requires a lot of vigilance on the part of mushroom farmers to ensure that no poisonous mushrooms ever get mixed in. As always, we strongly recommend against all items from China. This means avoiding all so-called "Asian mushrooms".

Organs as Food

One of the jobs of the liver is to safely remove toxins, or to store them whenever their removal is not possible. This explains why any successful cleansing protocol must begin with a liver cleanse; for without the help of a fully functional liver, other cleansing protocols will not work well. Any cleansing process involving a dysfunctional liver is like cleaning a dirty floor with a dirty mop and dirty water. The liver is the mop of the human body.

Some fringe health writers recommend that people eat organ meats, and most especially liver. A smaller subset of those people recommend eating the organs raw, intact with raw blood. They contend that liver is healthy because livers are extremely nutrient dense. Their advice is well intentioned, but equally foolish. These writers fail to account for the fact that the liver is also a body's long-term storage area for toxic materials. It is the wisdom of taking a lead pill with a multi-vitamin, and no amount of nutrition can compensate for the problems generated. The liver, along with fat cells, are the storage places for toxic materials that a body cannot eliminate. Consuming liver is the act of eating all of the toxins that an animal was unable to expel throughout its entire lifetime, and there are really toxic materials at farms nowadays.

Consumption of liver has been linked with increased rates of hepatitis E in the United States. Although, the condition is rarely reported. Liver consumption has also been repeatedly linked with clenbuterol poisoning in Spain, China, and Portugal. The symptoms of clenbuterol poisoning include muscle tremors, headaches, and nervousness. The condition can last for days, until the toxin is isolated by (and contained inside) the liver, where it will remain for the rest of a person's life, and impair his health forever after. Clenbuterol is a chemical that is illegally administered to livestock, for its ability to keep meat fresh for unnatural lengths of time. It is another reason to avoid products from the usual culprit: China.

People who eat liver need to weigh the benefits of some extra minerals against the risk of permanent poisoning; both from heavy metals and other poisons that the cow has been in contact with. The poisons can come from processed feeds, antibiotics, vaccine ingredients, pesticide over-spray, tainted water, and the synthetic hormones that are frequently given to farm animals. While organic liver is theoretically healthier than its extremely toxic counterpart, we strongly recommend against taking unnecessary risks.

Various toxins that we eat are stored in the liver, such as aflatoxin. It is something produced by molds that often appears on vegetables during their transportation or processing. It can also be ingested from antibiotics; which by the way, are still made from toxic fungal sources, despite the dishonest hype about 'breakthroughs'. Aflatoxin has been shown to massively increase the risk of liver cancer. It is important to note that studies in China have shown that this risk can be reduced by 55% with the help of chlorophyll, which naturally chelates many toxic materials out of the body.

Those who follow the most idiotic advice from the liver promoters, namely to eat it raw, have dramatically increased rates of parasitic infections and toxocariasis infections. These conditions are common for cats and dogs, but they are unusual for human beings, since toxocariasis is produced by roundworm infestations.

People should include some organic meats in their diets, but definitely avoid eating organs, and always cook meat thoroughly. Most of us need many more fruits and vegetables too.

Raw Meat and Fish

There are inherent dangers in eating uncooked food, because the bacteria on and inside the food is not killed before the food is ingested. There is a niché of people who proclaim that all foods (including meats) should be consumed raw. However, there is a huge likelihood of bacterial infection, and parasite infestation from eating raw meats. It is extremely dangerous, especially for children and the elderly. Raw fish ("sushi") presents the same dangers, and it should also be avoided. Any recipes which must contain raw eggs (such as homemade mayonnaise) should contain colloidal silver, to prevent sickness due to salmonella.

Iodine Drinking

There are people who drink iodine as a supplement, based upon the advice of scoundrels, or the quack book by Dr. David Brownstein. Taking iodine internally, except where naturally present in foods is reckless and dangerous. It will generally have an initial stimulating effect, which most users interpret to mean that an underlying deficiency is being corrected. This euphoric stimulation is actually a warning sign that the thyroid is being dangerously overdriven, and it will eventually fail. Other risks of oral iodine consumption include heart attacks and seizures. The fringe group that encourages iodine drinking is amongst the most fanatical and cult-like of the alternative medicine sects. They are so zealous that most health researchers cowardly avoid this topic altogether, for fear of inciting them. In comparison, the vegans and vegetarians seem like a calm and rational group. Iodine can safely be supplemented transdermally, or it may come from food sources. Information about the proper intake of iodine is inside the *Iodine* section of the *Supplements* chapter.

Green Coffee Beans

Following the popularity of green tea, the hyped fad of green coffee beans arrived on the market under the pretense that any green-colored thing must be beneficial. One of the primary claims is that green coffee beans can serve as a weight loss aid. Caffeine is a stimulant, and it aids weight loss; but this is not related to the beans being green. Roasted coffee beans have exactly the same property. An even more unscrupulous promotion regards products having extra chlorogenic acid extract added (at the chemical factory). The marketers boast of this product as being more of an anti-oxidant. Studies show that this unnatural combination causes diabetes.

Seaweed, Algae, and Other 'Super Foods'

We have Mike Adams to thank almost entirely for these scams, as much as Dr. Mercola got the krill oil supplement scam started, as with Dr. Weil's "Asian mushrooms".

Plants which grow in the oceans regularly clean the waters by absorbing contaminants, as bottom-feeders. Therefore, seaweed and algae are virtually always contaminated. These plants have been popularized as "sea vegetables" by some of the most unscrupulous. Those who eat such plants are consuming heavy metals and other pollutants. They are known for having PCBs. In the case of algae, some species contain their own bacterial toxins. The National Institutes of Health and Health Canada have issued warnings concerning blue-green algae, because their testing has shown that the bacterial toxins in common algae can lead to liver failure after long-term use. Their warnings applied to even the most commonly consumed algae types: spirulina and chlorella. Our recommendation is for humans to eat only human foods, instead of pond scum that is frequently found around the bottom of public toilets.

Copper Supplementation

Copper is a metal that is essential in trace amounts for good health. It is present in minute quantities in mineral-rich sea salt, and in produce. It is easy to get too much copper via supplementation, and even mild overdoses can cause organ damage. It is sold in pills and as a colloidal copper drink. The only way to supplement with copper safely is to use chlorophyll, or a topical copper lotion like the one that we produce. Oral copper supplementation is extremely dangerous, because overdosing is almost assured.

Detox Food Pads and Ionic Foot Cleanses

There are purportedly two types of foot cleanses: ionic foot baths and detox foot pads. Both are frauds. Detoxification foot pads were initially sold through infomercials and the Internet. They are now being sold inside major retail chains, including Walmart and Walgreens, with retailers smelling untapped cash flows. We have been researching long enough to know that their presence inside major retailers is allowed solely *because* they do not perform as claimed. Legitimate and effective alternative therapies have been categorically banned from retailers, without exception. Fraud products are allowed because they effectively satisfy the pharmaceutical agenda of destroying the reputation of alternative medicine.

Victims of the foot pad con are told to stick the pads onto the soles of their feet at night, and then the pads will almost magically pull toxins out through their soles, alongside removing candida (gastrointestinal yeast), mucous, and parasites. The pads become brown in most cases, which is claimed to be from the absorption of toxins. Yet, the pads turn brown even when moistened with 100% distilled water. This is an indication that the darkening is due to moisture from the feet. Some commercials have presented that the pads lighten in color every night, which supposedly proves that they are lessening the amount of toxins in the bloodstream. However, most users of the foot pads report no change in color from one night to the next. Their feet sweat about the same amount of salt water every night, in other words. The fact that there is a small portion of people who do actually get a reduction in color is a concern. For them, the pads are releasing a water soluble chemical that is absorbed into their skin, and it is toxic enough to impair the sweat glands. From what we know about antiperspirants, this means that the pads are releasing aluminum. Something very toxic is being put *into* the customers' bodies, instead of being removed. The F.D.A. silently blesses this sort of 'alternative medicine', because their petro-chemical industry partners could not ask for better malignment of their competition.

We searched for the ingredients of the foot pads, but we could only find partial lists. The product's marketers tend to boast about the presence of tourmaline. It is a boron silicate compound that always contains impurities, such as aluminum, iron, sodium, lithium, and potassium. Boron, by the way, tends to be especially toxic and inflammatory to the body.

Here is typical advertising from a seller of these pads:

> *"Utilizing only the highest purity of ingredients and the optimum blending ratios for maximum results - the Detox Foot Patch provides the one-two punch of the powerful detoxifying ingredients, in conjunction with tourmaline (the negative ion & far infrared producing mineral) to provide an unparalleled and effective external cleansing experience."*

We can read above that it creates "negative ions" and generates "far infrared" energy. The secret ingredient is obviously kryptonite. If these pads were really producing far infrared, then that type of energy is more appropriately called "microwave radiation". Even if these claims could be true, in some kryptonian parallel universe, do any of us *really* want our feet microwaved -- *for the sake of health*? What toxins do microwave radiation to the feet really cleanse?

The pads often contain mushrooms too, as if victims were not already getting enough heavy metals from the tourmaline. The mushrooms' metals will leach into the skin, but the mushrooms' usual natural antidote, selenium, is unlikely to be transdermally absorbed in enough quantity to help, as it normally does in foods. We can expect the usual result to be an amplification of heavy metal toxicity, and likely stimulated candida too. Fraudsters claim that the pads remove toxins from the body, but in actuality, they increase exposure to heavy metals and various chemicals. Most of the original Internet sales sites have disappeared, but the Internet is still riddled with foot pad cleanse products and smaller sellers. The imitations of the original Kinoki pads contain the same disturbing ingredients, and all of them have dishonest claims.

Ionic Foot Baths

The special ionic foot bath devices generally cost in excess of $1,000 (U.S.), and they are said to remove not only toxins from the body, but also candida, mucous, lung congestion, and joint pains. These devices consist of a basic D.C. power supply, wire, iron rods, and a plastic water container. Two 9-volt batteries and a piece of wire would do the same thing, so the manufacturers expend great efforts to make these devices look high-tech and medical enough to command a high price. Sessions with these 'medical' devices are available at some health food stores and chiropractic offices. If you are being *helped* by people who offer this service, then we recommend locating a more ethical practitioner.

In most cases, about a cup of salt is added to the water. Next, the victim is told to place his bare feet into the water, just before the device is turned on. It starts with bubbling, and a hazy material appears (which is explained to be "candida"). Over a period of about an hour, the water turns brown. To someone with no knowledge of electronics or chemistry, this carnival-like charade can seem very impressive. Victims are made to believe that toxins have been cleansed from their bodies, and they will often feel better due to the powerful faith effect. However, whenever the water from these sessions is actually tested, the only thing inside it is iron rust, and other metals in colloidal/hydroxide form. The same thing happens when feet are not submerged into the water.

The water becomes brown due to electrolysis (like electroplating). Electricity runs through the water, which is in contact with the conducting metal probes. This causes the probe metals to combine with the water; thereby turning it dark and hazy. Even in cases where salt is not added, there is salt on the skin and other naturally-occurring minerals that are released into the water, which makes the water conductive enough for this effect to be produced. The same result can be reliably obtained from a water container, two metal rods, salt, water, and a D.C. power supply. No feet are required.

Not only are toxins and candida not removed through the feet with these products, but these products actually increase the amount of foreign metals inside the body, due to skin absorption. These devices expose victims to large amounts of inorganic iron, and excessive iron is largely responsible for the high rates of heart disease in men. The iron that women and children need is much better obtained from dietary sources than ionic foot baths, and many people cannot properly use iron from inorganic sources. The inorganic iron saturating the water is generally more harmful to the human body than good.

The toxins of the human body rarely reside inside the feet, and they do not gravitationally fall whenever people stand up. Instead, the worst toxins tend to get stored inside fatty tissues and inside the liver. In order to truly cleanse the body, a legitimate heavy metal and liver cleanse needs to be done.

Silica Supplementation

Silica (silicon dioxide) is used in some powdered foods to ensure that they are free flowing. It is also used heavily in the manufacture of steel, thermal insulation, electronic circuit boards, semiconductors, and optical fibers. While its industrial uses are many, its health benefits appear to be nil.

Silica is a compound that is found in soil. There are people who have made the asinine assumption that it must be beneficial to health based on this. Another basis for the assumption about silica's benefits is the fact that trace amounts of it are found inside fruits and vegetables, which could produce some minor contributions to good health, but mostly to the health of those fruits and vegetables. Supplementing with silica has not been shown to provide any health benefit to humans, and all silica supplements contain far more silica than anyone could consume naturally.

Silica dust is a known carcinogen, lung irritant, and a central nervous system toxin. Although, it has been shown to be relatively neutralized when filtered through the human digestive system. This somewhat makes the point about how stupid silica supplementation really is. Since it is destroyed by the human digestive system, injections would be the only way to actually supplement with it. The website owners who profit from the fraud of silica supplements claim that it does all of the following:

Fraudulent Silica Claims

- Prevents Alzheimer's disease
- Prevents atherosclerosis (hardening of arteries)
- Strengthens bones
- Makes the skin "glow"
- Prevents hair thinning
- Increases mucosa during dehydration
- Improves circulation
- Prevents cancer

The list of supposed silica benefits goes on practically forever, so this is not a full listing of claims. It would be much simpler to list what its sales people do not make any claims about.

 Some companies have appeared on the market being dedicated to selling only silica, at prices which exceed those of real supplements. They are essentially selling sand as a high-priced dietary supplement, but it does not actually supplement any nutrient. Those who have a health condition can search the Internet for their ailment alongside the word "silica", and they will undoubtedly find accolades about it being the very "miracle" that they have been seeking. When silica is obtained for "supplements" from the horsetail plant (the standard process), it can actually cause a thiamine (vitamin B-1) deficiency. Thiamine is a real nutrient with real benefits. On the other hand, a silica (dirt) supplement simply is not going to be of much use to anyone, except the salesmen. A wise person should instead eat a balanced diet of natural foods, avoid refined sugars, and avoid chemicals. Sure enough, he will get trace amounts of silica in his diet too. Likewise, he will get trace amounts of other unnecessary elements that we would never recommend supplementing with, like arsenic.

> *"Studies in mice suggest that horsetail* [source of silica supplements] *may change the activity of the kidneys, causing abnormal control of the amount of water and potassium release. Low potassium, which in theory may occur with horsetail, can have negative effects on the heart."*
>
> -- U.S. National Institutes of Health

The above quote cites the only known effect of silica supplementation. Eventual heart attacks are hardly a desirable effect of any supplement. We do not know the effect of supplementing with small amounts of silica over an extended period of time. *No one knows*. All we know with certainty is that silica supplementation has never been proven to have any benefit for humans whatsoever, and we also know that it so thoroughly destroys the kidneys of laboratory animals that they become prone to having heart attacks.

Regular vitamins and supplements that contain tiny amounts of silica are not harmful; but the presence of silica will not present any therapeutic effect, either.

The H.C.G. Diet ("hCG")

In the 1950's, British physician Albert Simeons proposed that a hormone found in the urine of pregnant women could help to bring about weight loss. He believed that an injection of this hormone could allow people to survive on 500 calories a day, burn stored fat, and reduce appetite. Human chorionic gonadotrophin (H.C.G.) was tested extensively, but lost popularity until Kevin Trudeau wrote a book that advocated its use.

All studies on H.C.G. seem to follow the same pattern. Those who tested it alongside normal diets experienced no changes in weight, but those who followed Dr. Simeon's plan to restrict calorie intake to approximately 500 calories per day lost weight. Of course, it is really no scientific breakthrough to discover that starvation causes weight loss.

For some victims of this sham, the most bitter realization will be that this diet largely relies on the placebo effect, as will be explained in the next section. To understand this upcoming point, readers must note that true H.C.G. is only available by way of a prescription in the United States, which is what first clued us into something being amiss about the Internet and retail offers.

Most H.C.G. Is Glorified Water

The H.C.G. offered by the plethora of Internet scammers and retail stores is actually a *homeopathic* preparation. Homeopathic mixtures nowadays are based on the phoney theory of "water memory", including homeopathic solutions of H.C.G.

Due to real H.C.G. being available only by prescription, the non-prescription homeopathic preparations cannot contain any amount of the substance. Thus, the H.C.G. that is usually bought is homeopathic. It is only water, in other words. Luckily for the crooks, there is no way to test for the special homeopathic "memory" of their water products.

"Beyond questions about the effect of HCG, doctors also warn that the 500-calorie diet doesn't provide the body with enough carbs or protein and will send the body into a state called ketosis. Ketosis is a natural appetite suppressant."

-- Dr. Craig Primack, American Society of Bariatric Physicians

Ketosis is a dangerous condition, which leads to the blood pH becoming so extremely acidic that it is corrosive to internal organs. This state, induced by starvation, can cause long-term damage to the body. It has happened with both the homeopathic and the real H.C.G. versions of the diet, because people still attempt to survive from 500 calories. Ironically, a body will react to this perceived emergency state by attempting to metabolize everything into fat cells, because the diet triggers emergency starvation hormones. This can cause massive obesity problems for decades. Once the emergency starvation hormones have been activated, they are difficult to turn off. As far as the body is concerned, it is a live or die situation.

The Real H.C.G.

Prescription human chorionic gonadotropin is also an F.D.A. approved fertility drug, and it is listed in the Food and Drug Administration's Pregnancy Category X of drugs. That means anyone who takes H.C.G. while being pregnant is likely to have a child with birth defects. How is that for a known side effect of an approved *fertility drug*? Any serious research will produce a long list of potential adverse reactions. Most doctors, even those who specialize in weight loss, will not advocate or prescribe H.C.G. for these reasons. However, there are some dishonorable doctors who will, when they are pressured by ignorant patients. The following list is not complete, but it gives a glimpse into the reality of H.C.G. consequences.

Known Effects of Real H.C.G.

- Ovarian hyperstimulation syndrome (OHSS)
- Birth deformities, if taken during pregnancy
- Early puberty
- Prostate cancer
- Severe pelvic pain
- Swelling of the hands and legs
- Stomach pain and swelling
- Shortness of breath

- **Weight gain**
- Diarrhea
- Nausea and vomiting
- Headaches
- Depression
- Breast tenderness and swelling
- Edema
- Reduced penis size

Pharmaceutical H.C.G. is sometimes administered through a weekly injection, or in drops that are placed under the tongue. These are generally combined with the starvation diet to yield forced weight loss. One could just as easily substitute chemotherapy drugs for even faster weight loss. H.C.G. will cause a loss of muscle and organ tissues. A follower of the H.C.G. diet certainly will not be exercising, and he may have trouble with routine walking, due to the 500 calorie diet. The full effects of the protocol are sometimes only felt years later, when catastrophic damage surfaces. The delayed discovery of such side effects are usually not properly attributed to their real cause, so it is difficult to quantify how much damage the H.C.G. regimen does to its user population.

Most people who believe that they have tried H.C.G. are lucky to have only experienced the homeopathic memory water scam, and merely lost some money that would have been better spent on real dietary improvements. On the other hand, those who get a prescription for the real thing are getting much more than they bargained for. Our concern with the pharmaceutical is actually related to its efficacy. Starvation creates more fat in the long term, since a body will begin defending itself by storing everything as fat, in its emergency famine mode. Toxic pharmaceuticals frequently have the same fattening effect, because a body will protect itself by storing toxins that it cannot flush inside newly created fat cells. It is easy to lose *short-term* weight through poisoning, but this is hardly health wise. Instead, people should know that serious risks accompany this "wonder drug", and it is not part of legitimate alternative medicine. Its embrace by homeopaths seems to have created a bogus connection between H.C.G. and legitimate natural medicine, when no such association exists. Usage of this hormone comes with a high price. Read the *Dieting Right* section of the *Nutrition* chapter for an effective way to lose weight, without starving, and without any negative effects.

Unfortunately, natural and legitimate alternative medicines are sometimes incorrectly referred to as "homeopathic" by those who do not recognize the substantial differences. The same labeling problem occurs for legitimate herbalists and everyone else involved in legitimate holistic health therapies. It is segments like homeopathy, which lead to alternative medicine as a whole being dismissed as quackery. It is actually quite understandable, and sad.

DCA (dichloroacetic acid)

DCA is called dichloroacetic acid, dichloroacetate, and dichloroethanoic acid by chemists. It is essentially chlorine that is mixed with oxygen and acetic acid. This poisonous chlorine compound has been found in the tap water of some municipalities, which is something that even the World Health Organization has expressed alarm about. This toxic contamination occurs because bleaching agents are used to disinfect our drinking water. Oxygen would disinfect water better (e.g. hydrogen peroxide), and it would actually produce health benefits.

Symptoms of DCA Exposure

- Liver failure
- Decreased grip strength
- Neurotoxicity
- Kidney damage
- Limb paralysis
- Brain lesions
- Malignant tumors
- Inflammation of the pancreas

- Tremors
- Central nervous system damage
- Infertility
- Birth defects
- Hepatocellular carcinoma
- Sedation
- Muscle damage
- Diminished reflexes

Medicinal DCA

DCA does suppress some cancers, but it is a carcinogen itself. Using it as a cancer treatment requires even more than is needed for it to cause cancer. The amount necessary for it to have any effectiveness can kill a person, or lead to debilitating conditions. Proponents of DCA claim that it works by "turning on" the mitochondria, a crucial part of the DNA which regulates oxygen and cellular growth. However, dichloroacetic acid has been proven to cripple the mitochondria since the 1950's -- not assist it.

Judging from the effects of DCA on human health, it would appear that it *works* in the same manner as orthodox cancer treatments. It attacks the entire body, resulting in horrendous damage. It weakens all of the cells and the immune system. Mutated cancer cells are less resilient than healthy, respiration-using cells; so cancer cells are expected to die first when exposed to such poisons. Thus, the tumors may disappear, but it is important to remember that tumors are merely a symptom of cancer, which itself is merely a symptom of acidosis combined with toxicity, and possibly radiation damage. DCA actually stimulates the root causes of cancer: acidosis and toxicity. This leaves the patient with the same dismal chance of surviving cancer as if he had experienced standard therapies.

The parallels between this "alternative" and the mainstream are difficult to miss. This methodology of poisoning the whole body is identical to that of orthodox medicine, and it is why the long-term cure rates are so low. The methodology of poisoning a body into good health will be described as insanity by future generations, and rightly so. It will be mocked alongside other former 'miracles' of orthodox medicine, such as blood letting.

The trend of killing by medicine follows historical precedent. For example, while orthodox doctors of the not-so-distant past were using blood letting to kill people such as George Washington, natural physicians were prescribing herbal compounds, such as white willow bark extract that contained the active ingredient of aspirin. Eventually, the establishment *discovered* aspirin too.

When people read about alternative treatments, they generally assume that the treatments are natural and safer. These assumptions are well founded in the majority of cases. It is prudent to be watchful for alternatives that are actually dangerous pharmaceutical imitators. DCA is officially a part of orthodox medicine, but it has not yet become popular. Doctors provide it off-label, which is never the case for effective, natural, and safe alternative treatments. Allopathic doctors can be disbarred from practicing medicine if they recommend the Budwig Protocol, Gerson therapy, Hoxsey therapy, vitamin B-17, or mega-doses of vitamin C, as utilized by Linus Pauling. Yet they routinely prescribe dangerous and less effective chemicals, such as DCA, with no professional repercussions.

We were unable to find any dichloroacetate that is manufactured in the United States of America. The majority of DCA is produced in China. Therefore, it is likely to contain lead, cadmium, and worse.

There are safer, more effective, and natural ways to cure cancer and eliminate arthritis pain. There are proven methods that yield life-long cures: not just intermittent "remissions". Real medicine is cheap, painless, and without risk. Something is not medicine if it kills people. Fortunately, DCA does not have the same popularity as its weaker cousin M.M.S. However, if DCA becomes popular, not only will more people be harmed and killed by this treatment, but alternative medicine will be wrongfully blamed for their deaths. We, as a community, have a responsibility to both ourselves, and the prospective victims of DCA, to detach all associations between alternative medicine and it.

Magnet Therapy

Magnets are becoming popularized as a method for treating swelling and joint issues, with magnetic therapy growing to a billion dollar business internationally. This is due to massive marketing schemes. Magnet therapy advertisements plagued the June 2010 issue of *Carolina Country*, a free magazine that is distributed by the utility company, Energy United. The magnets were embedded into clothing, which allegedly relieves stiffness and fatigue. The product was essentially thick spandex underwear with embedded magnets. The manufacturer sells a large line of magnet-based 'therapies', and they hook their victims using products like the one described. That particular entry-level product was one of the cheaper ones ($9.97). It was merely designed to reel-in gullible people for future marketing.

Here is how the scam works. Customers are beguiled by the fact that the magnets *appear* to help, due to the tight and warm spandex wrapping; *not the magnets*. Attaching tight spandex bandaging to a swollen area will concentrate healing warmth, and its pressure will help to reduce swelling. This has absolutely nothing to do with magnets, and any sports coach can easily explain it.

It is important to note that the real agenda behind this particular product is simply to introduce victims to believable 'magnet therapy', so that they will eventually be purchasing magnetic bed covers too (above $100), magnetic jewelry, and even magnetic slippers. After all, a tight and warm bandage that helps to relieve a sore knee is indisputable proof that magnetic fields are beneficial to human health. It is the bogus connection that we are supposed to make.

Vendors take advantage of the fact that most people have no idea how magnets work. Thus, they can make claims which have no basis in reality. Here is an example from one of the magnet marketing web sites:

> *"Magnetic fields attract calcium ions in the blood, which then press against blood-vessel walls for a dilating effect that optimizes circulation. This improves oxygenation of injured tissue to promote healing."*

Magnets have no effect on calcium whatsoever, nor calcium ions. Magnets attract only iron and iron-containing compounds. They have an attraction to many of the commonly used steels and metals because they contain iron. The con men know that mesmerizing terminology like "calcium ions" sells products.

Studies have repeatedly shown that magnet therapy has no greater benefit than a placebo. That's not to say that the placebo effect isn't a powerful one, but it does mean that a lot of people are wasting massive amounts of money, and funding parasitic companies who fraudulently seek to profit from their continued suffering. The warmth generated by the aforementioned product will help to enhance the placebo effect, because the victim believes that he can actually feel it working via the bandage's warmth and pressure. Such victims are then likely to become life-long purchasers.

Copper bracelets with magnets have also become popular. They are alleged to assist with joint pains and arthritis, because they contain copper. While copper has been proven to help with these things, it is impossible for enough copper to absorb transdermally from a solid metal object to make any difference.

The Cult of Vegetarianism

Undoubtedly, many of our readers assume that we adhere to either a vegetarian or a vegan diet, because of issues concerning political correctness. In truth, we are strongly against such extremes. As people interested in truthful health reporting, it is our duty to inform our readers that vegetarianism is absolutely unhealthy and dangerous. This report may cost us some of our readers, but that is a risk that we are willing to take if it might save a few people from disease; and especially if it could save a few children from dying horribly. This is not a popularity contest for us. This is life or death, and the truth versus a cult.

There is nothing more perverse than when those who conform to such politics also dictate the same malnutrition upon their own children. News stories of children who have starved to death as a result of vegan diets continue to appear, and these diets are usually defended by the parents as being something good, all the way to prison. It is unknown how many uncounted vegan child deaths there have been, because such deaths are usually attributed to mysterious disorders; for regular doctors rarely examine nutrition.

Such parenting is based much more upon following a cult than it is about health, and we feel certain that there is a deep pocket in Hell waiting for such parents. Slowly starving one's children is the epitome of evil, regardless of whatever strained rationalizations are used to justify it. It is never justified. Such parents ought to be deeply ashamed, but few of them seem to be, even after the deaths of their own children. Their belief system overrides both their rational thinking and their consciences, and this is why we think of them as being cultish, in almost the same vein as the iodine drinkers. A child fed on a diet containing soy (the vegan protein substitute) is destined for impaired health for the rest of his life, with poor development combined with future thyroid and hormone issues. The lack of fats in a vegan diet makes just growing problematic. Red meat contains iron, which is desperately needed by growing children. Synthetic iron provided in supplements quickly becomes poisonous if allowed to accumulate, especially to infants and children, in addition to it being an extremely ineffective substitute for organic forms of iron.

Around twenty years ago, it was widely agreed in the scientific community that vegetarians do not get enough protein. This stance has since changed, because of marketing by the soy industry and political pressures exerted by the cult. Soy provides just enough protein for a vegetarian or vegan to survive, and it comes with great consequences. It is never adequate for a breastfeeding mother. Soy is always genetically modified, damages the thyroid, can cause infertility, causes deficiencies of zinc, deficiencies of iron, and scoliosis in children. Those who attempt a meat-free diet without soy usually fail, because they cannot get enough protein otherwise, even when nuts and legumes are used. For example, it would take 136 almonds, 239 peanut kernels, or 3.7 cups of kidney beans for a 140 lbs. person to get the bare minimal amount of protein needed each day. These conservative measurements are based on the R.D.A. (Recommended Daily Allowances), which have been repeatedly shown to be much lower than what is actually needed by healthy individuals.

Vegetarians often believe that they will have a longer lifespan as a result of their diets, but studies identifying any such relationship are scarce. There are two main studies that are used to show that vegetarian diets extend lifespan. The first study, *Diet, Metabolism and Lifespan in Drosophila,* is religiously cited as *the* "proof". It utilized fruit flies as the test subjects. Researchers gave the fruit flies a diet just slightly above malnutrition, and found that they lived longer than over-fed flies. Who would have expected that *fruit* flies could live best on fruit, or that over-eating harms health? The scientific methodology was more than a bit underwhelming. Should we give any credibility to such studies, which purport that malnutrition is beneficial, because it happens to be less harmful than gluttony, in the case of flies? This is clearly *F.D.A. science*, except this time, it's our side who is cooking the numbers. Fruit flies are hardly representative of humans, of course, and keeping one's diet just above complete malnutrition is not a wise long-term health plan. The research also showed that while the flies did actually live longer, they experienced more health problems, including infertility. The second study, which was conducted by the German Cancer Research Foundation, showed that those who lived the longest were those who consumed small amounts of meat and fish in their diet (balanced diet). Therefore, the real core finding (the very one being ignored) is that the under consumption of meat is as unhealthy as over consumption is. The latter study is also misquoted regularly for the sake of vegetarian propaganda. The two studies discussed in this paragraph are the alpha and the omega of "scientific proof". They have nothing else to stand on.

Carnosine is the Achilles heel of vegetarians, and this is especially true with the much more extreme vegan diets. Carnosine is a dipeptide which protects against aging, is a copper and zinc chelating agent, increases the lifespan of cells, is a pH buffer, assists in the contraction of the heart muscle, protects the brain from excitotoxins, and helps to prevent Alzheimer's disease (possibly through its extraction of heavy metals). Carnosine is only found in meat. Some vegetarians try to compensate with supplements, but such attempts are futile, due to the rate at which supplemental carnosine is excreted. When 248 mg. is consumed, it becomes undetectable within 5.5 hours. The minuscule synthetic 50 mg. supplements commonly used by vegetarians and vegans are useless.

It has become widely known that vegetarians do not get enough vitamin B-12. The luckiest vegetarians seem healthy for several years, before developing problems related to B-12 deficiencies. B-12 deficiencies result in a higher risk of heart disease and stroke, problems with the central nervous system, tingling in the hands and feet, fatigue, anemia, and it may eventually cause permanent blindness, deafness, or dementia. These problems are exaggerated in the elderly.

The health problems that vegetarians have associated with meat consumption only occur in meats which are laced with nitrates, antibiotics, and growth hormones. Even the hysteria surrounding saturated fats has been thoroughly debunked. We need those saturated fats, in moderation, of course. There are no valid reasons to avoid meats, because there are completely safe organic choices with animals that have been given their natural diets. The only typical meat that we avoid and recommend that others avoid is pork, for its overall help-to-harm ratio is poor.

Conclusionary Remarks

We do recommend juice fasting for short periods, especially for those who are suffering with certain chronic diseases. However, we would never recommend any permanent meat-free diet. We are aware that this chapter is likely to upset some people, but it is essential that these warnings are given. Vegetarian and vegan lifestyles have been embraced like a cult by those who refuse to listen to data that contradicts their religion. All of the justifications behind vegetarianism are bogus.

Dr. Andrew Weil

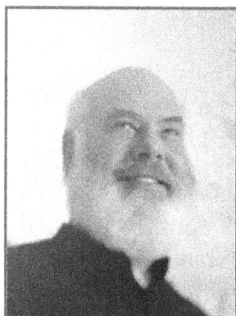

Andrew Weil (pronounced "while"), M.D., is a professor at the University of Arizona specializing in integrative medicine, which combines allopathic medicine with nutritional therapies. Dr. Weil is also a supplement spokesman, and a prolific author. The doctor is an icon for organic products and herbal supplements, a media darling, and a self-appointed leader of the alternative health movement. As if all that were not enough, Weil also has his own private medical practice, and is a proud graduate of Harvard University. Nowadays, one cannot stroll the aisles of most health-related retailers without seeing his face. These may be tough times for the rest of us, but business is great for Dr. Weil. At the beginning of his career, Weil lived on a South Dakota Indian reservation, where he studied herbal medicine and ritualistic healing with a Lakota medicine man named Leonard Crow Dog. In his 1972 book, *The Natural Mind*, Weil demonstrated his shaman influence by revealing his fondness for states of altered consciousness induced by psychedelic drugs, hypnosis, and meditation.

The backdrop of Dr. Weil's allopathic medical heritage causes us to wonder if he may be covertly aiding allopathic medicine by very publicly practicing alternative medicine in a manner which ultimately discredits it. He has been placed in an excellent position to do this by the long-standing enemy of alternative medicine, the mainstream media, whose funding from the pharmaceutical industry exceeds that from all other sponsors combined. We have been flabbergasted at how big media companies are so willing to aggressively promote Dr. Weil, when they have historically had a policy of mocking, suppressing, and marginalizing natural therapies. Our skepticism about the M.D. is founded upon an unmistakable pattern that is exposed herein.

"Keep your friends close, and your enemies closer."

-- Sun Tzu, *The Art of War*

General Sun Tzu knew that the surest way to destroy any enemy was from within, by undermining it with trickery and treason. The safest and easiest route for our publication would be, of course, to simply look the other way, as all of our cowardly peers have done. We are, however, striving for significantly higher journalistic ethics. To contrast the difference, Time Magazine featured Dr. Weil not once, but twice on the cover of its magazine; for issues which were dedicated to him. One of the articles confessed that Time Magazine was a partner corporation of Time New Media, which was bargaining with Weil for an affiliation contract.

F.U.D. and Industry

Not so long ago, during the so-called dot-com era, technology and Internet-based services were growing exponentially, at a rate never seen in any other modern industry. In the span of less than 10 years, we went from using the postal system and VHS video tapes to real-time streaming video, e-mail, and the mother of them all: the World Wide Web. Business in the technology industry was good; *really* good. Many of the meekly software companies quickly grew into titanic international corporations with billions of dollars flowing into them every year; and with no end in sight. It was an era fueled by incredible technological innovations by thousands of corporations and private projects. Foremost of the young mega-corporations was Microsoft. Greed got the better of them, and during the middle 1990's, Microsoft found itself in a court pile-on of epic proportions; fighting anti-trust charges concerning it having illegally used its monopoly power to destroy other companies. The charges were all true, and one of the most inflammatory of its predatory practices came to be known as "FUD".

The acronym F.U.D. referred to the dishonest practice of spreading <u>f</u>ear, <u>u</u>ncertainty, and <u>d</u>oubt about competitors' products, while pretending to be objective 3rd parties. Microsoft pioneered this despicable practice when it hired the marketing company, Waggener Edstrom, to pretend to be advocates of its top software rivals at various online technology forums. They half-heartedly pretended to promote the competing software at various Internet sites and in letters to editors, but they also simultaneously spread fear, uncertainty, and disinformation in these writings as a type of anti-marketing against competitors. They would post backhanded comments like, "Linux software is great, but they are still working on eliminating the hundreds of security weaknesses". Microsoft executives realized that fear and uncertainty are the most powerful weapons for destroying upstart competitors. Over time, this phenomena was noticed, because the questionable messages were traced back to the same locations, and it was noticed that all of them were written in a very similar manner. Unfortunately, Microsoft's campaign of F.U.D. against competition successfully ended the innovation of the dot-com era. Technological progress has been stalled for over twenty years, and that was the intent. Any new innovation is a threat to their monopoly position (the status quo), so Microsoft's executives consider meaningful technological progress as the company's greatest enemy.

The psychological warfare of F.U.D. is no longer just an issue of the software industry, and it is the surest way to protect established industry giants from innovative competition. Dr. Andrew Weil is an agent of F.U.D. and disinformation regarding the alternative therapies that he purports to espouse, as readers will come to understand.

Dr. Andrew Weil's Corporate Partner: Drugstore.com

We do not have much information about Dr. Weil's corporate partners, for Dr. Weil has made none of this information public. We became aware of Weil's business relationship with drugstore.com only because court-filed legal papers are public records. There is no way of knowing how many other pharmaceutical-industry business partners Dr. Weil has.

Casewatch.com reported the following from the records of the lawsuit of Brownstein Hyatt & Farber, P.C. on behalf of Drugstore.com in the case of *Drugstore.com, Inc. v. Dr. Andrew Weil, and Weil Lifestyle LLC.*

> "Drugstore.com is suing Andrew Weil, M.D. and Weil Wellness LLC for breach of a contract... the contact called for 'honorarium' payments totaling $1.6 million to Weil and minimum royalty payments totaling $12.4 million to the company from September 2003 through June 2008. Drugstore.com began featuring Weil's advice and products in October 2003, but the suit charges that he failed to 'make commercially reasonable efforts' to promote what was covered by the agreement. The 'Vitamin Advisor' uses an online questionnaire to promote 'personalized products' said to be 'based on your specific health concerns'."

According to papers submitted to the court, the Advisor Program was developed by drugstore.com, Weil, and members of his personal Science Advisory Board. The lawsuit further noted:

> "Pursuant to the Agreement, Weil Lifestyle and Weil agreed to promote various aspects of the parties' business relationship and to cooperate with Drugstore.com's operation and marketing of its online stores and services. In exchange, drugstore.com agreed to make monthly payments to Weil, Weil Lifestyle, and a foundation established by Weil Lifestyle ('The Foundation'). Pursuant to the Agreement, Drugstore.com pays Weil Lifestyle Monthly Sales Commissions and makes a monthly donation to the Foundation..."

Drugstore.com has paid in excess of $3.9 million in monthly sales commissions, donations, and quarterly true-ups (royalties). In addition to these amounts, Drugstore.com also pays a monthly honorarium directly to Weil.

> "I don't get money from the vitamins that I make. My after tax profits go to a foundation that supports integrative medicine."

-- Andrew Weil

The Weil Foundation

We have been led to believe that Dr. Weil does not profit from his sponsorships or his outrageously priced nutritional supplements, since he allegedly donates all of this income into the Weil Foundation. The Weil Foundation is registered with the I.R.S. as a 501(c)3 nonprofit charity, making it exempt from taxes. The name of this foundation is no coincidence; for all intents and purposes, Dr. Weil has been donating money to *himself*. He has stated that he pays taxes on his income before it is donated, but since he is required to pay income tax, this it is hardly the hallmark of philanthropy. This has been happening for many years, so it is likely that the high-profile doctor has some powerful friends in government. Meanwhile, he mentions that his proceeds go to a charity in his public appearances.

Publicly available financial records for the Weil Foundation are virtually nonexistent, which is something not found in the case of legitimate charities. We were able to gather some information from Weil's own Internet site for the year of 2007. The foundation's major benefactors for 2007 were the Arizona Center for Integrative Medicine at the University of Arizona in Tucson ($300,000), and the University of Arizona Foundation in Tucson ($250,000). The University of Arizona is Dr. Weil's employer. It is amazing what can be accomplished with creative accounting. We can be certain that Dr. Weil's job security with the University of Arizona is rock solid, and that he never misses a promotion.

> *"The Weil Foundation received nothing from Weil or his company in 2003 and 2004, according to the most recent tax returns the foundation filed with the Internal Revenue Service. Yet during that period, drugstore.com was contractually obligated to pay Weil and Weil's company some $2.5 million. Maybe the money was swallowed up in expenses before the after tax profits were computed. Or maybe when Weil says 'I don't get any money from the vitamins I make,' he's not including any salary or consulting fees his company may pay him. Or perhaps Weil is saving it all up to make a lump sum donation later. We tried to find out, but Weil didn't respond to repeated requests to his publicist, public relations firm, and foundation to talk about his marketing deals. In any case, Weil could have been more forthcoming about the foundation with the Today Show audience. When he said that 'my after tax profits go to a foundation that supports integrative medicine', he could have mentioned that the foundation's primary beneficiary is Weil's own program at the University of Arizona."*

-- Nutrition Action Health Newsletter

Dr. Weil's Backhanded Assault on Alternative Medicine

Andrew Weil hopes to eventually force all naturopathic practitioners to hold at least 4-year degrees, and to be *officially* licensed. Those who practice alternative health care would be forced to become the very people whom they have been trying to escape from. It would wrest control of alternative medicine into the hands of the American Medical Association if naturopathic and holistic healers were indeed required to be licensed by the same licensing boards. It would constitute Dr. Weil's greatest gift to Big Pharma and to the A.M.A.

The conflict of interest is massive, since Weil is the creator of integrative medicine, a college medical professor teaching it, and he is now promoting the mandatory integration of his own integrative medicine into the medical schools, while attempting to force all alternative practitioners to be licensed through this system. Despite the altruistic media image that has been constructed for Dr. Weil, it all looks a little too self-serving, and a little too much like a plan to make alternative medicine illegal.

Licensing means regulation, and alternatives would be soon regulated out of existence. Check and mate. Licensing would mean regulating therapies to be only those that are approved by Dr. Weil's future licensing boards, in the same crippling manner that is already seen throughout orthodox medicine. Not only would alternative health care providers live in fear of promoting "unapproved therapies" (even when these are just herbs), but additionally, average citizens could go to prison for "practicing medicine without a license" for merely helping neighbors with natural remedies. Dr. Weil was bold enough to boast about his plan during an online video entitled, *Naturopathic Medicine*.

> *"I think naturopathic doctors are well trained today and trained to operate within the scope of their practice. I also think there are natural partnerships between naturopathic doctors and medical doctors that are useful for both, and I see many opportunities for naturopathic doctors working in integrative medical clinics, which I think will be one of the forms of medical practice of the future. I think this is a natural partnership that can be useful. Many of the measures that naturopathic doctors are trained in, ahh, I think can lower health care cost, because the treatments are cheaper and safer than those used in conventional medicine."*

-- Dr. Weil, *Natural Medicine* video

Pay heed to the "operate within the scope of practice" part, which suggests that through licensure, alternative medicine will be controlled like the establishment's medicine. This would suppress unapproved methodologies, which would be a desired aspect of the "natural partnership" with the pharmaceutical industry. He uses some cunning tactics to promote licensing, including the usage of half-truths. Weil does indeed, "see many opportunities for naturopathic doctors working in integrative medical clinics", because he is the owner of integrative medicine, and he will be the final authority for naturopaths working in integrative medicine. While alternative medicine is practically always much cheaper than conventional medicine, having a license would not lower costs. The licenses would increase the costs of alternative practitioners, so that they would charge more to cover their exorbitant licensing fees that would be paid to enrich Dr. Weil further. He may not be much of a doctor, but he excels in law and business. Beware when anyone promises to help us by taking away our freedom.

Ivory Towers

The process of forcing licenses would once again ensure that only the wealthy could practice medicine, and history does not reflect kindly on the elite classes, like those from ivory towers who continue to dictate what is, and what isn't, allowed to be called medicine.

Weil's licensing scheme would be a repeat of the establishment, and more importantly, it would enable the establishment to control access to all health-related information by labeling alternative information as "unapproved claims" and treatments as "unapproved drugs", under the guises of licensing and regulations that are supposedly for our benefit. The F.D.A. has already threatened to remove cherries from the market as an "unapproved drug", due to accurate reports of how they eliminate arthritis pain -- so what is suggested here is actually standard procedure for how the pharmaceutical industry protects itself from alternatives.

In one discussion at his website, Weil suggests both surgery and radioactive iodine for those who have thyroid cancer, after admitting that it is a very slow-growing cancer. This would then be followed by a full year of birth control for women, due to the poisonous effects of the radioactive iodine upon the ovaries, which could cause birth defects. Despite the high risk of this therapy spreading cancer throughout the body, and in particular, causing leukemia; he remarked that he did not know of alternatives that were as effective. Our staff was able to find better alternatives to radiation with only a few hours of research, while he supposedly cannot with his three decades of training and his Harvard education. In fact, Dr. Weil is unique in the alternative community for making such suggestions, and for his appearance of blanket ignorance about standard alternative techniques for serious (the most profitable) health conditions.

The thyroid plays a critical role in the regulation of hormones and the metabolism. It absorbs the iodine that is found in our foods, and uses it to produce hormones that are paramount to the function of every cell in the human body. Cancer is a disease for which the alternative medical community has found cures, and it never recommends either radiation or poisonous treatments. Almost all of the alternative community mutually agrees that cancer can be cured through drastic changes in diet, avoidance of tainted water (e.g. tap water), internal food-grade hydrogen peroxide, omega-3 with sulfur proteins (The Budwig Protocol), key vitamins (in particular F.D.A. banned B-17), mega-doses of vitamin C, detox, and herbal supplements to help speed the process; since the root causes of cancers are internal fermentation combined with acidosis (low pH) and nutritional deficiencies. Instead of brutally attacking the entire body, the holistic process is one of correcting acidic body chemistry, so that the blood can again absorb oxygen at the rate it was intended to. This allows the immune system and the cells to begin functioning properly again. Alternative therapies tend to do much more than merely treat the symptom (tumors), and cancer cells are just a symptom of the real problems elsewhere. Dr. Weil seems not to understand these fundamental basics, and we cannot prove if his ignorance stems from his educational indoctrination, or if it is part of a manipulative charade that is intended to further marginalize alternative medicine.

Conversely, the orthodox use of chemotherapy and radiation as promoted by Dr. Weil are incredibly damaging to the entire body, and should be avoided, due to the way that these therapies attack all of the cells in the human body. The corruption of this system is shown by the fact that 20-90% of oncologists (cancer specialists), who were surveyed by the U.S. National Institutes of Health, would refuse their own treatments, dependent largely upon the specific type of cancer they had. Those treatments are fine for *us* and *our* families, however. The standard therapies actually fuel the internal fermentation process that triggers cancers; and therefore, standard treatments have long been documented to actually stimulate future cancers.

F.U.D. Allopathic Style

Dr. Weil strongly disagrees with holistic and naturopathic viewpoints. Although he founded integrative medicine, he is actually very reliant upon the standard treatments for serious conditions, and appears to support alternatives only in the area of nutrition, for lesser conditions which do not threaten the medical industry's cash cows.

> "[Dr. Weil] *cited such treatments as gene therapy, immuno-therapy* [chemically attacking and suppressing the immune system], *and anti-angiogenesis therapy, which involves blocking the development of new blood vessels that* [allegedly] *feed cancer. 'These hold the promise of being much less toxic treatments that I think may render chemotherapy obsolete, but at the moment chemotherapy is the best that we've got for certain kinds of cancers.'"*

-- C.N.N. (Cable News Network)

Most patients would prefer cancer over mutations in their genes, which could have horrific repercussions lasting throughout their family trees to all of their grandchildren's grandchildren, a total destruction of their immune systems, or the blocking of their critical blood vessels. He actually described these options as the "less toxic" *alternatives*.

No legitimate alternative practitioner would ever recommend these to even his worst enemy. We wonder what this could be other than an attempt to condemn alternative medicine with damningly faint praise, and these unique *alternative* treatments? In the typical M.D. manner, Weil made no mention of the real alternatives, and he merely recited some experimental biotechnology treatments that only effect tumors, instead of attacking the actual cancers. In the same interview, he parroted that many natural supplements (which compete with his own) are ineffective, yet he made no mention of the effects of his pharmaceutical recommendations, which cause heart attacks, diabetes, strokes, paralysis, seizures, stimulate more cancers; or how they are statistically less effective than nutritional therapies.

Perhaps Dr. Weil did not read the most recent U.S. Death Census, wherein adverse effects from pharmaceuticals are the 4th leading cause of death in the United States counting only the *properly prescribed* medications, and orthodox cancer *treatments* are the 2nd leading cause of death; because nobody actually survives long enough to die from the cancers anymore. The statistics indicate that pharmaceuticals shave 30 years from the average American's life. When comparatively combined, the industry's own records prove that it is the top killer in the United

States. How many people died of vitamin B-17 (anti-cancer) therapy last year? How many legitimate alternative practitioners would agree with Weil, who are not already a profiting part of his integrated medicine partnership? How many would subject themselves or their patients to his biotechnology experiments? How many of Weil's people would subject themselves or their families to Weil's "less toxic" recommendations?

Andrew Weil's F.U.D. Quotations

"I know of no effect of alcohol on tissue repair and no reason why you shouldn't drink alcohol (moderately, of course) after working out."

"I have always voiced the opinion that there should be a clear separation between a health care professionals recommendations and the potential to profit from those recommendations."

"Virtually every major US health organization has declared amalgam dental fillings, as they're known, safe, but some detractors remain unconvinced. Used to fill cavities, these dental fillings contain a mix of mercury, silver, tin, and other metals. Because elemental mercury and many mercury compounds can be toxic, some people worry that the dental fillings could be harmful."

"My advice is to stick with the antibiotic treatment your son is receiving. And what you might do -- what's better than using colloidal silver -- is investigate electromagnetic stimulation [radiation] *for bone healing, a treatment that is backed by scientific evidence."*

"Most doctors are taught to regard the placebo effect as a nuisance, but it's the meat of the medicine. Placebo responses are responses from within, elicited by belief."

"I'm not a proponent of the raw foods diet. First of all, when you eat everything raw, you lose much of the best flavor, texture and appearance of food. More importantly, however, is the fact that many of the vitamins and minerals found in vegetables are less bio-available when you eat these foods raw than when they're cooked. Another disadvantage stems from the fact that many of the natural toxins in edible roots, seeds, stems and leaves are destroyed by cooking. Although our bodies have natural defenses against these toxins, a raw food diet can add to the toxic load we're already dealing with. The latest word on raw food diets comes from a new study which shows that vegetarians who eat only raw foods have abnormally low bone mass, a sign that they may be vulnerable to osteoporosis."

"Sickness is the manifestation of evil in the body."

"It's unrealistic to imagine that you can never be sick. Health is cyclical: It breaks

down; it reforms. Being sick is part of being alive."

"Because autoimmune diseases tend to flare up in response to emotional ups and downs, I recommend some form of mind-body treatment hypnosis may be especially helpful (children are more easily hypnotized than adults)."

"The distribution of calories you take in should be: 40% to 50% from carbohydrates [sugars], 30% from fat and 20% to 30% from protein."

"It is more important to eat some carbohydrates [sugars] at breakfast, because the brain needs fuel right away, and carbohydrates are the best source."

"One claim holds that distillation removes all of water's beneficial minerals. While it's true that distillation removes minerals as well as various contaminants from water, we don't know that the human body can readily absorb minerals from water..."

"The underlying idea is that you can prevent disease by balancing your body's pH... None of these claims are true. Furthermore, your body needs absolutely no help in adjusting its pH. Normally, the pH of blood and most body fluids is near seven, which is close to neutral. This is under very tight biological control because all of the chemical reactions that maintain life depend on it. Unless you have serious respiratory or kidney problems, body pH will remain in balance no matter what you eat or drink."

"In general, I'm not a fan of products sold through multi-level marketing."

"The use of yage, or ayahuasca, in Amazonian Indian cultures is often credited with giving people visions that have valid content."

"You can lower your mercury levels over time by simply not eating fish likely to contain it."

"Children with autism can also benefit from probiotics, possibly because they decrease leakage of large molecules from the gut that can trigger immune reactions with effects on brain function."

"It's we who determine whether drugs are destructive or whether they're beneficial. It's not any inherent property of drugs."

"Early detection is key to winning the cancer battle. Once you reach the age of 50, the following tests should be done routinely... A digital rectal exam at the same time the sigmoidoscopy, colonoscopy or [radioactive] barium enema is performed... Consider taking aspirin therapy. Research suggests that taking a daily

low-dose aspirin over a period of years can cut colon cancer risk by as much as half."

"Some Essiac promoters irresponsibly advise against chemotherapy and other conventional treatments when using the tea. This is a reckless and dangerous recommendation... In fact, a 2004 study at the National Cancer Institute showed that Flo-Essence promotes the growth of mammary tumors in rats... can have unpleasant side effects... My advise? Avoid it."

Out of the Canola-Coated Frying Pan and into the Benzene

Dr. Weil was one of the pioneering proponents of canola cooking oil usage. The canola plant is the genetically modified offspring of the poisonous rapeseed plant, whose oil is an E.P.A. registered pesticide. The canola plant, in fact, did not exist prior to 1978. It was genetically engineered because its parent, rapeseed, had been banned in the United States for destroying people's hearts.

Upon its first appearance, Andrew wrote recipe books which emphasized canola oil, and claimed that it was the healthiest cooking oil. Dr. Joseph Mercola deserves credit for being one of the first people to uncover that canola oil is more-or-less a healthy cooking oil -- *until it is actually heated during cooking*. Once heated, canola oil becomes harmful to the body, and the rancid oil emits carcinogenic fumes. Whenever it is cooked, canola oil releases 1,3-butadiene, benzene, acrolein, formaldehyde, and other related poisonous compounds, which become infused into the foods being cooked.

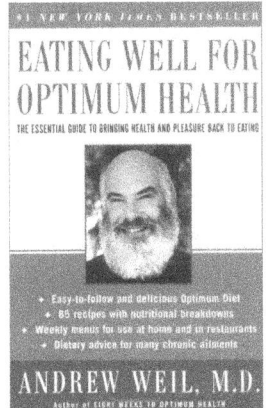

Dr. Andrew Weil Promotes CODEX

"I've had a lot of questions about Codex, often based on alarmist and erroneous information being circulated on the Internet. I'm happy to set the record straight. Here's the story: in 1963 the United Nations' Food and Agriculture Organization and the World Health Organization created the Codex Alimentarius Commission to protect the health of consumers and to ensure fair practices in the international food trade through development of food standards, codes of practice, guidelines and other recommendations."

-- Dr. Andrew Weil

Doctor and congressional Representative, Ron Paul, relayed the following on the Glenn Beck program (paraphrased). Codex Alimentarius, established in 1962 as a U.N. trade commission, serves corporate greed with no interest in health or consumer protection. The World Health Organization reported that Codex Alimentarius, "...has not made a contribution in human health in its 42 years of existence". Codex Alimentarius sponsors are Big Pharma, Big Medica, Big Chema (profitable toxic chemicals used on food and fields, including deadly pesticides banned in the U.S.), Big Agribiz (industrial factory farms that use antibiotics, drugs, and hormones to increase profits), and Big Biotech (creates dangerous genetically-modified organisms planned to become legal worldwide unlabeled). Codex Alimentarius has no actual legal standing, but it exerts enormous influence since it is used by the World Trade Organization to decide trade disputes. Codex-compliant countries win automatically; regardless of the merits of a case. Devastating trade sanctions result, so the U.S. is now racing to destroy protective laws that interfere with the implementation of Codex policies. The following list is what Codex has in store for us.

- Natural nutrients will be declared toxins that Codex will supposedly "protect" us from

- Ban virtually all natural health options

- High-potency supplements will be illegal

- Deadly drugs are sold unopposed

- Dangerous growth stimulants (hormones) made <u>mandatory</u> in all meat and milk (e.g. Monsanto's rBGH)

- Banned pesticides will be permitted in foods

- Untested, unlabeled, Frankenfoods (genetically-modified organisms)

- Free-radical enriched, radioactive foods (e.g. "cold pasteurized" or "irradiated")

- Weak and meaningless "organic farming" standards allowing dangerous drugs and chemicals in so-called 'organic' foods.

Conclusionary Remarks

Despite the seemingly insane advice of Dr. Weil, he is becoming increasingly popular amongst newcomers to the holistic movement, and his face has become an advertisement for many health products. His interest in becoming a walking commercial, and his zealous adherence toward promoting establishment protocols leads us to conclude that Dr. Weil is not as well-intentioned toward alternative medicine as he portrays. It is remarkable that he is being accepted as an expert, considering his own health. He boasts about his skin care products, while he has a terrible complexion, extreme hair loss, and is overweight -- all signs of severe acidosis -- something that genuine practitioners of natural medicine rarely experience. He is a walking example of a condition that he claims does not exist, but which is documented in even the standard medical literature. There are many out there who are just like him. They would love to monopolize supplements and alternative treatments, but Dr. Andrew Weil appears to be the most prominent of them.

We conclude that Dr. Andrew Weil is evil, for when he is not trying to sabotage alternative medicine from the inside, he is trying to corrupt us with his 'spiritual' teachings. As reported by the Organic Consumers Association, Weil's recent two million dollar donation to the Grocery Manufacturers Association will help to ensure that genetically-engineered foods remain unlabeled in the United States.

Mike Adams

The number of queries to The Health Wyze Report for information about fraudulent alternative medicines and unwise supplementation has increased dramatically during the past couple of years. Some of the requests included questions about the wisdom of eating mushrooms to cure cancer, *drinking* iodine for thyroid issues, and the supposed benefits of eating underwater plants. The questions might have been funny if the long-term implications of the misinformation had not been so tragic. As health researchers, we noticed unmistakable trends that could not be ignored concerning the increases in frequency of these requests. The spikes occurred especially after two events.

The first of the hallmark events occurred shortly after September 9th, 2008. It began with an article written by Mike Adams, and we immediately knew that it was something to be concerned about. The article related to a dramatic shift in his philosophy, and it was entitled, *The 7 Principles of Mindful Wealth*. In that article, Adams stated, "... it made me abandon five years of false beliefs and unlock a powerful new philosophy of financial abundance. I'm sharing that breakthrough financial philosophy with you here, but it's only something you'll find valuable if you're ready to let go of false limitations about money and welcome real, lasting change in attracting the money you deserve into your life... For nearly five years, I've been operating NaturalNews [formerly NewsTarget.com] in a way that practically guaranteed ongoing financial challenges. Because I never took money from the companies I wrote about -- and I never earned commissions on the products I recommended -- NaturalNews remained in a state of self-imposed financial stress." Mike noted that his new philosophy was based upon wisdom that he derived from a young girl who made homemade soaps. As his article dialogued their conversation together, Adams conveyed his attitude shift with the question, "Why shouldn't she be at least as wealthy as the executives at Proctor & Gamble who sell junk soap?". He pined in retrospect that he had operated Natural News like a charity, awhile earning the product companies that he had been previously plugging, "... tens of millions of dollars". Adams' financial epiphany purportedly happened when the young lady tempted him with the question, "... why are YOU the only one who doesn't benefit?". Mike's new guiding principle became, "Getting past self-imposed limits on wealth". He explained himself with the following dialog of what was purportedly spoken next. "'I explained to her that I could not earn anything from the products I recommended because that would compromise my integrity. People needed independent, objective recommendations, I insisted. My content had to be given away in order to be trusted.' She didn't entirely agree on that. '...It sounds to me like you've EARNED your credibility,' she said with a smirk. 'The only reason NaturalNews isn't earning more money is because you've voluntarily decided not to.'" At the conclusion of Mike's report about their conversation, which he commented was personally revolutionizing, he added, "But guess what? Karma doesn't pay the rent. Good karma isn't the recognized currency in modern society: Dollars are!".

The second event that preluded a noticeable flood in queries about health misinformation was the inclusion of Mike Adams as an official host of the Alex Jones Show. Mike Adams, the self-dubbed "Health Ranger" had greater ambitions than to merely remain the man plugging products for Natural News advertisers, so he found a way to reach millions by piggybacking the popularity of Alex Jones. In what might appear to be the result of yet another epiphany, Mike Adams remolded his persona into the image of Alex Jones to cement a mutually narcissistic union. The situation portrays a weakness that Mike has exploited to the maximum. Before their relationship began, the freshly patriotic Mike Adams had so despised the United States that he had relocated to Ecuador. With his new Alex-based personality, he's suddenly an all-American patriot who is fighting for American ideals.

Arial Software, Spam, and Telemarketing

Mike Adams is the C.E.O. of Arial Software. His clients include Microsoft, Zoom Airlines, Ebay, Gas Stations USA, DHL, XM Satellite Radio, and his company boasts to have 10,000 more customers. Thus, Michael Adams is hardly a lone ranger, who is battling against corporate giants and insurmountable odds. He is well-connected to some very powerful corporations. He should be exceedingly wealthy, because Arial Software's product is amongst the most expensive e-mail marketing options available, with many of his customers paying in excess of $5,000 for a single computer license. Even if all of his clients had only purchased the most minimalistic version of his software, which is priced at $985, he would have profited $9,850,000 (nearly ten million dollars) from his 10,000 clients; and of course, this estimate assumes that every company only bought a single license at the cheapest rate. If all of his customers had instead bought Adams' software at the maximum rate, his combined sales would have provided his company with a minimum of $50,000,000 (fifty million dollars). Arial Software has offices in the U.S. and Taiwan.

> "That's why today I still live in a modular trailer unit in Austin, I still drive a Toyota pickup truck, I dress like a rancher in blue jeans and flannel shirt, and nobody gives it a second thought when I'm out in public... Some people want to look rich and popular, so they wear a lot of bling, and they drive a high-end car they can't afford, and they live in a house they can't pay off, and they try to fool everybody into thinking they're rich and powerful. I'd rather fool people into thinking I'm NOT powerful."

-- Mike Adams

For years, programmers have worked tirelessly to find ways to block spam e-mails. Some systems block based upon keywords, while others search for sentence patterns in e-mails that are typical of spam messages. Mike Adams and Arial Software have been working to find ways around this spam detection. Our research indicates that Arial Software is solely a spamware company, meaning that its software is designed primarily to aid spammers. Arial Software has composed press releases, complete with quotes from Mike Adams, boasting about its ability to evade security.

> *"Once a personalized email message is composed, Campaign Enterprise Version 7.5 users can simply press the 'Anti-Spam Test' button to perform an instant check of their outbound email. The message is then instantly run through a pre-programmed checklist, which uses a set of evolving criteria to evaluate the outbound email message as anti-spam compliant. If any part of the email message resembles the traits of Spam, the user is alerted that the intended email message could be perceived as Spam by recipients or email filters."*

> -- Arial Software, Press Release

Arial Software's Campaign Enterprise software is designed to warn spammers when recipient spam filters are likely to intercept their messages, so that they can reword their messages to evade the Internet's mail security systems.

Mike Adams ironically owns SpamDontBuyIt.org, a web site that is allegedly aimed at instructing people not to buy from spammers. Yet this web site portrays that spam is a consistently profitable business, because some people actually purchase products that are advertised in spam e-mails. Mike wrote that it is this small percentage of people who truly bear responsibility for spam's continued existence. Mike Adams' anti-spam site appears to be created for the sole purpose of shifting blame from the responsible spammers onto the victims. The blame for spam should rightfully lie upon the spammers themselves, as well as those who promote and create specialized software for bypassing anti-spam security systems; companies such as Mike's own Arial Software.

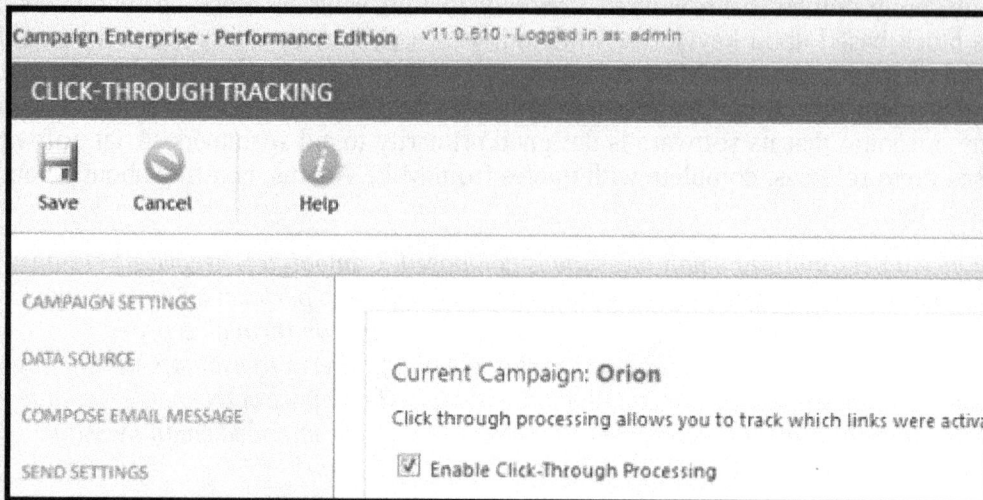

Above is a screen shot of Mike's Campaign Enterprise mailing software in action. Notice the nifty tracking feature? Secretly tracking people is always important when trying to monetize, and for building a list of suckers who will actually buy from spam.

In 2006, Mike set up hundreds of different domain names (Internet sites) providing thousands of web links back to Natural News. It reflects a practice that is used by spammers and so-called "viral marketers", which is meant to artificially improve a site's listing position in search engines. Internet search engines frequently judge the popularity of web sites by the number of other web sites that link to them. By creating lots of web sites with hundreds of links back to Natural News, Adams propelled his site to the top of the search engine results. It is a method which cheats the system, so that one's own site will be found more often on the Internet, in place of sites having better and more appropriate content. Such shenanigans have historically made it difficult for search engines to be effective in finding the best information. Eventually, search engine programmers began instituting countermeasures against this shady practice, and enacted punitive measures to lower the list positions for unethical web sites, such as Natural News. As a result of these search engine changes, the overwhelming majority of Adams' early web sites have now been shut down. Adams presently owns only a tiny fraction of the domains that he once did. Nonetheless, during a period of approximately five years, Natural News was able to artificially boost its Internet popularity through this unscrupulous practice.

We are still able to verify the records for 199 of Adams' former (450+) sites which contained Truth Publishing's address and contact information. The most commonly listed address in the whois records was:

```
Truth Publishing
12F-4, No.171, Sec. 4, Nanjing E. Rd,
Taipei, Songshan District,
Taiwan
```

Truth Publishing's official headquarters is at exactly the same address as Taiwanese telemarketing company, Enspyre. This address is still listed in the registration information for some of Adams' remaining sites, such as naturalpedia.org. For his flagship web site (naturalnews.com), Adams used the Domains By Proxy privacy service to make certain that nobody can look-up the information.

The Character of Mike Adams

On October 28th, 2008, Adams published an article entitled, *Green-Lipped Mussels Omega-3 Oils Join Moxxor*. The article explained that Adams had partnered with a direct sales (multi level marketing) company to sell green-lipped mussels as a supplement for omega-3. As part of this business partnership, Mike Adams promised to write friendly articles about the mussels, replete with links to sales sites.

> *"In fact, we've planned a whole series of articles on green-lipped mussel oil. And guess what? When you're on the NaturalNews Moxxor team, you can freely post these articles on your own web site or blog site, and replace our own enrollment link with YOURS."*

-- Michael Adams

Only one month after Adams' epiphany about wealth generation, he began writing articles expressing new beliefs in supplement methodologies, in order to sell products that personally profited him. He likewise encouraged his audience to promote the product line too. Adams was soon placed on Moxxor's Product Formulation Advisory Board in exchange for his willingness to play ball.

> *"The universe wants you to attract more financial resources when you're the right person to decide how to use it. And here I was, in the headquarters of the Moxxor company, being invited by the founders to participate in a potentially huge health-related financial opportunity being put right in my lap."*

-- Mike Adams

When the movie *Avatar* was released in late 2009, Adams promoted it:

> *"The concept of Gaia is also unleashed in the film, although it's never referred to as Gaia. At one point in the film when all hope seems lost for the natives, Jack Sully prays to Gaia to help save them, at which point the female character Na'vi says, 'Mother Nautre doesn't take sides. She only maintains the balance of life.' This demonstrates a much deeper understanding of the role of nature than most modern humans grasp."*

> -- Michael Adams

The phrase "Mother Nautre" was not actually a part of the dialog. It was later edited into the quote by Mike Adams, including the spelling mistake. Gaia was the name of a goddess from ancient heathen religions. She was the "Great Mother" because she was said to be the mother of all the other gods. It is from this mythology that the phrases "Mother Earth" and "Mother Nature" arose. With the growing thread of paganistic environmentalism in society, the term "Gaia" is being seen increasingly. The pagan religions have always been involved in nature worship, and they have long promoted that the Earth is a female figure, which should be worshiped. The pagan infiltration into the alternative health movement has led to a massive promotion of their belief system. These people typically believe that environmentalism should have a higher priority than human life. It is why carbon dioxide, which humans expel, has been vilified in recent years.

> *"In his book 'Her Hidden Children: The Rise of Wicca and Paganism in America' Pagan scholar Chas Clifton notes that the environmental awakening of 1970, the year of the first Earth Day, 'was a year when Wicca (in the broad sense) became nature religion, as opposed to the mystery religion or metaphorical fertility religion labels that it had brought from England.' Since then, modern Pagans of many stripes, particularly Wiccans and Druids, have placed a special emphasis on being religions that care for, and have concern about, our natural environment. A who's who of Pagans, both high-profile and not, have told the press, and the world, that we give special concern to problems facing our natural world, and further, that our faiths represent a positive shift away from abuse and towards sustainability."*

> -- Jason Pitzl-Waters

Alex Jones summed up the problem so well that we are quoting him:

> *"This film [Avatar] is pure propaganda... The U.N. has stated on record that they want to set up a global Gaia religion to sell the population of the Earth to have less resources, instead of developing their resources. And the movie says that earth is dead, and that humans are bad... It is total occultism, with Shaman ceremonies, with the horned god male and the goddess female... This film has come out now to push this global religion that Al Gore has openly pushed for."*

The religion that is being metaphorically encouraged by the global elites in the Avatar movie is one in which people worship the Earth and are willing to surrender all items which harm "her".

> *"Every pharmacy, health food store, shaman and medicine man openly talks about the anti-cancer properties of various herbs* [in Ecuador]... *Why would any nation want to lock up its healers?"*

> -- Michael Adams

Adams attempted to legitimize occult shamans and medicine men, calling them healers, instead of savages who get their mysterious 'knowledge' from spirits and hallucinogens. We noticed other indicators of Adams' *spiritualism* when reading about his interaction with Moxxor, the direct sales company that he partnered with.

> *"Furthermore, I specifically asked that before the harvest of the green-lipped mussels, the aquaculture fields be blessed with positive intention, and thanks be given to the oceans and Mother Nature for providing such abundance. They not only agreed; Noel invited me to New Zealand to bless the aquaculture fields myself!"*

> -- Michael Adams

Blessing or cleansing with "positive intention" is a pagan magic (witchcraft) practice. Modern day witches like to "clean" their magick crystals by rubbing their hands across the crystals whilst thinking so-called "positive thoughts". The fact that Adams wished to give personal thanks to Mother Nature further indicates that he believes Mother Nature to be a conscious, living deity, instead of merely a metaphorical phrase used to describe all life.

> *"And here's the philosophical contradiction in the liberty movement today: Too many of those who say they want the government out of their lives on issues like vaccines, parenting and local farm food are the very same people who demand government intervention on issues where someone else lives by a different moral code than their own (or a non-existent moral code, in some cases). Same-sex marriage, prostitution, abortion, recreational drug use you name it... Are you reacting to this story and thinking that people who engage in activity you don't morally agree with should be arrested or criminalized? If so, then you don't really believe in freedom. You believe in tyranny."*

> -- Mike Adams, Natural News

It is actually the core job of law enforcement to enforce morality, which is what our most fundamental laws are based upon. Morality is what tells us that it is unconscionable to kill another human being. The laws punishing murderers are in place because they give force to our most important morals. Adams contended that "tolerance is liberty" in the article's subtitle, but being unconditionally tolerant of the immorality of others would leave us in a world that nobody would want to reside in. For any nation to survive without a moral compass, it must become a police state to save itself from its own people. This has happened in nation after nation throughout history. Contrary to Mike's assertions, real freedom is not about the right to do wrong without consequences, which seems to be something close to his heart. Real freedom requires personal responsibility, and responsibleness is always a product of a moral code. Adams confessed his belief that a society could become more free by simply disregarding its moral values, but it is specifically a nation's moral ideals upon which the rights of its citizens are derived. His ideology of ignoring the destruction of one's neighbors and being selfishly concerned only for oneself is an accurate definition of immorality. Showing his anti-Christian bent again, Mike contended that morals are a type of slavery, but history proves the opposite. A non-existent moral code has been the basis of every communist regime, and we shall never find better examples of tyranny than those.

In 2008, Mike decided that it was time to abandon everything American, so he moved to Ecuador. He stated that he had become so concerned about corruption and poor health care in the United States that Ecuador was a wiser choice of homelands. Ecuador is a country that is plagued with poverty, kidnappings, disease, poor hygiene, and its citizens are often without access to clean water.

> *"In fact, I had many friends in law enforcement in Ecuador, and I spoke with them regularly. Sure, they were a little corrupt, but not in an over-the-top criminal way like with the FBI..."*

> -- Mike Adams

Ecuadorian immigration can be gained by anyone who purchases an expensive property in that nation. Citizenship in Ecuador can be literally bought. While in Ecuador, Adams partnered with a local real estate company to encourage his readership to join him. He even offered tours for interested parties. Adams regularly wrote articles about Ecuador, including tips to help visitors avoid theft. Then, after spending two years there, Mike decided to return the United States, stating that Ecuador did not provide him with enough privacy. So he naturally moved into a low-population area: Austin, Texas. At the time of this writing, Adams is still attempting to sell his Ecuadorian home for a measly $695,000, which comes with all of the Ecuadorian luxuries, including electricity from a gasoline generator.

When Adams distributes information about curing diseases, it is usually in the form of e-books, and the information is not free. For example, *How To Halt Diabetes In 25 Days* is available for $19.95. Adams claims to possess life-saving information, but then he acts as the gate keeper to that special knowledge. Even the mainstream medical establishment does not restrict vital information. While physical access to pharmaceuticals may only be available with a doctor's approval, the actual information is never restricted. We feel that withholding supposedly life-saving information until the victim of a disease pays a fee is wholly unethical, regardless of whether there is real value in the information. As researchers ourselves, we feel that if Adams were truly interested in helping people, then his allegedly critical information would be free. We made certain that our health information is always free on the Internet, including this chapter. Health information should never be used to bully whip people into choosing between paying or suffering consequences.

Health and Nutrition

On March 29th, 2011, Michael Adams published an article at Natural News titled, *Vegan parents charged in death of baby raised on mother's milk; facing 30 years in prison*. The article reported about an 11-month-old infant who had only been fed breast milk from a vegan mother. The child subsequently died from malnutrition. After the autopsy, it was predictably revealed that the child was extremely deficient in vitamin B-12 and vitamin A.

Mike Adams wrote:

> *"The baby died at 11 months of age, and when ambulance workers arrived and found the baby dead, instead of consoling the parents, they called the police. Why? Because the parents were vegans."*

Mike's detective-like analysis revealed that the emergency medical technicians were conspiring to keep the vegans down. When ambulance workers arrived, they found a child who was considerably underweight. Thus, the situation seemed very suspicious. The child had been suffering with a case of bronchitis, which was severe enough for a doctor to recommend that the child be hospitalized. The article at Natural News conveniently omitted this critical fact throughout its long glorification of the allegedly victimized parents. The parents had ignored their child's spiraling health issues, took their sick child home, and then they continued providing it with nutritionally-inadequate breast milk from the vegan mother. In contrast to this behavior, whenever people get sick, they require more fats and proteins in their diets, but the dead infant never got those.

Adams continued:

> *"Never admit to state authorities that you are raising your baby on a vegan diet. This immediately raises suspicion among the state child protective enforcement morons who have zero nutritional knowledge and probably still run their own fundraisers by selling donuts to families. If asked, just tell 'em you feed your baby a 'balanced' diet that includes a little bit of meat, a bit of cheese, and so on."*

Adams unintentionally admitted that a vegan diet is not balanced, and he recommended that vegan parents lie about what they feed their infants, in order to continue malnourishing their children unabated. Incredibly, Adams made these callous recommendations whilst reporting the death of a child, who died as a result of an inadequate vegan diet. Adams actually blamed the ambulance workers, and suggested that if junk food wrappers had been seen, then the paramedics would have had no problems with the child's terrible condition. He then self-righteously (and falsely) proclaimed that 7-year-old vegetarians do not get cancers. However, this young child never reached the age of seven because of a diet that was blessed by Adams, and it continued receiving Adams' blessing even after the child died from it. He blamed the emergency responders.

> *"And the third reason is because I would never want to be associated with the kind of people who live on steak and animal products as primary food sources -- those cigarette smoking, steak eating, pro-war, wife beating alcoholic numnuts who think global warming is a hoax and that that the whole world would be better off if we all just ate more beef and drank more milk."*

> -- Mike Adams

Adams' zealous anti-meat stance is something that he keeps private most of the time, especially when he is on the Alex Jones Show. Alex's audience is comprised of more astute people than Mike's regular audience, so they already grasp the nutritional importance of eating meats. Adams appears to hate meat eaters on a very personal level, but these personal problems disappear whenever he is partnering with Alex Jones, who is a "flesh eater". Adams is likewise careful to avoid mentioning the topic of global warming, because he is a true believer.

> *"So what to do? Well, for one thing, if you are on a vegan diet, don't forget the B-12 and the omega-3 oils -- two nutrients that do tend to be very low in many who pursue vegan diets. A vegan diet requires a lot of nutritional monitoring to make sure you don't leave out a few things."*

Vegans leave out more than just a "few things". Vegetarianism is like a bad religion, because there are only two types of vegetarians: those who know nothing about nutrition, and those who do know but nevertheless ignore the facts. A vegetarian diet is so unhealthy that they must regularly take nutritional supplements to compensate for their self-induced malnutrition. Without supplements, the drastic health implications are profound. Despite attempts by vegetarians and vegans to convince the world that their lifestyle is healthier, their vitamin B-12 deficiencies result in an increased risk of heart attacks and strokes. Adams typically neglects to mention most of the vegan deficiencies, but some further examples include carnosine, vitamin B-5, safe and effective iron, the most usable form of vitamin A, iodine, vitamin D, and of course, protein. The enormous nutritional deficiencies are why vegetarians must try (with varying success) to compensate by using toxic soy products. Even in the cases wherein soy products are capable of adequately compensating for the missing proteins, it still slowly destroys the person's overall health through its own inherent toxicity, and practically all soy is genetically engineered.

> *"There are a lot of negative effects associated with the consumption of red meat, and this is why more and more people are now giving up red meat and moving to healthier foods like fish, free-range chicken, or better yet, plant-based proteins like spirulina or soy products like soy milk and tofu. This is where you'll get your best protective effect and disease prevention, and you will be helping protect the*

environment at the same time. After all, it's far less stressful on the environment to produce food as plants than as animals."

Due to the lack of available proteins when no animal products are in the diet, Adams routinely recommends soy as a viable, healthy option for his vegan followers. The promotion of soy is one of the fastest and most reliable ways to distinguish when someone's advice cannot be trusted. The public has known about the dangers of soy for decades. Virtually all modern soy is genetically engineered. Soy contains toxins even in its original organic state, and it is always processed with genetically-engineered bacteria to lessen its toxicity, before they really start the chemical processing. Soy contains phytoestrogens, which are natural hormone disruptors that more-or-less mimic estrogen. These phytoestrogens produce severe hormonal imbalances, particularly in women; so soy consumption has greatly contributed to the epidemics of hypothyroidism and endometriosis.

Ironically, Mike's own Natural News features dozens of articles about the dangers of soy, but none of them were written by Adams, who continues to ignore soy's dangers. Adams acknowledged that pure soybean oil is used as a pesticide, but he still does not recommend against soy as a food. The phytoestrogens in soy are the plant's defense, which work to disrupt insect hormones to the degree that they cannot reproduce. Soy does the same thing with human fertility to a lesser degree.

In July of 2005, Adams released his backwards food pyramid, which he described as the "Honest Food Guide". It listed soy twice as a *health food*. Red meats were listed as the most unhealthy of all foods. In fact, meat was said to be far worse than donuts, soft drinks, or candy bars; but incredibly, diet products were the least harmful of the harmful items. Dairy products were rated in the middle, being unhealthier than candy bars. His top choices for human "superfoods" included seeds, kelp, and of course, soy. Many of Adams' recommended foods are not even foods at all. Algae such as chlorella and spirulina are prominently listed and recommended as healthier alternatives to food. Mike's "honest" food guide notes that eating meats will cause a person to become "easily injured", have "chronic pain", and to be "frequently sick". "Sea vegetables" (algae, kelp, etc.) on the other hand, were claimed to produce "mental clarity", "accelerated learning", and even prevent a person from becoming sick. These are the sort of false medical claims that could eventually land Adams in prison, since they specifically refer to products that he sells.

One of Adams' favorite words is "superfood". His superfoods ironically tend to be non-food items, or selected commercial products that are sold in the Natural News store. Mike's most commonly promoted *superfoods* are chlorella and spirulina. The biggest problem with these algae is that they are typically contaminated with toxins and heavy metals. The U.S. National Institutes of Health warns that contaminated algae products cause liver damage, and even certified algae is potentially contaminated. This is because algae can only be accurately tested whenever the testing laboratory already knows what contaminants to test for. It is impossible to test for random unexpected contaminants, and that is what is found in sea water. With most algae supplementation, ocean pollutants will accumulate inside the liver, doing cascading organ damage over time. When the symptoms of a dysfunctional liver become severe enough to get noticed, the unchecked damage is usually quite serious. Health Canada reported that almost all of the blue-green algae supplements that they tested contained organ toxins, and they strongly cautioned against their usage. It is truly ironic that those who are eating Mike's so-called "superfoods" are likely to develop liver dysfunction. Liver impairment makes a body much less effective in cleansing itself of future toxins. Red marine algae is the only underwater plant that is reasonably safe for routine supplementation, because it has a special tendency to not absorb most toxins, which is the opposite of most underwater plants. However, red marine algae is the only one not sold by Mike's online store.

A truth you will never learn from Adams is that most lean organic meats are absolutely harmless in moderation. All negative effects from red meats (such as beef and lamb) can be traced to industrial impurities. Examples are vaccines, artificial hormones, pesticides, antibiotics, metals, and most especially the nitrate compounds that are used to make the meats toxic enough for an extended shelf life. Those nitrate salts are extremely carcinogenic. Some of the meats even contain chemical colorants to prevent them from turning green or gray. None of the known disease issues exist for organic, range-fed animals, so why does Adams never mention *organic* meat? If he really wants to save the maximum number of people from cancers, then recommending organic meats is more likely to help people than recommending algae, which he already knows will be avoided by most people. He refuses to make a distinction between natural red meats and industry-tainted meats. Furthermore, he does not make distinctions between the types of red meat and their differing nutritional properties. These slight-of-hand tricks are political attempts to link harmful meats like pork with highly beneficial meats like beef, lamb, and venison.

> *"I sometimes blend it with fruit smoothies as well. We just happen to still have this at a significant discount at our store, by the way."*

> -- Mike Adams

On November 22nd of 2010, Mike Adams published the article, *The Top 10 Superfoods I'm eating everyday*. The article did not mention vegetables or other wholesome foods; but instead, he recommended product formulations that are available in the Natural News store. These formulations include such ridiculous ingredients as algae and pumpkin sprouts.

> *"I don't think people should eat animals at all, but if you're going to eat them, the brain is actually one of the most nutritionally-dense organs found in any animal. From a nutritional standpoint, the brain is the best source of healthy oils in all land animals... Those who eat more DHA have been clinically proven to be smarter in adulthood. And guess what's found in cow brains? DHA."*

> -- Mike Adams

Mike attempted to disgust his meat-eating readers; and in the event that this approach did not work, he encouraged them to get themselves killed. One of the reasons why people do not eat cow brains is because it causes Creutzfeldt-Jakob disease (mad cow disease). This is an incurable disease, whereby a human brain develops tiny holes and becomes sponge-like. *It is always fatal.* For this reason, few people eat cow brains, tonsils, eyes, or small intestines. Adams apparently despises meat eaters to such a degree that he recommended something that might induce a fatal illness in them.

People have renamed meats when discussing foods throughout history. For example, most people refer to a slab of cooked beef as a "steak" instead of a "cow slice". Instead of "deer", we say "venison". The only exception to this rule of civilized society is fish. Whenever Mike Adams writes about meat, he usually uses the phrase "animal products", and sometimes "flesh". Adams consistently refers to foods by their animal names, apparently in an attempt to disgust meat eaters. His word games can be noticed throughout most of his writings, and he infrequently even refers to steaks as "flesh steaks". Adams commonly refers to meats as "dead foods". Of course, the vast majority of all foods, meat or vegetable, are dead. Contrary to Mike's assertions, dead foods are not a bad thing. Food is usually cooked to make sure that everything, including bacteria, parasites, and various other pathogens are dead. Even Mike's top *superfoods* are sold dead.

The Natural News store features Nascent Iodine, an iodine product that people are expected to drink for the purpose of detoxification. The site describes it as a "transformative iodine in a bio-elemental nanocolloidal state". We are unsure about what it transforms into, or where bio-elements are found. Iodine is not a cleansing agent, but it can slowly neutralize accumulated fluoride. It does not remove heavy metals or other toxins from the body, which is what a real cleansing formula does. Even potassium iodide does not really cleanse the body. It simply saturates the thyroid and ovaries with iodine-like compounds to prevent radioactive iodine from being absorbed into these tissues during nuclear emergencies. Iodine can speed the metabolism, but that neither results in cleansing effects, which may be something else that Adams is confused about. He claims that his iodine product "maintains DNA integrity" and assists in "improving thinking". Iodine does neither. On multiple occasions, we have been contacted by people who have damaged their thyroids as a result of taking iodine orally, based on similar health shams.

We have written previously about the dangers of orally supplementing with elemental iodine. There are only two ways to safely supplement with iodine orally, and Mike's supplement utilizes neither. The preferred method is to have a diet rich in fish, which will solve a multitude of other nutritional issues. The other safe oral method of iodine supplementation is through red marine algae supplements, but they should be used with care. Transdermally supplementing with either iodine or iodide is usually safe, so long as it is not povidone iodine. Supplementing with iodine (especially orally) can be fatal in a person who has Hashimoto's thyroiditis. There is no warning given about this at Natural News.

One of the reasons why Adams encourages the intake of iodine and algae is because vegetarians and vegans are often deficient in iodine, but the reason behind these recommendations is never admitted -- namely that his other recommendations cause the iodine deficiency. The Slovakian study, *Iodine Deficiency in Vegetarians and Vegans,* showed that a quarter of vegetarians and 80% of vegans are iodine deficient, according to standards set by the World Health Organization. Most people obtain iodine from their consumption of chicken, fish, and beef. The severe iodine deficiencies that are seen in vegetarian mothers and their very young, protein-starved children lead to cretinism; a type of mental retardation. The iodine deficiencies that are caused by vegetarian diets can have permanent detrimental effects upon the intelligence of developing children.

> *"Sunbiotics' Daily Chewable Tablets are a potent probiotic supplement enhanced with Organic Yacon Root - a superfood renowned for its prebiotic properties... These FOS have been recently classified as 'prebiotics.' Since they are not digested in the human gastrointestinal tract, they are transported to the colon where they are fermented by a selected species of gut micro-flora (especially Bifidobacterium and Lactobacillus) and help to balance gut flora and aid digestion."*

> -- Mike Adams

This so-called superfood is poorly digested, which is presented as being advantageous. The undigested bacteria then admittedly ferments in the colon, and *that* is supposedly healthy. Poorly digested foods are a major contributor to our modern disease epidemics. In particular, rotting foods in the colon tend to produce colon cancer. The proper way to clean the colon is by eating fibrous foods. As is usual, Mike rejects mentioning the best and most natural probiotic of all, yogurt; because it is an animal product. Probiotics are supposed to benefit intestinal flora to aid digestion, but Adams' product places additional strain on the body by resisting digestive breakdown. Yacon root is actually a carbohydrate that is very high in fructose sugar, so it will multiply the pathogens in the gastrointestinal tract, causing the opposite effect of a real probiotic. It will cause dramatic yeast overgrowth instead of aiding the beneficial flora.

The Natural News store also sells Zeotrex, which is apparently, "The first and only product in the world using a combination of organic zeolites, herbs and minerals produced from a unique proprietary process". Zeolites are porous crystals that are made of aluminum and silica. They are extensively mined in some parts of the world, and are sometimes made synthetically. They are used by the nuclear and petrochemical industries. The Zeotrex product that is being sold by Natural News is marketed for its detoxing effects, but its primary ingredient is a heavy metal compound. Aluminum is one of the primary heavy metals that people who are detoxifying wish to eliminate, because of its tendency to contribute to neurological problems, such as Alzheimer's Disease. The Zeotrex supplement product is produced using a "proprietary process", which means that the company is unwilling to tell its customers how it is really made. Zeotrex also contains a "base of Humic and Fulvic acid", which are extracts of mud. The irony of detoxifying with dirt and aluminum is hard to ignore.

"And if you don't want to grow anything at all, you can just start juicing the grass as we have been doing for several months. The field grass mixes extremely well with pineapple juice to make a delicious, refreshing raw living juice right from the fields."

-- Mike Adams

There is nothing living about a grass juice, and promoting grass as a staple food is beyond irresponsible. During the Irish famine that occurred between 1846 and 1850, over a million people starved to death, due to a crop disease that wiped-out the potatoes. Potatoes had been a primary food source for the Irish. Many of them were found dead with green stains in their mouths, which they incurred from attempting to survive on grasses. Grass simply does not have enough nutrition to sustain human life. One of the biggest contributing factors to the Irish famine was that British law prevented the Irish from hunting or fishing, so their lack of meat greatly exacerbated the starvation. Due to the fact that the Irish were not able to get any access to proteins during this period, some historians refer to it as a genocide by the English.

In recent years, we have had numerous requests from people who wished to know what mushrooms we thought would be best for curing their cancers. We had assumed that this was the result of various health scams that litter the Internet. We recently discovered that in October of 2009, Adams published an article promoting the use of mushrooms to fight cancer. Cancer is fueled by yeast and fungus, due to the fact that cancer cells must derive their energy from a type of sugar fermentation, instead of respiration with oxygen. The waste products of this fermentation build in the tissues, causing cascading toxicity and increased acidosis. Mushrooms are fungi themselves, so they aid this fermentation process by providing the perfect nutrients for cancer cells. We discussed this topic in episode 25 and episode 16 of our audio shows, because the requests for mushroom information have been so frequent. Mushrooms are the vampires of the plant world. Their job is to clean up the wastes in soil. It would be more responsible and effective to recommend cigarettes and soft drinks to a cancer patient than it would be to recommend mushroom therapy.

In March of 2009, Adams' nutritional advice reached new lows when he published a video from Ecuador, featuring the squeezing of sugar cane through an oily, diesel-powered press. He then drank the unsterilized sugar juice, and claimed that "...because it's raw. It's not cooked. It's not processed. It's actually very good for you". At one point, he actually commented that freshly-squeezed sugar juice does not spike a person's blood sugar, because its naturalness somehow prevents it. He further noted that sugar juice contains phytonutrients, because the green liquid was "like a grass". Actually, the green color simply meant that it contained chlorophyll. Contrary to Mike's video suggestions, sugar should only be used to sweeten, and it should never be a staple of the diet. We have noticed Adams' fixation upon sugars and carbohydrates, so his behavior concerning the sugar juice is nothing new. It likely indicates that Mike never made a full recovery from his diabetes, or that his diabetes has been re-triggered by his absurd dietary products.

The Health Wyze Report was one of the first non-industry research organizations to discover the dangerousness of canola oil. The canola plant from which canola oil is derived is a genetically-engineered offspring of an equally toxic weed called rapeseed. The canola plant was engineered by the Canadian biotechnology industry to save Canada's faltering rapeseed oil industry, which had its oil banned in the United States, because rapeseed causes severe heart tumors. Canola's parent, rapeseed, had sometimes been a fatal cooking oil via inducing heart attacks, and the cooking fumes from it caused lung cancers. Besides the biotechnology industry, canola oil owes its life to help from the nuclear industry. The world's first canola plant was 'born' in a biotechnology laboratory in 1976. Canola is the most dangerous cooking oil, and we felt that the unnaturalness of it would get the attention of Natural News.

In the summer of 2008, we made multiple attempts to contact Mike Adams and other representatives from the Natural News web site, concerning the topic of canola oil. Natural News was promoting canola oil to its readers as the healthiest cooking oil. All messages from Health Wyze Media about this topic were ignored, except for one of them. We desperately wanted to change Mike's position on canola oil. We so wanted to get the message out that we offered our canola research with the copyrights waived, if they would only run with the story. We offered to let Natural News take full credit and break the story. One of Adams' handlers finally replied, stating that Mike was too important to have his time wasted, and that he might entertain our message if we summarized everything into a small paragraph. In other words, beg.

A year later, *Adams discovered* that canola oil is bad, and suddenly other alternative health sites agreed in chorus, as if all of those health sites had always reported it; instead of promoting canola. It is similar to the situation with soy. One of Mike Adams' pro-canola articles from October 4th, in 2005, is still online; so not all of the evidence has been removed. That article parroted the F.D.A. position and republished official statements from the biotechnology giant, Dow AgroScience. In this last remaining pro-canola article from Adams, which is entitled, "*Canada moves toward healthier cooking with canola oil*", Adams actually wrote:

> "*Trans fat-free Natreon(TM) canola oil provides an alternative to hydrogenated oils used for restaurant frying, and the heavy marketing of this food seems primed to move the Canadian food industry toward healthier solutions for a population riddled with heart disease... A new generation of canola oil developed by Dow AgroSciences is a growing solution to a healthier Canada... Natreon canola oil is trans fat free and contains the lowest amount of saturated fat of any vegetable oil on the market. Natreon is abundant in 'good' mono and polyunsaturated fats. It's natural stability makes it ideal for food service applications, such as frying, and for products that require extended shelf-life, such as baked goods and snack foods... Dow AgroSciences Canada is an affiliate of Dow AgroSciences LLC, a global company based in Indianapolis, Indiana.*"

At the end of the article can be found, "Adams is an independent journalist with strong ethics who does not get paid to write articles about any product or company". The quote above came from an official corporate press release from Dow AgroSciences, which could be seen parroted

462

at other health sites having similar ethics. After his canola turnaround, Mike has since published articles such as, *Canola Oil is a Classic Example of Food Fraud*, and *Canola Oil is Another Victory of Food Technology over Common Sense*. We believe that his turnaround largely happened because our audience rightfully made this topic an embarrassment. It could be argued that doing the right thing late is better than never, but doing the right thing should not have taken him a year, and there is no way to know how many of his own people were harmed by his promotion of Dow AgroSciences and its genetically-engineered canola oil.

Terrorism - Mike Adams Style

In 1998, Mike Adams started Y2K Newswire, a web site that was instrumental in stirring up hysteria regarding the upcoming year 2000 software failures. It is widely reported to have been the most popular web site for information about the allegedly impending crisis. Adams also used this distribution medium to publish press releases about his humanitarianism, which included him quoting *himself*:

> *"Y2K Newswire, the Internet's most popular Y2K news site, saved the public half a million dollars in just two days by working with two large food distributors to offer below-wholesale prices on long-term storable food. One-year supplies of storable food were made available for just $479, less than half the $1000 retail price and even lower than most annual grocery bills... 'We moved half a million dollars in food and didn't make a dime,' said Mike Adams, creator of Y2K Newswire and engineer of the food deal."*

He released another press release comparing the supposedly impending Y2K disaster with NBC's thriller, *Thirst*. It is a fictional film about a crisis in which public water supplies are contaminated in the midst of a heat wave. Adams commented:

> *"Y2KNEWSWIRE's analysis points out that 'Thirst' teaches viewers a dangerous lesson: that the good guys will always find a last-minute solution and everything work out in the end."*

Adams argued that people should panic instead of being calm. His solution to the apocalypse was for people to get a Y2K Newswire subscription, for a fee. In November of 1999, Adams shut down Y2KNewswire.com; claiming that he was afraid of being blamed for creating panic.

> *"Americans always panic in the final moments before any coming crisis for which they are not prepared, whether it be a hurricane, war, or -- I believe -- Y2K. When this happens, officials are going to look for someone to blame. They will never take responsibility for the situation they have caused. Instead, they will attempt to blame the only people who actually tried to prevent the problem: the Internet Y2K skeptics and those people who took action to prepare."*

Mike committed a Freudian slip (above) by admitting that the only people who were making a positive difference and trying to prevent problems were those who disagreed with him: the

Y2K skeptics. Adams then pre-emptively attempted to shift the blame for panic onto those who had worked to keep the public calm about the year 2000 switch-over.

Following the Fukushima nuclear disaster in Japan, Adams again elevated his fear mongering in March of 2011. He wrote that the Japanese radiation, "spans oceans and continents", panicked his audience, and then shamelessly tried to sell them products that were supposed to save them from yet another disaster that wasn't. Adams is almost certainly the person who convinced Alex Jones that the radiation coming from Japan was a real threat to Americans living on the mainland. On March 11th, Jones reported that he believed there was a serious radiation exposure problem in North America, and then Mike followed with his own story the next day. It was a 1-2 punch that sent most of the alternative media into a hysterical frenzy that lasted for months. During this period, Mike and his peers cashed-in on the hysteria with the explosive iodide sales, which became obvious from the product questions that we received.

Healthy people who have had no significant exposure to radiation should never take potassium iodide (the main product) because there is a risk of thyroid damage, respiratory distress, and heart attacks. The toxicity issues concerning overuse of oral iodine/iodide supplementation epitomizes why we endlessly recommend improving diet as the ideal way to eliminate nutritional deficiencies, instead of retroactively fixing a bad diet with supplements. Mike's audience was indeed at risk; not from the Japanese radiation, but again from his recommendations.

> *"In a world where a Fukushima-style disaster could happen any day, potassium iodide is an FDA-approved supplement that's scientifically proven to help protect your body from radiation... Click here to get potassium iodide discounted at the Natural News Store."*

-- Mike Adams

Mike Adams respects F.D.A. science whenever it helps him to sell a product. Potassium iodide does not actually protect the body. It only suppresses the entry of radioactive iodine into the ovaries and thyroid, which may provide *some* protection for those organs but *only* those two organs. Concentrated chlorophyll extract is more effective for overall radiation protection, as shown by U.S. Army research. Chlorophyll, the dark green pigment found in some vegetables, is significantly safer and better suited for resisting whole body radiation damage, but it is not sold in the Natural News store.

> *"The food and water in Japan is already contaminated, the oceans are radioactive, the air is radioactive, neutron beams are jetting out of the nuclear facility, it's raining yellow water, workers are being hospitalized with radiation burns... Always have extra food available, just in case. Next week on NaturalNews, by the way, we will be announcing the launch of a new line of long-term storable superfoods... The NaturalNews Store has potassium iodide back in stock today."*

-- Mike Adams

Accomplishing one's agenda through fear is the very definition of terrorism, and such behavior is the antithesis of journalism. Now that Y2K is over, and the Japanese radiation hype has passed, Adams has shifted to parroting whatever Alex Jones reports about the risks of martial law and potential food shortages. His rants about gun ownership rights have an unconscious effect upon his audience, so that they feel a persistent sense of dread that something terrible is going to happen. Adams knows that fear sells, and after all, "The universe wants you to attract more financial resources when you're the right person to decide how to use it".

Adams continually promotes his vegetarian, low-fat, storable foods as the solution to any future food crisis; but in a true survival situation, high-fat foods and proteins would be essential. Vegetarian diets were not even possible before industrialization, because vegetarians quickly develop health conditions without supplements. This is especially true for regions with extreme climates.

> "It takes 10 acres to produce the same amount of red meat protein as it does to produce one acre of soy beans. And producing spirulina yields a tenfold increase over the production of soybeans. So think about it: one acre of farmland used to produce spirulina can produce 100 times as much protein as beef and red meat. That will be very important to realize as our world population grows and it becomes increasingly difficult to produce the protein required by the population."

-- Mike Adams

Actually, a diet of algae would leave a person with extreme protein deficiencies. Truckloads of algae are required to get the protein of one steak. He has also been willing to terrorize people with the scam of over-population to push his vegetarian religion. We are not running out of food or land. The United States discards 40% of its food, because much more food is produced than can be sold. With wiser and more ethical food management, America alone could feed the world. At the end of World War II, it almost was.

Natural News and Truth Publishing: Made in Taiwan

Natural News is based in Taiwan, as is Truth Publishing International, its parent company. Mike has a history of promoting American companies which outsource jobs to foreign countries. He attacked a legislative bill from the U.S. Congress of 2004 that was meant to penalize such companies. The bill was entitled, *The Defending American Jobs Act of 2004*.

> "The real problem here isn't that companies are trying to save a buck by moving jobs overseas, the real problem is that U.S. workers simply aren't competitive these days thanks to a failing national education system that churns out dopey students who can't do math except when it comes to figuring out how high their salary should be."

-- Michael Adams

According to Adams, Asian workers are more qualified to perform American jobs than the ignorant Americans are, and this is the real reason for outsourcing. Americans cannot even perform simple math, he contends. He conveniently ignores the topic of slave labor being cheaper, that outsourced jobs are often performed by children for almost no pay, and that health and safety laws are virtually non-existent in the non-Western countries. Mike Adams wants us to believe that corporations are just looking for better educated people, which leads them toward seeking employees in countries like China and Taiwan. In actuality, our Asian replacements are frequently children, who skip an education to work 14+ hour days in factories. Due to Asian child employment policies, Chinese and Taiwanese children tend to have more work experience than our college interns do.

In March of 2009, Mike posted a video of a business in Ecuador. The video featured the production of sugar cane juice. Children were shown assisting in manufacture. In his accompanying article, Mike seemed confused by the outrage that was generated by his video, which essentially featured child slaves. He excused the affair by saying that it is normal for children to be actively involved in family businesses in South America.

> *"The site's* [Natural News] *expansion into multiple languages is part of the global vision of editor Mike Adams, also known as the Health Ranger, who speaks some Mandarin Chinese as well as Spanish."*

> -- Natural News

None of the international languages at Natural News are Western languages, such as German, Spanish, or French. Chinese and Japanese are featured. Meanwhile, Adams assures his readers that:

> *"Some of the best product brands in the world are all designed and made in Taiwan: Acer, Asus, Giant (bicycles), Trend Micro (anti-virus software), D-Link (network computing gear) and many others. Many quality brands that you think of as being American are actually manufactured in Taiwan then rebranded in America."*

> -- Mike Adams

In the above tirade, Adams somehow forgot to mention his own companies. Truth Publishing and Natural News are both headquartered in Taiwan. Perhaps he forgot.

> *"The cost of living in Vilcabamba, Ecuador is surprisingly low, even if you're hiring a lot of help. A typical garden worker makes from $10 - $15 per day, and locals are always looking for more work."*

> -- Mike Adams

When Mike lived in Ecuador, he took advantage of the impoverishment he found. He ensured that it stayed in the same condition, instead of fueling the economy. Adams admitted that the streets were void of street lights and that there was no reliable source of sanitary drinking water. His new Alex Jones-like persona now chastises the U.S. Government for similar exploitative behavior. Meanwhile, he is still exploiting the economics of outsourcing to Taiwan and taking advantage of its lack of legal regulations. An example of legal regulations that could be avoided by relocating to Taiwan are laws against medical fraud.

Everything is Wrong

It is no exaggeration to report that most of what Mike Adams writes about alternative medicine is woefully wrong, and in some cases, dangerous. We conclude that Michael Adams sorely lacks the skills needed to research the materials that he writes about, and most of what he teaches people about traditional medicines appears to be poorly researched at best. What follows are examples of misinformation taken from Adams' e-book, *Secret Sources*. This section is included to help readers grasp the breadth of the problem.

The disclaimer of *Secret Sources* begins with, "The information should be used in conjunction with the guidance and care of your physician. Your physician should be aware of all medical conditions that you may have, as well as the medications or supplements you may be taking". Why must Adams' readers get permission from their doctors just to use vitamins or his advice? It is a rather odd disclaimer for someone who is supposedly fighting the system; especially since it asked readers to trust the establishment as the final authority in all health matters. The disclaimer need not exist for legal concerns, since his Taiwan-based operation should help him to avoid most messy legal issues.

> *"One final point on all this is that I make absolutely no money from the sales of the products I mention here. None of the companies paid to be listed here. This is not a giant advertisement. Many of the companies here are not even aware they are being listed, and won't know until this is published... You can get close to that experience today by using this freeze-dried berry blend product from Emergency Essentials. For $26 you get a can full of a blend of freeze-dried berries that are absolutely loaded with antioxidants and health-enhancing phytonutrients."*

> -- Mike Adams

The switch-over from promising not to advertise products to advertising products happened quickly. At the time of writing *Secret Sources*, Adams had always disclaimed getting compensation from his advertised companies. The products listed in his book, for which he is supposedly receiving no compensation, include detailed pricing lists for products, and information about where they can be purchased from specific companies.

The word "phytonutrients" deserves special attention because it is one of Adams' favorite words. Phytonutrients is a word that actually has very little meaning except with people like Adams, who liberally use it as a buzzword to impress everyone with their finesse regarding health research. Mike cannot have a good understanding of phytonutrients, because the research about them is in its infancy. In theory, these poorly-understood trace compounds exist only in plant-based foods, and they are not considered to be essential nutrition. Adams likes to sprinkle this word for two reasons: 1. to seem impressively brilliant, and 2. to promote his vegetarian agenda; since phytonutrients do not exist in meats.

Ironically, the nutrients that are found in meats are generally superior to comparable phytonutrients. Take for example that some researchers have labeled beta-carotene as a phytonutrient, which is the source of vitamin A found inside carrots. While there is nothing wrong with getting some vitamin A from carrots, it is important to know that the vitamin A derived from beef (retinol) is absorbed by the body at a level that cannot be obtained through vegetable consumption. It is one of the reasons why vegetarians have a greatly increased chance of developing terrible eyesight. These are the sort of nutritional facts that Adams goes to great lengths to avoid.

> *"Blueberries have been clinically proven to lower cholesterol better than statin drugs."*

> -- Mike Adams, *Secret Sources*

Adams did not bother citing evidence, because there are no credible, third-party, peer-reviewed, independent studies yielding any evidence of this. As alternative health researchers, the whole premise of Mike's statement is appalling, because any decent alternative medicine practitioner would never consider the existence of excessive cholesterol as a disease in itself; but it is instead a symptom of a more serious problem. Cholesterol is actually a good thing, at least in the short term, because it aids a body in protecting itself from serious inflammatory damage; and thus from both internal bleeding and drastic arterial damage. Cholesterol saves lives. It is not necessarily the evil villain that Adams and the medical establishment would have us believe. Blueberries *might* decrease certain types of inflammation, and that would be a good thing. If that is the case, then blueberries *might* also help to reduce elevated cholesterol levels.

It needs to be mentioned that Adams has a terrible habit of implicitly supporting the bad (and somewhat disproven) cholesterol science that is still influencing modern medicine, which contends that any diet containing what Adams calls "animal products" may be harmful by way of introducing saturated fats into the body. It conveniently ignores that a balanced diet containing some natural fats is vital for decreasing whole-body inflammation, and to thereby decrease the "bad" cholesterol levels. Adams does not accept the newer findings that verify what humans had already known for thousands of years prior. Namely that the human body needs real protein and some natural fats. Serious cholesterol issues come from not having a properly-balanced diet, but Adams' typical solution is to imbalance the diet of his audience even further through vegetarian therapies. More vegetarians have contacted us about elevated cholesterol problems than normal people have, because a body will produce much more of its own cholesterol if a person's diet is lacking in beneficial fats. This is why the cholesterol problem cannot be cured in most cases, because the recommended fat-free therapies themselves will cause a body to produce more in ever-increasing levels to defend itself from the inflammation caused by the deficiencies of those diets. It is like nature's revenge.

> *"Broccoli - Contains an assortment of phytochemicals clinically shown to prevent the growth of tumors."*

-- Mike Adams, *Secret Sources*

Adams somehow forgot to cite those clinical studies again. Broccoli is indeed a powerhouse for health, but no tumor has ever been halted with broccoli. This sort of despicable misinformation leads to people dying horribly from cancer. Adams transitioned from the silly "phytonutrients" to the even sillier "phytochemicals". It is a concept that he borrowed from the American Cancer Society. Only alternative health 'gurus' and the American Cancer Society suggest that cancers might be stopped with phytochemicals, despite the fact that we barely have any understanding of them. There are no documented cases of cancer patients ever being helped by either broccoli alone or by isolated phytochemicals. To state otherwise is patent dishonesty.

> *"As a service to www.NewsTarget.com readers, I've negotiated an exclusive discount with Emergency Essentials. Type 'newstarget' in the promo code box of the shopping cart at http://BePrepared.com, and youll get free shipping on any order more than $20 inside the united states."*

-- Mike Adams, *Secret Sources*

Adams repeatedly insists that he is providing this information to people because of the importance of helping others, but the product plugs and price lists are withheld inside a book that costs $29. A skeptic might conclude that he is double-dipping.

> *"Secret source #2 is a company called Walton Feed. Visit their web site at www.WaltonFeed.com. I have been using Walton Feed for many years. I learned about this company years ago when I was helping people with preparedness and nutrition. Walton Feed is absolutely the best source for affordable healing foods such as whole grains and quinoa. At Walton Feed, you can feed yourself and your family at a fraction of the price you've been spending at the grocery store... You should also avoid all milk, butter, margarine, shortening and sugar products."*

-- Mike Adams, *Secret Sources*

No reason was given for the above recommendation against dairy products, but we know by now. Milk and butter are unacceptable because they are "animal products", as Adams calls them. Butter is almost an essential item for perfect dental and heart health. Natural butter can actually reverse cavities through a process known as remineralization, but butter's heart effects are too complex to cite here. We agree with Adams about industrial monstrosities, such as margarine and shortening; but the harmfulness of sugar is completely dependent upon the source and the amount. For example, people should not drink large glasses of unclean sugar water and expect to become healthier, which is something that Mike promoted in one of his videos. He has repeatedly demonstrated that he will spread misinformation about so-called "animal products", even at the detriment of his follower's health. There were good reasons for dairy products being categorized into an official food group, because there are incredible benefits to consuming (non-homogenized) organic milk and natural butter. To drive the point home: dairy products are a critical part of alternative medicine's best anti-cancer therapy, the Budwig Protocol. This is a topic that Adams has always personally avoided, despite the protocol being all natural and despite it being the most successful anti-cancer treatment known.

> "Secret Source #3 is a wonderful company called the Amazon Herb Company. It sells what may very well be some of the most medicinally useful herbs in the world: rainforest herbs... These aren't just standard rainforest herbs, either. These are the most medicinally powerful herbs I've ever tasted."

> -- Mike Adams, *Secret Sources*

The herbs come from the rainforest and have what Mike Adams considers to be the special medicinal taste, so we can be very certain that they are indeed powerful medicines. It's really hard to argue with science and logic like that. The special herbs are actually more powerful than the standard rainforest herbs, and that really is saying something.

> "In other words, these 8 ounces of liquid contained the same concentration of herbs that could have easily cost $160 if I had purchased them as tinctures from another company. Yet the Amazon Herb prices were quite reasonable -- just a fraction of that $160... Amazon Herb products are based on truly miraculous medicinal herbs. It's no exaggeration to say that these herbs can prevent and even reverse chronic diseases like cancer, heart disease and diabetes."

> -- Mike Adams, *Secret Sources*

If the F.D.A. ever proved a financial tie, then Adams might find himself in prison for these claims, for a very long time. This could be why he so frequently reassures his readers that he receives no compensation from the companies that he advertises. Falsely stating that a product cures cancer, and then profiting from the sale of that item is a very serious offense in the United States.

> "Call it homeopathic influence if you want, but the truth is that the emotions and intentions of the people producing these products really do have an impact on your health."

> -- Mike Adams, *Secret Sources*

That homeopathic influence explains much, but it is more important to note that mistreating the human body with fraudulent medicine is far more harmful than any amount of intentions. The positive intentions thing has a deeper, hidden meaning that was revealed inside the *character* section of this chapter, reflecting what Mike considers to be his spirituality.

> *"The Amazon Herb Company goes even further and uses what they call a spagyric process for transferring the healing power of the harvested herbs into a consumable product... Nothing gets thrown away, and the full energy of the original plant is reconstituted back into the liquid or capsules that customers purchase. This spagyric process, which is only practiced by a few companies around the world, may help explain why I have personally found these Amazon Herb products to be so potent and medicinally valuable."*

> -- Mike Adams, *Secret Sources*

We would love to view the official research about that spagyric process. Perhaps it would explain Amazon Herb Company's techniques for transferring healing power. Some of our readers may have been thinking that Mike's marketing attempts were just hokey pokey, instead of the product of serious health research. Let the lesson be learned. How do they manage to reconstitute the vital plant energy with their special spagyric process? The spiritual plant energy is obviously more significant than the energy from animal products, and it betrays a heathenistic belief system.

> *"These herbs are so powerful that if I had a family member who was diagnosed with cancer, for example, I would immediately send them a combination of products from Amazon Herb Company, including Cat's Claw (Una de Gato) and Gravizon."*

> -- Mike Adams, *Secret Sources*

Mike Adams must be very unpopular with his relatives. Cat's claw -- that's another solution for cancer? Perhaps cat's claw should be used when the phytochemicals are not strong enough.

> *"Quinoa Flour... A versatile 'healing food' flour that can replace flour in most recipes. Quinoa is an ancient grain, used extensively by the Incas. It offers the highest protein of any grain, even boasting a complete protein (all essential amino acids)."*

> -- Mike Adams, *Secret Sources*

Hemp is the only plant containing all recognized amino acids; but a body would still become malnourished if hemp were used as a total replacement for meats, due to the lack of symbiotic proteins and fats, certain vitamins, and perhaps other nutrients yet to be discovered. The various proteins in meats are the building blocks of the human body. Flour is never an adequate substitute. The fact that Adams hinted that real proteins might be replaced with (and we shudder) flour -- left us stunned. Containing a protein does not make any flour a special healing food. He suggested that diseases can be treated by a food item that is known to convert into sugar inside of the body; when in actuality, inflammation from excessive sugar is the single biggest cause of disease world-wide, and the aftermath cannot be halted with blueberries or phytochemicals.

> *"As your body digests the quinoa, it will eventually figure out that there weren't a lot of calories in the meal. But by that time, you've already won the appetite battle. The meal is over. You've already fooled your stomach into thinking you've had a huge serving. This is a little trick to get around your ancient appetite control system -- the one we're all pre-wired with as human beings."*

-- Mike Adams, *Secret Sources*

Adams' advice encourages his readers to diet via self-imposed malnutrition and carbohydrate consumption. It is not exactly the wisest health advice that we have ever encountered. What is most amazing is that such a diet will cause massive weight gain into the future, because the self-imposed malnutrition will trigger emergency survival hormones (ketosis). It will cause a body to hunger much more often and store significantly more food as fat for years. Of course, any diet consisting largely of flour-based carbohydrates is also a diet of mostly sugar. Such terrible advice is why most diets (particularly starvation diets) fail. The most successful diets have people eating more often, for the purpose of deactivating those hormones, which are already active in most of us, due to our less-than-ideal 1-to-2 meal lifestyles. Five or six small and healthy meals are ideal for the human body, and such exemplary diets are the reason why body builders have almost no body fat. Astute readers may also realize that body builders and others with low body fat do not consume flour of any kind. Mike's flour-based suggestion for how to lose weight is truly a Natural News original.

> *"The Health Ranger (Mike Adams) is a holistic nutritionist with more than 5,000 hours of study on nutrition, wellness, food toxicology and the true causes of disease and health. He is the author of The 7 Laws of Nutrition, Grocery Warning, Spam Filters for Your Brain, and many other books available at www.TruthPublishing.com."*

-- Mike Adams, *Secret Sources*

As an ethical journalist, Adams did not simply fabricate that 5,000 hour thing, and he did in fact, time himself. There is no such thing as a holistic nutritionist. We wish our readers good luck in getting a college degree for that. It is a self-endowed title meant to impress, and his secondary education is actually a degree in technical writing.

An Editorial

We debated whether this report should ever be written for years. We knew that there were some disturbing facts about Michael Adams, but we always weighed them inside his overall help-to-harm ratio. We measure the help-to-harm ratio in everything that we do, and in every recommendation that we make. Being ethical requires finding and embracing the lesser of evils, and journalism is no exception. Above all, we must first do no harm.

We finally reached agreement that Mike Adams has become heavily tilted towards being more harmful than helpful, and that he has been so for a number of years. The ratio recently became much worse. With much reservation, we decided that this had to be written, and none of our colleagues would ever muster the courage to do it for us. So now we take the lead, because we have to.

As reporters of health issues that particularly highlight the methodologies of alternative medicine, we have monitored the work of Mike Adams from his earliest writings, and we have likewise monitored the works presented at Adams' main web site, Natural News. During earlier times, we had recognized so much bursting potential in Michael Adams that we gave him free advertising in Naturally Good Magazine.

We eventually realized that Adams' business is like that of Kevin Trudeau's. The policy consists of being obscure about critical details concerning alternative disease treatment methods, for which individuals are encouraged to pay money to obtain the official media. Such media tends to be little more than marketing itself, because even the included health suggestions tend to be plugs for more products, in addition to the more blatant marketing for additional media that is found at the end of the documents. Incredibly, Mike has a history of writing that he does not do it for the money, even inside those commercial books themselves. He seems to have carefully molded his business strategy after Kevin Trudeau's extremely profitable marketing empire. Regardless of whatever readers might feel about either Adams or Trudeau, it cannot be denied that both of them are truly brilliant marketers. The biggest difference between Kevin Trudeau and Mike Adams is that the latter boldly takes it a few steps further. Adams actually gives harmful health advice, whilst railing that the F.D.A. is unfairly persecuting people like him. In actuality, Adams is not being persecuted at all. The F.D.A. could put Adams away in a heart-beat, so his entire lone ranger routine is little more than marketing that is meant to generate karma and credibility for himself amongst the disenchanted. He is alternative medicine's pied piper.

Adams has never truly been anti-establishment, because he *is* the establishment. Adams is a proud businessman with his own online health store, a sizable media empire, the owner of a lucrative software company, a mass-marketing genius with affiliates, owner of a web site that is somewhere near the 700th position for web sites in the United States, and now Michael is routinely getting free advertising for himself to millions of people by way of his new connection to Alex Jones.

We conclude that Michael Adams is severely ethically challenged, but he compensates with his cunning. He is doing quite well for himself, despite his persona of a meekly lone ranger involved in fighting corporate Goliaths on our behalf. We have become convinced that his "Ranger" routine is a slight-of-hand trick that is designed to improve his marketing efforts and to discourage this sort of factual exposure. Most of our alternative media colleagues would consider this report as journalistic suicide, because Mike Adams has marketed himself so well as the uncaped crusader. His crusade to rid the world of globalists and unethical corporations would best begin with a hard look in a mirror.

We are concluding this report with a public confession about our complicity in the rise of Mike Adams. What comes next is the most painful paragraph of this document, because it exposes a failure at Health Wyze Media. Let us preface by stating that our intentions were always good, but our policy was flawed. We have debated Adams' merits as a researcher and as a human being for many years. These things could still be debated now. However, we always knew that there was something about Mike Adams that could never be debated. This special quality is his marketing skill. He is a master marketer at a level that we can barely grasp. In fact, this is the one thing that we envy about Mike. Early on, we recognized that we could never market alternative medicine as well as Adams did. The particular items that he marketed were often questionable, but we felt that his marketing at least helped people to realize that there might be viable options to the hellish pharmaceutical treadmill. We felt that perhaps through our silence that some people would ultimately find better sources of alternative information; like The Health Wyze Report, for example. In retrospect, our former policy was like making a deal with the Devil. We recently discovered that there was something terribly wrong with our policy of silence, based upon the continual messages from people who have worsening cancers, which have included questions about why mushrooms were not helping. We must wonder how Adams responds to such questions, and if he is willing to simply let those people die. We realized that we could not do it anymore. I told my colleague, Sarah Corriher, "Damn-it, this is going to stop, and we're not going to be silent anymore". Her reaction was the "It's about time" one.

I am continuing with the most disturbing of all the topics herein. It encompasses something vitally important that the overwhelming majority of our readers will have missed. We missed it ourselves until recently, despite having been dedicated health researchers for over six years. Going back to our early history, the pervasive carnage and corruption that can be seen within the modern medical establishment was one of the guiding factors that prompted our initial work. Believe it or not, Mike Adams was one of the people who inspired us to begin it. Many things have changed throughout that six-year period, and we have grown in wisdom. Since the beginning, one of our core ideals has been to become the most politically incorrect of all alternative media sources for health; and thereby, to be the most honest of all sources. We knew that political correctness is always a corrupting factor, regardless of the particular politics involved; because political correctness means hiding facts or rewording them to avoid popularity problems with one's peers. We believed that we would never be guilty of it, until we realized that we were already guilty.

It is an expression of a much greater problem that goes far beyond Health Wyze Media and Natural News. Our epiphany is that all of the people behind the alternative sites about health are working together: either directly or indirectly. There is no independent research that is ethically peer-reviewed amongst the others. Even the most absurd findings are analyzed through a politically-correct lens, and marketability is usually the only factor concerning which treatments are valid. The situation grotesquely mirrors the bad science and corruption of the medical industry. Sometimes the motive is financial gain, and it is popularity at other times; but truth cannot be found amongst those who do not possess ethics. Despite our admitted flaws and mistakes, we still believe that our alternative health research is the most independent, and thereby the most honest.

The bigger problem was revealed when we noticed that our formerly esteemed peers at the Weston A. Price Foundation had begun using the term "superfoods". We immediately knew that they had been *Miked*. We took a quick scan of their site to verify; and verify it we did. The next thing of notoriety was an article by Sally Fallon Morell, which was entitled, *The Great Iodine Debate*. There was actually very little debate. The article promoted drinking ever-increasing amounts of elemental iodine, as if it were a healthy elixir. Take the following quotation from the article as an example of the new age and politically correct science that most of our peers have embraced:

> *"Abraham and Brownstein argue that the iodine requirement is 1,500 mcg per day (1.5 mg), which is difficult to achieve without using a species of seaweed high in iodine, iodized salt or supplementation."*

We never expected to see the Price Foundation including material that promoted underwater plants as food for human beings, or the intake of excessive amounts of processed salt, but these things have become politically correct amongst our peers. The important thing to notice from the previous quotation is that iodine toxicity is actually being encouraged in the fact that the admittedly high amount of iodine cannot be gained from any normal human diet; and therefore, it is trivial to deduce that the human body was not designed to process that much iodine. The article essentially catalogs a shameful process of experimenting on humans to see what happens; and while that could be called science, it most certainly is not ethical medicine. The test subjects of these grand experiments are not given the informed consent that they are being used as test subjects for a substance with known toxicity issues. Instead, readers are told the lie that their health is being helped. If Weston Price were alive today, he would be deeply ashamed of Sally Fallon and the colleagues whom she has come to admire. Fallon is not some random lady from Blogspot. She has been involved in some serious research in the past, and we quoted her work in previous times. Of course, we can no longer quote her as a credible source of information. Such politically-correct articles are why so many iodine drinkers have written to us about miserably failing health; including serious, life-endangering issues, like difficulty breathing and heart rhythm abnormalities. We get lots of those "help me" messages as a result of such advice. We also get plenty of attacks, because either we are wrong, or everybody else is. We wish it were the former, for we could easily fix the problem between our chairs and keyboards. It is unfortunately not so easy.

To spell it out, there is an elite club that is made up of the who's who in the alternative health media. They work together, profit together, and nobody gets out of line. They are a chorus, sometimes spouting truth, and sometimes lies, but the chorus always sings unanimously. Except us, that is. We are not welcome in the club, and the problem that this reveals is a serious one. The fact that there is unanimous agreement about what is to be promoted amongst the club members means that there really is no independent alternative media covering health issues, and this is a very disturbing realization. Some of you will not be able to believe it at first, and we will understand that. It is nonetheless the truth, and it is a truth that we cannot run from forever. Take for example the highly esteemed Dr. Russell Blaylock. He absolutely ignores us, and he's just one of dozens who do. If Blaylock disagrees with something that we published, then we would expect for him to jump at the opportunity to correct us. We're shunned instead. All of the gurus likewise ignore us, because we tell the truth, even when it makes our own community look bad. That makes us the problem. Thus, we do it alone, because we have to, because they won't do what we do.

There are no other open, honest, objective sources, or real independent research within our community. I'm sorry, but it is the truth. The things that the F.D.A. says about our community... well... they're sadly true. Our leadership is comprised of con-men and other opportunistic manipulators, whose suggestions will often hurt you more in the long term than doing nothing at all. Even those who have character (and these people never make it to the top) rarely have the research skills needed to do the job.

The members of the elite club will continue sticking together tightly, and now more than ever, they will privately (and maybe publicly) label Health Wyze as the problem, alongside anyone else who threatens their dogma. We should expect to see even more reports from them promoting mushrooms to treat cancers, urine-based therapies, M.M.S. (chlorine dioxide), and drinking elemental iodine; despite the fact that these things tend to have the opposite effect upon health than what is advertised.

Real science is a good thing, but its perversion is equally terrible. Whether bogus science comes from the establishment or from people who falsely present themselves as truth seekers; bad science is still bad science. It is a dangerous fabrication that is built upon a foundation of lies. It is the sort of thing that we intend to fight, regardless of its source. Political correctness shall not get in our way again.

I'll go deeper into the source of the problems, even at the risk of totally demonizing my efforts. There is a singular dark and sinister force behind our problems in obtaining truthful health reporting, and I do mean literally. The anti-Christian religions, including the Wiccans (witches), other pagans, and flat-out Satan worshipers have embraced what is legitimately God's medicine. Our community is infested with that human trash, so we needn't look far to find evil. That junk about us not eating animals and saving the environment from humanity isn't a new thing. These are ancient principles of Earth worship going back thousands of years. It's why you see the words "Natural", "Earth", "Mother Earth", and "Gaia" being thrown around so much at alternative medicine sites. Hidden in plain sight, they are worshiping the "Great Mother" (also known as "Mother Earth"). The people of these religions don't really want to help us with our health, despite their embrace of alternatives. In fact, the dark religions promote hurting others for self-gain. They mainly want to stop us from offending their goddess, "Mother Earth", and that starts with us no longer eating *her* animals. What follows is tricking us into offending the one true God, by disregarding our rightful dominance of nature. He commanded us to eat meats after the great flood, but the pagans tell us that we are to become subservient to the beast(s). We have studied the dark religions, and the patterns are unmistakable. It's why you'll only find the truth here.

> *"If you will listen carefully to the Lord your God and do what he considers right, if you pay attention to his commands and obey all his laws, I will never make you suffer any of the diseases I made the Egyptians suffer, because I am the Lord who heals you."*

-- Exodus 15:26

M.M.S. - "The Miracle Mineral Solution"

M.M.S. was an acronym for "Miracle Mineral Supplement", but it was changed to "Miracle Mineral Solution" to evade media attention and F.D.A. actions. If you are not already cringing from the marketing, you may be when you discover that it is chlorine dioxide (oxygenated chlorine). The marketing of this product is so dishonest that even its name was based upon lies. It was never a mineral nor a miracle, or even a supplement. Chlorine deficiencies do not exist in any living creature. The name change happened because the product had been well exposed as a dangerous fraud, in much the same way that a career criminal will change his name to inhibit police investigations and arrests. A similar product is called "MMS2", and it is sold by the same people.

Chlorine dioxide is the compound that is used to bleach flour, and disinfect municipal water supplies. This bleaching process is one reason why processed carbohydrates are so destructive to the human body. In addition to being nutritionally destroyed by the bleaching process, food exposure to chlorine leaves behind dioxin compounds in the food, as chlorine reactions tend to do.

Promoters of M.M.S. claim that it cures A.I.D.S., herpes, cancer, malaria, tuberculosis, and "many more diseases". Snake oils never had it so good. The M.M.S. fraud would be amusing if it weren't so dangerous. It is primarily being promoted by Jim Humble and Adam Abraham. It is not surprising that the same people who sell chlorine dioxide as a dietary supplement, also sell detox food pads. The pads, by the way, simply turn brown when any moisture is applied to them.

Consumers of M.M.S. are told to mix sodium chlorite with citric acid to produce chlorine dioxide. This is due to the fact that concentrated chlorine dioxide is explosive, and therefore illegal to ship to customers, so they must complete the finishing chemical process themselves. Customers are advised to take several drops per day, inside an acidic fruit drink. They are sometimes warned by sellers (sometimes not) that they should expect to become extremely ill soon after using it, and that their symptoms of poisoning just indicate that the "healing" has begun. Then customers are told to begin reducing the amount of drops that are used daily, until the "miracle" solution stops making them violently ill. This self-poisoning is supposed to continue perpetually for a lifetime. Its sellers claim that it kills all pathogens, parasites, diseases, and it even removes all heavy metals too!

Chlorine bleach is very effective for cleaning toilets of fungi and other undesirable pathogens, but it should never be consumed. Bleach kills pathogens by first poisoning them, and then corroding them.

> *"Amazing as it might seem, when used correctly, the immune system can use this killer to only attack those germs, bacteria, viruses, molds, and other microorganisms that are harmful to the body...*
>
> *"It has been used in stock yards to kill pathogens on meat, and on slaughtered chickens; it has been used to sterilize hospital floors and benches, and to kill pathogens in water works without killing friendly bacteria for over 70 years...*
>
> *"If you notice diarrhea, or even vomiting that is not a bad sign... It is not real diarrhea as the body is just cleaning out, and it is not caused by bacteria or virus. When the poison is gone, the diarrhea is gone."*

-- themiraclemineralsupplement.com

The mastermind behind the M.M.S. con, Jim Humble, actually tells his victims to ignore their diarrhea, since their diarrhea is not *real* diarrhea. Bleach compounds are poisonous to all living organisms, regardless of size or function, so M.M.S. does not just kill the harmful pathogens. Chlorine dioxide may be used on dead meats and farm equipment to sterilize them, but no farmer would ever feed it to one of his living animals. The above quotes express an extremely manipulative personality, who wishes for potential customers to think of M.M.S. as being as pure and organic as the range-fed animals on old McDonald's farm. There is no such thing as "friendly bacteria" on the surface of dead meat or the bloodied surfaces of slaughter houses, where bleaching agents such as chlorine dioxide are used.

If a solution such as chlorine dioxide did work as Humble claimed, then it would work in the same despicable manner as chemotherapy. It would poison the entire body, and *hopefully* kill-off the weaker (diseased) cells first; but it would also have the side-effect of damaging all healthy cells too. Chlorine is used to sterilize hospitals and slaughter houses because it is so effectively toxic. The very term sterilization means to kill everything, which is something the fraudsters are apparently unaware of, as is shown by their claims. The same is true for water chlorination. If chlorine dioxide were effective as a medicine, then tap water would be ideal for our health, along with bleached white flour, white sugar, and bleached white rice, but those who most consume these bleached carbohydrates are the unhealthiest in society. The one common thread amongst the unhealthy carbohydrates is bleaching with chlorine. The chlorination of water in the United States, in the early twentieth century, happened at the beginning of the heart disease and cancer epidemics. It is no coincidence.

This product (M.M.S.) is particularly dangerous, because those who sell it are encouraging people to ignore the symptoms of poisoning. Vomiting and diarrhea are clear indications that the body is being made unwell, and that something really bad is making it violently ill -- not healthier.

The Health Effects of Chlorine on the Body

The U.S. Environmental Protection Agency website explains that chlorine dioxide reduces activity in laboratory rats, and produces neurological disorders. However, there have been very few studies on the effects of orally-consumed chlorine dioxide, because governmental agencies do not expect for people to be drinking a chlorine bleach as a supplement.

Chlorine has been known for years to both cause and worsen respiratory problems, including asthma and pneumonia. As a thyroid-crippling halogen, chlorine damages enzymes across the board to decimate the immune system upon ingestion or inhalation. Chlorine causes magnesium deficiencies, which can cause almost any symptom imaginable, including migraine headaches, high blood pressure, chemical sensitivity, and in severe cases: sudden death, according to Mark J. Eisenberg, M.D. When such magnesium deficiencies are combined with MSG intake, it sometimes leads to sudden and unexpected heart failure; even amongst young people. Chlorine also decreases the absorption of calcium and phosphorus while increasing their excretion. This loss of calcium into the urine leads to bone-related problems including osteoporosis. Chlorine has been known to irritate the skin, the eyes, and the respiratory system. It has a tendency to react with other chemicals (especially acids) to produce even more toxic byproducts. Some of chlorine's byproducts are known as trihalomethanes (THM's) and they are typically found in municipal water. An example of a THM is chloroform, a documented cancer-causing agent. Studies have repeatedly demonstrated that chlorine and THM's are leading causes of colon and bladder cancers, as well as diabetes, kidney stones, and sudden heart attacks.

Chlorine-tainted water changes the preferred HDL cholesterol into LDL cholesterol, creates free radicals inside the body that require more anti-oxidant vitamins to neutralize, and it destroys fatty acids that are needed by the heart. According to the book, *Coronaries Cholesterol Chlorine* by Dr. Joseph M. Price, chlorination was first suspected of causing heart disease during the Korean War, because the men who had canteens with the highest amounts of chlorine also had the greatest damage to their arteries. Physically fit soldiers in their twenties had arteries reminiscent of their seventy-year-old grandfathers.

M.M.S.: Part II - The Debate Between HealthWyze.org and Jim Humble

On the 30th of July in 2010, we received a message from none other than the infamous Jim "M.M.S." Humble. Humble was upset about the unflattering findings that our research uncovered about his cash cow.

His message thusly began:

> Thomas and Sarahlcain
>
> In looking this site over I find quite a lot of useful information. Thus I wondered if you might be interested in opening a dialogue concerning what I am doing since there is a lot of inaccuracies in you information about my stuff, M.M.S., that is if you know who I am.
>
> I have no animosity towards those of you who talk as you do. Possibly we could have an amiable dialogue.
>
> up to you
>
> Jim Humble

Thomas replied with:

> Mr. Humble,
>
> Yes, we did plenty of research into M.M.S., so we are familiar with you. There are two possibilities that I see here: 1. You really believe in what you are doing or 2. you have real guts. It is possibly both.
>
> We take our work very seriously. Seeking the truth is one of our highest objectives: just behind "first do no harm". We would never print anything that we were not absolutely certain was true. Not only are there moral issues at play; but moreover, our credibility is always on the line.
>
> If you would like a chance to debate us, in order to demonstrate that we have been wrong, then I suggest we do it out in the open. Let's not debate privately in the shadows, because complete openness and honesty are

principles that we value, and because this issue has the potential to have a massive impact on the lives of our readers. We normally would not make such an offer to someone who we so strongly feel is harming people, but I get the overwhelming impression that you sincerely believe in what you are doing. Your noble intentions have earned you some karma in my opinion.

If an open and public debate seems agreeable to you, then we will need to agree to some basic rules, like how long our debate should last, and how long the replies may be. I will do no editing on your replies, unless you want me to. Perhaps I could use a picture of us and a picture of you at the top, if that's okay. Readers really like that sort of personal touch, and it draws them into the story.

-- Thomas Corriher

Jim Humble accepted the challenge, so here we are with the debate for all to see. We play no games and have very few secrets here. Unfortunately, Mr. Humble did not do the same. Immediately after accepting our challenge, we suddenly and *coincidentally* began getting flooded with pro-M.M.S. e-mails and article comments, from people pretending to be concerned average Joes and regular readers of The Health Wyze Report. Mr. Humble and his sock puppet partners apparently believe that we are as naïve as M.M.S. customers are, despite the work that we have already done in exposing him. This M.M.S. brigade has flooded countless online forums with deceptive astroturf messages in an attempt to convince everyone that M.M.S. is a legitimate medicine, and that people all over the world are using it safely every day to cure any and all ailments. Some of these postings even claimed that it is doctor recommended by phantom doctors, who do not seem to exist, even though it is not approved for human consumption (much less medicine) in any country in the world. Until we began getting such messages, we wanted to believe that he meant well, and might actually conduct himself in an honorable manner. Further aggravation was caused by the fact that we have a personal problem with anyone who makes a habit of insulting our intelligence.

We should have expected the behavior that he demonstrated from his well-known reputation as a con artist; but whenever someone writes that he wants to begin a peaceful and friendly relationship, then we really want to believe it. In regard to Humble's infamous reputation, just look him up on the Internet for yourself. Readers will notice that he, and his business partners, are flooding forums with dishonest astroturf messages in an attempt to convince everyone that M.M.S. is legitimate medicine. The number of messages from people clearly hiding their identities and exaggerating claims grows every time that we look. The usual pattern is that you don't need anything except M.M.S., because it cures everything from cancer to A.I.D.S. The M.M.S. claims are flabbergasting, but they barely compare to Humble's claims about himself.

Apparently, Humble is single-handedly wiping out malaria in Africa. All that the Africans had to do was drink his bleach-like 'miracle' solution, and suddenly their malaria symptoms were not so noticeable anymore. Isn't that like hitting oneself on the toe with a hammer in order to forget about a tooth ache? We have been waiting for the proof of Humble's 'miracles', but that scientific data is just too censored to ever get out; according to Humble. In the meantime, we'll have to bank on his integrity.

Believe it or not, that's not all that Humble has accomplished. According to one of his marketing sites, "Jim" is a former aerospace engineer for N.A.S.A., but that's not all! He also helped the moon missions by designing the lunar rovers. That was just the beginning of Jim's glory. He helped design the first atomic bombs too, so he was likely to have been personal friends with Albert Einstein. We must wonder if he constantly insulted Einstein's intelligence. Humble also made the first satellite remote control digital logic circuits at Hughes Aerospace Corp., and then he innovated analog electronics too, by documenting how foregone vacuum tube computers work. He completed that last task for the less gifted, little people.

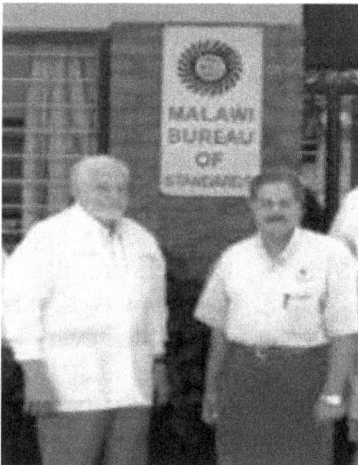

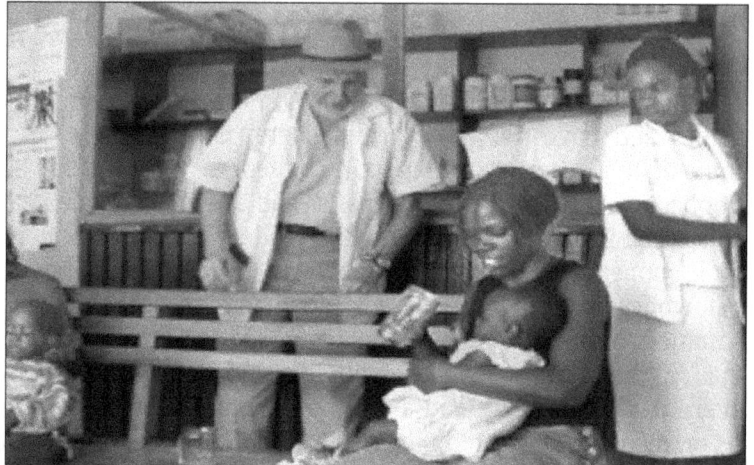

On the topic of his M.M.S. web sites, there are some unique patterns to them. All of them pretend to be made by independent 3rd parties, yet virtually all of them are hosted with Bluehost. If that were not enough for coincidences, then how about the fact that each of these sites hides the person who registered the D.N.S. by using the anonymous Domains By Proxy service? A skeptical person might get the impression that all those independent sites were produced and paid for by a single person, who is trying to hide his identity.When he's not building spacecraft for N.A.S.A., one of Humble's favorite hobbies is image editing, to make it appear as if he has done things that he has not really done, or been to places where he has never been. Closely inspect these forgeries from his sites, which are purportedly showing Humble wiping out malaria. In these photos, he's playing doctor again, and he is even sporting improperly fitting lab coats. Notice the glow around the guy's head, and around the two ladies' heads on the right? That isn't The Force we're seeing. These are remnants of cut and paste operations from photo editing software. Jim may be the world's best aeronautical engineer, computer engineer, and atomic weapons expert, but his graphics skills leave much to be desired. Skeptical people could get the impression that Jim is not a completely honest person.

Anyway, Thomas specified the rules of the debate with Humble. The rules specified a 500 word limit for each side's replies, and a single argument per day, which was to last for a period of 2 weeks. Of course, Mr. Humble did not abide by the rules. He pretended like he was too confused to understand our previously agreed upon rules of conduct, once he began sending us his tirades. Considering his alleged intellectual accomplishments, we found his sudden *confusion* to be rather intriguing, and it is what we would expect from a sociopathic manipulator. We have seen Humble's type of arrogance before, and we studied Humble's *modus operandi* enough to anticipate that he would flood us with overwhelmingly lengthy, circular arguments, in an attempt to wear us down. The confirmation of our predictions about him told us that Mr. Humble had no comprehension whatsoever of what, or whom, he was up against. We were okay with that. He was welcome to make a noose and insert his head. So be it.

Round 1

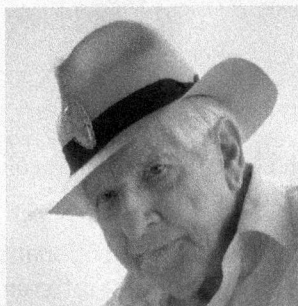

The first mistake that you enter into your Criticism of M.M.S. is that you think that Chlorine Dioxide and Chlorine are the same thing and that they would thus have the same result in the human body. So let me address that point first.

The fact is, there is no available chlorine in chlorine dioxide. It's sort of like table salt, there is no available chlorine in table salt, if there were, you would have been dead long ago. Do you see? Table salt is made of chlorine and sodium. Yet it doesnt kill you. The same situation exists with chlorine dioxide.

Let me suggest a little bit of chemical technology reading. Lenntech a Corporation that sells many kinds of chlorine for various purification purposes has published a technical article on chlorine dioxide that is quoted in many Colleges and Universities around the world. The name of the article is "Disinfectants Chlorine Dioxide." Let me quote just a couple sentences in the paragraph labeled Chlorine Dioxide as an oxidizer: "As an oxidizer chlorine dioxide is very selective. It has this ability due to unique one-electron exchange mechanisms. Chlorine dioxide attacks the electron-rich centers of organic molecules. (I hope everyone understands that pathogens are made of organic molecules) "First, chlorine dioxide takes up a single electron and this causes it to reduce to chlorite: The chlorite ion is oxidized and becomes a chloride ion and that during this reaction it accepts 5 electrons. The chlorine atom remains, until stable chloride is formed from it." I hope you understand what that means. It means that no chlorite or chlorine is formed. It turns to chlorite first, but only for milliseconds and then to chloride (which is table salt.)

To explain those quotes a little bit if it is too technical, the "Chloride" that is mentioned that is formed is table salt (sodium chloride). The chlorine atom remains until chloride is formed. No free chlorine ever becomes available from the chlorine dioxide. The Lenntech.org article goes on to explain that chlorine dioxide has a very low oxidation potential (under .95 volts), much lower than chlorine which is (over 1.4 volts), or oxygen which is (about 1.3 volts), or hydrogen peroxide which is (1.8 volts) and thus cannot oxidize many of the microorganisms in water supplies and other plants where selective oxidizers are needed. And to then explain that in terms of M.M.S., chlorine dioxide in very low concentrates cannot kill some of the beneficial organisms located in the stomach and intestines that are required for digestion.

This data is available from many different educational sources in the world. Don't take it from me. Look it up for yourself. You may not be aware of the fact that sodium chlorite has been sold in Health food stores for 80 years in the US and was brought to America from Germany about 1930. Only the name was different it is called stabilized oxygen. Hundreds of thousands... [**Word limit exceeded**]

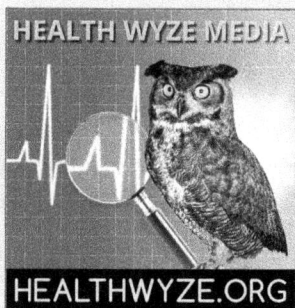

Thank you for not getting too technical for our feeble minds. We appreciate your concern for us.

Mr. Humble, it has been you who has been intentionally blurring and confusing the lines between the different compounds that chlorine can form. On one hand, you claim M.M.S. is as harmless as salt, while on the other hand, you speak of how powerfully reactive the chlorine is, which supposedly enables it to "kill everything". By the way, we actually agree on that last part. So which is it? Is the chlorine neutralized, so your customers are buying glorified table salt, or is it the powerful reactive chlorine that is well known for its toxicity? Either way, it's called "fraud". You cannot have it both ways, but nice try.

Just so you know, table salt is not harmless either, as I'm sure a great world-changing engineer like yourself knows. The only salt that is almost harmless is sea salt, because it contains minerals that counteract the toxic effects of the chloride. Table salt is well known for its toxic effects, so even if your safety claims were true, you would still be arguing from an eroded position. You also recommend M.M.S. for people with heart disease and high blood pressure, so if your product is safe "like salt", then you are part of their health problems.

As far as its safety, first let us state that your chlorine dioxide is identical to that used for pool decontaminations, and the effects of intentionally consuming it are well known. For one thing, it is an E.P.A. registered pesticide. According to the E.P.A., "Chlorine dioxide is an antimicrobial pesticide recognized for its disinfectant properties since the early 1900s. Chlorine dioxide kills microorganisms by disrupting transport of nutrients across the cell wall."

We already looked it up, and that's why we wrote the original article. The burden of proof is upon you to prove us wrong, if you can.

There is no chlorine dioxide in stabilized oxygen. There is a small amount of table salt inside it. Nice try, but we're well-versed in your slight-of-hand tricks.

I'm standing here with Thomas' electronics multimeter, with its probes inside some hydrogen peroxide, and frankly, I'm just not getting any voltage reading from it. Should we recalibrate the meter? We are a little slow, after all. Seriously, we can talk about your atomic theories all you want, and go into as many circles with those as you want, but the fact that matters is that the effects of your product upon the human body are already well known, and the electrons really don't care. Let's stick with the real issues here, and you can impress us with your fancy-smancy nuclear knowledge later.

Round 2

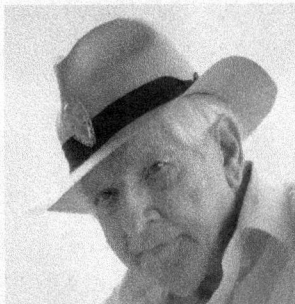

In the criticism of M.M.S. the writer continues to confuse the technologies of chlorine and chlorine dioxide not realizing that there is a life and death difference in the two technologies. So let me use the same heading on my article as is used in a section of the Critical article on M.M.S..

The effects of Chlorine on the Body.

In reading the Healthwyze write up concerning this subject I notice that the problems concerning ingestion of chlorine seemed to be pretty much according to the research of the literature that I also found. Chlorine is an oxidizer and in order to destroy most any compound found in the body, it must in the process of oxidation combine with that compound forming a totally new compound and these new compounds are often carcinogenic in nature. This kind of oxidation is known as chlorination. This is one of the main reasons that most new water purification plants employ chlorine dioxide. It does not combine with the item being oxidized, but rather it steals the electrons that hold the item being oxidized together. With the electrons being removed the item, pathogen or heavy metal or other poison, flies apart into its compounds which can be neutral or a poison. The electrons then change the chlorine dioxide components into a chloride which is the basis of table salt, sodium chloride. There is no chlorine dioxide in Clorox or any of the chlorine bleaches, only chlorine.

You may remember in my last article I mentioned that chlorine dioxide actually has no chlorine available at any time during the chemical oxidation cycle and that includes the degeneration cycle into chloride. The chemical oxidation cycle with any pathogen and chlorine dioxide consists of the chlorine dioxide stealing 5 electrons from the cell walls of the pathogen. The sequence goes like this. First a single electron is drawn off of the cell wall and onto the chlorine dioxide ion changing it to a sodium chlorite ion, but that only lasts for a millisecond or two. Then the newly formed sodium chlorite ion exerts a much heavier attraction and thus 4 more electrons are instantly drawn off. No other ion in pathogen chemistry has this unique sequence. The chlorine dioxide doesn't have the power until it converts to a chlorite and then it blows a hole in the side of the pathogen and thus killing it.

In the case of chlorine dioxide there are a number of conditions that the pathogen must meet in order to be destroyed. The most important condition is the ORP (Oxidation Reduction Potential) voltage of the cell walls of the pathogen. It must match the voltage of the chlorine dioxide in the proper way to be destroyed. Chlorine kills (oxidizes) everything in its path, but as mentioned above, by chlorination, but chlorine dioxide is very selective. It does not combine; it destroys by disassembling the biological components of the cell walls of the pathogen by removing the electrons that hold it together.... [**Word limit exceeded**]

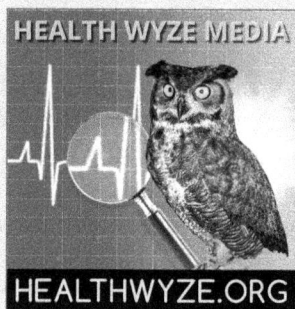

Stealing electrons? That is some bad, bad, naughty chlorine.

Maybe we could get back on topic now. We answered most of this in our previous rebuttal. All of your irrelevant atomic theory smoke screens will continue to get ignored. You may discuss those at a physics or chemistry site. Perhaps they'll even be impressed. We're not. We're concerned only with the health implications of M.M.S., and your attempts to distract our readers away from that topic will fail.

We agree that chlorine kills everything in its path, and so does chlorine dioxide. There is nothing "selective" about either. When your product is used as an E.P.A. registered pesticide, for instance, it does not merely kill the bad pathogens inside termites. It kills them. All of them. A poison in small doses is still a poison, regardless of whatever the electrons are doing. It is also worth noting that we, as humans, have cell walls too, so chlorine is also bad for us. What's worse is those scientific studies, like the one below.

Meggs et al. (1996) examined 13 individuals (1 man and 12 women) 5 years after they were occupationally exposed to chlorine dioxide from a leak in a water purification system pipe. The long-term effects of the accident included development of sensitivity to respiratory irritants (13 subjects), disability with loss of employment (11 subjects), and chronic fatigue (11 subjects). Nasal abnormalities (including injection, telangectasia, paleness, cobblestoning, edema, and thick mucus) were found in all 13 individuals. Nasal biopsies taken from the subjects revealed chronic inflammation, with lymphocytes and plasma cells present within the lamina propria in 11 of the 13 subjects; the inflammation was graded as mild in 2 subjects, moderate in 8 subjects, and severe in 1 subject.

I really liked this statement, "The chlorine dioxide doesn't have the power until it converts to a chlorite and then it blows a hole in the side of the pathogen and thus killing it." Wow, that must be impressive. Could you give us a peer-reviewed, 3rd party, independent study that proves this is exactly what your product does, while not harming human tissues and blood? I mean, I'm sure your contentions are backed with credible scientific evidence, after all. Otherwise, you would just be pulling this stuff out of your butt.

You actually state in one of your movies that your product kills only the weaker cancer cells, which would put your formula in the same category as chemotherapy; if this were indeed true. Didn't you also claim that your product would not harm human tissues (like chemotherapy does)? Aren't the cancer tumors made from human tissues? Oh, I forgot: it's "selective". I suppose the moral here is to never underestimate the intelligence of chlorine, at least not atomically, and always underestimate the intelligence of the Health Wyze Report staff.

Round 3

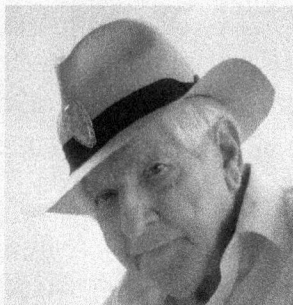

It would seem only fair that someone being sarcastically critical of someone else's work should at least know their chemistry so that they can adequately explain the mistakes that persons is making. So let me correct their writing about how pathogens are killed so that later you the reader will be able to understand what really happens to diseases if you should take a drink of M.M.S..

My critic says, "Bleach kills the pathogens by poisoning them, and then corroding them." But you see that really isn't the chemical process at all. Actually the chlorine in the bleach actually attracts the electrons that hold the pathogen together and the pathogen and chlorine mix together to form a new compound and the pathogen is killed in the process of forming a compound with the chlorine. But although wrong, that really isn't important to us as M.M.S. uses chlorine dioxide and no chlorine is available. Chlorine dioxide kills in a different way. As I already explained the chlorine dioxide removes the electrons that hold it together and it flies apart or at least part of it does.

Then the critical writer asks for a list of bleach resistant good bacteria, and then he says we know that they do not exist and of course I have to agree. But then again I am not talking about bleach and chlorine. I am talking about chlorine dioxide a substance as different from chlorine as is table salt.

The next paragraph the critical writer mixes chlorine bleach and sterilization and chlorine dioxide sterilization so thoroughly together that I cannot explain what he is saying. They are not the same thing. They are not used in industry for the same thing except on occasion Yes chlorine is poisonous to most everything, but there is no chlorine in chlorine dioxide. This is confusing because it has that same word in it "Chlorine," but a chemist quickly comes to understand that they are not the same. If they were the same, then table salt would kill you.

So last year 975 thousand people in the US died after taking a dose of one drug or the other ALL OF WHICH WERE FDA APPROVED. During that same time more than one million people used M.M.S. and not a single one died and many reported getting better quickly. More than 5 million people have downloaded my free M.M.S. book. I have personally given more than 5000 sick people drinks of M.M.S.. Most of them became well in a few hours. I make no money from the sales of M.M.S.. I don't manufacture it, or sell it, or receive royalties from the sale of it. I am just trying to make Earth a better place to live.

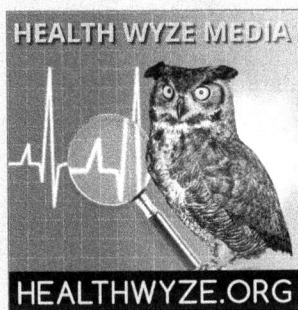
HEALTH WYZE MEDIA

HEALTHWYZE.ORG

We *really* don't care about your Chemistry 101 homework. Likewise, none of our readers care whether you believe that an electron moves this way, or that. Some people believe gremlins are under their beds, but that has nothing to do with the <u>health effects</u> of chlorine dioxide, or the price of eggs in China.

As far as nobody dying from M.M.S., perhaps you should review the news articles at: http://www.smh.com.au/national/death-in-paradise-20100108-lyxv.html and http://www.smh.com.au/national/deadly-chemical-being-sold-as-miracle-cure-20100108-lyvl.html.

You already knew about Silvia's death, because you publicly berated her grieving husband for telling the press about the horrific details of her death.

Most people won't immediately die from M.M.S., but from long-term secondary conditions such as cancers, which will be difficult to trace to their real causes. It usually takes a large amount to die quickly, so most M.M.S. deaths will be conveniently blamed elsewhere.

O.S.H.A. has this to report about chlorine dioxide:

"Chlorine dioxide is a very unstable material even at room temperatures and will explode on impact, when exposed to sparks or sunlight, or when heated rapidly to 100 degrees C (212 degrees F). Airborne concentrations greater than 10 percent may explode... Chlorine dioxide reacts with water or steam to form toxic and corrosive fumes of hydrochloric acid... Chlorine dioxide is a severe respiratory and eye irritant in experimental animals... Chlorine dioxide dissolves in water to produce chlorate and chlorite ions. Chlorite has been shown to produce methemoglobin in rats and cats"

Methemoglobin, a particular type of hemoglobin is useless for carrying oxygen to tissues. Since hemoglobin is the key carrier of oxygen in the blood, its wholesale replacement by methemoglobin can cause cyanosis (a slate gray-blueness) due to suffocation.

The National Institutes of Health reported, *"The results indicated that CIO2 may have central neurotoxic potential."*

One of the material data sheets from a chlorine dioxide manufacturer states that chloride dioxide is:

"CORROSIVE to the eyes and skin. Can cause damage to vegetation. Inhalation: Severe respiratory irritant. May cause bronchospasm and pulmonary edema, which may be delayed in onset. May also cause severe headaches. All symptoms may be delayed and

long lasting. Long term exposure may cause chronic bronchitis. An LC50 value of 500 ppm/15m3 (rat) is quoted in the literature. Skin Absorption: May be absorbed, causing tissue and blood cell damage. Ingestion: Not applicable except for solutions, in which case the symptoms would be expected to parallel those for inhalation. Hazardous Combustion Products: Chlorine, oxygen, and hydrochloric acid."

Pay attention to: "Ingestion: Not applicable except for solutions, in which case the symptoms would be expected to parallel those for inhalation." Thus, interested parties should investigate the identical inhalation results. (Your own work says its gas is released during product preparation.) We hope those electrons don't mind.

Closing Arguments

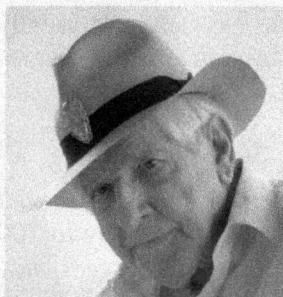

Instead of believing you guys are chemists and especially you Sarah, you should spend a little money with a professor of chemistry at a university. You guys are not chemists. You haven't a slightest clue as to the facts here. You are sailing along in la la land. You should have read that paper I suggested.

More than 5 million people have downloaded my basic free book. My total book is printed in 15 different languages. I have done lectures to hundreds of people all over Europe and other parts of the world with many actual chemists in the Audiences. Again you don't have a clue as to the chemistry. I have personally treated 5000 people and another 5000 over the internet all free of charge. More than a hundred thousand malaria victims were treated by people I trained and they were OK in less than 4 hours. Normally 400 out of that many would have died, but there were no deaths. I have seen more people cured of more diseases than any other person on Earth, you you guys are denying thousands of people the chance to overcome their suffering or to live a longer healthier life.

Please tell me why would I do this. I don't sell M.M.S.. I get no income from anyone who does sell M.M.S.. Why would I spend the time in the jungle. Can you possible believe that I just want to stand up in front of people and lie to them for no reason?

I am sorry. I was merely trying to help. All I have gotten out of you is sarcasm and hate. I am going to have to let you poor that out on someone else as I am not going to even bother reading the rest of your rebuttal. The last paragraph I have read is where you have laughingly tried to measure the oxidation voltage of hydrogen peroxide (Round 1). That is so dumb I can't believe you expert chemists could possible prepare the formula for an apple pie. You all have less knowledge of chemistry than a 6th grader and you then you call me names with sarcasm and hate. Frankly I don't see why you don't apply for a nice job at the FDA as you all have the same mentality. Here is a guy trying to help mankind so lets just see if we can make him look like shit. And you can, for a little while, then you will find that you were wrong about everything. I offered to help you and you just treated me worse that a cow.

I must not understand me. Maybe you can help. Why am I spending 18 hours a day doing all this for no income for the last 14 years. People didn't listen at all for the first 10 years, just the last 4 years. I spent all my retirement money and sold everything I own and gave my house trailer away to one of those homeless girls... [**Word limit Reached**]

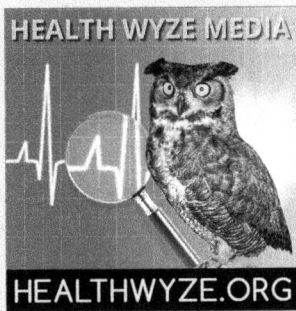

Firstly, chemistry is not the solution to the diseases that plague our society. It's the cause.

Your success statistics are only available from you: an uncredible and self-serving source of information. We have given you chance after chance to provide real evidence that M.M.S. has some benefit, and that it is indeed safer than the bleach that it is. With thousands of purported "miracle cures" worldwide, we would expect for at least one credible, independent, verifiable, 3rd party somewhere to actually document it.

If we ever decide to begin a business of poisoning already sick people (for instance with bleach) then we'll accept your advice about getting proper chemistry degrees. Until then, we'll suffice with our inferior educations.

Unlike yourself, real saints do not boast about their own greatness, stroke themselves publicly, or falsify information. You're far from the altruistic, selfless saint that you have consistently paraded yourself as being. It is unnecessary for truly righteous people to tell us of their greatness, and real saints have no desire to brag about themselves. You are hurting people, and you have willfully chosen to continue hurting people indefinitely. That is the opposite of saintly, as far as we are concerned.

Your allegation of not making money from your M.M.S. scam is cunning. You know that the one thing we cannot verify is your financial records, and therefore we cannot prove that you are lying about it. Be aware that this will quickly change if you are ever prosecuted in the U.S. for your crimes, because the incriminating evidence would become public records. When it happens, you can count on us to be one of the first to publish it. We noticed you moved to Mexico, which is a smart move. I likewise noticed that you said elsewhere, "I live in Mexico, just in case." Would a saint cowardly flee to another country, and would he even have a reason to?

Your personality closely matches a sociopathic boyfriend from when I was age 14. He was a convict and a pedophile in his middle thirties. This boyfriend followed the familiar sociopathic pattern of first reigning me in with fantastic fabrications about his history that made him appear heroic and saintly. Later, when he felt that his position and power had diminished somewhat, he began beating my spirit down by telling me about how inferior I was morally, and about how intellectually crippled I was. We know people like that, don't we, Mr. Humble? Finally, when all else failed, and he had become really desperate from his manipulation failures, he appealed to my conscience with guilt games about how I was hurting a modern day messiah. Sounds really familiar, doesn't it?

You are too arrogant to realize that you were beaten long ago, Mr. Humble, and you're too prideful to ever admit that we read you like a book from the very beginning. I hope this stands as a testament to your modus operandi, so that others will not be taken in by your slick games in the future.

Mr. Humble, you are in ours and many others' opinion, an inherently evil man.

May we call you "Jim"?

The wildly popular Signs of The Times (SOTT.net) site has backed The Health Wyze Report on the M.M.S. issue, and has reprinted both of our special reports about M.M.S. in their entirety. Because of this, Mr. Humble moved onto trying to manipulate the people behind SOTT. He apparently felt that they would be easier targets considering how effective his manipulations have been with us. Mr. Humble has discovered that they are no easier. His newest claims about his own holiness are so incredible that we feel compelled to mention them.

Humble wrote:

> *"This church* ['Spiritis Church', a.k.a. 'Liberal Catholic Church'] *has come to us down through the centuries from the original apostles of Jesus Christ. There is an unbroken lineage of succession of Bishops for 2000 years to now. The name of each Bishop is recorded. The first apostles were Bishops. The Catholic Church broke off from this first Church 325 years AD, but the Original Church continued until now. You have never heard of it because it is small. It embraces all denominations of Christianity and actually all religions of the world and always has for 2000 years. I became a minister, a Deacon, a Priest, and finally a Bishop. So let me introduce myself again. I am Bishop James Humble...*

"Let me introduce myself to you again, I am Bishop James V Humble concecrated [sic] into the lineage of Bishop leading back to Jesus Christ at Antioch when he gave the command, "go ye into the world and Heal the sick." As a Bishop I am expected to form a church which I have. The Genesis 2 Church of Health and Healing. That is what we do. We do healing. We do healing free at no cost and support the church on donations. We do not teach religious truths, but rather leave that up to other churches while we concentrate on healing the sick. Our Ministers, of course, do the same."

With Jim Humble being the swindler that he is, we believe that we know where he is going with this. He is eventually going to try to hide behind Americans' right of religious freedom by declaring that M.M.S. is his holy healing elixir, which is necessary for the practice of his "faith", as soon as he finds himself arrested in the U.S., or his sales become too crippled by legal actions.

Additional Frauds

There are many more frauds, including green lipped mussels, healing bracelets, oil pulling, and earth walking ("grounding"). We could never hope to list every scam that exists. In the interest of brevity, we have opted to report about only the most common frauds.

Biotechnology

G.E. Patented Swine Flu

The U.S. Patent and Trademark Office has a patent for, *Genetically Engineered Swine Influenza Virus and Uses Thereof* (patent #8124101). It was filed in 2005 for approval. The makers of the human variant of the swine flu virus waited until the patent was finally approved in January of 2009, before unleashing the virus into the wild. The makers of the swine flu vaccine had begun the lengthy patenting process long before the swine flu supposedly existed, which means that the outbreak was no accident, and the virus is clearly not natural. Patents only apply to man-made items, and natural things cannot be patented. The virus conveniently went public only after its vaccine patent was approved, after patiently waiting 3 years for that to happen. The pandemic was declared just five months after the patent was approved, in June of 2009. The tremendous hysteria following the outbreak was promoted by the same groups who had *invented* this genetically-engineered virus. The word "invented" was actually used to describe the virus in the patent application.

The patent application states:

> *"The present invention relates, in general, to attenuated swine influenza viruses having an impaired ability to antagonize the cellular interferon (IFN) response, and the use of such attenuated viruses in vaccine and pharmaceutical formulations. In particular, the invention relates to attenuated swine influenza viruses having modifications to a swine NS1 gene that diminish or eliminate the ability of the NS1 gene product to antagonize the cellular IFN response. These viruses replicate in vivo, but demonstrate decreased replication, virulence and increased attenuation, and therefore are well suited for use in live virus vaccines, and pharmaceutical formulations."*

This human-infecting variant of the virus was not first discovered in the wild. It was invented. Without genetic engineering, animal viruses seldom infect humans, because human DNA varies too greatly from animal DNA. There were rare cases of cross contamination with certain diseases, such as cow pox, but these infections require contact with the animal and are not contagious between humans. This has been the situation throughout almost all of history. That is until animal viruses were given biotechnology and biowarfare industry help.

The patent ownership is claimed by the Mount Sinai School of Medicine (New York University), St. Jude Children's Hospital, and the U.S. Secretary of Agriculture. Under the inventors section of the patent, the following people are listed.

- Palese, Peter (Leonia, NJ)
- Garcia-Sastre, Adolfo (New York, NY)
- Webby, Richard J. (Memphis, TN)
- Richt, Juergen A. (Ames, IA)
- Webster, Robert G. (Memphis, TN)
- Lager, Kelly M. (Colo, IA)

Why would an attenuated (weakened for the purpose of vaccines) genetically-engineered virus exist, and then be patented prior to any outbreaks in history -- when it doesn't even exist outside the laboratory? When we first reported on the swine flu in our audio show, we mentioned the implausibility of it having occurred naturally. For swine flu, avian flu and human flu, DNA cannot naturally mix without destroying themselves. It does not happen in nature.

If the patented version of the swine flu virus now being put into vaccines failed to be identical to the version that is now being found in humans, then it would be completely useless for creating immunity. Therefore, since the above patent is for a genetically-engineered virus, the virus that spread throughout the population had to be genetically engineered in an identical fashion, and it must have originated from the same facility.

The very existence of the patent demonstrates that it was intentionally produced for a commercial endeavor. The only question that remains is, was this germ warfare attack against the U.S. public accidental, or intentional? Considering that they had this vaccine ahead of time, and then coordinated a media cover-up, yields a depressing answer to this question.

This virus became weaker the longer that it existed in the wild. It was initially killing a lot of people in Mexico, but then the virus quickly mutated, and it became much less harmful. Due to the virus' rapid mutations, the swine flu vaccine is ironically unlikely to be helpful against current strains. What was initially unleashed upon the public was horrific, and the weakening of this virus through natural mutation was never intended by its manufacturers at the medical schools, and within the U.S. Government. The fact that this virus essentially neutralized itself over time is an indicator that God has not yet completely abandoned us.

Genetic Engineering Horrors

For many years, independent health reporters have been warning the public about the dangers of genetically modified foods. Meanwhile, consumer awareness groups have consistently campaigned for honest labeling on all G.M.O. (genetically modified / genetically engineered) foods. However, organizations like the F.D.A., who are friendly with the biotechnology industry, have mocked ethical concerns as being "irrational" fears about bio-engineering. A truly independent study between the universities of Rouen and Caen, in France, demonstrated that the consumption of Monsanto's genetically-engineered foods can cause organ failures.

Genetically-engineered foods are now in an estimated 80% of processed foods in the U.S., without any labeling whatsoever. In fact, the United States is one of the few civilized countries in the world that does not require labeling for G.M. foods, and we have routinely warned our readers about the dangers of soy, canola, cottonseed, and corn. These foods are almost always genetically engineered (unless they are "organic"). Make special note that there is no organic canola, because the canola plant was *invented* in 1976 through genetic engineering. Equally there is no truly organic soy for human consumption, because soy in its raw organic form is poisonous. Therefore, we strongly recommend boycotting companies that pretend to sell "organic canola" or "organic soy" in food products.

The Huffington Post reported that the F.D.A. had approved Monsanto's genetically-engineered produce using only Monsanto's own 90-day study. Monsanto had limited the study to just 90 days, despite the fact that most chronic problems will not be evident in that length of time, which was of course, Monsanto's intent. In addition, they flatly dismissed all of their own data which was linked to the sex of the test subjects, because sex traits are usually closely linked to genetic disorders. It was another example of *F.D.A. science*. Official responses indicate that we are expected to believe that Monsanto's dismissal of all its unflattering test data was merely coincidental.

Monsanto uses its seed patents to prevent independent research into its genetically-engineered seeds: employing the courts and the patent system to suppress meaningful scientific investigations. We would instead expect for Monsanto to encourage independent research, if it had any confidence whatsoever in the safety of its genetic monstrosities. There have been no independent 3rd-party verification processes, until recently. The researchers involved with the aforementioned French study made this conclusion:

> *"Effects were mostly concentrated in kidney and liver function, the two major diet detoxification organs, but in detail differed with each GM type. In addition, some effects on heart, adrenal, spleen and blood cells were also frequently noted. As there normally exists sex differences in liver and kidney metabolism, the highly statistically significant disturbances in the function of these organs, seen between male and female rats, cannot be dismissed as biologically insignificant as has been proposed by others. We therefore conclude that our data strongly suggests that these GM maize varieties induce a state of hepatorenal toxicity... These substances have never before been an integral part of the human or animal diet and therefore their health consequences for those who consume them, especially over long time periods are currently unknown."*

While we now know some of the potential dangers of G.M. foods, we still have no idea what results we will see in 20 years from now, or what genetic malformations will be seen in our grandchildren. When more so-called "genetic disorders" inevitably appear in the population at large, we will have no way of knowing how they manifested, because genetically-engineered foods continue to remain completely unlabeled. This fact removes all traceability and all accountability, which is entirely by design. The American public (and its unborn grandchildren) are the test subjects of Monsanto's genetic engineering. The lack of consumer labeling and the deceptions about our new Frankenfoods appears to be intentional. Our food regulators are trusting those who gave us dioxins and Agent Orange, and who presented fraudulent studies to prove the safety of those products.

Monsanto is not the only guilty biotechnology company, but it is the biggest and the worst of the offenders. It has a murderous history that dates back to the days of DDT and Agent Orange. As its so-called "terminator" pollens continue to infect organic species of crops and wipe out colonies of pollinating bees, Monsanto is poised to cause the greatest famine that the world has ever experienced. For these reasons, it is widely regarded as the most evil corporation in the world.

> *"If a company can control the research that appears in the public domain, they can reduce the potential negatives that can come out of any research"*

> -- Ken Ostlie, University of Minnesota

Monsanto's rBGH Milk

There has been massive controversy over rBGH (recombinant bovine growth hormone), and the arguments have not been limited to the safety implications surrounding this artificially-produced hormone. Involved corporations and corrupt regulators have worked to stop us from knowing which milk contains growth hormones. The war over rBGH labeling is mostly lost. Monsanto (the manufacturer) fought hard to prevent us from knowing how most milk is produced. Thankfully, many dairy farmers and some major companies stood up for what is right. Walmart, Kroger, PET and certain other major companies pledged to sell only milk that has never been exposed to rBGH. It is rare that we have an opportunity to applaud large corporations, but the above group earned it.

State lawmakers, particularly those in Pennsylvania, tried to prevent any labeling of milk that did not contain rBGH. They knew that companies using rBGH would certainly never label their milk as such. They knew that consumers would avoid the rBGH-tainted milk, and some of the governmental cronies involved wanted to help Monsanto and friends ensure that we were not able to avoid it. They colluded to make tainted milk the greatest part of the milk supply before the public had any opportunity to refuse it, so that its use would be practically impossible to undo. Public outrage managed to stop such laws from being signed.

As a result of lengthy legal battles, milk products which bear the purity labels must also bear an F.D.A. disclaimer stating that there is no difference between the two forms of milk. The required labeling actually claims that the milk containing the ingredient that was intentionally added to manipulate hormones is identical to milk that is absolutely pure of this artificial hormone, which it isn't. It should be very clear who the F.D.A. is working for, and that the biotechnology damage control apparatus is in full motion.

Fox television station WTVT in Tampa, Florida almost aired an investigative report about the health implications of rBGH-tainted milk, but it backed-down at the last minute, and desperately tried to silence its own reporters. Journalists Jane Akre and Steve Wilson were fired after refusing to change their investigative report on Posilac, a reconstituted bovine growth hormone (rBGH) made by Monsanto. They had documented the health risks of drinking milk containing the synthetic hormone, but when threatened with legal action from Monsanto, the Fox station demanded that all negative effects be edited out (a whopping 83 edits) so that the story would become a Monsanto advertisement. A court eventually threw out Akre's whistle-blower lawsuit after deciding that falsifying news is not actually a violation of any U.S. law. Fox News then ran a story about how it had been "vindicated", because it had been given approval to falsify news. We recommend watching the documentary, *The Corporation*, for the whole story.

In a sense, we lost the war over rBGH, because companies must now lie on their products to protect Monsanto profits, a corporation which routinely buys our news media and rents governmental agencies.

The convenient claim that there is no significant difference between tainted and untainted milk is patently false, and the effects upon human health are why rBGH is banned throughout most of Europe, Australia, New Zealand, Canada, and Japan. Monsanto's rBGH causes cancer in human beings. It is worth noting that its effects are also cruel to the animals. This rBGH affair is just one of dozens of reasons why Monsanto is widely regarded as the most evil corporation in the world.

Health Wyze Media would support a ban on rBGH, but more importantly, we support full and honest labeling of all products. We would love to see the better companies placing "fluoride free" labels on their "from concentrate" juices and soft drinks. Honest labeling is about a basic right of all people to have freedom of choice.

PLU Numbers and Genetically Engineered Produce

Foods that are G.M.O. (genetically modified organisms) are always grown using modern, non-organic farming methods. The combination can easily become less nutritional than a diet of processed carbohydrates and cola.

There is a means to differentiate the good produce from the Frankenfoods in U.S. retailers, despite the fact that the F.D.A. does not require that G.M. (genetically modified) foods be labeled in any way that would be easily understood. This is, of course, intentional.

Fruits and vegetables in the U.S. usually have a small sticker on them. This sticker will include a "PLU" number. The first digit in that number is significant.

The Meaning Of The PLU Number (First Digit)

8	The product is genetically modified, and almost any chemical may have been used on it. It is a verified Frankenfood. Please boycott all companies producing and distributing it.
3	The product is *likely* genetically modified, and almost any chemical may have been used on it, at any time. The genetic heritage is unknown or not disclosed.
4	The product was grown with synthetic fertilizers and chemical pesticides.
9	This is organic. It is the highest quality produce, most nutritious, most natural, and the most safe.

If you are wondering why the system is made to be so confusing, it is because our regulators are encouraging us, on behalf of their industry partners, to eat the new chemically-laced, G.M.O. Frankenfoods, without our consent or knowledge.

The Bee Genocide

Bees have been slowly declining in number since 1972. The drop in bee populations was traditionally called "fall dwindle disease", which is cited here for the aid of future research; even though the word disease is not applicable. In 2006, a far more rapid bee population decline ensued. The problem was renamed to "colony collapse disorder", or less frequently "honey bee depopulation syndrome". Despite the various mentally-challenged naming conventions of this problem, it nevertheless is becoming a very serious problem for all of us. Prior to 2006, the gradual decline was attributed to a number of causes, including pesticide use and Varroa mites. By early 2007, the decline had reached new proportions. Bees simply disappeared, instead of dying in their hives. Large bee hives became miniature ghost towns, and there is still no official explanation for the disappearance of the bees.

> *"Beekeepers on the east coast of the United States complain that they have lost more than 70 percent of their stock since late last year, while the west coast has seen a decline of up to 60 percent."*

-- Spiegel Magazine (2007)

What Changed?

Many people blame pesticides, but it is important to remember that conventional pesticides were used for many decades prior, and they had never caused such a dramatic depopulation. Although, there is a new generation of pesticides that are sprayed onto the soil, resulting in toxins being incorporated into every cell of the plants via the roots. The effects of these new fumigants on the dwindling bee populations are unknown, but our research indicates that there exists an even greater threat than these new-age pesticides.

In late 2002, so-called "Bt corn" was approved for commercial use. Its safety record was based solely on studies that had been done by its manufacturer, Monsanto. B.T. is an abbreviation for Bacill thuringiensis, a bacterial toxin that kills the main predator of corn (a caterpillar). Through genetic modifications, Monsanto incorporated this toxin into the genetic structure of its genetically modified corn product. Monsanto's herbicide resistant, Roundup Ready varieties of crops are already widely known, but few people are aware of their toxic corn that has been genetically engineered to kill all of the insects that eat it. The corn plants were genetically altered to be inherently poisonous, so it is not possible to wash the produce clean of the pesticide. Technically, the plant is not actually corn anymore, and it would likely fail a DNA test for corn. It looks like corn, but it acts as an insecticide bait within the growing fields. It is also on the dinner tables of millions of people who were given no warning. Monsanto's B.T.

"corn" is a genetically engineered, corn-like product that was designed to be an insecticide delivery system that naturally germinates internal bacterial toxins.

The bacterial disease, Bacill thuringiensis, was historically sprayed onto plants prior to its direct incorporation into every plant cell by Monsanto's engineering. Genetically-engineered plants containing B.T. were approved for use under the agreement that there could be no health risk to non-target insects. There has been no serious consideration of human health implications by U.S. regulatory agencies at any point. B.T. was briefly studied for its effects upon bees, but only an immediate and direct correlation was studied. The test bees were exposed to B.T. in a controlled setting, and had the bees died within a few days, then a direct correlation would have been inferred. However, this is not how the toxin actually works, so the usual industry 'science' was employed to get the 'right' test results. The sub-lethal effects that cause massive fatalities from long-term side effects were categorically ignored; even though this is how the toxin is supposed to eliminate insects. Monsanto itself was allowed to perform and fund all of its own testing, without any pesky independent 3rd parties to ruin their *scientific* results. Their "corn" product is now in the food supply for both humans and bees.

> *"The* [Monsanto] *study concluded that there was no evidence of a 'toxic effect of Bt corn on healthy honeybee populations'. But when, by sheer chance, the bees used in the experiments were infested with a parasite, something eerie happened. According to the Jena study, a 'significantly stronger decline in the number of bees' occurred among the insects that had been fed a highly concentrated Bt. poison feed."*

-- Spiegel Magazine

There has been evidence of Varroa mites attacking bees in the United States for decades. They are a type of parasite that sucks hemolymph (a fluid from the circulatory system) from bees, leading to diseases and deaths. It has been attributed to causing fall dwindle disease. However, some beekeepers have noticed that their bees can survive in the presence of these mites, particularly when the beekeepers did not use antibiotics or gases inside the hives. Only bees with weakened immunities cannot survive Varroa mites. It is the combination of these natural parasites *and* genetically-engineered B.T. pollen that is proving to be especially fatal. When bees have historically died from parasites, diseases or pesticides, the beekeepers saw piles of dead bees outside the hives. The dead had been carried outside by the worker bees.

> *"Colonies can die so fast from high Varroa infestations that thousands of dead bees will pile in front of the hive."*

-- Dr. James E. Tew, Associate
Professor of Entomology

The historical patterns are no longer being witnessed in recent cases of colony collapse disorder. Bees are simply vanishing without a trace. Scientists are having trouble explaining the cause of these disappearances; and beekeepers are typically horrified whenever their hives suddenly become empty. In recent cases of colony collapse disorder, the adult bees disappear, leaving behind only young bees to complete the tasks of adults. The queen always remains.

Bacterial toxin Bacill thuringiensis is known to provoke an immune response in both humans and bees. The immune response in a bee prevents proper memory formation, and causes overall confusion. One of the initial symptoms of impending colony collapse is a bee's decreased navigational ability. During the summer, bees have enough available pollen to be able to tolerate weakened immune systems. However, in the winter months, when pollen becomes scarce, and the bees have to travel much further, then their decreased navigational ability becomes fatal. They never find their way home. Thus, many beekeepers find their colonies to be vacated when they check in the spring. The aftermath is vanished bees, and a lonely queen.

A preliminary report that was published by the Colony Collapse Disorder Working Group mentioned that they had found crystalline compounds in dead bees. B.T. is specifically designed to form these crystals, which fatally create holes in insects' gut membranes. The same report also found scar tissues that were attributed to immune responses. It is the fingerprint of B.T. damage. This is exactly how Monsanto's B.T. "corn" was designed to kill.

> "It is particularly worrisome that the bees' death is accompanied by a set of symptoms which does not seem to match anything in the literature."

> -- Diana Cox-Foster, C.C.D. Working Group

More research into the effects of Bacill thuringiensis on bee populations is ongoing; but meanwhile, the bees are dying at an alarming rate, and genetically-engineered crops are still growing in the wild. This is yet another example of serious research being done only after the harm has been found, and with none of it actually being done by the groups who are legally and ethically required to do it. It may now be impossible to completely eliminate Monsanto's genetically engineered, toxin-laced, Frankencrops, due to cross-pollination, which was almost certainly intended. In fact, Monsanto routinely sues farmers for having crops that have been tainted by its genetically-altered pollens, as if those farmers had stolen from the company by just being down wind. What is most amazing is that Monsanto wins these cases. Monsanto always wins, and it even has its former attorney as a judge in the U.S. Supreme Court (Clarence Thomas).

Despite assurances by the guilty parties that Bacill thuringiensis does not have any effect upon non-target insects, a slew of independent studies have shown otherwise. One showed that B.T. can poison streams, reducing the growth and increasing the mortality of a variety of insects. The study expressed concern over the long-term ecological impact of killing insects on such a widespread scale. In a clinical trial performed by E. J. Rosi-Marshall (et al.), in 2007, it was concluded that:

"Laboratory feeding trials showed that consumption of Bt corn byproducts reduced growth and increased mortality of nontarget stream insects. Stream insects are important prey for aquatic and riparian predators, and widespread planting of Bt crops has unexpected ecosystem-scale consequences".

Even Organic Growers are Killing Bees

Whilst researching Bacill thuringiensis, we discovered that even organic growers are using this toxin. B.T. is a bacterial toxin, and thus it is allowed to be called "natural". Organic crops are not genetically engineered unless there has been a pollination contamination, but B.T. is often sprayed onto the crops as an "all natural" pesticide. This is particularly disturbing, because very few people who purchase organic products would find such bacterial contamination to be acceptable or honest.

What You Can Do

- Spread the word, and harass organic companies about their use of this toxin. Only public pressure will convince companies to stop killing the bees and poisoning our foods. The more that people are aware of this problem, the more pressure that will be put on growers.

- Planting flowers or crops that produce pollen will help local bees. It has been proven that bees only choose corn as a last resort.

- Start a backyard hive. This may not be possible for many readers, but those who can, should.

Supplements

Flax Seed Oil and Omega-3

When untainted and unadulterated by the food industry, flax seed oil seems to have virtually countless miraculous health-generating properties, which are falsely believed to stem from the oil's omega-3 content. Technically, flax seeds and flax seed oil do not contain omega-3's. They instead contain alpha-linolenic acid, which a body's enzymes use as a raw material to synthesize its own EPA and DHA (omega-3 oils) in exactly the amounts needed to balance the inflammatory omega-6 and 9 oils that are so common in our diets. These facts make flax seed oil superior to fish oil supplements for getting both the exact amount of needed omega-3's, and for getting absolutely pure omega-3's into the body. For these reasons, we have always recommended that only flax seed oil be used for omega-3 supplementation. It may be the most important supplement that a person can take, with it racing closely against vitamin C. It literally is a cure for cancer and it substantially fights heart disease and other inflammatory disorders.

The polyunsaturated fats include vegetable oils such as soy, corn, safflower, canola, sesame seed, sunflower, and flax seed oil. Unfortunately, they all produce an undesirable repercussion whenever they are used for cooking, due to the fact that they are easily altered with exposure to light, heat, or oxygen. They quickly become rancid and carcinogenic.

Flax seed oil is especially sensitive. Supplemental flax seed oil is usually stored in dark bottles and refrigerated for this reason. If exposed to heat, light, or oxygen, then the oil can quickly become rancid. Polyunsaturated oils become trans fats and worse through break-down. Flax seed oil may develop a profuse odor, and it can become toxic to the point of becoming a carcinogen. The odor is caused by rancidity. It is the reason why dangerous fish oil supplements smell so terrible. That smell is usually much more than just the smell of the fish, and fish oil, in particular, is usually rancid from the extra processing that is required. Highly-processed fish oil is precisely the omega-3 supplement that is prescribed by the medical establishment, and it is certainly good for business. The rancid trans fats that are produced with shoddy or over-processed oils actually neutralize the useful omega-3 that is already in the body, so the consumption of them is like taking an anti-omega-3 supplement.

> *"...I investigated the high temperature treatment for fish oils, for the purpose of making them keep longer, and killing their fishy taste. I came to the conclusion that these oils do great harm to the entire internal glandular system, as well as to the liver and other organs and are therefore not suitable for human consumption."*
>
> -- Dr. Johanna Budwig, *Flax Oil as a True Aid Against Heart Infarction, Cancer and Other Diseases*

Flax seed oil has become famous for fostering improved health, so the food industry is offering a plethora of flax seed-based foods. There are a variety of food items such as cereals that are marketed for having health benefits, due to the inclusion of *baked* flax seeds. Remember what heat does? Surely these companies must know what they are doing to people, for these food empires have huge R&D departments.

What is even more incredible is that some products contain whole flax seeds, such as granola bars. Whole flax seeds are extremely difficult to digest, unless they are first ground. This must be done just prior to consumption, in order to avoid rancidity. Whole seeds just pass without any digestion, which merely burdens the digestive system, instead of providing health benefits. The destroyed omega precursors neutralize iodine too.

Once again, the food industry has found a way to toxify an otherwise healthy food, and then it tricks health-conscious customers into consuming it. These harmful products are even in health food stores.

Our Omega-3 Recommendations

We recommend that omega-3 supplements be consumed in the form of individual, light-resistant capsules to protect the oil from heat, light, and oxygen. It should also be cold pressed. Buy it and all other supplements from health food and herbal retailers, unless you are shopping by way of the Internet. The products found in regular retailers have serious quality control and potency issues. Especially avoid U.S.P. supplements, which are made by, and approved by the pharmaceutical industry. Flax seed oil should be combined with a source of sulfur proteins (such as cottage cheese, quark, or yogurt) for optimal benefits. This is described in more detail in the *Budwig Protocol* section of the *Cancer* chapter.

Natural Stimulants

We recommend caution concerning the use of stimulants for those with unresolved heart problems or high blood pressure. Use caution when combining stimulants. For people of reasonably good health and common sense, stimulants can be like a God-send; especially for those who have slowed metabolisms. Of course, we recommend dealing appropriately with whatever underlying issues might be causing a slowed metabolism, but sometimes a multi-pronged attack is prudent. Appropriately used stimulants can help a person to get into better shape, while providing the necessary energy to do so, at the same time. Again, common sense and responsible usage are prudent to ensure that more good is done than harm.

Our official recommendation is that people start slowly discovering how these various stimulants effect them independently. As Confucius once stated, "Never test the depth of the water with both feet at the same time". If used excessively or unwisely, these stimulants could cause serious health issues. The first major problem will be kidney stress for most individuals who use this information unwisely.

The Stimulants List

Guarana	We have written about guarana, and described it as the natural Ritalin. A common misconception is that guarana simply provides caffeine, but its more active ingredient is actually guaranine. One study tested improvements in cognitive function from the guarana plant and it concluded that, "The effects cannot be attributed to caffeine alone". The Human Cognitive Neuroscience Unit conducted another study, showing improved memory, concentration, and increased task performance. Researchers concluded that "the effects are unlikely to be attributable to its caffeine content". Unlike caffeine, guarana does not usually cause jitters, and its effects typically last for 8-10 hours, instead of the usual 2-3 hours as experienced with caffeine. Instead of just stimulating, it enhances all cognitive functions. Guarana is currently being tested for post-cancer therapy, in an attempt to provide energy and improved cognitive function in those who are suffering from "chemo-brain".
Ginseng	Before guarana became popular, ginseng was the most common herbal stimulant. Korean ginseng (*Panax ginseng*) is believed to be much more stimulating than American ginseng (*Panax quinquefolius)*. The ingredients label on ginseng supplements will reveal which type it contains. Korean ginseng has been shown to reduce blood sugar levels and improve cognitive performance. American ginseng has likewise been shown to lower blood sugar and appears to be useful for the treatment of attention deficit disorder, particularly when combined with ginkgo biloba. Studies have shown that it boosts the immune system. According to the University of Maryland, American ginseng is an adaptogen, which means that it helps the body to better deal with various types of stress. Ginseng is also an appetite suppressant, which makes it ideal for dieters. The quick summary is that overall, American ginseng is better for health, but the Korean variety is more stimulating. Beware of "Asian ginseng", for it is likely to come from China and be unsafe.
Gotu Kola	Gotu kola is a mild stimulant that improves circulation. It has been found to augment the memory, improve mental clarity, and reduce anxiety. It also strengthens the veins and capillaries. It is popular amongst people with varicose veins, and was historically used by the Chinese to reduce scarring when applied soon after a wound. Like ginseng, it is an adaptogen, which means that it boosts the immune system in times of stress.
Fo-Ti	Fo-ti stimulates a portion of the adrenal glands, which provides energy. It

	is often used to help with erectile dysfunction, and is used as an aphrodisiac. In addition, the root of the plant has been shown to lower cholesterol levels and reduce hardening of the arteries. Its effects mimic those of Korean ginseng, but the body develops a tolerance to both. Therefore, we recommend taking only one on a rotating schedule with the other, and switching every two weeks.
B Vitamins	Vitamin B-12 is special. Be sure to get B-12 in the form of methylcobalamin, if possible. Hold it in the mouth or chew until it dissolves. Avoid the so-called "food-based" vitamins, which are usually yeast based and genetically engineered.
Chlorophyll	Chlorophyll is responsible for the pigmentation of green plants. Chlorophyll extract can be purchased in health food stores, and it is sometimes so concentrated that it may actually look black until diluted. Chlorophyll provides mental clarity and physical energy by increasing the rate of oxygen absorption into cells. This is important for the prevention of cancer, as oxygen deprivation is a primary cause. The Linus Pauling Institute discovered that chlorophyll speeds the healing of wounds when applied topically.
Coconut Oil	Organic coconut oil can be purchased from a health food store or online. It provides energy rapidly, warms those who have cold-sensitivities, and it even kills candida. You can cook with it, or eat it plain. In many cases, a quarter of a teaspoon is adequate to get a dramatic energizing effect. An improvement will be felt both mentally and physically. There are very noticeable quality differences between organic, cold-pressed coconut oil, and the highly-processed coconut oil that is sold in most grocery stores. The cold-pressed organic coconut oil is much more effective in providing energy and health benefits.
Taurine	Taurine is an amino acid, which has been shown to improve athletic performance, energy, and stamina. It is responsible for regulating the mineral salts in the body. It is used with magnesium to regulate the pulse. It also protects against damage to the central nervous system. It is naturally found in all proteins. In another section, we wrote about how taurine is an effective antidote for monosodium glutamate (MSG). Taurine has been shown to be depleted in people with diabetes, so supplementation will be particularly helpful in those cases. One of the most interesting facets of taurine supplementation is that it has been shown to reverse some of the damage caused by smoking. Taurine has been known to stop heart attacks, especially when combined with cayenne pepper.
DHEA	DHEA has been extensively studied, and has been shown to provide

DHEA (Continued)	energy, improve mood, reverse aging and improve memory. It has become very popular for its ability to improve sexual stamina and for its use as a weight loss aid. DHEA supplementation should be avoided in those who have adrenal fatigue, heart problems, or male pattern hair loss. Extreme doses in women can lead to the growth of facial hair.
Ginkgo Biloba	Ginkgo biloba is known primarily for its beneficial effect upon circulation, and it is through this function that it increases the energy of those taking it. At the same time, it can actually increase the oxygen capacity of the blood and improve mood. According to the U.S. National Institutes of Health, ginkgo has been shown in numerous studies to alleviate the leg pain that is caused by clogged arteries. It has also been shown to be very beneficial for those with early-stage Alzheimer's disease. It improves the vision of those with normal tension glaucoma.
Hoodia	Hoodia is used primarily as a weight loss aid. It is a powerful stimulant that does not cause jitters. This cactus-like plant from South Africa naturally suppresses the appetite and provides energy. Always read the ingredients on hoodia supplementation packages, and be sure to avoid chemical additives. Deceptive advertising is frequently used to trick people into taking minute amounts that are too small to be effective.
Iodine	Iodine deficiencies are rampant in the U.S., which is largely due to fluoride poisoning. Fatigue is a symptom of both. Fluoride neutralizes iodine and simultaneously causes a body to need more iodine. Iodine supplementation should be used carefully and cautiously. Before supplementing with iodine, please read the *Iodine* section of this chapter. Supplementing improperly with iodine can be dangerous and even fatal.
Arginine	Arginine is a mild stimulant for most people, but it tends to be more helpful for people aged over 40. This amino acid is produced by the body less with age. In men, arginine can be a very helpful supplement for both increasing energy and for remedying erectile dysfunction. It is also useful for preventing heart attacks, clearing blood clots, and for strengthening the heart. However, as a strong notice of caution, arginine should never be used in the months following a heart attack, because it increases the chance of another heart attack during this period.
Kola Nut	Kola nut has psychogenic effects and it contains some caffeine. Kola nut extracts are used by the pharmaceutical industry in products that are formulated to suppress nausea and migraine headaches. In Jamaica and Brazil, kola nut is consumed as a sexual stimulant and to treat erectile dysfunction. It can be chewed before meals to promote better digestion and to enhance taste. It is also used to heal superficial cuts throughout Brazil.

	Because it increases metabolism in the body while causing appetite suppression, kola nut can also be used as an aid in losing weight. Keep the dosage small, because kola nut can overdrive the heart.

Chamomile

Chamomile (sometimes pronounced with a silent "h") has not only been popular with modern alternative medicine practitioners, but its medicinal roots can be traced back for centuries. It is famous for its ability to ease discomfort in the digestive tract. It has also been used for:

- Allergies
- Indigestion
- Anxiety
- Migraines (resulting from allergies)
- Colic
- Crohn's disease

- Diarrhea
- Insomnia
- Irritable bowel syndrome
- Peptic ulcers
- Skin irritations
- Minor wounds

Chamomile is effective as a mild sedative, and for promoting restful sleep whenever it is infused into tea, or otherwise taken internally. It is ideal for anyone who suffers from insomnia, because it is very unlikely to cause drowsiness the following morning, so long at it is taken at a reasonable time in the evening. For readers who suffer with insomnia, we urge them to deal with the cause; whether it is emotional or physical. In the meantime, chamomile would certainly help.

Chamomile is a useful remedy for insect bites when topically applied. It eliminates itching better and more rapidly than any pharmaceutical or retail product that we have found. Insect bites often disappear completely within hours of chamomile application, and the itching usually stops within minutes. We were so impressed with how rapidly chamomile alleviates common insect bites, that we decided to incorporate it into one of our products (Byte Back Itch Remover).

Topical applications of chamomile decrease the healing time necessary for wounds. To make a topical solution, mix ground chamomile powder with vodka. These are the two methods of manufacture that we recommend. Method 1 is to blend chamomile flower heads with vodka, and then strain after several weeks. Method 2 is to purchase chamomile as a supplement, and empty the chamomile powder from the capsules into the vodka. It will be ready after a thorough mixing, but it will become much stronger with time. It is wise to make the solution long before it is needed, for maximum efficacy. It remains useful for a year.

Chamomile is known in some gardening circles as the "plant doctor", due to its ability to help the health of other plants growing nearby. It is also said to increase the production of essential oils in those nearby plants.

Chamomile contains a natural anti-histamine, so it helps to treat allergies and asthma. Be aware that large amounts will cause drowsiness.

Warning: Chamomile is a relative of ragweed, so those who suffer from ragweed allergies should use it with caution. If any allergic symptoms occur, then discontinue. As with all things, it is wise to begin by using a small amount until you are certain of how it will effect you.

Iodine

Most of us never consider the link between diet and chronic fatigue or insomnia. A body produces negative warning reactions when it has too much or too little of any given thing. Most of us lack vital nutrients like the B vitamins, which are found in most vegetables. They are weakened by cooking, and they are destroyed whenever they are microwaved.

Iodine is an element that is found in trace amounts throughout the human body. It is the foundation of all nutrition, since cells need it to regulate their metabolism. When lacking iodine, people are known to suffer from swollen glands in the throat, thyroid diseases, increased fluoride toxicity, decreased fertility, increased infant mortality, sugar regulation problems, and (with severe deficiency) mental retardation. It has been theorized as a cause of A.D.H.D. for newborns of iodine deficient mothers. Iodine is the only substance known to neutralize fluoride stored inside the body, and it can shield against some radiation damage.

A New York Times syndicate reported:

> *"Besides causing unsightly goiters, iodine deficiency slows all the systems of the body: The digestive system becomes sluggish, nails grow more slowly, skin and hair become dry and dull, tendon reflexes stiffen, sensitivity to cold increases, and the pulse slows. Iodine helps form who we are to such an extent that a deficiency can lead to a dulling of the personality, deterioration of attention and memory, increase in irritability due to fatigue and extreme apathy."*

Iodine deficiencies, soy consumption, and fluoride exposure are all causes of the hypothyroidism epidemic. Hypothyroidism generally strikes women, causing fatigue, weight gain, and cancers amongst many other problems. Therefore, we recommend topical applications of iodine, because there is no known toxicity whenever it is absorbed through the

514

skin into the blood. Low to moderate amounts of iodine are harmless when absorbed transdermally.

Organic iodine is found in some foods naturally, including eggs, fish, beef, sea salt, cheese, asparagus, garlic, beans, and spinach. As is usual with all of the critical minerals, iodine is found in higher amounts in organic foods. There is no comparison between organic iodine, and the synthesized versions in retail products, or those sold by quacks. People do not die from the iodine in fish and meats. The difference is another glaring example of the difference between God-made and man-made nutrients.

The Iodine Speed Test

Most people are deficient in iodine, and there is a simple test that can be used by anyone to determine if he is deficient. Here is the simple procedure:

1. Apply standard 2% topical iodine in a circular area that is about the size of a silver dollar (2 inches) on the abdomen, and allow it to completely dry before redressing.

2. Check to see if it almost completely disappears in 12 hours.

If the iodine disappears within 12 hours, then the test subject is iodine deficient. This test works due to the fact that the skin absorbs iodine at the rate at which it is needed. We do not pretend to understand the whole process, but the results accurately and reliably reflect iodine consumption in the diet. Whenever a person is ill, transdermal iodine will absorb especially rapidly, because iodine is used to produce the hormones that fuel the immune system. In our own testing, we have witnessed a 4 to 5 times absorption rate increase during periods of high stress or illness. Apply it cautiously, because it will stain almost anything.

Hashimoto's Thyroiditis

There is a lot of conflicting information on the Internet regarding the application of iodine for those with Hashimoto's, with much of it being entirely wrong. Iodine dosage is especially important in Hashimoto's thyroiditis cases, since an overdose can destroy the patient's thyroid. However, a small amount of iodine does actually help this condition. Problems tend to occur for those who consume potassium iodide supplements, and those who internally consume iodine drops. There is greatly reduced risk with iodine applied topically, as we generally recommend. Remember that topical applications allow a body to better self-regulate iodine absorption.

If you feel that you must consume iodine orally, then get it through supplementing with red marine algae. It is the safest natural source for oral iodine supplementation, and other underwater vegetation generally contains toxins, such as heavy metals and PCB's. You can also safely get iodine by eating fish. Potassium iodide is a much safer alternative to iodine for those who are careful not to overdose, but people should beware of companies that include additives such as sodium benzoate. Potassium iodide should never be used by those with Hashimoto's disease.

The Insanity of Ingesting Iodine

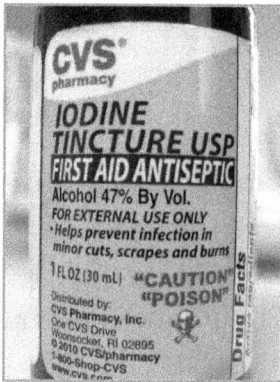

Lugol's iodine is a special formulation of iodine that is sold by quacks, who proclaim it to be a supplement for internal consumption. They suggest that it is a medicine for an endlessly growing plethora of diseases, but they are careful to never actually call it a medicine, lest they risk imprisonment. They present Lugol's iodine as the gold standard of iodines for drinking. The formulation is 5 g. of chemically-extracted iodine, and 10 g. of potassium iodide per 100 milliliters of distilled water. There are rogue people who advocate drinking as much as three teaspoons of chemically-extracted iodine daily; to supposedly cure and prevent countless illnesses. In some cases, they are even orally giving it to small children in what is blatantly child abuse.

Dr. Guy E. Abraham and his close partner Dr. David Brownstein have been repeatedly quoted and cited by the quacks of iodine drinking as "the experts" on this topic; so it is worth a moment to discuss them. Brownstein wrote an entire book about drinking iodine, and Abraham's faithful point to his credentials as a professor and a former M.D. However, their therapies are not even endorsed by their own establishment. In previous times, they were both a willing part of a medical system that routinely gives children radioactive iodine to virtually destroy any chance of them having a long and healthy life.

> "Want to join the experiment? If you are already taking iodine click here to become a member, or Order a bottle for $40 to try it out for yourself!"

-- Dr. Guy E. Abraham

Elemental iodine is quite useful as a topical antiseptic, and topical applications eliminate a plethora of health issues wrought by iodine deficiencies. However, elemental iodine can quickly become toxic when orally consumed, for it is so difficult to not overdose. It is always safe whenever it organically occurs in foods, such as fish. The effects of an overdose with elemental iodine mimic the central nervous system problems that are caused by well-known poisons; for instance, the metallic taste that is caused by arsenic poisoning. The iodine that is found in typical retailers is always toxic in any amount if taken orally.

The poisonous short-term effects of ingested iodine are well known, but the consequences of tiny amounts being ingested over a period of years are unknown. We have written this hoping that those considering following such asinine advice will research enough to find the truth prior to hurting themselves, or their children.

Symptoms of Iodine Toxicity

- Abdominal pain
- Coughing
- Delirium
- Diarrhea
- Fever
- Metallic taste
- Mouth and throat pain
- Inability to urinate
- Seizures
- Shock
- Shortness of breath
- Stupor
- Excessive thirst
- Profuse vomiting
- Death

Some misguided followers of Abraham and Brownstein allege that iodine itself is not toxic, and that the toxic effects only result from methanol being inside the over-the-counter products. They usually follow with boasts about how Lugol's iodine lacks methanol, while ignoring all of the other toxicity facts about it. However, the U.S. National Institutes of Health specifically cites Lugol's iodine as being poisonous, and even its fumes are dangerous whenever it is heated. The official medical term for toxic overexposure to iodine is "iodism", and this condition is virtually always the result of oral consumption. No other supplement requires environmental protection suits in its production process, because iodine synthesis is a dangerous and chemical-laden production process.

Some of those who are consuming synthetic iodine (and even giving it to their children) believe that it must be safe because iodine is added to salt and bread. This is actually not true. It is normally trace amounts of potassium iodide (not iodine) that is added food items. It is a significantly less toxic relative of iodine that somewhat helps to compensate for iodine deficiencies. While the safer iodide can be found inside the Lugol's solution, and inside of other supplemental iodine solutions, it is still dangerously easy to overdose. It is so dangerous that it is absolutely irresponsible to supplement with it or recommend it.

It is worth noting that iodine is much safer when combined with carbohydrates like bread, because starches are known to neutralize it. Thus, even if real iodine were inside breads, then the breads would neutralize that iodine. The excessive carbohydrate consumption of our Western diets is one of the many reasons why so many of us are lacking iodine. For this reason, victims of iodine poisoning are told to eat bread by iodine manufacturers and poison control centers.

There has been a philosophical debate that has raged for eons about whether a people should be protected from themselves. However, there is no debate about whether children should be protected from bad adults. All of us in society have a shared duty to protect children from harm. It is our moral duty to report any parent who is poisoning a child with iodine, or any other toxic substance, to child protective services or other relevant governmental agencies. Contact us if you know of this happening to a child, if you are too afraid to get involved.

Poisoning a child is a symptom of the mental illness, Munchhausen by proxy, so the abuse will only get worse in time if there is no intervention. For some really bad parents out there, the book from Brownstein is the excuse that they need.

Safe Ingestion Methods

The safest supplement for iodine is red marine algae, which can be purchased in capsule form. Other marine plants have toxins, such as heavy metals and PCB's. The ideal food source for iodine is baked fish. Beware of bottom feeders and shell fish, for they have the same toxins that most underwater vegetation does. Pure potassium iodide is an acceptable solution for those who are careful not to overdose, but people should beware of impure products that include additives like sodium benzoate. Potassium iodide should never be used by those with Hashimoto's disease, nor any other oral iodine supplements.

The potassium iodide that is added to table salt is not adequate to compensate for most iodine deficiencies. It is usually sufficient to stop goitrous boils from swelling in the neck, which are caused by an extreme deficiency. However, not enough iodine can be obtained from table salt to maintain optimal health, unless a dangerous amount of salt is consumed. Naturally-occurring iodine is present in unadulterated sea salt, with naturally-occurring complimentary minerals, but even the vastly superior and healthier sea salt option might not be enough for a tiny fraction of people having extreme iodine deficiencies, which are caused by fluoride toxicity and other mitigating factors. The safest way to intake more iodine is to increase the amount of healthy seafood in the diet, but this excludes bottom feeders.

Avoid Povidone Iodine

It is becoming increasingly difficult to know what sort of iodine to use, and a new form of iodine is being sold in stores. It is called Povidone iodine, which is a mix of polyvinylpyrrolidone (PVP) and elemental iodine. The compound is similar to PVC plastic.

There is no need to add a chemical to iodine as a preservative. The classic formula (water or alcohol, potassium iodide, and iodine) is always sterile, and comes with less side effects. Pure iodine is itself a disinfectant, so the addition of toxins to supposedly preserve it is merely another instance of useless chemical tainting. PVP (the "povidone") is said to simply pass through the body when taken orally, but is admitted to cause problems when injected. It is reported to cause pulmonary vascular injury in the latter case. Observant readers will have noticed that polyvinylpyrrolidone contains vinyl. After all of the controversy surrounding such plastics as PVC, can you imagine the effects of chronic exposure?

PVP has some technical applications:

- An adhesive in hot melt glue sticks
- An additive for batteries, ceramics, fiberglass, inks, inkjet paper and in the chemical-mechanical planarization process
- An emulsifier and disintegrant for solution polymerization

There have been a disturbing number of cases in which people have gone into anaphylactic shock due to an allergy to the povidone in this iodine. It is considered hazardous by O.S.H.A. (U.S. Occupational Safety and Health Administration) due to it causing respiratory distress and eye irritation. For the same reason, fire-fighters wear self-contained breathing apparatuses before they enter into buildings containing this substance. There is also evidence to indicate that there is a cancer link.

Zinc Supplementation

According to many pharmacists, zinc is the single greatest dietary supplement. Chemists, pharmacists, and doctors alike glorify zinc supplementation. Some of them maintain that zinc will ward off all sickness. While this is not entirely true, zinc does nonetheless fight the rhinovirus, which is responsible for about a third of the common colds in adults, along with many other illnesses which exhibit flu-like symptoms. Zinc boosts the overall immune system to fight infections and speed recovery times. It is therefore a useful supplement for almost everyone. Deficiencies of zinc lead to decreased thyroid hormone levels, and possibly hypothyroidism. Zinc supplementation is absolutely vital for pregnant women. If zinc were given to every mother-to-be, then a large portion of birth abnormalities, pre-eclampsia occurrences, and deformations could be avoided. Give zinc the same respect that you would give to folate (the superior version of folic acid) and calcium during pregnancy.

Symptoms of Zinc Deficiency

- White spots (cuticles) in the fingernails.
- Pale, rough skin, dry hair, and acne
- Unhealthy weight loss caused by loss of appetite
- Dandruff
- Slow wound healing occurs in particularly bad cases of zinc deficiency.

The primary ingredient in anti-dandruff shampoos is zinc. While there is nothing wrong with putting zinc in the hair, it would be much more prudent to simply supplement with it orally.

Not All Zinc is Created Equal

Zinc sulfate and zinc oxide are among the most popular types of zinc to be sold, but they are definitely not the best. These two zinc varieties simply flush out of the body without much cellular absorption, and may increase a body's burden, instead of lightening it. In the particular case of zinc oxide, it is a widely-known carcinogen that is used in sunscreens. This is a dirty industry secret, and sunscreens are the main reason why sunlight has been falsely accused of causing skin cancers, for those with the most sun exposure use the most sunscreen. Always avoid zinc oxide.

Chelated zinc is partially absorbed by the body. There are different types of chelation, but most zinc manufacturers do not cite which form they use. For companies which do, zinc gluconate and zinc citrate are among the best forms of chelated zinc. Zinc orotate is a chelated form of zinc that is more readily absorbed by the body than any other zinc supplement available. Manufacturers of it will usually boast about having this type, because they have good reason to. Zinc orotate passes through the membranes of cells easily, and it pulls the highest amounts of accompanying minerals into the cells, which leads to higher tissue concentrations of zinc and other beneficial nutrients.

Excellent food sources of zinc include cashews, almonds, kidney beans, flounder, and eggs. Zinc is also present in oysters, pork, and crab, but we do not recommend these latter items as foods. See the section of our nutritional chapter, *God's Nutrition: From The Big Guy Himself* for more information about why one should avoid the latter group.

Zinc is one of the few supplements that the medical establishment actually recommends. For some people, especially pregnant women, it is absolutely essential. We do not recommend zinc supplementation for vegetarians, because zinc will reduce their absorption of iron, and thereby increase their already elevated chance of developing anemia. However, the U.S. National Institutes of Health disagrees, and suggests that vegetarians get 50% more zinc than non-vegetarians, because zinc is one of the many things that vegetarians tend to have a deficiency of. Never take zinc supplements while having an empty stomach, or the zinc may cause nausea and stomach pain. In the very least, follow zinc supplementation with a glass of water.

The Copper Connection

The human body needs copper to properly utilize zinc, so zinc supplementation will yield poor results during a time of copper deficiency. Unfortunately, it is unsafe to supplement with copper directly. It is far too easy to overdose and to cause serious liver problems with direct copper consumption. There are unscrupulous individuals who sell colloidal copper for internal consumption on the Internet, but we warn readers to beware of such scoundrels. They are found astroturfing Internet forums with miraculous stories, and stories are just what they are. The safe way to supplement with copper is to get it indirectly through chlorophyll supplements. Chlorophyll contains enough copper to make a huge difference, and it includes compounds that work with the copper for its best utilization. It is virtually impossible to get an overdose through chlorophyll, and it helps health in many other ways.

Chlorophyll

Chlorophyll is what gives plants their green pigment. It is also responsible for channeling the sun's rays into chemical energy for photosynthesis in all plants. Photosynthesis is the transformation of carbon dioxide and water into useful carbohydrates and oxygen. In human beings, chlorophyll is one of the few substances that pulls more oxygen into the cells, while simultaneously protecting them from oxidative (free radical) damage.

During the 1950's, it was used in certain U.S. toothpastes, due to it being only toxic to harmful bacteria and yeasts, such as candida. It was a remarkable breath freshener that also stimulated gum repair in people with gum disease. The Colgate company had its own line of chlorophyll toothpaste. There was also Palmolive's chlorophyll soap for improved skin complexion. These products worked better than their modern equivalents, because they came before products were required to use toxic chemicals to preserve them for extremely long shelf life. It was before the poisoning of the public was required by official regulations.

There was a period when scientists actually believed that chlorophyll could not be absorbed into the human body, since no trace of toxicity could be detected from it. Modern chemists in the food, pharmaceutical, and cosmetics industries have sadly become that unaccustomed to non-toxic substances. When a controlled study discovered chlorophyll inside the blood plasma of those supplementing with it, serious studies into the health benefits of chlorophyll finally began. Nevertheless, there still remains gross misunderstandings of the absorption and bio-availability of chlorophyll today.

Chlorophyll has the rare tendency of binding with certain carcinogenic chemicals, preventing them from causing damage, and aiding their excretion from the body. This includes aflatoxin-B1, known for causing liver cancer, benzo[a]pyrene, known for causing lung cancers, dioxins, and components of typical tobacco products. These facets of chlorophyll are still being researched. Chlorophyll should eventually be recognized as the major cancer preventative that it is, because it reduces the cellular damage done by all carcinogens, including radiation. Moreover, chlorophyll actually removes benzene from the body, which is produced in proteins whenever they are exposed to radiation.

There are studies ongoing about chlorophyll's ability to prevent liver cancers in subjects who have had aflatoxin exposure. Aflatoxin-B1 is produced by a fungus which lives on moldy grains, beans, and corn. There are some areas where this exposure is unavoidable, so human studies have been conducted in these Chinese regions. So far, it appears that chlorophyll supplementation provides massive protection for those who consume this carcinogen. Conclusive studies are expected to take about 20 years, but there is already enough research for any reasonable person to see an unmistakable trend.

Supplemental Chlorophyll

Chlorophyll is present in all green vegetables, and thus it could be obtained through diet if we were to eat enough vegetables. However, the great majority of people never get enough vegetables in their diets. This trend, in combination with deficient soils that no longer produce nutrient-dense foods, generates the modern need for supplementation. Chlorophyll is best purchased as a liquid concentrate. Multiple drops may be added to drinks or swallowed straight. Supplementation with chlorophyll provides a long-lasting boost of energy, by somehow increasing the overall oxygenation of cells to enhance respiration, but this process is not well understood.

Almost every bodily process is somehow related to oxygen usage. As a result, chlorophyll has shown to help its users resist not only cancers, but also diabetes and heart disease. According to the Linus Pauling Institute, chlorophyll has historically been used to speed the recovery of bruising, and as an internal deodorant. Chlorophyll is sometimes mixed in ointments, and applied topically to wounds, but we recommend against eliminating bruises with pure chlorophyll drops, because concentrated chlorophyll stains skin a greenish-black. Nevertheless, chlorophyll was well recognized as the most effective way to quickly eliminate bruising in the mid-twentieth century, likely due to its high concentration of copper.

Despite 50 years of study, chlorophyll has never shown any toxic effects. Through the act of providing more oxygen to the cells, chlorophyll increases energy, improves concentration, boosts the immune system, aids the body to cleanse itself, and prevents some cancers. It contains magnesium and copper, which are minerals that the overwhelming majority of Americans are deficient in. Magnesium deficiencies lead to heart attacks, migraines, depression, insomnia, and irritability. Copper is necessary for a body to utilize zinc.

Most people should supplement with a small amount of chlorophyll daily. There are no side-effects, and it is essential for the proper functioning of the body. It is fairly tasteless when mixed with juices. The improved energy and concentration derived from it are remarkable. Kids will love the fact that chlorophyll drops will make their mouths green when it is placed directly on the tongue, which is the fastest way to absorb it. The concentrated form is more natural and effective than the weaker solutions, which have additives.

Niacin

The need for niacin (vitamin B-3) is often marginalized, even amongst the health conscious. Multi-vitamins and B-complex supplements typically contain only negligible amounts of it. Ensuring an adequate intake of niacin should be paramount considering that about one out of every three people die from heart disease in the industrialized world, and clinical depression effects about one in every ten adults.

Niacin is an essential nutrient that we typically do not get enough of through our diets, due to depleted soils and processed foods. It is found in dairy products, poultry, fish, lean meats, and nuts. Niacin is vital for the proper digestion of foods, as well as maintaining nerve health and repair. It likewise maintains healthy skin.

Pellagra and Associated Diseases

Pellagra is a disease state that is synonymous with niacin deficiencies. It occurs amongst poor populations having niacin deficiencies. This condition impairs memory and mental health in as much as it contributes to various chronic diseases.

Symptoms of Pellagra

- Diarrhea
- Dermatitis
- Dementia
- Hyper-pigmentation
- Thickening of the skin
- Inflammation of the mouth and tongue
- Digestive disturbances
- Amnesia
- Delirium
- Depression
- Death

Pellagra (pel•lag'•ra) *noun.*

A disease caused by a deficiency of niacin and protein in the diet and characterized by skin eruptions, digestive and nervous system disturbances, and eventual mental deterioration.

Taken from The Free Dictionary
(thefreedictionary.com)

In modern times, it is extremely rare for deaths to be attributed to pellagra, but niacin deficiencies are still a key factor in causing chronic diseases. A deficiency of niacin will cause digestive problems (malnutrition), slow the metabolism, and decrease one's tolerance to cold temperatures. Niacin is utilized for DNA repair, and it assists in the production of natural steroid hormones inside the adrenal glands.

Niacin is also very helpful for the treatment of depression and anxiety, in part because the body converts it into L-tryptophan. Pellagra sufferers have historically displayed the classic symptoms of dementia (which is not to be confused with the modern, redefined version of "dementia", which is actually a variant of Alzheimer's disease). Therefore, niacin is critical for maintaining mental health. A dosage of 500 mg. has been shown to enhance short-term memory by 40%. The overall effect upon long-term memory maintenance may be even greater, but this is more difficult to test.

As in the case of scurvy (vitamin C deficiency), death from this condition is much slower in this modern age, and such deficiencies manifest themselves in the form of heart disease. Niacin protects the arteries from inflammatory damage, which dramatically reduces cholesterol levels; since cholesterol is produced by a body to patch arterial damage. Therefore, niacin can significantly decrease the risk of heart attacks, since it eliminates the conditions that place undue stress upon the heart.

The Coronary Drug Project did a study, wherein 8,000 heart attack victims were issued 3 grams of niacin daily for six years. They reported that there was a reduced incidence of subsequent heart attacks by 27%, and strokes by 26% (compared to the placebo group). A third of the heart attacks and a third of the strokes were prevented by the supplementation of niacin, with no other dietary or lifestyle changes. The combined percentages equates to about half of the at-risk subjects having their lives saved with niacin supplementation alone.

Supplementation Suggestions

Flushing is a condition that is often experienced after niacin supplementation; especially with beginning users, people who use tobacco products, or those who drink alcoholic beverages. Parts of the body (usually the face and upper chest) become rosy red for people experiencing niacin flushes. Niacin flushes may produce the sensations of hot flashes. Severe itching may occur, or the sensation of a mild sunburn. Flushes may last for two hours. Flushing does not cause pain, but it can be a great annoyance.

Purchasing an optimal niacin supplement may not be a simple task, because several forms are available. There is plain niacin, no-flush niacin, and time-released niacin. Time-released niacin can be dangerous. It has been known to cause terrible side effects, including hallucinations and insomnia. We strongly recommend against using time-released niacin because of these risks, and due to its inexcusable toxic impurities.

No-flush niacin is simply a fraud, because it does not even contain niacin. It should be avoided. It is actually niacinomide, which is believed to be one of the compounds that is metabolized by the body from niacin. It is believed that the conversion process from niacin to niacinomide is what causes flushing. No-flush niacin attempts to skip this important biological step. The natural conversion of niacin to niacinomide is what reduces cholesterol and protects the arteries. Therefore, this lab-created bio-chemical does not help to reduce cholesterol or protect the arteries. In addition, it is likely to cause liver damage with long-term usage. In other words, no-flush niacin is actually a dangerous chemical with no benefits, and it is not even niacin.

Niacin Recommendations

The wisest approach is to use plain niacin, and to cope with any initial flushing issues. Flushing does not occur for everyone, and it usually stops occurring after about two weeks of daily supplementation with a consistent dose. The flushing is not dangerous, but it can scare first-time users. There is no need to panic or to confuse it with an allergic reaction. The redness occurs due to the widening of the blood vessels near the skin, which dramatically increases the blood flow to the outer tissues. Regionalized itching will indicate that niacin is flushing toxins from a particular area. Due to our toxic lifestyles, most people will experience this for up to several weeks. Some people may benefit from taking niacin prior to sleeping, so that they may sleep through the flushing. Both nicotine and alcohol greatly intensify the flushing reactions.

Of course, be watchful for rashes, swelling, or difficulty breathing, which could indicate a true allergic reaction that would likely be caused by an impurity within the supplement. It is one reason to avoid supplements from notorious countries such as China, and it is becoming difficult to locate supplements that are not.

Always keep some activated carbon (*Emergency Medicine* chapter) for such emergencies, and decide if a hospital visit is necessary using common sense. Supplement reactions are much less likely when they have been purchased from a reputable health food or herbal supplies store. Never buy supplements from general retailers or grocery stores.

We recommend against supplementing with more than 1,500 mg. (1.5 grams) of niacin, due to the risk of liver damage with extreme dosages. It is wise to start with small doses like 100 mg., and gradually increase as needed. Of course, this is an adult recommendation, so children should be given less.

Cayenne Pepper

Cayenne pepper is a herb which should be added to foods whenever possible. Cayenne's benefits to the digestive system, circulatory system, and the heart have earned it the nickname "miracle herb". Some have used it to aid with weight loss, due to its ability to boost the metabolism. Cayenne pepper was first used as a stimulant by the Cherokee Indians. It is most notable for its effect upon the cardiovascular system. Cayenne has been known to stop heart attacks within 30 seconds, when taken orally.

The benefits of cayenne usage were first reported by Dr. David Christopher, a naturopathic doctor who spent most of his life discovering and promoting alternatives to pharmaceutical medications. He spent his career being persecuted for challenging the establishment. He is the most noted pioneer in the use of cayenne pepper as medicine. Dr. Christopher was so instrumental in promoting cayenne in the naturalistic, nutritional, and herbal communities that he is sometimes referred to as "Dr. Cayenne".

> *"Recent clinical studies have been conducted on many of the old time health applications for this miracle herb. Again and again, the therapeutic value of cayenne pepper has been medically validated."*

-- Dr. Patrick Quillin

Most nations outside the Americas use such herbs as part of their standard protocols. These countries always have better results. In fact, the U.S. is ranked 38th in life expectancy, which places the U.S. health care system below Cuba's, South Korea's, Costa Rica's, Guadeloupe's, Singapore's, and 32 other nations, according to an investigative report by Mother Jones Magazine. It is worth noting that these countries do not have an organization like the F.D.A. to suppress truly conventional medicine on behalf of the pharmaceutical industry.

Why Everyone Should Use Cayenne Pepper

Cayenne should be used daily by anyone who has problems with his heart or blood pressure, because it is beneficial to both. Unlike pharmaceuticals, cayenne pepper helps blood pressure regardless of whether it is initially high or initially low, because it relaxes blood vessels, while causing the heart to beat more efficiently. These dual actions practically guarantee circulation improvement, regardless of the pre-existing condition. It is the difference between man's and God's medicine. Cayenne does what the 'experts' claim is impossible.

Its main medical applications are: weak digestion, chronic pain, shingles, heart disease, sore throats, headaches, high cholesterol levels, poor circulation, blood pressure issues, heart attacks, and toothaches. The use of cayenne has been attributed to the following benefits in patients: dissolving plaque in the arteries, improving heart efficiency, relaxing blood vessels, increasing metabolism, it helps the body to eliminate scar tissue after heart attacks, eliminates pain when applied topically, produces endorphins to enhance mood, eliminates shock, eliminates cluster headaches and in some cases, treats migraine headaches, fights cancer, provides partial relief of sinus problems and congestion, is anti-inflammatory, causes weight loss, prevents blood clots, reduces serum cholesterol, reduces triglycerides, reduces platelet aggregation, alleviates muscles spasms, cramps, and bowel pain, and it will rapidly cure sore throat infections when used in a gargle. It is a gift from God, in other words.

Cayenne pepper can be purchased in convenient capsule form at health food stores for people who wish to use it as a supplement. If cayenne supplements cause a burning sensation in the stomach, simply consuming parmesan cheese will minimize it. We always recommend avoiding regular retailers for supplements.

It is popular to use cayenne that is infused in warm water. Some people add half a teaspoon of cayenne to 8 ounces of water or tea, and then they gradually increase the amount of cayenne as their tolerance grows. In sufficient amounts, it can kill gastrointestinal parasites.

For the best emergency treatment of heart problems, cayenne should be mixed with taurine and held in the mouth, before swallowing. Do not forgo immediate emergency medical attention in the event of a heart attack.

Cherry Supplements

Cherries are considered to be among the most powerful disease-fighting foods available, largely because of their high anti-oxidant content. Cherries are becoming well known for their ability to improve the circulation, along with possessing anti-aging and anti-carcinogenic properties. The title of an enlightening U.S.D.A. report was, *Arthritis hurts. But fresh cherries may help*. Of course, the F.D.A. eventually noticed this report after it began getting quoted at Internet health sites such as ours, so the article seems to have now *disappeared*, but we archived it at our site. The evidence of this governmental admission can also be found by plugging the report's title into an Internet search engine, but the entire report has become difficult to find. At one point, the F.D.A. threatened to use the Federal Marshals to arrest cherry farmers, and even confiscate the entire U.S. cherry crop if farmers continued quoting the scientific findings about the medicinal properties of cherries from the government's own reports.

Cherries are famous amongst naturopathic practitioners for their ability to relieve the pains of arthritis and gout. Researchers from Michigan State University found that anthocyanins, the same chemicals that give cherries their color, have powerful anti-inflammatory effects. The study showed that these anthocyanins inhibit COX-2 enzymes, which play a key role in the body's production of prostaglandins -- natural chemicals involved in inflammation. Another study affirmed that tart cherries have anti-oxidant and anti-inflammatory effects that are comparable with prescription drugs.

Unfortunately, cooking cherries is known to kill many of the beneficial compounds found inside them. Therefore, eating cherry pie would probably produce very little benefit. Cherries may be eaten raw, or concentrated cherry supplements can be purchased for higher potency and convenience. Concentrated cherry supplements have been shown to be more effective in reducing arthritis pain and inflammation than pharmaceuticals.

High concentration cherry supplements can also be used for general soreness and joint issues like carpal tunnel syndrome. They are very effective; especially when combined with MSM and vitamin B-6.

Guarana

The most common complaints amongst those suffering with routine illnesses are fatigue and the inability to concentrate. When the immune system is weakened, it uses up all of its reserve energy trying to fight off the threat. Likewise, due to our modern eating habits, the immune system of the average person is under constant stress, leading to chronic fatigue.

Guarana is an all-natural stimulant that contains a substance called guaranine, which is often mistaken for caffeine. Guaranine is safer, and yet more potent as a stimulant. Guarana also contains large amounts of theophylline, theobromine, and tannic acid. It is rich in saponins, which reduce the risk of cancer and boost the immune system. Guarana seed is not water soluble, so absorption is usually slow. While the effects of caffeine only last for around 3-4 hours, the effects of guarana can last for 8-10 hours. Other than elevating the blood pressure slightly, guarana has proven to be harmless.

Studies in rats have shown that guarana increases memory retention and physical endurance in comparison to a placebo. In 2007, a double-blind study assessed behavioral effects of four doses (37.5 mg., 75 mg., 150 mg., and 300 mg.) of guarana extract. Memory, alertness and mood were increased, which confirmed a previous study finding cognitive improvements following just 75 mg. of guarana. Surprisingly, the two lower doses produced more cognitive improvements than the higher doses, so sometimes less is more.

The Human Cognitive Neuroscience Unit, which conducted the four phase study concluded that, "the effects cannot be attributed to caffeine alone". Caffeine is found inside the nuts that produce guaranine, and it has been impossible to chemically separate caffeine from guaranine, so it is commonly believed that guaranine is caffeine. The people making this claim should acknowledge that guaranine and caffeine have different strengths, are found in different plants, and have somewhat different effects. The confusion demonstrates how primitive modern science is at understanding these kinds of nutritional substances.

Guarana is ideal for dieters, because it somehow releases and uses energy primarily from fat cells. This process is not understood either, but it has been repeatedly observed and documented. In a study published in the June 2001 issue of the *Journal of Human Nutrition*, guarana extract induced weight loss for over 45 days in overweight patients who were taking a mixed herbal preparation containing yerba mate, guarana, and damiana. Body weight reductions averaged 11.22 pounds in the guarana group, compared to less than one pound in the placebo group after 45 days.

It is difficult to find something that compares with guarana. It enhances mood, improves concentration, improves memory, dissolves extraneous fat cells, and provides abundant energy for about 8 hours, without jitteriness or side effects. There are many properties of guarana that remain unexplained by science, and the true chemical makeup is misunderstood. Some studies cited anti-oxidant and anti-bacterial effects, and fat cell reduction in mice when it was combined with conjugated linoleic acid (found in real butter).

In summary, guarana enhances moods, helps with weight loss, and provides a much needed energy boost for most people. If you doubt the power of alternative medicine, then this may be the supplement that you need to become a believer. Guarana is not recommended for those with chronically high blood pressure. We also precaution women against using it during pregnancy, due to a lack of testing with pregnant women.

Hemp Supplementation

In the 18th century, the hemp plant was used extensively for everything from clothing to ship sails. It is extremely strong and lightweight, so there is a plethora of industrial applications. America's Founding Fathers grew it, and the U.S. Constitution was written upon hemp paper. Yet it is now illegal to grow in the United States. It is nonetheless making a comeback. Hemp-made clothing is now available, and hemp bricks are being used to built select homes. Hemp oil is the easiest and most renewable oil in existence; so it could therefore solve many of our economic problems, including our dependence on petroleum. Furthermore, it does not produce severely toxic fumes as petrochemical products do. When burnt, it produces only carbon dioxide (not carbon monoxide), which benefits plants, and thus the overall environment. Its financial threat to the petrochemical industry plays a large role in why it is illegal to grow in the U.S.

Along with its industrial uses, hemp is incredibly beneficial for maintaining health. We have already recommended that vegetarians use hemp instead of soy, because of its superior protein content. Hemp is the only plant in existence that contains all twenty-one known amino acids that are needed by the human body. It provides an almost complete source of nutrition, and thus we recommend hemp fiber as a routine supplement. It has become difficult to get all of the nutrition that we need through our foods, due to depleted soils and chemical fertilizers. This generally forces healthy individuals to rely on supplementation to augment even good diets. The usage of hemp is an exceptional beginning for any protocol of dietary supplementation.

Despite the health benefits of hemp, Americans are not currently allowed to grow their own. It is federally regulated, although some states have ignored the federal law, and made the cultivation of hemp legal under licenses. However, none of the state governments have been bold enough to issue licenses before reaching compromising agreements with the Drug Enforcement Administration.

To be sold legally, hemp must be completely free of THC, the narcotic of "marijuana" (cannabis). THC is a natural part of the plant, and it has health benefits of its own. Contrary to the propaganda of the prohibition crowd, THC will actually boost the immune system and improve health. Unlike tobacco smoking, the smoking of cannabis actually strengthens the lungs, increases air capacity, and decreases a person's chances of cancer. Like in the case of hemp, cannabis is primarily illegal because of what it can do for us at the expense of the disease industry. There is nothing that works better or faster to eliminate nausea and migraine headaches than cannabis. It has anti-cancer properties too.

Affirm Your Rights

Due to U.S. federal laws, all hemp sold in America as a supplement is currently imported into the States. Thus, instead of supporting the U.S. economy, hemp has become a drain on it.

These plants were not created for the sole purpose of getting us "high". Governments have no right to claim that God did not know what he was doing, and to mandate that natural medicinal plants be banned. The contention that plants should be banned or chemically changed before people may have access to God's medicines is blasphemous at best, and it runs contrary to our rights. The people should stop tolerating it, because we are supposed to be making the rules -- not every pharmaceutical company that fears a competitive threat. The medicinal benefits of plants are still being discovered. It is inherently wrong for a small group of elites to make our health decisions for us and enforce a type of slavish dependence.

Those who suffer from herpes should be cautious when using hemp, because of its high L-arginine content. It is prudent to compensate with lysine supplementation simultaneously. We recommend avoiding hemp completely whenever a herpes outbreak is present, and this includes relatives of the virus, such as shingles, chicken pox, and Bell's palsy.

Indian Tobacco

Some readers will be surprised by our endorsement of any herb that is to be smoked; especially one that is called a "tobacco". We endorse the medicinal use of Indian tobacco (lobelia inflata). Smoking truly natural substances is not necessarily harmful. Even real tobacco does not need to be dangerous, but it is made dangerous by the industry. Commercially-made cigarettes are harmful because of the additives, the glues, the radioactive fertilizers, and the papers that are used -- not the tobaccos themselves. The American Indians smoked organic tobacco for a thousand years before the Europeans arrived, without cancers. They get cancers now, for the same chemical reasons that everyone else is getting cancers.

Both the seeds and the dried leaves of Indian tobacco contain alkaloids which yield its effects.

Indian tobacco is mostly used for its beneficial effects upon the lungs, although it is also believed to boost the overall immune system. It has the unusual property of being a stimulant to the respiratory system, whilst being a general relaxant for the rest of the body. It has been found to be very helpful for asthmatics, with some asthma sufferers substituting it for their inhalers.

Indian tobacco has been traditionally used to effectively suppress common colds, bronchitis, and pneumonia. The smoke from Indian tobacco reduces phlegm, and kills infections in the lungs. It thins mucus, which increases recovery time, and causes many infections to be less symptomatic. When people use it for this purpose, it is often smoked with the herb mullein. Mullein was once used to soothe the coughing associated with tuberculosis, and to cure it. Mullein has no "flavor", and is a very light smoke. Most people feel like they are breathing pure air when smoking mullein. It mixes well with Indian tobacco. The two tend to work well together to amplify the benefits of each. We recommend an ideal ratio of 2:1 in favor of Indian tobacco.

Indian tobacco has been used by many people who were trying to quit smoking, but it was banned in such products in 1993 by the F.D.A., even though the agency had no legitimate jurisdiction. The agency claimed that Indian tobacco was ineffective. The F.D.A. did not bother to fund any studies to test its effectiveness at all; which leads us to conclude that the ban was to protect both the pharmaceutical industry and the tobacco industry. Americans can still freely buy Indian tobacco, but sellers are not allowed to inform people that it greatly helps with smoking cessation or of its medicinal benefits.

One of its constituents, isolobelanine, helps to relax people whenever they are experiencing stimulant withdrawal symptoms, which includes nicotine withdrawal. Indian tobacco contains lobeline too, an alkaloid that helps to clean the lungs. When a person's lungs are clean, smoking becomes disagreeable, causing the smoker to become dizzy or nauseous, like when he first began smoking. This will generally aid someone who is trying to quit smoking, by serving as a deterrent. Studies have widely-varying results regarding the benefits of Indian tobacco, but most of the negative studies were illegitimate, because they used orally-consumed extracts that had been chemically altered. It exemplifies the sort of data shopping that the F.D.A. routinely conducts to get the 'right' research results.

Researchers have been studying the effects of Indian tobacco on amphetamine addictions. Lobeline counteracts excessive dopamine, which occurs in people suffering from methamphetamine addictions. Some people have successfully used it to treat alcoholism. Studies on rats have shown that one of the active constituents in Indian tobacco actually improves the memory of rats, even 24 hours after its usage.

Indian tobacco was historically smoked, but people have begun swallowing the dried leaves and making herbal teas from it, in recent times. The newer methods of oral consumption are unwise, even though they are ironically intended to make it safer. For those who decide to use Indian tobacco medicinally, we strongly recommend smoking it via a pipe, instead of ingesting it. This is because the dosage is extremely important, and people have a tendency to overdose with ingestion. Large amounts will induce vomiting, so smoke only a pinch, and use more if needed. Dizziness is an early symptom that too much has been used, and the person could become ill if it is continued after that. Old herbalist books refer to Indian tobacco as "pukeweed" for its tendency to induce vomiting.

Do not use Indian tobacco alongside pharmaceuticals, because it has a tendency to interact with drugs. It especially amplifies the effects of medications that are given to control blood pressure, but it counteracts drugs given to control diabetes. It increases the loss of potassium from the body if it is taken alongside diuretics or corticosteroids. Aspirin and NSAIDs may increase the risk of overdose reactions to lobelia, leading to vomiting and other illness symptoms.

Purchasing Indian Tobacco

Sellers of this herb often refer to it by its botanical name, lobelia inflata, instead of Indian tobacco. This is because they are avoiding the stigma and regulations that are associated with tobacco products. Searching for the plant by its botanical name will make sellers easier to locate.

General Supplement Recommendations

We are constantly asked by readers which vitamins they should use. For years, we recommended that people choose food-based vitamins, because they have the potential to be much safer, and nutrients are much more readily absorbed in the organic form. However, we recently re-evaluated the multi-vitamins that are available, and came to the depressing realization that things have drastically changed since our original research. The changes in the supplement industry happened at a very fast pace.

The food-based vitamins that are currently available are actually worse than their synthetic counterparts. Almost all of the food-based vitamins that we recently evaluated were fermented in yeasts and bacteria. Usually these were genetically-engineered yeasts and bacteria to make them toxic enough to accelerate their pathogenic life processes. This manufacturing is a way to cheat using bacteria and yeasts to break the foods down instead of using chemicals. In actuality, neither the process nor the end product is natural or food-like. The biotechnology industry found a way to trick us all into making genetic engineering a part of our "natural" supplementation. We wrote this because we have had repeated calls from people who were having allergy problems or sicknesses that increased with multi-vitamin usage. In every case, it was caused by one of the multi-vitamin products that was allegedly food-based, but which was not actually made from foods. A diet of yeast will, in fact, attack the immune system to make both allergies and illnesses worse. These so-called "multi-vitamins" are worse than no vitamins at all.

"The food industry has used genetically engineered bacteria and yeasts for more than 20 years to produce vitamins and nutritional supplements."

-- Agricultural Biotechnology,
The University of California

Customers are actually ingesting rotten vegetable matter that is produced with biotechnology assistance, for health benefits. Of course, the companies have not studied whether this fermentation process produces toxic byproducts, as most fermentation does, because the priority is profit. Such studies would actually make them more liable, because until they have evidence that demonstrates harm, they can simply claim ignorance. The few food-based multi-vitamin products which did not contain yeast had other questionable ingredients, such as oyster extract, various algae, and seaweeds. These items should never be considered foods, and especially not health foods. The real foods in the "food-based" supplements have been replaced with non-food, bottom-feeding scavengers from the oceans and pond scum, which are known for a huge variety of toxins. Some of these vitamins will prove deadly for people with shellfish allergies, and the cause of death will never be traced to the vitamins.

We must reverse our prior recommendations about supplements, and we are now recommending synthetic vitamins instead. In the past few years, a lot has changed in manufacture, and it is obvious that the biotechnology industry has made in-roads into supplement manufacture. We previously recommended food-based multi-vitamins on the basis that synthetic vitamins are much harder for the body to absorb, and there is a chance of simply causing stressed kidneys when using high quantities of them. However, there is no good choice for supplementation anymore, so it has become a matter of choosing the lesser of evils. The current situation is that if one does not use vitamins from the chemical industry, then he must instead use the "food" vitamins from the biotechnology industry, which are considerably worse. While we hope and expect that this will one day change, it is the current deplorable situation.

The fact that we are reversing our position should help to explain why we are usually so careful not to make specific supplement recommendations. Any recommendations that we make could become invalid within weeks or months, and thousands of people might act upon those recommendations, so we are cautious.

The most important long-lasting recommendation is to read the ingredient labels, and learn to spot the unacceptable ingredients. The following is a list of common vitamin ingredients that should always be avoided:

- Yeasts, including brewer's yeast.
- Algae, such as spirulina and chlorella.
- Mushrooms and other fungi.
- Organs, such as liver and kidneys.
- Seaweeds. Kelp is a common addition.
- Titanium dioxide

Brewer's yeast and so-called nutritional yeast feed candida, which is the fungus in the gastro-intestinal tract that is responsible for allergies, frequent headaches, and mood swings. When there is an excess of candida, the body becomes unable to properly absorb nutrients from foods. So, there is an incredible irony when yeasts are added to supplements, only to prevent proper nutrient absorption.

We cannot recommend multi-vitamins, for they seem to be the worst category. A good dietary supplement should provide a nutrient that heals a known condition, or corrects a likely imbalance, but multi-vitamins provide a shotgun approach to supplementation that has become increasingly dangerous. This is especially true now that most companies are getting ingredients from China. What you do not know can kill you, slowly and horribly. Whenever a person takes a vitamin, he is making a gamble that the vitamin will help him more than it impairs him. Multi-vitamins pose an irrational level of elevated risk, for minimal convenience. With multi-vitamins, it is especially hard to find a company that is willing to document where it obtained every ingredient, or whether the vitamins come from a disreputable country, such as China, which has a history of poisoning us. The risk of multi-vitamin contamination is much higher than for regular supplements.

People who want (or need) to get extra nutrients daily can achieve this by using hemp protein powder as a natural source for all of the amino acids and dietary fiber. Another option is to mix fruits and vegetables together in a blender to make juices. Such natural approaches do not come with the same level of risk as unnaturally-extracted nutrients, and purely organic nutrients work much better.

Vitamin B-12

Vitamin B-12 is necessary for good cognitive function and mental alertness. It can only be found naturally in meats, so it is always lacking in vegetarian and vegan diets, but it is sometimes lacking even in those with reasonably balanced diets. Cyanocobalamin is the most common type of vitamin B-12 added to supplements, but it is very poorly absorbed. Its manufacturing process is cheaper, so it is preferred by the less-ethical supplement manufacturers, which is the majority of them. Methylcobalamin is much better absorbed, and its absorption is improved if it is held inside the mouth and allowed to dissolve into the mouth tissues, instead of through normal digestion. Most of the ethical companies which sell methylcobalamin (B-12) supplements provide them in a lozenge form for maximum absorption. We likewise encourage this method.

Conclusionary Remarks

The best vitamins are always those from foods as God made them. There is no pill substitute for a good diet. Supplements are able to somewhat "supplement" a diet that is lacking in a specific nutrient, but they will never be able to replace good nutrition. The reality is: No one has been able to identify all of the nutrients that are in our foods, so any attempt to replace a good diet with supplements is both futile and foolish. The people who choose to eat processed foods and then take supplements to compensate are likewise on a fool's errand, because their overall gastrointestinal health is typically too impaired to properly absorb and utilize the nutrients from the supplements.

When attempting to improve the diet, be aware that organic foods have a higher density of nutrients. In addition, they do not contain pesticides that weaken the immune system, cause diseases, and make it more difficult for the body to absorb nutrients. Organic foods are not 'enhanced' by the biotechnology industry either. You may listen to our discussion about yeast-based vitamins in the audio show, *Parts is Parts* (episode 26), which may be found in our audio archive at our site, healthwyze.org.

Consumer Lab

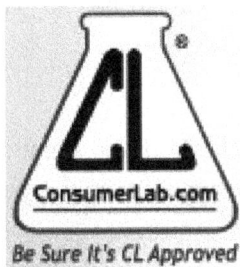

"Our Mission: To identify the best quality health and nutritional products through independent testing."

-- www.consumerlab.com

We were contacted to evaluate an organization known as Consumer Lab. They have been cited numerous times in mainstream news publications as experts in appraising nutritional supplements. They have a reputation for targeting specific companies aggressively. We normally embrace any group that is seeking higher standards and accountability concerning supplements and alternative medicine, but something seemed terribly wrong about Consumer Lab.

Consumer Lab claims to be working for the public; similar to Consumer Reports. It tests the concentration and purity of supplements, and it then reports its findings to paying customers. Individuals who want to know its results must subscribe to Consumer Lab for $30 a year, when we last checked pricing. In addition to getting money from the consumers, it also gets money from the supplement companies themselves. Companies pay them thousands of dollars for favorable product reviews and certifications. Recommendations from Consumer Lab have expiry dates, so manufacturers must pay again every 12 months, if they wish to continue using the certified "CL" seal. On one hand, companies are paying Consumer Lab for favorable reviews, while individuals are paying them for what they believe is objective reporting.

"Also try the vendors below, as each sells some of the products tested... We have not, however, tested nor approved all of the items that they carry, so check our Reviews. These vendors pay a fee to be listed below but we receive no revenue from purchases made. We have reviewed the advertisements for accuracy but do not review or endorse editorial information appearing on their websites. Click here for more information about advertising on ConsumerLab.com."

-- www.consumerlab.com

The above quote appeared on their official "Where To Buy" (supplements) web page. Those statements comprised a slip that revealed their financial double-dipping.

Marc Ullman, writing for *Natural Foods Merchandiser* magazine, previously reported how this is an extreme conflict of interest. It is impossible to be a paid client of the industry, while providing an objective analysis; like the third-party watchdog that they pretend to be. So we decided to dig a little deeper into Consumer Lab.

Consumer Lab's C.E.O.

The president of Consumer Lab is Tod Cooperman, M.D. While in medical school, he spent a summer working at an investment bank in New York City, where he evaluated new health care companies. His first job following graduation from medical school was with Bristol-Myers-Squibb pharmaceuticals, where he remained from 1987 to 1993.

He then founded CareData Reports, which rated insurance plans and H.M.O.'s; purportedly based on customer feedback. The company continued to expand until it covered everything from pharmacy benefits to dental care. At which time he sold CareData to J.D. Power and Associates, and remained there as an employee until 1999. We found the company's explosive growth to be puzzling; considering that it profited solely by providing consumer reports. However, we have been unable to prove that CareData Reports profited from the same payola scheme that fuels Consumer Lab.

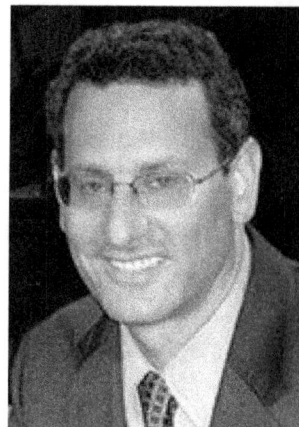

Consumer Lab's website claims that one of Cooperman's first actions, when starting consumerlab.com was to hire one of the "world's leading experts on dietary supplements", Dr. William Obermeyer. Dr. Obermeyer had been working as an upper-level Food and Drug Administration chemist for nine years before undertaking his business partnership with Cooperman. We investigated Obermeyer based upon speculations about why someone with a cushy, well-paid, governmental job at the F.D.A., with likely no accountability whatsoever, would suddenly give up that secure position in favor of a risky job venture in a new business that had never been explored.

Dr. Obermeyer's work at the F.D.A. had been limited to investigating contaminations in dietary supplements, and watching for *unapproved* claims from competing treatment methodologies. It is documented that Obermeyer complained that the F.D.A. did not have the necessary funds to persecute people who reported competing cancer treatments, whilst investigating supplement companies at the same time. Obermeyer's comments have led us to conclude that his resignation was prompted by the F.D.A. not being aggressive enough in suppressing information about successful alternatives, instead of sincere concerns about product safety.

The Agenda of Consumer Lab

Consumer Lab claims to have tested approximately 1,600 products, including making the rather ambitious claim that it has tested 95% of all supplements sold in the United States. Cooperman claims that one quarter of the products failed his company's testing, which is probably about the number of companies that categorically refused to pay for the "independent" testing or a U.S.P. certification. It reflects despicable business policies that could be called blackmail, and the uncertified companies are therefore more ethical because of their non-compliance. As an ex-employee of Bristol-Myers-Squibb, and someone who actively seeks F.D.A. advice on nutritional supplements, we have a fairly clear idea of Cooperman's agenda.

Cooperman's partner, Dr. Obermeyer, spent nine glorious years inside the F.D.A., seeking problems with dietary supplements, before continuing the same work at Consumer Lab. The very name of this company reminds us of The Center For Consumer Freedom, a P.R. front for Monsanto and "hundreds of companies that wish to remain anonymous". While such cute names are designed to be disarming; such organizations are usually paid by the very industry that they are supposed to be policing. In the case of Consumer Lab, they likewise appear to be team players.

> *"In a recent test of multivitamins, ConsumerLab.com found that Equate-Mature Multivitamin 50+ sold by Wal-Mart was just as good as the name brand Centrum Silver, but at less than a nickel a day is half the price."*

> -- New York Times (Dec. 4th, 2009)

The deception is their covert placing of Centrum Silver as the gold standard of supplements in the minds of readers, without them noticing. In our educated opinion, we believe that neither product is actually fit for human consumption, nor does either provide more benefit than harm in the long term. Both supplement companies likely paid a great deal of money to both the New York Times and to Consumer Lab for such 'objective' reporting.

> *"What does Consumerlab.com charge to participate in its 'voluntary certification program'? One of the comments posted after my first letter noted that the fee charged for testing products containing Glucosamine, Chondroitin and MSM was $4,650.00 for the tests completed in the early summer 2009. Is this the standard fee that Consumerlab.com charges companies that wish to ensure that your test results are proprietary to the manufacturer?"*

> -- Marc Ullman

Marc Ullman is chair of the Legal Advisory Council for the Natural Products Foundation. He pinned-down Mr. Cooperman in a public discourse, wherein his questions became a little too uncomfortable for Mr. Cooperman to answer. The term "proprietary" means that the test results are owned by the manufacturer buying the study, so that all negative findings may be stricken from public disclosure. Any organization that truly serves the public and operates under scientific principles does not keep secrets about its results. Consumer Lab is the anti-thesis of principled scientific research.

There are times when being endorsed by a certain group is actually an indication of dishonor. This appears to be the case for Consumer Lab certified companies. We recommend avoiding all vitamins that have either the C.L. seal or a U.S.P. certification. The vitamins that are recommended by Consumer Lab are known as U.S.P. vitamins. The C.L. seal marks an approval from an organization that is run by those, who in the very least, have vested interests outside of what they fully disclose. While we generally have no disagreements with groups seeking to benefit the public by providing honest information about supplements, there are far too many coincidences for us to ignore here. The Food and Drug Administration is the last place that one should ever search for honest and accurate advice about herbs and supplements. It is very much like seeking advice from a drug dealer about how to break free from a drug addiction. Likewise, seeking advice from Consumer Lab appears to be just as irrational, since its owners have been heavily immersed in the pharmaceutical cartel for most of their careers, and even directly employed by the F.D.A. itself. They are part of a good-ole-boy network from a chemical industry that profits from sick care, but never healing. It is an industry that openly mocks supplementation and nutritional medicine.

A System Designed to Protect Itself from Threats

If the F.D.A. needed to put more resources into a particular area, surely it would be the area that is resulting in the most deaths. We never see emergency rooms filled with those who are experiencing horrendous vitamin B-12 reactions, or vitamin C overdoses. Instead, the majority of people are there for life-threatening reactions to *properly prescribed* drugs; so the F.D.A. should spend more time checking the safety of drugs that are already on the market. If they were as rigorous in enforcing recalls for pharmaceuticals as they are for dietary supplements, then medicine as we know it would cease to exist. Ephedra was banned by the F.D.A., after concentrated doses of the stimulant had been taken by people who were also using hypertension medications; resulting in roughly 200 deaths. Of course, it was the herb that was blamed. In contrast, Vioxx caused 27,000 deaths before it was *voluntarily* recalled. The *voluntary* recall means that the pharmaceutical manufacturer *still* has full F.D.A. approval to put Vioxx back onto the market at will. Be watchful for that to eventually happen, under a new and more marketable drug name.

Quick Tips

Food Poisoning

Those who eat at restaurants on a regular basis are certain to occasionally experience food poisoning. The symptoms can appear within three to four hours. They include diarrhea, vomiting, headaches, and fever. The symptoms can be violently extreme. An individual will typically suffer with food poisoning for 24 to 36 grueling hours. Most of the so-called "stomach bugs" are actually minor cases of food poisoning, but they are rarely recognized as such. Food poisoning is a much more common problem than most people realize.

Staphylococcus aureus is a very common food poisoning bacteria. It is killed by normal cooking, but it is frequently found in hand-made products that are left at room temperature for a long time, such as potato salad or sandwich spread. Salmonella is the most infamous food poisoning agent, but it is easily destroyed in temperatures above 150 degrees Fahrenheit. The presence of listeria in meats has resulted in a large number of meat recalls. It breeds in the unhygienic conditions of factory farms. It causes flu-like symptoms, and it has the unusual trait of becoming contagious in an infected individual. It can be deadly to children and people who have weakened immune systems. The botulism toxins are caused by the clostridium botulinum bacteria. Botulism poisoning is rare. It is only responsible for 1 in 400 cases of food poisoning, but it is more likely to result in death. Cl. botulinum can exist as a heat-resistant spore, and may grow to produce a neurotoxin in under-cooked, home-canned foods. Incredibly, botulinum poison therapy ("Botox") is an approved *medical therapy*, which is used to temporarily hide wrinkles through its central nervous system toxicant effect, which paralyzes patients' faces like venomous snake bites. Incredibly, the establishment is testing the effects of injecting botulism into the brains of those with neurological disorders, in its quest to find innovative ways to poison patients.

Pepto-Bismol is a popular option for symptom relief in the Americas; but ironically, it is itself one of the most toxic remedies available. Along with being radioactive, the inactive ingredients range from saccharin to benzoic acid (a benzene derivative), to aluminum compounds. Therefore, Pepto-Bismol will actually contribute to long-term health problems.

There are natural options which greatly reduce the recovery time, and they come with no dangerous side-effects.

- **Ginger**: Even some pharmacists will recommend this herbal option for nausea and vomiting. For faster absorption, it can be held in the mouth, and allowed to sink through the tissues into the bloodstream. Ginger pills can be purchased cheaply from health food stores. The media and medical establishment expressed shock when ginger was successfully used to eliminate nausea from chemotherapy poisoning. It is very effective.

- **Activated Charcoal**: Having astounding properties, activated charcoal is able to neutralize the overwhelming majority of toxins, from Prozac to arsenic. It is the world's best general-purpose filtering agent. It is all natural (made from burnt coconut shells). It has been a staple of poison control centers since their inception. A consequence of using it is that it will stop an individual from absorbing his food nutrients and medications. It will usually stop a case of food poisoning from progressing, and do so rapidly. See the *Activated Carbon* section of the *Emergency Medicine chapter* for detailed information about its unique qualities. Never use charcoal briquettes, like those used for outdoor cooking. Activated charcoal is an essential first aid item, so every family should keep some that has been pre-emptively ground into powder and stored inside an air tight container, for poison emergencies.

- **Colloidal Silver**: When food poisoning is caused by bacteria (it usually is), then colloidal silver will kill it. Some people use colloidal silver as a natural and non-toxic preservative.

- **Cannabis** ("Marijuana"): Cannabis has a vast array of medicinal uses, and it may be the most beneficial plant known to mankind. One of its properties is its incredible suppression of nausea. It is especially useful whenever a person is too sick to swallow. Some studies demonstrate that it is more effective than its pharmaceutical equivalents in stopping nausea. Contrary to the propaganda, it has no known adverse effects, and it is safer than aspirin. It actually improves the lung capacity in those who smoke it, making both their hearts and lungs stronger.

It would be wise to keep these items available in preparation, because food poisoning is never planned. It happens suddenly, and leaves no opportunity for its victims to go shopping. You should begin collecting these items now, because you will not have time to prepare in an emergency. Be prepared, because emergencies are not a matter of *if* they happen, but of *when* they happen.

It is possible that the victim will lose the colloidal silver and the charcoal through vomiting, at least during the first attempt to use them. Work to control the nausea, and then try again shortly later. Be advised that almost every medicine will be completely neutralized by the activated charcoal.

Remedying Hangovers

Home remedies for hangovers have been circulating for years, but they are invariably ineffective. To eliminate a health condition, we must first isolate the true causes. In the case of hangovers, the causes include dehydration, a sugar crash, and chemical poisoning. Modern alcoholic beverages are far more likely to produce hangovers than those available decades ago. Many wines now contain nitrates, which are known to cause headaches and grogginess, whilst reducing oxygen flow in the body to yield extreme acidosis. Some alcoholic drinks contain artificial flavors and colors, and are barely comparable to the beverages of yesteryear. Drinking large amounts of these beverages is the equivalent to having a huge binge on chemically and genetically-engineered ConAgra foods. To make the point about toxicity clear: taking a teaspoon of powdered activated charcoal prior to drinking these toxic products will usually prevent a hangover, since activated charcoal prevents the absorption of most poisons, while not effecting alcohols.

Most people already know that drinking water during a hangover is important, because alcohol causes dehydration. However, they do not realize that one of the main reasons for a hangover is an extreme sugar crash. Alcohol is little more than fermented sugar, so the aftermath of it is drowsiness, poor mood, headaches, and a general feeling of weakness. All of which are associated with both hangovers and sugar crashes. Consuming a small amount of sugar (1-2 teaspoons) during a hangover will speed recovery time dramatically. As always, we recommend the use of evaporated cane juice instead of the bleached and refined sugars whenever possible. Of course, honey is always fine.

Some people recommend vitamin B-12 during a hangover, which assists with concentration and energy. Vitamin B-12 can be taken daily in the form of methylcobalamin, but never use cyanocobalamin. You should either chew up your B-12 vitamins, or hold them under the tongue to get direct absorption into the blood. Otherwise, normal digestion will destroy most of the B-12.

Of course, we are not encouraging people to drink large amounts of alcohol, as it may produce long-term health consequences, and it has a tendency to make some people violent or depressed. It is important to remember that with routine heavy drinking, some individuals will develop a severe addiction to alcohol. Drinking moderate amounts of organic red wine, however, can actually benefit the health.

Tylenol Warning

Tylenol is extremely poisonous when it is combined with alcohol. It is likely to have killed a large number of college students, who were recovering from hangovers, and later their deaths were blamed on "binge drinking"; not the Tylenol. It is difficult to know how many people this has happened to, because Tylenol liver toxicity is not tested for during the autopsies.

Eye Drops

Most people experience periodic eye problems, including infections, dryness, and injuries. Eye drops are usually the first response to these situations, but the eye drops that are sold in pharmacies normally contain thimerosal ("thiomersal"). It is an allergy-inflicting, mercury-containing preservative that has rightly sparked outrage for its use in vaccines. Standard eye drops contain a plethora of other toxic ingredients, which were designed to ensure that they never have bacterial growth. The chemicals were chosen specifically because they are poisonous.

After becoming aware of these problems, we decided to formulate our own eye drops; with safety, simplicity, and effectiveness as our guiding principles. Our simple formulation is more effective at relieving conditions such as conjunctivitis (pink eye) than over-the-counter medications. The base for the eye drops is colloidal silver, which is a safe, natural antibiotic, and anti-microbial.

A small amount of sea salt is added to the colloidal silver to resupply the saline that the solution washes away. Sea salt should always be used instead of table salt. Sea salt specifically results in less burn, and it further helps to kill infections with both its sodium and its trace minerals. Normal saline (made with table salt) will usually cause some discomfort in the eyes, regardless of how well the solution is made. Table salt is slightly toxic because of the way that minerals are stripped from it during processing, and ironically, these same minerals are often later resold to vitamin companies. Despite the visible mineral particles that are found in some sea salts, which can seem initially frightening, a person is very unlikely to experience any irritation.

The Recipe

- 3 fluid ounces of colloidal silver (6 U.S. tablespoons)
- A pinch of sea salt (about 1/8 of a teaspoon)

We recommend that the solution be discarded after three weeks, since the silver particles are eventually destroyed by the salt. It is a good idea to write the date on the bottle, or the future disposal date. Almost everyone knows that silver is extremely resistant to corrosion, but this solution contains almost atomic-sized silver particles that are kept in salt water for an extended period. Salt will destroy all colloidal-sized metal particles in time. In the meantime, the solution will transform into silver chloride. Silver chloride is not usually recommended for medicine, but it is actually better for outer tissue absorption (like the eyes) than colloidal silver is.

Those who must use eye drops routinely, due to contact lenses, should know that it is possible to improve, and in some cases, actually correct poor vision with improved nutrition. Sprouts (as in baby plants, not brussel sprouts) seem to be particularly helpful for the eyes. In addition, retinol, the most absorbable form of vitamin A, is found in animal sources including eggs, fish, and especially beef.

Whitening Teeth

You can safely bleach your own teeth using a natural substance: oxygen. Simply rinse and gargle with oxygenated water, more commonly known as hydrogen peroxide, every time that you brush your teeth. In a matter of weeks, a tremendous change will be seen in the color of the teeth. The oxygen from hydrogen peroxide will safely bleach teeth white. If caught early enough, gargling with hydrogen peroxide can sometimes wipe-out a sore throat infection. Unlike fluoridated toothpastes, it can even be swallowed without the necessity of a visit to a hospital. Ingestion of low doses is actually good for the body. The main side effect is a reduced cancer risk. The ideal peroxide is 3% strength or weaker of food grade hydrogen peroxide. Normal hydrogen peroxide contains chemical stabilizers and other additives, which may get absorbed into the body.

For the best teeth, real butter should be added to the diet. Butter can actually eliminate small cavities, and it provides fat-soluble vitamins that are hard to find elsewhere. There is extensive information about this in the *Dental Health* chapter. Toothpastes containing monocalcium phosphate are ideal, because they can help to remineralize damaged teeth. Avoid any toothpaste that contains sodium lauryl sulphate or sodium laureth sulphate. These industrial degreasers are terrible for the health. Fluoride should always be avoided too, and it is specifically known to darken teeth.

Lemon Pineapple Drink for pH

There is a link between body pH and many diseases. Health conscious people often attempt to maintain a higher-than-normal body pH (being alkaline). Those eating a healthy diet will naturally become alkaline from their diets, but it is very easy to become acidic from a relapse of processed foods. Soft drinks have a pH of around 2.5, and the effects upon pH are dramatic. It is always much easier to become acidic than to become alkaline. However, there are methods to dramatically speed up the process of becoming alkaline.

Acidic fruits often have an alkalizing effect upon the body. It is important to remember that the initial acidity of a food is not important in regard to its alkalizing effect. It is actually the minerals that matter, not the food's initial acidity. Ironically, the most acidic fruits tend to have a mineral composition that causes the human body to become more alkaline when they are metabolized.

Lemon juice and pineapple juice are extremely useful for helping a person to quickly regain some balance. If these are drank regularly, then we guarantee that you will feel the difference.

Some people choose to drink homemade lemonade everyday throughout the winter, in order to prevent the illnesses which are common throughout the colder months. Along with alkalizing and thereby making it difficult for pathogens to live, lemons contain vitamin C and potassium. When the body is alkaline, the oxygenation of the blood is increased, which provides extra energy and health improvements.

To make homemade lemonade, squeeze the juice from two small lemons into a 16 ounce glass, and add two teaspoons of evaporated cane juice (or honey) and water (preferably spring or well water). Do not use carbonated water, for it has an acidifying effect on the body.

We generally combine the lemon juice with pineapple juice. This yields the benefits of both, and it removes the need for a sweetening agent. The product of the two is better than either juice alone. It tends to have a nice sweet-sour taste that is unique, and remarkably delightful.

Sore Throat Remedy

Whether people are suffering with the common cold or bronchitis, a sore throat is often one of the first symptoms. There are very few useful pharmaceutical options, so even doctors frequently recommend home remedies. We have found a cure for some cases of sore throat. It can dramatically reduce pain in a matter of minutes.

Mix one teaspoon of powdered cayenne pepper with one teaspoon of sea salt, in an 8 ounce glass. Fill with water and mix well. Gargle with this formula, and then refrigerate it. You should re-use it whenever the throat becomes painful again. It does not need to be warmed. It will quickly break-up the coating in the throat, so expect to be profusely spitting for a few minutes afterward. Discard it after a day, and remake it as necessary.

While most people are familiar with gargling salt water, combining it with cayenne massively boosts the efficacy. Contrary to what most people will assume, the cayenne does not burn, nor is it unpleasant. In the right conditions (like a raw throat), cayenne pepper actually acts as a numbing agent. It will be a welcome relief from the suffering. Cayenne is an extremely useful herb, regulating the blood pressure, helping with the heart, acting as a numbing agent, relieving shingles suffering, assisting weight loss efforts, stimulating the body, and of course, relieving sore throats.

In addition, standard hydrogen peroxide (3% strength) can be extremely useful. Turn the head sideways (best done whilst laying down sideways) and use a medicine dropper to squirt a small amount of it in both ears. Wait until fizzing stops before standing up. It should take about 5 minutes. Roll the head slightly in all directions while it is sideways, to ensure that the hydrogen peroxide reaches its maximum depth inside the ear canal. This kills bacteria deep inside the ear, making it much easier to recover from the infection. Be warned that with bad infections, the tickling sensation from the bubbling hydrogen peroxide can make laying still a challenge. Have a towel ready to catch the hydrogen peroxide for when you become upright again. You may also periodically gargle with the peroxide if you have a sore throat, and this should help to hasten the recovery time.

With a little luck and quick timing, you can normally kill a sore throat infection before it becomes a serious problem. A little colloidal silver helps too; both in the gargle and ingested.

Tea for Coughing, Sinuses, and Lungs

The following recipe should help to arrest coughing and improve breathing. It is especially helpful during cold and flu infections. Several of the herbs have a numbing effect which soothes lung and throat pain. For especially bad lung irritation, this tea may be used in conjunction with mullein that is smoked, but this will rarely be necessary. Readers should not underestimate the effectiveness of this herbal formulation. It is as powerful as any cough syrup, and faster acting. Moreover, this remedy has a therapeutic effect overall, while the chemicals of commercial cough syrups impair the immune system.

- 1 green tea bag *
- 1/2 teaspoon cloves
- 1/2 teaspoon turmeric
- 1/2 teaspoon thyme
- 2 teaspoons honey
- Juice of half a lemon

    * Green tea is preferred, but regular tea can be used as an inferior substitute.

Prepare this remedy by placing the tea bag and herbs into a coffee mug with boiling water. Let them seep for three minutes, then strain before adding the honey and lemon.

Chronic coughing and lung inflammation problems may indicate candida overgrowth in the gastrointestinal tract. For more information about this, see the *Allergies and Candida* section of the *Alternative Medicine* chapter. Doctors will usually test people with chronic coughing issues for lung cancer, but the testing itself is prone to causing cancers. Thereafter, the doctors congratulate themselves for their early cancer detections. Patient beware.

Diarrhea Remedy

Diarrhea is not the most pleasant topic to read about, but sooner or later, it is an issue that everyone is forced to take an interest in. We have all been there, and none of us want to return. This gentle anti-diarrhea formula works impressively well. The ingredients may be surprising; because in a homeopathic sense, they normally have the opposite effect. We understand how the ingredients manage to fix the problem; but frankly, most readers do not want the details. The important thing is that it works very well. In the worst cases, it can take up to 2 hours for it to fully activate, so there may be one or two final trips to the restroom. When it does activate, it works better than anything else, and it is unlikely to be needed again for the remainder of the illness.

The Formula

- 8 ounce glass of orange juice (needed for potassium)
- One heaping tablespoon of hemp fiber
- 10 drops of concentrated chlorophyll
- 2 opened licorice supplement capsules (900 mg.)
- 1 tablespoon of finely ground activated carbon (*Emergency Medicine* chapter)
- 2 opened ginger supplement capsules (1,000 mg. / 1 gram)

Several tablespoons of colloidal silver may be added to kill problematic bacteria. Creating this formula is more work than most remedies, but it is both safer and more effective than other diarrhea treatments. In most cases, a single use of this drink will end the issue completely, and leave the person feeling significantly better than before. It works best on an empty stomach.

We would like to warn readers that they should obtain the ingredients beforehand (like now), because it is too late to go shopping when diarrhea strikes, and it has a tendency to happen at the worst times, like in the middle of the night.

Indigestion and Heartburn

Almost everything that you have been told about heartburn, indigestion, and common stomach ailments is wrong. Indigestion is not caused by excessive acid in the stomach, nor is acid reflux. In fact, the worst treatment for these problems is taking an antacid, whether prescribed or not.

Being acidic is the natural state of the stomach, so there is no such thing as an excess of acid or acid buildup regarding the stomach. It is like claiming that the lungs suffer from excess oxygen, or the blood has an excess of red cells. Attempting to neutralize stomach acid to treat an uneasy stomach is as wise as treating an excess of blood cells with leaches. Both cases are demonstrations of using poor medicine to treat only the symptoms of nonexistent medical conditions, of which the establishment either cannot accurately diagnose, or it is too unprofitable to do so.

The truth about most stomach disorders is that they are caused by not having enough acid, so the pharmaceutical industry has made fools out of most of us. The true reason behind acid reflux and indigestion is that whenever the stomach is lacking in acid, it must churn violently to make the best use of its limited acid. This in-turn causes pressure and back-flows of the existing acid. The combination of the back-flows into the esophagus and the stomach's cramping action is what causes pain.

Antacids *seem to work* because they render the acid being spewed by the churning stomach as even less potent, and therefore, less painful. In the rare cases when acid is actually being overproduced by the stomach, it is virtually always a body attempting to compensate for antacids having been routinely administered. The effects of taking antacids eventually snowball, preventing proper digestion, temporarily eliminating only the symptoms, and eventually causing the very excess acid problem that they had been meant to stop. To recreate acid which has been neutralized, the body must carry out a set of complex chemical reactions that stress the body and cause it to develop an acidic pH. The process is quite unhealthy.

Why Stomach Acid Deficiency Happens

The end result of our accumulated toxicity from the factors mentioned throughout this book, is that our body chemistry has been artificially altered to become acidic. The relationship between an acidic body and illness has long been established, and the medical term for this condition is "acidosis". It ironically leads to an acid deficiency in the only organ requiring acid: the stomach. The toxicity of the majority of foods in a typical diet causes the body to become more acidic during digestion, and this includes the shoddy water. An acidic body (which is most) destroys its own cells, has a crippled immune system, ages rapidly, experiences skin and hair problems, has metabolic and weight regulation problems, is disease prone, is prone to allergies, cannot effectively absorb nutrients, cannot effectively flush toxins, cannot properly cope with cholesterol, cannot properly regulate minerals such as calcium, and most importantly, cannot maintain a high level of oxygen.

The Aftermath of Weak Stomach Acid and Antacids

Donna Gates explained the problems with low stomach pH better than we could. Readers are notified that this is not a blanket endorsement of her work, because she sells health frauds, such as pond scum (algae) as a healthy food item *for human beings*. Nevertheless, Donna actually did very well in understanding and explaining the issues of this particular topic, so she is quoted below.

> *"There are two main consequences of low stomach acid: 1. You become protein malnourished. When your stomach acid is low, you are not able to digest protein. Improper digestion of protein creates toxins in your intestines that can set the stage for illness and disease. Improper digestion of protein also creates acidic blood, since protein is by nature acidic. 2. You become mineral deficient. As your blood becomes more acidic, it will look for minerals from anywhere in your body, in order to get your blood to its more ideal alkaline state. Acidic blood robs your body of minerals, even taking minerals from your bones (which is important to know if you want to prevent osteoporosis).*

> *"Low stomach acid eventually creates a vicious cycle: low stomach acid = low minerals = acidic blood. This cycle continues because acidic blood further creates low minerals and low stomach acid. Once this vicious cycle has started, there is a cascade of consequences:*

> *"You could eat plenty of protein and still be protein malnourished. This raises cortisol levels (stress or death hormone), thereby raising your blood glucose (blood sugar levels). Elevated cortisol adversely affects your behavior and temperment.*

> *"Eventually, your adrenals become depleted (adrenal fatigue) and DHEA, the youth hormone, is suppressed, leading to premature aging.*

> *"Low DHEA and high cortisol affect your brain and behavior, but that's not all. The vicious cycle of low stomach acid affects your inner ecosystem too. Low stomach acid can lead to more bad guys (pathogenic bacteria, candida and viruses) than good guys (healthy microflora), thus lowering your immunity.*

> *"Here are some of the common symptoms and disorders caused by low stomach acid: Bloating, belching, and flatulence immediately after meals, heartburn (often thought to be caused by too much stomach acid), Indigestion, diarrhea, or*

constipation, undigested food in stools, acne, rectal itching, chronic candida, hair loss in women, multiple food allergies, iron deficiency, weak, peeling, or cracked fingernails, chronic fatigue, adrenal fatigue, dry skin, various autoimmune diseases."

A Natural Remedy

The next time that you have indigestion problems, try an experiment that gives your stomach the acid that it needs. Take a tablespoon of apple cider vinegar, and chase it with a glass of water. All stomach churning and pain should subside within minutes, unless the problem is ulcers. The results are amazing.

We recommend avoiding apple cider vinegar whenever it is packaged inside of clear plastic bottles, because such plastics are prone to leaching chemical contaminants. This is especially likely to happen with acidic solutions. The ideal container is glass, as is the case for most food products. Read the *Poisonous Plastics* section of the *Poisoned World* chapter for detailed information about this.

No pharmaceutical company will make billions from this, and none of them will ever be able to become the gate keeper of this remedy by getting a patent to monopolize apple cider vinegar. Regulatory agencies will not be able to profit from this either. Therefore, do not expect to read about this in any of the medical journals, or to ever hear it reported in the mainstream media.

Curing Stomach Ulcers

Over the years, the medical establishment has repeatedly changed its list of suspected causes for stomach ulcers (peptic ulcers). It has been like a soap opera to monitor. At various times, ulcers have been blamed on stress, excessive alcohol consumption, extended use of pharmaceuticals, a weakened immune system, bacterial infections, and of course, it is now genetic too. They really have no idea. Ulcers continue to be a great enigma that is beyond the bounds of modern doctors.

Ulcers are a surprisingly common condition. Most people know of at least one person who has suffered with ulcers, and who was placed on the usual pharmaceutical treadmill. The prognosis of pharmaceutical treatments is bleak. Some argue that doing something for a suffering victim is always preferable to doing nothing, because at least the doctors are trying to help. It is tempting logic, so long as the assumption is maintained that there are no known alternatives to the current protocols of experimental medicine. With that in mind, consider the following carefully.

While researching an unrelated topic, we came across an enlightening study from the year 1949. It included:

> *"The average crater healing time for seven of these patients who had duodenal ulcer was only 10.4 days, while the average time as reported in the literature, in 62 patients treated by standard therapy, was 37 days... The average crater healing time for six patients with gastric ulcer treated with cabbage juice was only 7.3 days, compared with 42 days, as reported in the literature, for six patients treated by standard therapy."*

The study, *"Rapid Healing of Peptic Ulcers in Patients Receiving Fresh Cabbage Juice"* was simply ignored by the medical establishment. Two more studies were later done in 1952 and 1956, with identical outcomes.

The ulcer-healing factor of cabbage (S-methylmethionine) is often referred to as "vitamin U". What is astounding is that this natural therapy has been known for over six decades, yet the public has never been told about it. The initial study used a quart of raw cabbage juice, which was consumed throughout each day. Based upon the results of the studies, we recommend a protocol lasting 10-13 days.

It is well known throughout alternative medicine and amongst naturopathic doctors that ulcers are caused by an imbalance of the stomach pH. Therefore, we recommend alkalizing the body, because virtually all modern pH issues consist of a body being too acidic, and a stomach that is too alkaline. Following an alkalizing diet should eventually help a patient to regain a natural balance. See the *Body pH and Disease* section of the *Wellness* chapter for detailed information about this. Severe indigestion is sometimes confused for ulcerations, and this can sometimes be corrected in the same manner.

Radiation Poisoning

In the 1950's and 1960's, experiments were done by the United States Army, showing that the consumption of broccoli and other dark green vegetables protects a body from radiation damage to a surprising degree. This led to further research into the most common factor of such vegetation: chlorophyll.

Chlorophyll (the green pigment of plants) cleanses the body of many toxins, including aflotoxin, benzo[a]pyrene, and dioxins, all of which are known carcinogens. It is worth noting that radiation exposure produces benzene compounds within humans, such as benzo[a]pyrene. Chlorophyll is also able to directly shield a body from radiation damage, which has been demonstrated in multiple studies including, *Breast Tissue Dosimetry of PhIP at Human-*

Relevant Exposures, by the U.S. Army.

Given the U.S. Military's refinement of atomic weapons, there is not a more credible source than it. Studies such as, *Effect of Dietary Supplementation With Broccoli on X-Irradiation-Induced Enzyme Changes*, used conventional cabbages and broccoli as a small chlorophyll source. It enabled test subjects to show dramatic recoveries from radiation poisoning. Therefore, concentrated liquid chlorophyll, like that which is available at most health food stores, should be expected to yield impressive results.

The Linus Pauling Institute demonstrated that vitamin C taken after medical radiation reduced radiation sicknesses, and subsequent cellular damage. No more than 3 grams (3,000 mg.) of vitamin C should be taken daily to suppress radiation sickness, for an average adult.

Apple pectin is a food-based supplement which neutralizes radioactive particles inside the body. It was used following the Chernobyl nuclear disaster with stunning results. The dosage was 800 mg. for every 100 pounds of body weight.

We also recommend that people consume flax seed oil. It is more effective when it is combined with something containing a sulfur protein. This mixture is a core component of the anti-cancer Budwig Protocol. For more information about proper usage, reference the *Budwig Protocol* section of the *Cancer* chapter.

Potassium iodide is the only remedy for protecting against radiation poisoning that is mentioned by other sources, but it will only partially protect the thyroid and the female reproductive organs. While its usage may be a good idea, it is important to remember that the rest of the body will still be completely unprotected. Potassium iodide is sold commercially to protect people from radiation, but it is only an option for people who plan ahead of time. The following dosages are recommended by the U.S. Centers for Disease Control.

Potassium Iodide Dosages

- Newborns from birth to 1 month of age should be given 16 mg. (1/4 of a 65 mg. tablet or 1/4 mL. of solution).

- Infants and children between 1 month and 3 years of age should take 32 mg. (1/2 of a 65 mg. tablet or 1/2 mL. of solution).

- Children between 3 and 18 years of age should take 65 mg. (one 65 mg. tablet or 1 mL. of solution). Children who are adult size (greater than or equal to 150 pounds) should take the full adult dose, regardless of age.

- Adults should take 130 mg. (one 130 mg. tablet or two 65 mg. tablets or two mL. of solution).

- Women who are breast feeding should take the adult dose of 130 mg.

There is an alternative do-it-yourself approach as follows. Apply a large patch of iodine to the abdomen area, several hours before exposure, if possible. This alternative treatment should protect both the thyroid and the ovaries somewhat. One should also consume some potassium. Unfortunately, the amount of potassium needed is greater than can be gained from diet. A great deal of potassium is needed for radiation shielding. You can effectively utilize a salt substitute that is made primarily of potassium. About half of a teaspoon should provide plenty of potassium from a salt substitute.

Extra Risks and Countermeasures

Be forewarned that there are inherent dangers to excessive potassium intake. Excessive potassium in a body will dramatically increase blood thickening and blood clotting. You may get an increase in blood pressure, and perhaps some symptoms of kidney stress. Increased potassium equals an increased chance of strokes and blood clots. Thus, we encourage readers to use common sense in weighing the help-to-harm ratio before using a potassium salt. We recommend supplementing with gotu kola, ginkgo biloba, cayenne, vitamin E, omega-3 (flax seed oil), and American ginseng to thin the blood and increase oxygen intake during the stressful period of using potassium. Red wine is also helpful in small doses.

The use of iodine or iodide can be dangerous for people who suffer with Hashimoto's thyroiditis. Birth control pills greatly increase the dangers of potassium consumption.

Juice Concentrate

Whenever a juice is made "from concentrate", there is reason to beware of it. Such juices are first concentrated by high heat over a relatively long period, which is prone to destroying all nutritional value; but this is hardly the worst aspect. The worst part is that the juices are then recombined with tap water. This tap water composes about 90% (or more) of the fluid of reconstituted juices. Therefore, you may be drinking more impurities by drinking juices that are made from concentrate than if you drank your local tap water, due to it having been shipped to multiple locations and the excessive processing. The quality of the resultant juice is a product of the tap water quality at the bottling plant, which could be worse than your local tap water. The final product may still taste like delicious juice, but it is often little more than flavored tap water by the time that it reaches your local retailer, and it is likely to be less pure.

The most popular brands of orange juice in the U.S. are owned by PepsiCo Inc., and The Coca-Cola Company.

Gnat Control

Households employ different methods to eliminate insect pests, such as gnats. These range from banning all fruits to spraying pesticides. There is a natural and safe method for eliminating gnats.

In a dish or container with a wide top, combine the following:

- 1 Tbsp. liquid dish detergent
- 8 Tbsp. apple cider vinegar
- 1/4 cup water
- 1 heaping Tbsp. sugar

Leave this solution in an area where gnats congregate. It generally takes a couple of days for it to take effect, but when it does, it will begin killing large numbers of gnats. They will be attracted to it, and die in the mixture.

Morning Nausea

Morning nausea has a singular and easily remedied cause in the overwhelming majority of cases. It is usually caused by simple dehydration. Many factors can contribute to this, including snoring. Alas, the cure to most cases of morning nausea is a cold glass of water. If there are other stomach problems, such as indigestion or heartburn, then precede the water with apple cider vinegar. Of course, morning nausea can sometimes indicate a health condition, but if the water and the apple cider vinegar are enough to remedy it, then it was merely dehydration.

Poison Oak and Poison Ivy

Jewelweed (*impatiens capensis*) could become your best friend in the woods, in the garden, and wherever you go camping. This little flowering weed is responsible for alleviating untold amounts of suffering. It does something that only powerful steroids can do. It completely neutralizes the histamines that are produced by poison oak and poison ivy. While there are various commercial creams and treatments for suppressing the symptoms of poison plant exposure, they are fairly ineffective, and they must be routinely reapplied until the immune system completely finishes dealing with the "poison". Conversely, jewelweed completely neutralizes the allergens, meaning that jewelweed usually needs to be applied only once, and there are no effects from the poison plants if it is used soon enough.

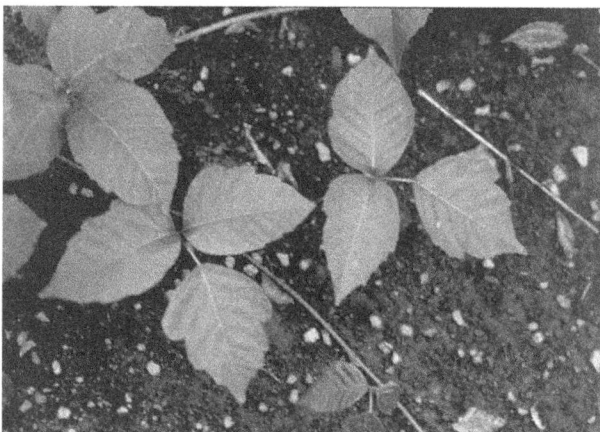

Photo of Poison Oak

Beware of the three leaf pattern that is seen on both poison oak and poison ivy. Also beware of burning these plants, because the smoke can cause swelling in the throat and suffocation.

Jewelweed soap can be purchased on-line and from health retailers for cleaning oneself after poison plant exposure. Timing is critical. Jewelweed must be applied in the first couple of hours after exposure to prevent the histamine oils from sinking through the outer layers of skin. The sooner it is applied, the more effective it is. Waiting until the next morning to wash will make the jewelweed ineffective. We advise our readers not to underestimate this natural remedy.

Emergency Medicine

Activated Carbon

Activated carbon, in powdered form, should be in every medicine cabinet and first aid kit. It is also known as activated charcoal. It is used around the world as a universal antidote for hundreds of poisons, including arsenic, mercury, pesticides, strychnine, warfarin, hemlock, E. Coli endotoxin, and gasoline. Over 4,000 chemicals, drugs, plant and microbial toxins, allergens, venoms, and wastes are effectively neutralized by activated charcoal, when it is given in sufficient quantities. Activated charcoal is also an effective detox for practically any drug overdose if administered in time. It counteracts ingested aspirin, barbiturates, Prozac, paracetamol (Tylenol), phenobarbital, amphetamines, cocaine, morphine, opium, and the list continues endlessly.

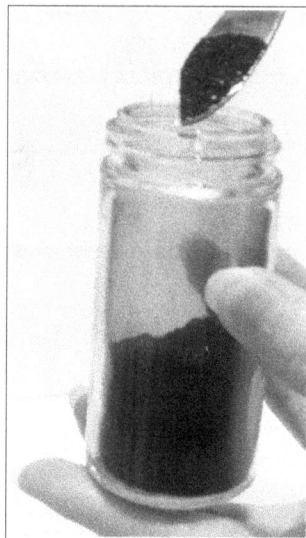

In 1813, French chemist Michel Bertrand swallowed five grams of arsenic trioxide: 150 times the lethal dose. He had mixed it with activated carbon beforehand. He experienced no nausea, no vomiting, no diarrhea, no excruciating cramping, no severe burning in the mouth or throat, no collapse, and no death. In a dangerous but dramatic way, he had avoided certain death while publicly demonstrating charcoal's phenomenal ability to neutralize poisons.

In 1831, in front of his distinguished colleagues at the French Academy of Medicine, Professor Pierre-Fleurus Touéry drank a deadly cocktail of strychnine and lived to tell the tale. He had combined the deadly poison with activated charcoal. It demonstrated how powerful activated charcoal is as an emergency decontaminant. Activated charcoal is still the most potent and rapid-acting general detoxification agent available.

We witnessed the saving power of activated charcoal ourselves, when one member of our household experienced a severe allergic reaction to an unknown ingredient from a restaurant. We orally administered two teaspoons of dampened activated charcoal powder, followed by a glass of water. The allergic reaction began subsiding rapidly, and completely dissipated within thirty minutes. Activated carbon may have saved our patient from a visit to a hospital, an injection of steroids (and only God knows what else), a stomach pump, and possibly the need for the victim to remain in the hospital for several days.

Manufacture and Storage

The best and cheapest option for obtaining quality activated carbon is to powder aquarium filtration charcoal with a mortar and pestle. Aquarium charcoal has the same purpose for aquarium water: to extract various toxins from the water, including organic wastes. It is also found in some pharmacies. Regardless of where it is obtained, it should be powdered before it is stored, and dampened when used. It should be stored in an air-tight container, because it will absorb impurities from the air. Swallowing it damp prevents the powder from being inhaled into the lungs, where it could become dangerous. A glass of water should be consumed immediately afterward.

Exceptions: Activated charcoal is less effective in neutralizing cyanide, alcohols, ethylene glycol, iron, lithium, mineral acids, and alkaline substances (usually lime or cleaning agents). Alcohols, in particular, appear to be immune to activated carbon.

Risks: Charcoal significantly decreases a body's absorption of nutrients and medications. Because of this, frequent use of it is strongly discouraged. Activated charcoal may also cause abdominal pain or swelling in rare cases. If this occurs, contact a doctor immediately, since this could be an indication of intestinal bleeding or blockage. For mild cases of charcoal-induced constipation, a person may self-treat with a hemp fiber supplement.

Other Uses

- Colon cleanse: activated charcoal binds intestinal toxins and unfriendly microbial growth and helps the body excrete them.

- Eliminates diarrhea, gas, and bloating.

- Prevents hangovers: hangovers are usually caused by the chemical toxins put into beverages, and are not usually the result of alcohol consumption.

- Neutralizes food poisoning.

- Neutralizes venomous bites (such as the brown recluse spider bite) - taken both internally and externally.

- Toothache pain - make into a paste around the tooth.

Note: Charcoal briquettes, like those used for outdoor grilling, should never be used to make medical activated charcoal, and no part of them should ever be ingested.

Bee, Wasp, and Hornet Stings

If a stinger is left embedded in the body, then remove it as soon as possible. This should be the first step. Use whatever tools are immediately available to dig it out. You could use a knife, credit card, pliers, tweezers, or a needle. Sterilize the tool if possible, but do not waste time. For maximum absorption, clean the area with soap and water before applying remedies, otherwise the oils on the skin will repel them.

Wasp and Hornet Stings

Vinegar - Wasp and hornet venom are powerfully alkaline. Use an acid such as vinegar to neutralize them. It can be applied via a piece of cloth or bandaging. Make sure to keep the sting sites soaked for at least 15 minutes. Some vinegar will absorb through the skin, and it should greatly help to eliminate the discomfort.

Bee and Yellow Jacket Stings

Baking Soda - In the case of bee stings, baking soda will help to neutralize the acidic venom. Make a paste by combining baking soda with water. Leave this paste on the sting site for at least 15 minutes. Some of the dissolved baking soda will leach through the skin to neutralize the venom somewhat. After applying it, and cleaning the sting area of residue; a chamomile tincture may be repeatedly applied for any residual itching or swelling.

Allergic Reactions

If there is difficulty breathing, extreme dizziness, or nausea after a sting, then there is a high probability that it triggered a dangerous allergic reaction. In these cases, we recommend quickly consuming a large (i.e. quadruple) dose of chamomile. Chamomile is related to ragweed, so those with ragweed allergies should skip this step. A large amount of echinacea is also strongly recommended, if available. If pulse irregularities are experienced, then try to take some taurine, even if that means just holding the powder in the mouth. Then immediately get to the nearest hospital. The allergic reaction may stop by the time that you arrive at the hospital, but you should definitely make the trip in case it does not. In these unfortunate latter cases, a steroid injection may be required to save your life.

Misinformation about Sting Remedies

Treating most bee, wasp, and hornet stings is easy, but that may be difficult to believe if you have spent any time researching this topic on the Internet. Researching natural treatments for stings is revealing about how much misinformation there is on the Internet. Some of it is laughable.

The Incredibly Stupid Sting 'Treatments' That We Discourage

- Meat tenderizer
- Onion
- Potato
- Mud (literally dirt and water)
- Garlic
- Ammonia
- Vinegar combined with baking soda (neutralize themselves)

Brown Recluse Spider Bites

Brown recluse spiders migrate into homes in the autumn, where warmer climates may be found. These spiders reside in places with regular human movement, but they are not usually aggressive. They are known to bite when they feel threatened or trapped. Bites often occur when a spider is trapped between a piece of clothing and the human body. It is believed that they enjoy human dwellings because their nocturnal lifestyle benefits from artificial light.

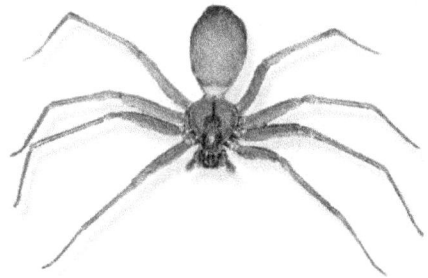

Brown recluse venom contains at least 9 distinct poisons; making it similar to rattlesnake venom. It effects blood vessels in the bite area to potentially cause massive tissue destruction. The result can be horrific. A bite that is left untreated may require an amputation of the limb, and it can lead to death. The bites cause kidney failure in some people.

Avoiding Brown Recluse Bites

Since bites often occur whilst people are sleeping, it is not always possible to avoid them. We recommend that bedding be fully checked before going to sleep, and that clothing be violently shaken before it is worn. These little devils love the insides of shoes, so beat your shoes together, and inspect the insides of them before wearing them. Keep all dresser drawers tightly closed, because they will hide in the underwear too. We normally recommend against the use of chemicals (especially poisons), but it is wise to spray a long-lasting insect repellant around windows and doors in the autumn. Please take all precautions, including wearing splash-resistant goggles, and a respirator, if you do.

How to Know if You Have Been Bitten

A brown recluse victim is not always aware that he has been bitten; at least not immediately, when treatment would be the most beneficial. Sometimes the bites immediately cause extreme pain, but in other cases, there is no sensation at all. There may be visible fang pits at the bite site, but this is not always true either. Sometimes there is itching at the bite site, or a generalized fever. The general rule is that there are no general rules for brown recluse spider bites in the early stage. Some victims do not realize that they have been bitten until several days have passed.

Between one and three days after being bitten, an untreated brown recluse spider bite is likely to form one or more blisters. The bite site may become bluish colored at this time, and it may begin forming a crater.

Seeking Emergency Medical Care

A brown recluse spider bite could easily be considered an emergency condition, so a hospital visit may be essential to ensure that the victim is stabilized. Be forewarned that there is very little that orthodox medicine can do to stop the regional damage that is caused by a bite. Doctors typically give antibiotics and anti-histamines in the hope that regionalized damage can be somewhat minimized. These are truly desperate measures that yield very little success. Therefore, we recommend that you follow our alternative treatment recommendations, which are listed next.

Self Treatment - Stage 1

If you have been bitten by this spider (or any other spider), the first thing that you should do is apply activated charcoal directly to the wound. This is something that should always be kept in the medicine cabinet for poison emergencies. You can find it inside capsules that are sold at health food stores, or you can buy it in the aquarium department of a grocery store. Either way, the charcoal must be finely ground before it is used. Apply a thick paste to the bite area that is made from the fine charcoal powder and water. Tape the charcoal and water mixture to the bite, and leave for four hours. Using it again, or for longer periods is unlikely to help.

Take large amounts of echinacea supplements until the bite wound completely disappears. Echinacea was used by the American Indians to heal snake bites, which is where the phrase "snake oil" originated. Some reports indicate that echinacea is very effective for treating venomous bites.

Self Treatment - Stage 2

After the first few hours, charcoal will no longer be useful. Purchase bentonite clay powder from a health food store, and mix it with enough water to form a paste. Apply this paste onto the wound, and cover it with medical tape. Use colloidal silver instead of water if it is available. This paste should be left on the skin for at least two hours, several times a day. The skin should be washed before the clay is applied to remove any oils. A mild hand soap should be adequate. Avoid moisturizing soaps and lotions.

Topical bentonite clay has yielded some amazing results for victims of brown recluse bites. Internal use of bentonite clay is not advised. For best results, mix a small amount of echinacea with the bentonite clay powder. The clay will typically remain useful for about a week, but every bite will be different. Continue for a couple of weeks.

Brown recluse spider bites usually take 6-8 weeks to heal, but this treatment method should speed the process dramatically, and reduce suffering in the meantime. Hopefully it will help victims eliminate, or at least reduce the crater scars for which these spiders have become infamous.

Be Prepared

You may not be able to get bentonite clay from local retailers, so every family that is at risk of being bitten by brown recluse spiders should purchase it as soon as possible, and keep it ready in storage. Once bitten, a person may not be able to obtain it from online sources in time to be useful. Seriously, order it now, along with the activated carbon.

Snake Bite Treatments

Snake bites can be very dangerous. We recommend immediately seeking emergency medical treatment, if it is available. Hospitals are the only source for getting antivenin. However, there are scenarios when emergency medical assistance is hours, or even days away. This section catalogs some treatments that may help in these situations.

Apply dampened activated charcoal to snake bite fang wounds as soon as possible. With some snake bites, making a small slit in the fang lesions is necessary, while other bites leave large enough holes for the activated charcoal to absorb well. Use a band-aid, cotton with medical tape, or anything else that is available to firmly hold the dampened charcoal onto the wound. Check periodically, and re-dampen the charcoal if it has dried out. Do not use DMSO to increase absorption, for it will cause the venom to sink deeper into the body.

We found that there are varying results in the use of tourniquets. The medical establishment is preaching to never use them nowadays, and we likewise acknowledge that there are inherent dangers to using them. As such, it is necessary for people to use their best judgment in deciding whether a tourniquet should be applied. Tourniquets can lead to the loss of a limb, but this is an acceptable risk in some instances. If you decide to use a tourniquet, you should write "TK" and the time on the victim's forehead, so medics will know how long it has been applied, in case you get separated or injured yourself.

Some people use a tourniquet that is just tight enough to slow the circulation, instead of entirely stopping it. This method is designed to allow treatments to take effect before the venom spreads throughout the body. If done correctly, it eliminates the risks associated with tourniquets.

Echinacea oil is known to help neutralize snake bites. This property of echinacea was first discovered by the American Indians. In addition, echinacea boosts the immune system, and thus it helps to fight infections. In the event of a snake bite, we strongly recommend taking a large dose of echinacea supplements, and repeating every 6 hours. If swallowing is difficult, then hold it in the mouth for as long as possible to allow for blood absorption through the cheeks and tongue, before attempting to swallow. Get supplies ready beforehand, because it is too late to go shopping during a poison emergency. Only purchase echinacea from herbal or health food stores, due to supplement quality issues. Please read the previous section about *Activated Charcoal* for its safety and preparation instructions.

After the first 24 hours has passed, activated charcoal will be largely ineffective. You may wish to topically apply moistened bentonite clay at this time. Bentonite clay is known for removing outer-tissue toxins, and it is also advised for treating spider bites. For best results, mix echinacea powder with the bentonite clay and water. Apply this paste to the wound. You may simply open echinacea supplement capsules to obtain the powder. As with the other items, have the bentonite clay ready beforehand in storage. Bentonite clay is not found in most retailers, and it must usually be purchased online, so get it now.

Always remember to seek medical attention at the earliest opportunity, because snake bite victims should get an antivenin as soon as possible. These techniques are virtually guaranteed to help a victim, but they may not be enough to save a person from a fatal snake bite.

There are four types of poisonous snakes in the United States, and they all tend to be temperamental, despite what the politically correct, new-age nature lovers would have us believe. These vicious monsters include the copperhead, cottonmouth, rattlesnake, and the coral snake. It is important to be able to recognize the different types of poisonous snakes, so that you can get the best medical treatment. Being treated with the wrong type of antivenin can be fatal. If possible, it is best to kill the snake, and then take it with you to the hospital, in order to get a verified identification of its species. The snake's head should be severed, in order to be certain that it is dead. Be cautious of the fangs, which could convulse at any time to inject venom.

Broken Bones

There is a simple method for determining if a bone is broken, without the use of any instruments. A bone will reliably maintain a certain degree of stiffness, unless it is broken. Utilizing the inherent stiffness differences between broken and unbroken bones, a light pain response test can be used to check a bone's integrity.

When an injured bone is unbroken, acute pain will be observed directly at the impact site. The pain rapidly decreases in proportion to the distance from the injury. Gentle poking with a finger is all that is needed for this test.

On the other hand, if a bone is severed, then the pain will be almost uniform across the entire bone. This is because poking produces unnatural shock waves throughout that part of the body, because there is no intact bone to resist it. The pain distribution from a broken bone will be virtually the same anywhere along the bone.

There are cases in which two bones exist together to maintain a region's stiffness, such as those of the forearms and lower legs. It is more difficult to accurately perform this test in these cases. Nevertheless, a highly observant person should be able to accurately deduce if one of the bones is broken by using the basic methodology given herein. It should be obvious in cases where both bones are broken.

Even when a bone is just fractured or bruised, care should still be taken to protect it from further injuries. Be aware that a fractured bone may become broken with only a light impact. Be paranoid in the care of injured ribs, because a break in these can rupture an organ.

Dental Health

Brushing and Sugars

For decades, dentists have insisted that one of the best ways to avoid cavities is to brush the teeth immediately after consuming anything that contains sugar. New evidence shows that they were wrong. One should be mindful that modern dentistry also promotes mercury ("silver") fillings and fluoride in drinking water. The dental industry is one of the most destructive toward health.

After consuming sugary foods or drinks, the enamel of a person's teeth becomes weaker; especially within the first hour. Brushing the teeth during this period leads to increases in abrasive damage. This damage usually becomes significant by the time that a person reaches middle age.

Soft drinks are especially detrimental to tooth enamel. The average pH of soft drinks is 2.5, while the mouth should remain at about neutral (7.0). It has been religiously cited by dentists that the low pH of soft drinks is the singular causative factor of weakened tooth enamel. They claim that the teeth should be immediately scrubbed clean after soda consumption, or the ingestion of anything containing sugar. However, there are multiple factors which make immediate brushing unwise. Soft drinks typically contain fructose, in the form of high fructose corn syrup. A soft drink's fructose neutralizes the phosphates in teeth, making them softer and more vulnerable to abrasive damage. Furthermore, ascorbic acid (vitamin C) and citric acid are usually added to soft drinks, which are both known to likewise soften enamel. The combination of fructose, acids, vitamin C, and the sugars that are routinely in soft drinks causes tooth enamel to become extremely vulnerable. Most candy will produce the same long-term risk to tooth enamel if brushing is an immediate follow-up. Contrary to popular consensus, waiting at least an hour before brushing, and always using a "soft" bristled tooth brush, leads to the best lifetime dental health. Immediately rinsing the mouth with clean water is a much better option than the official recommendation.

Despite the influence of groups like the American Dental Association (A.D.A.), a stunning 59% of American children aged 12 to 19 have at least one cavity in their adult teeth.

Vitamin C Problems

We encourage daily supplementation of vitamin C for everyone. It protects against everything from sudden infant death syndrome (S.I.D.S) to scurvy, heart disease, and in some cases, cancer. Two-time Nobel Prize winner, Linus Pauling, recommended a whopping 3 grams of vitamin C every day for the average healthy male, and 6 grams for those at risk of heart disease. There are many methods of vitamin C supplementation, in the form of capsules, powders, and syrups. For decades, parents have been providing their children with chewable vitamin C pills.

Vitamin C is destructive to tooth enamel, so chewable pills may lead to increased cavities, particularly in those who are lacking minerals, such as calcium and phosphorus. Vitamin C should never be taken in a manner which leaves residues of it on the teeth for an extended time. Some well-intentioned toothpaste manufacturers have misguidedly added vitamin C or "citrus" to their formulas, without realizing the dental problems that this presents. Similarly, some alternative medicine sites on the Internet recommend cleaning the teeth with lemon-based solutions. Citrus acids have the tendency to make the teeth feel clean. This occurs partly because the acid strips the teeth of everything, including the minerals bonding with them. It can cause long-term enamel damage; especially when it is combined with abrasives or stiff bristle brushes.

Vitamin C actually strengthens teeth when taken internally, and the rest of the body. However, it should never be kept in direct contact with the teeth. We strongly recommend for those who are brushing their teeth with citrus formulas to discontinue immediately. Fluoride-free toothpastes which contain calcium carbonate are ideal for long-term dental health and for tooth whiteness. Toothpastes containing phosphorus (phosphates) are even better. Therefore, we recommend that aluminum-free baking powder be used as the primary ingredient for any homemade toothpaste.

Tooth Nutrients

Those who suddenly start experiencing tooth decay should know that it is often a symptom of a phosphorus deficiency. It is a common problem for vegetarians. Phosphorus is best obtained through meats, fish, and dairy products. It is in seeds and some nuts, but not in sufficient quantities. Fructose causes a decrease in phosphorus, which is one reason why sugar seems to cause cavities. Technically, sugars and carbohydrates can be harmful too, but the greatest factor is the connection between phosphorus depletion and the intake of fructose.

Those suffering from periodontal diseases such as gingivitis should look in the direction of CoQ10. Gingivitis sufferers are invariably deficient in co-enzyme Q10. It has shown good success with topical application, so mouth rinses are now available with this ingredient. In addition, CoQ10 is created by the body during exercise. Chlorophyll can also reverse gum disease, and it was once an ingredient of popular toothpastes.

Tooth Remineralization

While traveling to some of the most remote regions of the world, Dr. Weston Price discovered that some groups, which had no access to modern medicine, had extremely low incidences of cavities. He discovered that the cultures which consumed foods that were high in fats and minerals had the best dental health. Some of those groups did not even brush their teeth.

When people are malnourished, dental problems are often the first indicator. Most people from the Western world believe that teeth naturally decay with age, so everyone will inevitably get cavities. Popular consensus is that teeth self-destruct. However, a person's diet primarily determines his dental health. The myth that people have no control over the deterioration of the teeth is one of the justifications for the fluoridation of water supplies, because it is tacitly contended that human teeth disintegrate without help from the chemical industry. In truth, cavities and dental malformations occur as a result of malnutrition, which is actually exaggerated by chemicals, such as pharmaceuticals and fluoride. Western foods are not only deficient in vitamins and minerals, but they also contain chemicals that impair the utilization of nutrients in the body. Tooth decay is more common in pregnant and nursing women, because these women have greater nutritional needs.

Fluoride, in particular, pulls calcium and phosphorus into areas of the body where they would not normally travel, such as the pineal gland and the arteries, so that these minerals are not properly used for strengthening the bones. Teeth too are bones. Fluoride can prevent the healing of cavities, because it disrupts the proper mineral usage of the human body.

> "It is most remarkable and should be one of the most challenging facts that can come to our modern civilization that such primitive races as the Aborigines of Australia, have reproduced for generation after generation through many centuries -- no one knows for how many thousands of years -- without the development of a conspicuous number of irregularities of the dental arches. Yet, in the next generation after these people adopt the foods of the white man, a large percentage of the children developed irregularities of the dental arches with conspicuous facial deformities. The deformity patterns are similar to those seen in white civilizations."
>
> -- Dr. Weston Price, *Nutrition and Physical Degeneration*, 1939

Healing Cavities

When provided with the right diet, cavities can heal. This healing process is known as remineralization, because it is a process of giving the teeth the minerals that are needed to repair them. The two minerals that are most important for dental health are calcium and phosphorus. To use calcium properly, the human body needs adequate amounts of vitamin D from sunlight or fish (not the chemical type found in milk), and the body also needs magnesium from vegetables and nuts. In addition, the fat-soluble vitamins are invaluable. Fat-soluble vitamins include A, D, E and K. These vitamins can be found in butter, eggs, dairy products, and meats. A healthy diet that heals cavities is the opposite of the low-fat diets, which are most often promoted by the media. The ideal dental diet is reminiscent of the Atkins Diet. The best food for tooth remineralization is real butter. This is especially true if the butter is dark yellow, which is an indication that it is rich in minerals.

Foods High in Phosphorus

- Meats
- Real butter (yellow-orange butter is best)
- Cheese (especially parmesan)
- Oats
- Pumpkin seeds
- Sunflower seeds (contain vitamin E, magnesium, and other fat-soluble vitamins)
- Nuts (especially brazil nuts, cashews and walnuts)
- Flax seed oil *

  * Flax oil must be processed, packaged, and handled properly to be safe and effective. Reference the section about *Flax Seed Oil* in the *Supplements* chapter for more information.

Items to be Avoided

- Artificial foods, chemical additives, and pharmaceuticals invariably impair the body's ability to absorb nutrients, and they lead to an increased excretion of nutrients, by being toxic to the beneficial bacteria of the intestinal tract.

- Soy should always be avoided, because the high level of phytic acid that it contains reduces the assimilation of magnesium, calcium, copper, iron, and zinc. Soy also imbalances the hormones, which exaggerates issues that are caused by malnutrition.

- Tea and coffee contain some naturally-occurring fluoride, so those who currently have cavities should limit their intake until the cavity is healed. Iodine intake cannot counteract fluoride that is in contact with the teeth.

Do not brush or attempt to clean the teeth with lemon juice or acids. Similarly, abrasives such as baking soda should not be used whilst attempting to heal a cavity, and these things should only be used occasionally by people with good dental health. The ideal toothpaste will include both calcium and a phosphorus-containing ingredient, such as monocalcium phosphate. It should never contain fluoride.

Antibiotics cause tooth decay in multiple ways. They reduce the assimilation of nutrients by triggering an artificial immune response with their mold-based bio-toxins. Antibiotics additionally kill the beneficial bacteria. The mouth is similar to the gastrointestinal tract in that there is always the presence of two types of microorganisms. Candida albicans (or just simply "candida") is the yeast that ferments sugar inside the human body. It is known for eroding the teeth with its acidic wastes. It is also responsible for bad breath and a plethora of health issues cataloged in the *Allergies and Candida* section of the *Alternative Medicine* chapter. Sugars stimulate yeast growth. In a perpetual war with candida is a beneficial bacteria that is known as flora. It is much easier to kill, and when it dies, candida flourishes. Flora is killed by a variety of chemicals and toxins, and it is vital in helping a body to digest its food.

Sugars should be avoided as much as possible, and carbohydrates should be reduced while attempting to heal cavities. Fructose specifically causes a decrease in phosphorus, which is one of the reasons why sugar contributes to cavities. Cavities are certain to occur whenever there is phosphorus depletion, because contrary to popular belief, the teeth (like everything else in the human body) are always in a process of being slowly destroyed and rebuilt.

It is not possible to heal cavities on a vegan diet, and it would be quite challenging on a vegetarian diet. The nutrients that are needed for good dental and bone health do not exist in adequate quantities in vegetable sources. In fact, persistent dental problems are the most common reason why vegetarians and vegans return to healthy diets.

When a cavity is healed, the pit where it previously existed often turns black. This is purely cosmetic, and there are no health implications. The discoloration is likely to be permanent. Any dentist who notices it will drill it, if you are foolish enough to let him.

Toothache Remedies

The remedies being provided are meant to help people in obtaining temporary relief from toothache pain. If these steps are used perpetually, but no effort is made to heal the cavity, then it may eventually become impossible to heal. This could result in serious complications; for example, a brain infection.

- Clove oil applied directly to the the troublesome tooth is known to be very effective. If clove oil is not available, a paste can be made using ground clove powder and olive oil. The paste can then be applied directly to the tooth.

- Vanilla extract, applied directly to the tooth using a cotton ball. Ensure that it is real vanilla, not an artificial flavoring.

- If the toothache is the result of wisdom teeth entrance, simply using menthol-based cough drops may be enough to reduce the swelling and provide pain relief. Read the ingredients in such products to avoid artificial sweeteners or other unacceptable ingredients.

Teeth Grinding

Teeth grinding (bruxism) usually occurs at night while the sufferer sleeps, and normally it is first noticed by the person's spouse. In children, teeth grinding is likely to go unnoticed until significant damage has occurred. Bruxism should be considered a serious health condition, because a sufferer's tooth enamel may be eventually destroyed, leaving effected teeth extremely vulnerable to decay. The cosmetic consequences can be terrible too. In the worst cases, the aftermath of bruxism requires the complete removal of teeth.

The dental and medical establishments usually recommend that sufferers wear mouth retainers (night guards) during sleep periods, to protect against further damage. While this is a wise option for some sufferers of bruxism, it is nonetheless important to note that this reflects an institutional policy of categorically ignoring all causes of the condition. The standard approach is, at best, a temporary suppression of a single symptom of some potentially-serious underlying issues. It is like removing the batteries from a smoke detector, instead of fighting the fire that is causing the alarm. Teeth grinding is always a symptom of another health issue, so masking the symptom with a retainer should only be a short-term solution.

In some cases, teeth grinding is related to the presence of an underbite. It is unknown why an underbite increases the risk of bruxism. Nutritional therapies may not be enough to completely eliminate the problem in these cases. In a small subset of cases, bruxism can be the result of nerve damage, infection, or other factors that cannot be determined.

Nutritional Factors

Teeth grinding normally occurs because of nutritional deficiencies, so it can usually be corrected nutritionally. Since the condition typically indicates that the patient is malnourished, the wisest initial treatment option is to change the diet. It is unwise to merely compensate with supplements, or just mask the problem with a mouth retainer. Supplementation is somewhat effective, but supplementation is never truly an adequate replacement for a healthy (preferably organic) diet.

Scientific research of bruxism is sorely lacking, which is largely because mouth guards are considered to be an adequate treatment measure, and it is believed that there is little pharmaceutical money to be made from this disorder. Due to the lack of financial incentives, practically all available bruxism research is conducted outside of the United States, and most of the testing is based upon animal studies.

Recommended Supplementation

Vitamin B-5	This vitamin is found naturally in fish, chicken, and eggs. It is often sold in supplement form by its scientific name, pantothenic acid.
Magnesium and Calcium	Magnesium and calcium always work together, and are nearly useless alone. In many cases, a magnesium deficiency is the root cause of bruxism. Magnesium is found in green, leafy vegetables, and nuts (especially cashews and walnuts). For certain individuals who do not eat enough vegetables, our *Green Drink* from the *Nutrition* chapter may be enough to solve the problem if it is drank regularly. Vitamin D is also necessary for proper absorption of magnesium and calcium, and it may be obtained by both sunlight exposure and by eating fish. Some individuals will not be able to get enough vitamin D, due to liver impairment, which is usually a result of pharmaceuticals or heavy metal toxicity.
Potassium	High levels of potassium can be found in bananas, tomatoes, potato skins, oranges, or orange juice. It is in green leafy vegetables to a lesser degree.
Vitamin C	This exists in almost all fruits, and it is in the highest amounts in citrus fruits.

Vegetarian and Child Victims

Vegetarians do not get an adequate amount of vitamin B-5 (pantothenic acid), so bruxism is one of many diseases that plague them. Vegetarians attempt to correct their chronic malnutrition with supplementation, but dietary supplements are only capable of augmenting an adequately nutritious diet. They can never replace it. Oral problems are often the first indication that a vegetarian's or a vegan's health is suffering from malnutrition. There are a disproportionate number of vegetarians with teeth grinding issues, which is unexpectedly high; even when their chronic vitamin B-5 deficiencies are compensated for with supplements. It is likely that there are necessary nutrients in meats and fish, which have not yet been identified by researchers. Ironically, whenever children experience bruxism, it is most often related to their refusal to eat vegetables. Therefore, an ideal diet is balanced.

Unusual Cases

There are some cases wherein a dietary problem is not the root cause of bruxism, but the diet is virtually always a factor. For example, teeth grinding is sometimes caused by anti-depressant drugs or other medications, because the drugs deplete the body of magnesium and other vital nutrients.

Nerve damage can also cause people to grind their teeth, even during their waking hours. This too is caused by anti-depressants, and also artificial sweeteners. In such cases, efforts should be made to stimulate nerve repair or regeneration. Effective techniques include supplementation with MSM and the B vitamins, especially vitamin B-6 and B-12, which gained fame for their seemingly miraculous effects upon nerves. Healthy fats should also be incorporated into the diet, such as butter. The goat cheese and flax oil blend that is described in our Budwig Protocol (cancer) chapter is ideal. For further tips about how to repair nerve damage, reference the *Bell's Palsy* section of the *Alternative Medicine* chapter.

Wisdom Teeth and Memory

There was a time when the great majority of children had their tonsils removed, in the name of disease prevention. The medical establishment maintained that the tonsils had no purpose, and that they should therefore be removed to prevent future health problems. Then the polio epidemic occurred, and only those who had their tonsils removed were severely impacted. It was discovered that the tonsils are the only organ which produces polio antibodies.

In the present, the wisdom surrounding wisdom teeth is likewise lacking. They are removed as preventative medicine, because they are felt to be another unnecessary part. If a dentist sees wisdom teeth appearing during a routine check-up, he will usually schedule to have them removed. This may be a legitimate necessity in certain instances, but it is not for the majority of cases. Studies are beginning to show that all teeth have a special function, including the wisdom teeth.

It has been shown that there is a direct correlation between the number of teeth that a person has and his memory capacity. The more teeth that an individual has, the longer he can retain information. In particular, healthy mouths are closely correlated with people having excellent short-term memory. Researchers are baffled by this. The main hypothesis is related to the fact that dentists cut the nerves that rest behind the teeth during extractions. These nerves are believed to be directly connected to brain tissues, and cutting them may kill, or at least injure certain regions of the brain.

"While carrying out their experiments on animals, our Japanese colleagues managed to prove that whenever a doctor extracts a tooth, he also pulls out the nerve that stretches to the brain."

-- Prof. Ian Begdahl, University of Umea

Studies of rats have shown that tooth transplants do not return lost memory, lending credence to the presiding hypothesis. Perhaps most interesting is that the loss of memory does not occur when a tooth falls out naturally. It only occurs when a tooth is forced out through brute force trauma, whether that be from a brawl or dental work. The current research shows that memory problems are increased for every tooth that is pulled. Dental procedures may be responsible for most of the memory problems that are attributed to aging.

Reducing the Pain

The most common reason for removing the wisdom teeth is not because they present a health risk, but because they can become a painful inconvenience. Some wisdom teeth point in the wrong directions or get trapped under adjoining teeth, but they eventually correct themselves in the overwhelming majority of cases if they are left alone. It is completely normal to experience some pain from incoming wisdom teeth. There are less psychotic ways to cope with them, instead of getting butchered.

Remedies

- **Menthol** -- An extremely helpful painkiller, which can be found in a wide variety of cough drops. Natural cough drops are available at some grocery stores, and health food stores. Be sure to read the ingredients, and take care to avoid artificial sweeteners. Cough drops that are sweetened with honey actually help to prevent cavities through honey's natural anti-microbial properties, and it will help regulate blood sugar too.

- **Devil's Claw** -- A known anti-inflammatory herb that reduces swelling and pain. Studies have repeatedly shown that it is more effective than pharmaceuticals for certain pain conditions. It also helps alleviate carpal tunnel and arthritis pain.

- **Diatomaceous Earth** -- This a mineral-rich drying agent. Apply a pinch directly, when the tooth has become visible. This reduces inflammation and pain. Be sure to dampen diatomaceous earth slightly, because the dust should never be inhaled.

- **Cherry Extract** -- Cherry has natural anti-inflammatory properties. Concentrated cherry extract contains large doses of natural COX-2 inhibitors, and it does not come with the side effects that its pharmaceutical counterparts do (e.g. heart attacks). You can purchase cherry concentrate supplements.

- **Cloves** -- These have been used for centuries as a natural remedy for tooth aches. Simply apply clove powder to the offending tooth and pain will usually disappear rapidly. While this has been used for centuries by herbalists, Western studies have just recently begun to confirm the ability of cloves to numb tooth pain.

These methods should help to make the pain of emerging wisdom teeth much more tolerable. If you keep these teeth, then you are likely to experience improved memory, and possibly other benefits which have not yet been discovered.

Fluoride Lies

The presence of fluoride in U.S. tap water has increased in recent years, but it has not reduced cavities. In fact, the Fluoride Action Network issued a press release in 2001, which showed that whenever fluoridation is discontinued, the rate of cavities declines. The U.S. Government's statistics also confirm the inverse relationship between cavities and ingested fluoride: that ingesting fluoride fuels cavities (and many other diseases). However, there has been success in reducing cavities when fluoride was applied directly to the teeth, but never from ingesting it. The results of topical applications are heralded as proof that fluoride is beneficial, but they do not actually use data from ingestion tests.

Water fluoridation is not actually done in the interest of health, but for some very twisted politics. For more on the link between fluoridation and the pacification of the public, read the *Hidden Dangers of Tap Water* section of the *A Poisoned World* chapter. That section catalogs how fluoride was first misused by placement in the water of people who were conquered by the NAZI's. The NAZI's used it as a social control and population control drug. Fluoride destroys fertility, and pacifies populations having dissent, through its unique narcotic effect. It is meant to ensure that Americans never truly fight against their government.

Water fluoridation in the U.S. began life as part of a sham that was designed to benefit the nuclear, aluminum, and fertilizer industries. Feeding sodium fluoride to the public was a way to rid industry of its toxic waste product, at our expense. It all began with a fanciful public relations campaign by Edward Bernays, who was a hired gun for the U.S. atomic weapons program in World War II. His job was to convince the public that the tons of radioactive waste products from nuclear weapons processing were so safe that they were okay for human consumption. It is worth noting that in his private job, he also convinced regulators and the public that lead was safe in our gasoline, construction materials, clothing, and even our foods. As the nephew of Dr. Sigmund Freud, Bernays knew everything about manipulating the public. He is known as "The Father of Public Relations".

If a truckload of fluoride were spilled, it would initiate an emergency cleanup that would restrict all traffic within miles, and require a small army of spacesuit-wearing emergency workers. Even the fluorine fumes are deadly, in the event that it is heated.

Water fluoridation is doubly convenient for the chemical companies who are unloading this waste into our bodies, for they benefit financially whenever we get chemotherapy and radiation treatments for the cancers that were caused by their fluoride. Fluoride is verified to be one of the most potent carcinogens ever discovered.

Fluoride also directly attacks the thyroid, and it neutralizes precious iodine. It is the main reason for the current epidemic of hypothyroidism, and for hormonal problems for women throughout the United States. Fluoride is a major factor in osteoporosis, due to the fact that it causes brittle bones; especially over extended periods.

> *"Hydrofluorosilicic acid is also known as fluorosilicic acid or fluosilicic acid. It comes as a liquid and so it is easier to add to water than crystalline sodium fluoride and fluorosilicate. All of these chemicals are derived from pollution scrubbing operations. A common source is the processing of phosphate rock to make phosphate fertilizers. The rock also contains fluoride, silica and traces of heavy metals such as uranium, radium, radon and lead. When the phosphate rock is treated with sulfuric acid, silicon tetrafluoride and hydrogen fluoride gases are given off. These gases pass through scrubbers and react with water to form hydrofluosilicic acid."*
>
> *-- Fluorine Recovery in the Fertilizer Industry: A Review*

Juicing Recipes

The juicing experience can be an enjoyable one. Feel free to experiment with different combinations, and search for additional recipes. Try to ensure that most of the ingredients are organic, because conventional produce contains pesticides and is significantly less nutritious. Constant fruit juice can be too high in sugar for some diabetics, so they should concentrate on emphasizing vegetables.

Blood Cleanser

- 2 bunches of red grapes or 2 cups of dark grape juice
- 6 oranges or 2 cups of orange juice
- 4 lemons or 1/2 cup of lemon juice
- 1/4 cup of honey

Blend all of the ingredients in a blender. If you decide to use the whole fruits, instead of buying juice, then you may wish to run them through a juicer too, in order to remove the pulp. This is the favorite juice at Health Wyze Media. It is very tart, and especially good on summer days. The taste is like liquid sweet tarts, but there is no need for guilt with this treat.

This drink somehow cleanses the blood, and the lemon will greatly help to alkalize the body. The honey provides its own sugar, while simultaneously balancing blood sugar, in addition to crippling candida, and infusing the body with natural anti-histamines. This is the closest thing to the perfect energy drink. It is like raw octane without any jittery side effects. Expect an enormous energy rush within twenty minutes of drinking it, and the energy boost will typically last for more than eight hours.

Hormone Regulator

- 1 apple
- 1 pear
- 2 peaches

Blend these together, and run them through a juicer or strainer to remove pulp, if desired.

History: This combination is recognized throughout Traditional Chinese Medicine (T.C.M.) for being especially helpful for women with hormone irregularities. This will calm a woman with hormone imbalances and help her to feel at peace.

Tangy Delight

- 1 mango
- 2 carrots
- 2 granny smith apples
- 7 strawberries
- 1/2 cup orange juice

Juices such as this one, which contain lots of fruits, can be used periodically to quell sugar cravings.

Tomato Combo Juice

- 1/2 cup baby spinach
- 2 cups cherry tomatoes
- 1/2 cup diced carrots
- 1 stick celery
- 1/4 lemon
- 1 apple

Sugar Regulator

- 1/2 cucumber
- 1/2 green apple
- 1/2 bitter melon
- 1 stick of celery
- 1/2 red bell pepper
- Small handful of baby spinach

This is known for being particularly helpful for regulating the blood sugar.

Tasty Spinach Juice

- 1 bunch baby spinach
- 2 apples
- Juice from 1/2 lemon

A very good tasting, yet nutritious juice. This is good for people who are new to juicing.

Yummy Fruit Vegetable Blend

- 1 avocado
- 1 whole peeled orange
- 1 banana
- 1 celery stalk
- 1/2 apple

Super Nutrient Combo

- 1 green bell pepper
- 3 carrots, peeled and sliced
- 1-2 stalks of celery
- 1 beet, cleaned, peeled and chopped
- 2 dozen baby spinach leaves
- 1 bunch of parsley

Asparagus Swirl

- A handful of parsley
- 1/4 cucumber
- 1 or 2 asparagus stalks
- 4 carrots

Sweet Zucchini

- 1/2 zucchini
- 4 carrots
- 1/2 apple

Garden Tonic

- Handful of baby spinach
- 3 stalks of celery
- 2 stalks of asparagus
- 1 large tomato

Produce Delight

- 8 carrots
- 1/2 large beet
- 1/2 turnip
- 1/2 parsnip
- 2 celery stalks
- 1/4 rutabaga
- 1/8 head red cabbage
- 5 radishes
- 1 large apple
- 1 cup cranberries (optional)

V Dinner

- 2 large carrots
- 3 stalks celery
- 1/2 cup parsley
- 3/4 cup baby spinach
- 1/2 beet root
- 1/2 cup alfalfa sprouts

Green Drink

The best juice is not listed here. For the best of the best in nutrition, reference the *Green Drink* section of the *Nutrition* chapter.

Socialized Medicine

American health care is abysmal, and this sorry state is used as one of the primary justifications for implementing a nationalized health care system, under the pretext that the medical situation cannot possibly get worse. For instance, the U.S. currently has the highest infant death rate of the civilized world, despite virtually all births being performed at hospitals, and its infants getting the most prenatal care. The socialized 'solution' would force Americans to funnel even more money into this greed-ridden pit of death and destruction, which is already considered world-wide to be the worst of the worst, despite what Americans like to believe. To put the true carnage into perspective, every country with working telephones has better survival rates, and in fact, the U.S. is ranked 38th in life expectancy. This is why the people of other countries tend to laugh whenever they hear Americans bragging about having the best medicine in the world. Just properly prescribed medicines kill more Americans every year than any war in its history, and this information comes from the medical industry's own mortality statistics. That does not account for the mistakes, the botched surgeries, or the cases wherein the establishment refused to take any responsibility. It is an exercise in sociology to understand how the American society can convince itself that it has superiority in an area where all of the data shows that it is clearly amongst the most inferior.

Therefore, the real problem with America's death rate is not that Americans are getting too little medicine, but that they are already getting too much. Americans are medicated more than any other people in the world, and there is something terribly wrong with the result. The only thing providing any checks against this catastrophe is the fact that doctors know that people can shop elsewhere. American doctors know that people are not beholden to them, and that it is their customers (not governmental agencies) who have the final decision in their own welfare. If any 'successful' nationalized health care system is adopted by the U.S., then the situation will get considerably worse, not better. Success in one regard will mean failure in another way that will literally be impossible for many patients to live with. The principal of "first do no harm" will be only a memory of the past that is linked to decadent capitalists by the comrades of the future.

Important Considerations

1. The current socialized system in the U.S. (a.k.a. Obamacare) illegally applies tax penalties to citizens who are too poor to buy health insurance. It is an extremely immoral and thinly-veiled policy of taxing the poor, but it has been disingenuously promoted as a way to help them.

2. In England, the richest socialized country in the world, one in ten parents are skipping meals to feed their children. Is this the quality of life that Americans should be seeking?

3. How has socialism helped America in other areas? Remember education before the teacher's unions and governmental regulations? How about when America had manufacturing, and it was the best in the world? Now America's education and manufacturing industries are unionized welfare systems, and are ranked amongst the worst in the world.

4. Will we ever get our rights back once the medical system becomes a taxing agent of the U.S. Government?

5. Has any governmental agency peacefully surrendered any of its power back to the people in the entire history of the world?

6. Didn't every communist nation begin exactly this way -- with bogus pleas to help suffering people, which is only obtainable if everyone surrenders his rights?

7. As is the case with medicare and medicaid already, what happens when you suddenly and unexpectedly must pay a bankrupting hospital bill when coverage was retroactively terminated because you didn't obey the orders of your doctor? Who do you appeal to?

8. If the poor are actually monetarily helped by socialized health care, then how does that money help them, since they will be told exactly how they'll spend it? Doesn't that just enslave the poor even more, as well as everyone else?

9. Will the greed, corruption, and the medical carnage really stop once we are enslaved to a system that has the ability to perpetually tax all of us at will? Isn't that like paying mafia protection money, in the hope that the mafia doesn't ever become greedier?

10. Will the medical establishment charge us more or less once it has unlimited health taxation power?

11. Why did the White House use Big Pharma consultants to help draft the Bill if it really is meant to cut our expenses? How exactly is that going to work out for us?

12. Isn't that why the Bill is about 3,000 pages -- to prevent us from reading or understanding it?

13. Will the industry's greed really be stopped by governmental hand-outs, and will our health care suddenly become safe and effective?

14. What happens once we run out of *other people's* money? Can you name a country with socialized medicine that this hasn't happened in?

15. If the expense is really the issue to be solved, then how does creating even more expense make the poor wealthier?

16. Isn't the government already the problem by blocking cheaper, safer, and more effective alternatives in its efforts to financially prop-up the very system that helped to

write the Bill?

17. How do we opt-out whenever we find better alternatives? Where is that freedom in the Bill?

18. If governmental take-overs are really a positive factor in a nation's quality of life, then can you name any communistic nation with a superior quality of life?

19. What happens when you are refused treatments because you are on some type of "no fly" list, or when the government mandates certain treatments that the doctors know will kill you, because something qualified you as a trouble-maker. This is not merely conjecture. Reference the *Shane Geiger* section of the *Victims* chapter to read an actual instance of medically murdering a trouble-maker.

20. What happens to the patients who are too expensive? Will they start refusing to give medicine to the elderly as has happened in England, or will they cut costs like Greece, by amputating the limbs of diabetics who do not need amputations?

21. You can fire your doctor. Will you be able to fire socialized medicine once a doctor is assigned to you?

22. If Obamacare is about promoting smarter, preventative care, then how do I get my refunds for my supplement purchases and organic foods? Does our money actually just go back into Big Pharma, as if this is how they planned it all along?

Legal Notice

Open Sans and Tinos (Fonts)

The chapter titles of this book utilize the Open Sans font from Google Corporation, which was designed by Steve Matteson of Ascender Corporation. The paragraphs use the Tinos font, from the same designer. They are licensed under the Apache License, version 2.0. You may not use these fonts in your own creative work, unless you comply with their license. You may obtain a copy here: http://www.apache.org/licenses/LICENSE-2.0. Unless required by applicable law or agreed to in writing, software distributed under the license is distributed on an "AS IS" BASIS, WITHOUT WARRANTIES OR CONDITIONS OF ANY KIND, either express or implied. See the license for the specific language governing permissions and limitations.

The Authors

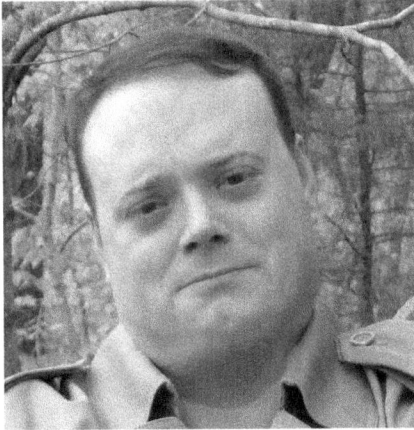

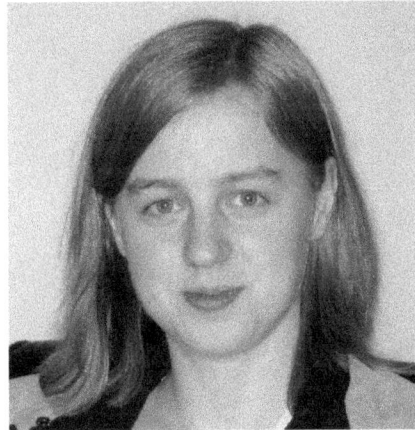

We (Thomas Corriher and Sarah Corriher) are the detectives from Health Wyze Media. We attempted to provide everything that you will need in this book. It is up to you to do what is health wyze for yourself and your family. We will be here if you ever need us. Our contact information can be found at HealthWyze.org. We never charge for consultations or interviews, but we accept unconditional donations with great appreciation.

Throughout the seven years leading to this book's authorship; we have been involved with media concerning health care alternatives, and we contrast them with standard care. We began with a print magazine for retailers that was called *Naturally Good Magazine*, and we later created *The Health Wyze Report* (HealthWyze.org), which is the *de facto* online encyclopedia of legitimate alternative therapies. We also work on documentaries. We produced *The Cancer Report*, the most comprehensive video about the history of cancer and the treatments that actually work. It shall forever remain freely available, like most of our work. Finally, we have an online archive containing about 40 hours of audio shows from the last seven years. These unique audio reports tend to be the favorite media amongst our fans.

Neither of us has special credentials to boast about, nor would we cite such. We believe that the writings of investigative journalists should speak for themselves, and that our modern obsession with credentials demonstrates that something is usually lacking in the writings and thinking of modern writers. Both of us are extensively self educated in the materials of which we write, and both of us are "drop outs" of failed educational systems. Had we been more typical, then we would be of no use to you, or any of the other people that we have helped.

We're Health Wyze. Have you told your friends about us?

Notes

www.ingramcontent.com/pod-product-compliance
Lightning Source LLC
Chambersburg PA
CBHW061828260326
41914CB00005B/914